Ignatavicius · W

MEDICAL-SURGICAL NURSING
Concepts for Interprofessional Collaborative Care

Ignatavicius ▪ Workman ▪ Rebar

MEDICAL-SURGICAL NURSING

Concepts for Interprofessional Collaborative Care
9th Edition

NICOLE HEIMGARTNER, MSN, RN, COI
Former Associate Professor of Nursing
Kettering College;
Subject Matter Expert, Author, and Consultant
Louisville, Kentucky

CHRIS WINKELMAN, PhD, RN, CNE, CCRN, ACNP,
FCCM, FAANP
Associate Professor
Frances Payne Bolton School of Nursing
Case Western Reserve University;
Clinical Nurse
Trauma/Critical Care Float Pool
MetroHealth Medical Center
Cleveland, Ohio

ELSEVIER

ELSEVIER

3251 Riverport Lane
St. Louis, Missouri 63043

CLINICAL COMPANION FOR MEDICAL-SURGICAL NURSING: ISBN: 978-0-323-46170-2
CONCEPTS FOR INTERPROFESSIONAL COLLABORATIVE CARE,
NINTH EDITION

Notices

Knowledge and best practice in this field are constantly changing. As new research and experience
broaden our understanding, changes in research methods, professional practices, or medical
treatment may become necessary.

　　Practitioners and researchers must always rely on their own experience and knowledge in
evaluating and using any information, methods, compounds, or experiments described herein.
In using such information or methods, they should be mindful of their own safety and the safety
of others, including parties for whom they have a professional responsibility.

　　With respect to any drug or pharmaceutical products identified, readers are advised to
check the most current information provided (i) on procedures featured or (ii) by the manufacturer
of each product to be administered and to verify the recommended dose or formula, the method
and duration of administration, and contraindications. It is the responsibility of practitioners,
relying on their own experience and knowledge of their patients, to make diagnoses, to determine
dosages and the best treatment for each individual patient, and to take all appropriate safety
precautions.

　　To the fullest extent of the law, neither the Publisher nor the authors, contributors, or
editors assume any liability for any injury and/or damage to persons or property as a matter of
products liability, negligence or otherwise, or from any use or operation of any methods,
products, instructions, or ideas contained in the material herein.

Executive Content Strategist: Lee Henderson
Senior Content Development Manager: Laurie Gower
Senior Content Development Specialist: Laura Goodrich
Publishing Services Manager: Deepthi Unni
Project Manager: Apoorva V
Design Direction: Brian Salisbury

Printed in United States of America

Last digit is the print number: 9 8 7 6 5 4 3 2 1

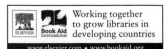

Working together
to grow libraries in
developing countries

www.elsevier.com • www.bookaid.org

Welcome! The new edition of *Clinical Companion for Medical-Surgical Nursing: Concepts for Interprofessional Collaborative Care* has been updated and streamlined to match content changes in the most current Ignatavicius, Workman and Rebar textbook. Many changes reflect the increased emphasis in health care on implementing strategies for patient care that have evidence for both safety and effectiveness.

Part One has been revised to emphasize concepts in nursing education and reflects many of the ideas developed in the Ignatavicius and Workman textbook.

Part Two, the core of the *Clinical Companion*, provides A-to Z synopses of more than 250 conditions, along with collaborative care. Part Two retains the format consistent with that of the Ignatavicius and Workman textbook.

Throughout Parts One and Two, important aspects of care are highlighted, such as Genetic/Genomic Considerations 🧬, Considerations for Older Adults, Gender Considerations, and Cultural Considerations 🌐. These considerations help nurses and nursing students offer focused and individualized assessment and intervention. Canadian brand name drugs are represented by a maple leaf icon 🍁, and Nursing Safety Priority boxes ❗ highlight important information that nursing students and nurses can use to avoid patient harm. These boxes are further categorized as Drug Alert, Action Alert, or Critical Rescue. New QSEN boxes have been created to reflect nursing roles in the health care system, such as actions that improve quality and safety. These **QSEN** boxes reflect both competencies described by the Quality and Safety Education for Nurses website (QSEN.org) and quality measures from the Centers for Medicare and Medicaid Services (cms.gov). Effective, safe, efficient, and patient-centered care is delivered individually and across settings. Also, new to this edition is the Exemplar icon ❖ used to highlight exemplars found in the Ignatavicius and Workman textbook. There are now three appendixes. Each appendix is designed to provide brief, concentrated capsules related to medical-surgical nursing care.

This content provides information about both common and specialized skills that cross settings, diseases, and conditions. Medical-surgical nursing is a demanding specialty, often considered the foundation of all nursing. Most adults will receive care from a medical-surgical nurse sometime during their life. We hope this book supports our readers' efforts to provide comfort, avoid error, and promote high-quality patient-centered care.

ACKNOWLEDGMENTS

Thank you, Donna, Linda, and Cherie for your mentorship and continual support. Many thanks to Elsevier for transforming this manuscript into publication.

I am grateful for the support and love of my husband and beautiful twin girls—you all inspire me each day.

Students, I am so thankful for you and excited for the journey that lies ahead for you in the profession of nursing!

Nicole

As always, I acknowledge the patients and their families who REALLY teach us how to be great nurses!

The editors at Elsevier perform miracles in ensuring content in this text is clear, accurate, and visually pleasing.

And my family is acknowledged as fun and a constant source of wondrous support.

Chris

PART ONE

Overview of Professional Nursing Concepts

Medical-surgical nursing, sometimes called *adult health nursing,* is a specialty practice area in which nurses promote, restore, or maintain optimal health for patients from 18 to older than 100 years of age (Academy of Medical-Surgical Nurses [AMSN], 2012). Medical-surgical nursing is practiced in many types of settings, such as acute care agencies, skilled nursing facilities, ambulatory care clinics, and the patient's home, which could be either a single residence or group setting, such as an assisted living facility. The roles of the nurse in these settings include care coordinator and transition manager, caregiver, patient educator, leader, and patient and family advocate. To function in these various roles, nurses need to have the knowledge, skills, attitudes, and abilities (KSAs) to keep patients and their families safe.

QUALITY AND SAFETY EDUCATION FOR NURSES (QSEN) CORE COMPETENCIES

QSEN competencies are based on the Institute of Medicine (IOM) report, *Health Professions Education: A Bridge to Quality*, which identified five broad categories of care. The QSEN Institute validated the IOM competencies for nursing practice and added the concept of safety. In addition to the concepts identified by the IOM and QSEN, the authors have selected four professional nursing concepts to integrate throughout the clinical companion. The ten concepts reviewed in Part One are:

- Patient-centered care
- Safety
- Teamwork and interprofessional collaboration
- Evidence-based practice
- Quality improvement
- Informatics and technology
- Clinical judgment
- Ethics
- Health care organizations
- Health care disparities

Each of these concepts plays an integral role in safe, effective management of care within the clinical setting. Chart 1.1 provides a brief overview of each competency along with tangible clinical application examples. These competencies will be addressed throughout this resource allowing focus on the knowledge, skills, and attitudes that are needed for safe nursing care. Keep in mind that these competencies do not exist in isolation. Rather, they are interdependent to form the foundation for safe nursing care. For more discussion of the competencies, review Chapter 1 in Ignatavicius, Workman, & Rebar's *Medical Surgical Nursing: Interprofessional Collaborative Care, 9th edition.*

Chart 1.1	Quality and Safety Education for Nurses (QSEN) Core Competencies	
Competency	**Overview**	**Clinical Application Examples**
Patient-Centered Care	The patient is "the source of control and full partner in providing compassionate and coordinated care based on respect for the patient's preferences, values, and needs" (QSEN, 2011).	Integrative Therapies: Massage therapy, guided imagery, music therapy, acupuncture Care Coordination Case Management Transition Management
Safety	Safety is the ability to keep the patient and staff free from harm and minimize errors in care.	National Patient Safety Goals The Joint Commission: Culture of Safety Best safety practices: Assess unit protocols, memory checklists, medication administration systems, such as the bar-code administration systems.
Teamwork and Interprofessional Collaboration	To provide patient and family-centered care, the nurse "functions effectively within nursing and interprofessional teams, fostering open communication, mutual respect, and shared decision-making to achieve quality patient care" (QSEN, 2011).	To improve communication between staff members and health care agencies, procedures for hand-off communication were established. An effective procedure used in many agencies today is called *SBAR* (pronounced S-Bar) or similar method. **SBAR** is a formal method of communication between two or more members of the health care team. The SBAR process includes these four steps:

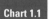 **Chart 1.1**	**Quality and Safety Education for Nurses (QSEN) Core Competencies—cont'd**	
Competency	**Overview**	**Clinical Application Examples**
		• **Situation:** Describe what is happening at the time to require this communication. • **Background:** Explain any relevant background information that relates to the situation. • **Assessment:** Provide an analysis of the problem or patient need based on assessment data. • **Recommendation/Request:** State what is needed or the desired outcome.
Evidence-Based Practice	Evidence-based practice (EBP) is the use of the best current evidence and practices to make decisions about patient care (QSEN, 2011).	The best source of evidence is research! Health care organizations receiving Medicare and/or Medicaid funding are obligated to follow the evidence-based interprofessional Core Measures to ensure that best practices are followed for selected health problems.
Quality Improvement	Quality improvement (QI), sometimes referred to as continuous quality improvement (CQI), is a process in which nurses and the interprofessional health care team use indicators (data) to monitor care outcomes and develop solutions to change and improve care. This process is also sometimes called the evidence-based practice improvement (EBPI) process because the best sources of evidence are used to support the improvement or change in practice.	When a patient care or system issue is identified as needing improvement, specific systematic QI models such as the **Plan-Do-Study-Act (PDSA)** may be used. The steps of the PDSA model include (Sutton & Suhayda, 2015): 1. Identify and analyze the problem (Plan). 2. Develop and test an evidence-based solution (Do). 3. Analyze the effectiveness of the test solution, including possible further improvement (Study). 4. Implement the improved solution to positively impact care (Act).

Continued

Chart 1.1	Quality and Safety Education for Nurses (QSEN) Core Competencies—cont'd	
Competency	**Overview**	**Clinical Application Examples**
Informatics and Technology	Informatics and technology are the access and use of information and electronic technology to communicate, manage knowledge, prevent error, and support decision making (QSEN, 2011).	Safety and quality of health care are the major purposes of informatics and technology Be mindful of patient and family privacy in the clinical setting. For example, it is a violation of patient privacy and confidentiality for staff and students to take photos of patients to show their family and friends. In some cases, these photos are posted on social media such as Facebook. *This action is a violation of patient privacy and confidentiality.*
Clinical Judgment	Clinical judgment is the process that nurses and other members of the interprofessional team use to make decisions based on interpretation of the patient's needs or problems. The nursing process, critical thinking, and a variety of reasoning patterns help the medical-surgical nurse make clinical decisions while being respectful of the patient's and family's cultural diversity, age, gender, and lifestyle choices.	Clinical judgment involves specific reasoning and critical thinking skills. Throughout the clinical companion, each of these skills is paired with the steps of the nursing process for all exemplar health problems as follows: Assessment: Noticing Analysis: Interpreting Planning and Implementation: Responding Evaluation: Reflecting

Chart 1.1	Quality and Safety Education for Nurses (QSEN) Core Competencies—cont'd	
Competency	**Overview**	**Clinical Application Examples**
Ethics	According to the American Nurses Association (ANA), ethics is "a theoretical and reflective domain of human knowledge that addresses issues and questions about morality in human choices, actions, character, and ends" (ANA, 2015, p. xii)	There are six essential *ethical principles* that nurses and other health care professionals should use as a guide for clinical decision making. **Respect:** Implies that patients are treated as autonomous individuals capable of making informed decision about their care. This patient autonomy is referred to as *self-determination* or *self-management.* **Beneficence:** Encourages the nurse to do good for the patient **Nonmaleficence:** Emphasizes the importance of preventing harm and ensuring the patient's well being **Fidelity:** The agreement that the nurse will keep their obligations or promises to the patient **Veracity:** The obligation of the nurse to tell the truth to the best of his or her knowledge **Social justice:** Refers to equality and fairness, that all patients should be treated equally and fairly.
Health Care Organizations	Health care organizations (HCOs) are purposely designed and structured systems in which health care is provided by members of nursing and interprofessional teams (Giddens, 2016).	Generally, the delivery of care outlined in this clinical companion is expected to take place in an acute care setting within a health care organization that promotes safe, effective health care.
Health Care Disparities	Health care disparities are differences in patient access to or availability of appropriate health care services.	Special needs of older adults Special needs of ethnic minorities Special needs of the LGBTQ population

OVERVIEW OF HEALTH CONCEPTS FOR MEDICAL-SURGICAL NURSING

Nurses care for adults in a variety of settings to help them meet a multitude of biopsychosocial needs. When these needs are not met, the nurse plans and implements care in collaboration with the interprofessional health team. The clinical companion presents diseases and disorders alphabetically that are commonly seen in adults. Selected diseases and disorders have been identified as exemplars, with expanded assessment and interventions presented with a conceptual focus.

The health concepts included in this text are:
- Acid-Base Balance
- Cellular Regulation
- Clotting
- Cognition
- Comfort
- Elimination
- Fluid and Electrolyte Balance
- Gas Exchange
- Immunity
- Mobility
- Nutrition
- Perfusion
- Sensory Perception
- Sexuality
- Tissue Integrity

ACID-BASE BALANCE

Acid-base balance is the maintenance of arterial blood pH between 7.35 and 7.45 through control of hydrogen ion production and elimination. Blood pH represents a delicate balance between hydrogen ions (acid) and bicarbonate (base) and is largely controlled by the lungs and kidneys.

Assessment: Noticing

Assess patient health history. Ask about recent signs and symptoms such as excessive vomiting or diarrhea that could predispose the patient to acidosis or alkalosis.

Intervention: Responding

Managing a patient with an acid-base imbalance depends on which type of imbalance is present. When possible, the health care team aims to diagnose and treat the underlying cause(s) of the imbalance.

CELLULAR REGULATION

Cellular regulation is the process to control cellular growth, replication, and differentiation to maintain homeostasis. Cellular *growth* refers to division and continued growth of the original cell. Cell *replication* refers to making a copy of a specific cell. Cell *differentiation* refers to the process of the cell becoming specialized to accomplish a specific task.

Assessment: Noticing

Assess for common risk factors of impaired cellular regulation such as smoking, poor nutrition, physical inactivity, environmental pollutant exposure, radiation, and genetic risk.

Intervention: Responding

Interventions include primary and secondary prevention techniques. *Primary prevention* includes minimizing the risk of developing impaired cellular regulation. *Secondary prevention* includes proper and regular screening to identify early any risks or hazards that could be present.

CLOTTING

Clotting is a complex, multi-step process by which blood forms a protein-based structure (clot) in an appropriate area of tissue injury to prevent excessive bleeding while maintaining whole body blood flow (perfusion). An inability to form adequate clots can result in bleeding and threaten a person's life.

Assessment: Noticing

Assess for common risk factors for inadequate clotting such as immobility and smoking. Observe patients for signs and symptoms of *decreased* clotting, especially purpuric lesions such as ecchymosis (bruising) and petechiae (pinpoint purpura). Notice if bleeding is prolonged as a result of injury or trauma. Check urine and stool for the presence of occult or frank blood. Observe for frank bleeding from the gums or nose.

Intervention: Responding

Teach patients with *decreased* clotting ability to report unusual bleeding or bruising immediately. For many adults at increased risk for clotting, *anticoagulants* or *antiplatelet drugs* (also called *blood thinners* by many patients) are prescribed either in community or inpatient settings. Examples of medications that require frequent laboratory testing are sodium heparin and warfarin.

! **NURSING SAFETY PRIORITY: Critical Rescue**

An *arterial* thrombosis is not locally observable and is typically manifested by decreased blood flow (PERFUSION) to a distal extremity or internal organ. For example, a femoral arterial clot causes an occlusion (blockage) of blood to the leg. In this case, the distal leg becomes pale and cool; distal pulses may be weak or absent; *this is an emergent problem requiring immediate intervention.* If these changes are present, notify the primary health care provider or Rapid Response Team immediately. If this condition continues, the leg may become gangrenous and require amputation. A mesenteric artery thrombosis can cause small bowel ileus and gangrene if not treated in a timely manner. A renal artery thrombosis can cause acute kidney injury.

COGNITION

Cognition is the complex integration of mental processes and intellectual function for the purposes of reasoning, learning, memory, and personality. *Reasoning* is a high-level thinking process that allows an individual to make decisions and judgments. *Memory* is the ability of an individual to retain and recall information for learning or recall of past experiences. *Personality* refers to the way an individual feels and behaves, often based on how he or she thinks.

Assessment: Noticing

Assess for common risk factors for inadequate cognition such as loss of short- and/or long-term memory; disorientation to person, place, and/or time; impaired language or reasoning; inappropriate or uncontrollable emotions; and delusions and/or hallucinations. Refer to Chart 1.2. Conduct a mental status assessment using one of several

Chart 1.2	Differences in the Characteristics of Delirium and Dementia	
Variable	**Dementia**	**Delirium**
Description	A chronic, progressive cognitive decline	An acute, fluctuating confusional state
Onset	Slow	Fast
Duration	Months to years	Hours to less than 1 month
Cause	Unknown, possibly familial, chemical	Multiple, such as surgery, infection, drugs
Reversibility	None	May be possible
Management	Treat signs and symptoms	Remove or treat the cause
Nursing interventions	Reorientation not effective in the late stages; use validation therapy (acknowledge the patient's feelings, and do not argue); provide a safe environment; observe for associated behaviors, such as delusions and hallucinations	Reorient the patient to reality; provide a safe environment

available mental health/behavioral health screening tools such as the Confusion Assessment Method (CAM).

Intervention: Responding

Nursing interventions focus on *safety* to prevent injury and foster communication. For adults with delirium or mild dementia, provide orientation to person, time, and place. Collaborate with the interprofessional team to determine the underlying cause of delirium, such as psychoactive drugs or hypoxia. Patients with moderate or severe dementia cannot be oriented to reality because they have chronic confusion.

COMFORT

Comfort is a state of physical well-being, pleasure, and absence of pain or stress. This definition implies that comfort has physical and emotional dimensions. A primary role of the nurse is to promote basic care and comfort.

Assessment: Noticing

Assess for common risk factors for decreased comfort such as physical and/or emotional discomfort. Ask patients if they are comfortable. If pain is the source of discomfort, assess the level of pain and plan interventions to manage it.

Intervention: Responding

Assess patients at risk for discomfort and plan interventions to alleviate it, depending on its source and cause. Collaborate care with members of the interprofessional health care team as needed.

ELIMINATION

Elimination is the excretion of waste from the body by the gastrointestinal (GI) tract (as feces) and by the urinary system (as urine). *Bowel* elimination occurs as a result of food and fluid intake and ends with passage of feces (stool) or solid waste products from food into the rectum of the colon. *Urinary* elimination occurs as a result of multiple kidney processes and ends with the passage of urine through the urinary tract.

Assessment: Noticing

Assess for common risk factors for changes in elimination such as incontinence, diarrhea, and urinary retention. Monitor the frequency, amount, consistency, and characteristics of urine and stool. Listen to bowel sounds in all four quadrants for presence of adequate bowel sounds.

Intervention: Responding

Maintaining normal elimination requires adequate nutrition and hydration. Teach adults to ensure a diet high in fiber, including eating fruits, vegetables, and whole grains, and drinking 8 to12 glasses of water each day unless medically contraindicated. Adults with diarrhea or constipation need medical attention to determine the underlying cause. Adults who experience urinary incontinence need frequent toileting every 1 to 2 hours. Patients with urinary retention may require straight urinary catheterizations to empty the bladder until the usual voiding pattern returns.

FLUID AND ELECTROLYTE BALANCE
Fluid and electrolyte balance is the regulation of body fluid, fluid osmolality, and electrolytes by processes such as filtration, diffusion, and osmosis. To maintain balance or homeostasis in the body, fluid and electrolyte balance must be as close to normal as possible.

Assessment: Noticing
Assess for common risk factors for fluid and electrolyte imbalance such as acute illness (vomiting and diarrhea) or serious injury or trauma. Monitor vital signs, especially blood pressure, pulse rate and quality, fluid intake and output, and weight. *Changes in weight are the best indicator of fluid volume changes in the body.* Assess skin and mucous membranes for dryness and decreased skin turgor.

Intervention: Responding
Priority nursing interventions include maintenance of patient safety and comfort measures when managing fluid or electrolyte imbalances. For patients with a *fluid deficit,* the primary collaborative intervention is fluid replacement, either orally or parenterally. Depending on the cause of *fluid overload,* patients may require a fluid restriction (e.g., for those with chronic kidney disease). Diuretic therapy is often used for patients with fluid overload caused by chronic heart failure to prevent pulmonary edema, a potentially life-threatening complication.

GAS EXCHANGE
Gas exchange is the process of oxygen transport to the cells and carbon dioxide transport away from the cells through ventilation and diffusion.

Assessment: Noticing
Take a complete health history and perform a focused respiratory assessment. Ask the patient about current or history of lung disease or trauma. Assess the patient's breathing effort, oxygen saturation, capillary refill, thoracic expansion, and lung sounds anteriorly and posteriorly. Monitor for the presence of a cough and/or sputum; report of shortness of breath, dizziness, chest pain, presence of cyanosis, or adventitious lung sounds such as wheezing, rhonchi, or crackles.

Intervention: Responding
Teach patients the importance of using infection control measures (primarily proper hand washing), smoking cessation to prevent

chronic obstructive pulmonary disease (COPD), and getting vaccinations as recommended to prevent influenza and pneumonia. Managing decreased gas exchange requires understanding the underlying cause and treating it, often with drug therapy.

IMMUNITY

Immunity is protection from illness or disease maintained by the body's physiologic defense mechanisms. *Natural active* immunity occurs when an antigen enters the body and the body creates antibodies to fight off the antigen. *Artificial active* immunity occurs via a vaccination or immunization.

Assessment: Noticing

Assess for common risk factors for changes in immunity including but not limited to low socioeconomic groups, older adults, nonimmunized adults, adults with chronic illnesses, and adults with substance use disorder. A thorough history of the individual and the family is necessary to determine any of the previous risks associated with an immune problem.

Intervention: Responding

Avoiding infections, hand washing, and having recommended immunizations are essential for promoting healthy immune function. Patients with a *decreased* immune system for any reason are very prone to infection. Remind them to wash their hands frequently and use hand sanitizer when water and soap are not available. Patients with an *excessive* immune function have hypersensitivity reactions. Interprofessional collaborative management of these adults depends on the type and severity of the reaction.

MOBILITY

Mobility is the ability of an individual to perform purposeful physical movement of the body. When a person is able to move, he or she is usually able to perform activities of daily living (ADLs) such as eating, dressing, and walking. This ability depends primarily on the function of the central and peripheral nervous system and the musculoskeletal system and is sometimes referred to as *functional ability*.

Assessment: Noticing

Observe patients within the environment to determine their mobility level. The mobility level of the patient is adequate if he or she can move purposely to walk with an erect posture and coordinated gait and perform ADLs without assistance.

Intervention: Responding

The nurse has a major role in promoting mobility and preventing immobility. Assessment of patients who are most at risk for decreased mobility is critical. For patients who are immobile or have decreased mobility it is important to perform passive range of motion (ROM) exercises, turn and reposition every 1 to 2 hours, keep the patient's skin clean and dry, and encourage deep-breathing and coughing exercises. Interprofessional collaboration with a registered dietician, physical therapist, and respiratory therapist should be anticipated.

NUTRITION

Nutrition is the process of ingesting and using food and fluids to grow, repair, and maintain optimal body functions. Nutrients from food and fluids are used for optimal cellular metabolism and health promotion. Examples of nutrient groups are proteins, carbohydrates, fats, vitamins, and minerals.

Assessment: Noticing

Conduct a complete patient and family history for risk factors that could cause impaired nutrition. Ask about current or recent GI symptoms such as nausea, vomiting, constipation, and diarrhea. Obtain the patient's height and weight and calculate body mass index (BMI).

Intervention: Responding

Collaborative interventions to improve nutrition depend on the cause of decreased nutrition. For those with weight loss or low weight, common interventions include high-protein oral supplements, enteral supplements (either oral or by feeding tube), or parenteral nutrition. Collaborate with the registered dietitian for specific instructions regarding enteral feedings; consult with the pharmacist to administer parenteral therapy.

PERFUSION

Perfusion is adequate arterial blood flow through the peripheral tissues (*peripheral* perfusion) and blood pumped by the heart to oxygenate major body organs (*central* perfusion). Perfusion is a normal physiologic process of the body; without adequate perfusion, cell death can occur.

Assessment: Noticing

Conduct a complete patient and family history for risk factors and existing problems with perfusion. Assess for signs and symptoms of central perfusion, including dyspnea, dizziness or syncope, and chest pain. Signs and symptoms of decreased cardiac output include hypotension, tachycardia, diaphoresis, anxiety, decrease in cognitive function, and dysrhythmias.

Intervention: Responding

The nurse plays a vital role in promoting adequate perfusion and preventing impairment. Inadequate perfusion can cause serious and life-threatening consequences. For patients who have decreased perfusion, the primary health care provider may prescribe vasodilating drugs to promote blood flow.

SENSORY PERCEPTION

Sensory perception is the ability to perceive and interpret sensory input into one or more meaningful responses. Sensory input is usually received through the five major senses of vision, hearing, smell, taste, and touch.

Assessment: Noticing

Conduct a thorough patient and family history to determine risk factors for vision or hearing loss. Ask the patient about the use of eyeglasses, contacts, or a magnifier to improve vision. Inquire if he or she uses one or more hearing aids or amplifier.

Intervention: Responding

Primary and secondary preventive interventions are used to promote vision and hearing and prevent sensory deficits. *Primary* measures focus on avoiding risk factors that cause vision and hearing loss or using protective devices to minimize risk. The purpose of *secondary* prevention is to perform screening and diagnostic tests for early detection of beginning sensory loss.

SEXUALITY

Sexuality is a complex integration of physiologic, emotional, and social aspects of well-being related to intimacy, self-concept, and role relationships. It is not the same as *reproduction,* which is the process of conceiving and having a child. Sexuality involves sex, sexual acts, and sexual orientation; these terms are *not* the same as gender identity.

Assessment: Noticing

Discussing sexuality, sexual health, and sexual intercourse is often difficult for both the patient and nurse. Ask patients about their perception of their sexuality, including both sexual activity and intimacy behaviors. Determine if they have sex and/or intimacy with one or more partners. Ask about protection measures and any history of sexually transmitted infections (STIs) or problems during sexual intercourse.

Intervention: Responding

Interventions include STI screening and physical examinations to determine any physical cause of changes in sexuality. For patients with changes in sexuality, interventions depend on the cause of the sexual impairment.

TISSUE INTEGRITY

Tissue integrity is the intactness of the structure and function of the integument (skin and subcutaneous tissue) and mucous membranes. The skin is the largest organ of the body and has multiple functions, including protection from infection, fluid preservation, and temperature control.

Assessment: Noticing
Take a thorough health history of previous and current chronic health problems and current medications (prescribed and over-the-counter [OTC]). Assess for change in skin color, moles or lesions, excessive skin dryness, bruising, and hair loss or brittle nails (indicating decreased tissue perfusion).

Intervention: Responding
The primary health promotion focus is on proper hygiene and nutrition to enhance tissue health. Teach patients at risk for impaired tissue integrity to inspect the skin every day. Keep the skin clean and dry; when needed, moisturize the skin to prevent excessive dryness.

CLINICAL COMPANION OVERVIEW

Remember, a concept is an organizing principle. Using concepts to organize your care in the clinical environment will help you to recognize similarities and apply general concepts to individualized patient-centered care. Throughout the clinical companion, concepts will be identified in small caps.

In Part Two, you will find disorders that are commonly seen in adults. Each disorder will follow a format in which you will see an overview followed by Interprofessional Collaborative Care. Exemplars will follow an expanded format with the addition of care coordination and transition management. Be sure to organize care with concepts in mind, while still personalizing care based on each patient's individual needs.

PART TWO

Diseases and Disorders

A

ABSCESS

OVERVIEW

An abscess is an enclosed collection of pus. Swelling, erythema, and pain (induration) are common symptoms. This local infection is surrounded by inflamed tissue and can occur in a variety of sites. Almost all abscesses require an intervention of systemic antibiotics. The most common sites and interprofessional collaborative care are identified in Chart 2-1.

| Chart 2-1 | Abscess: Interprofessional Collaborative Care |

Location	Interprofessional Collaborative Care
• **Anorectal Abscess:** Results from obstruction of the ducts of glands caused by feces or rectal trauma.	• Most common sign and symptom: rectal pain. • Most anorectal abscesses can be excised and drained with local anesthesia. • **Priority Care:** Maintain comfort and promote perineal hygiene by providing sitz baths and analgesics. Avoid constipation through the use of stool softeners and bulk-forming agents.
• **Brain Abscess:** Occurs as encapsulated pus in the brain, most commonly in the frontal or temporal lobes.	• Most common signs and symptoms are associated with increased intracranial pressure, including but not limited to headache, fever, lethargy, confusion, seizures, aphasia, and focal neurologic deficits.

Continued

Chart 2-1 Abscess: Interprofessional Collaborative Care—cont'd	
Location	**Interprofessional Collaborative Care**
	• **Priority Care:** Antibiotics, typically administered intravenously or intrathecally. Antiepileptic drugs, as prescribed, to prevent or treat seizures. Surgical drainage or an exploratory craniotomy may be performed.
• **Liver Abscess:** Result of invasion of the liver by bacteria of protozoa. Liver abscess is uncommon; however, associated mortality is high.	• Abscesses can result from acute cholangitis, liver trauma, peritonitis, or sepsis, or an abscess can extend to the liver after pneumonia or bacterial endocarditis. • Most common signs and symptoms: right upper quadrant pain with a tender, palpable liver; anorexia: weight loss; fever and chills; jaundice; nausea and vomiting; and shoulder pain. • **Priority Care:** Surgical drainage is required.
• **Lung Abscess:** Result of subacute infection and necrosis that is generally associated with pyogenic bacteria.	• Common causes are tuberculosis, fungal infections of the lung, pneumonia, aspiration of mouth or stomach contents, and obstruction as a result of a tumor or foreign body. • Most common signs and symptoms: recent history of pulmonary infection, fever, fatigue, unplanned weight loss, cough, foul-smelling sputum, pleuritic pain, decreased breath sounds on affected side, and abnormal chest x-ray. • **Priority Care:** Interventions are similar to those for pneumonia. Management includes percutaneous drainage of the abscess and antibiotic therapy.

| Chart 2-1 | Abscess: Interprofessional Collaborative Care—cont'd |

Location	Interprofessional Collaborative Care
• **Pancreatic abscess**: Result of infected, necrotic pancreatic tissue and may follow acute necrotizing pancreatitis.	• Most common signs and symptoms: fever with temperature spikes as high as 104°F (40°C). Hyperglycemia can occur if insulin-secreting beta cells are destroyed with the infection. • **Priority Care**: A pancreatic abscess must be drained (percutaneously or laparoscopically) to prevent sepsis, and multiple drainage procedures may be necessary.
• **Peritonsillar abscess**: Results as a rare complication of acute tonsillitis. The most common cause is infection with group A beta-hemolytic streptococci.	• Most common signs and symptoms: collection of pus behind the tonsil, pushing the uvula toward the unaffected side. The swelling can cause severe throat pain, a muffled voice, fever, and difficulty swallowing. If difficulty breathing occurs (i.e., stridor, signs of obstructed airway), treat emergently. • **Priority Care**: Percutaneous needle aspiration to drain and culture the abscess; antibiotic therapy; intravenous corticosteroids can be used if the airway is compromised.
• **Renal Abscess**: A collection of fluid and cells resulting from an inflammatory response to bacteria in the renal parenchyma, renal fascia, or flank.	• Most commons signs and symptoms: flank pain, general malaise, and fever unresponsive to antibiotic therapy with an established kidney infection. • Priority Care: Broad-spectrum antibiotics and drainage by surgical incision or needle aspiration.

ACIDOSIS: ACID-BASE BALANCE CONCEPT EXEMPLAR

OVERVIEW

In acidosis, the acid-base balance of the blood and other extracellular fluid (ECF) is upset by an excess of hydrogen ions (H^+). This is seen as an arterial blood pH below 7.35. The amount of acids present is greater than normal compared with the amount or strength of bases.

Acidosis is not a disease; it is a condition caused by a disorder or pathologic process. It can be caused by metabolic problems, respiratory problems, or both.

METABOLIC ACIDOSIS

- Four processes can result in metabolic acidosis: overproduction of hydrogen ions, underelimination of hydrogen ions, underproduction of bicarbonate ions, and overelimination of bicarbonate ions.
- Reflected by the following arterial blood gas (ABG) values: pH below 7.35 and bicarbonate (HCO_3^-) values below the normal range (below 22mEq/L [mmol/L]).
- Metabolic acidosis often is accompanied by potassium excess (hyperkalemia).
- Common causes of metabolic acidosis include:
  1. Conditions that overproduce hydrogen ions:
     a. Diabetic ketoacidosis
     b. Fever
     c. Heavy exercise
     d. Hypoxia, anoxia, or ischemia as a result of lactic acid production (anaerobic metabolism)
     e. Starvation, carbohydrate-free diets
     f. Aspirin or other salicylate intoxication
     g. Ethanol, methanol, or ethylene glycol intoxication
  2. Conditions that cause underelimination of hydrogen ions (renal failure)
  3. Conditions that underproduce bicarbonate ions (liver failure, pancreatitis, or dehydration)
  4. Conditions that overeliminate bicarbonate (diarrhea)

RESPIRATORY ACIDOSIS

- Respiratory acidosis results when respiratory function is impaired and the exchange of oxygen (O_2) and carbon dioxide (CO_2) is reduced. This problem causes CO_2 retention, which leads to the same increase in hydrogen ion levels and acidosis (McCance, et al., 2014). Unlike metabolic acidosis, respiratory acidosis results from only one cause—retention of CO_2, causing increased production of free hydrogen ions.

- *Acute respiratory acidosis* is reflected by ABG values indicating a pH below 7.35, normal HCO_3^-, and high partial pressure of arterial carbon dioxide ($Paco_2$) values above 45mm Hg.
- *Chronic respiratory acidosis* is reflected by ABG values indicating a pH below 7.35, high HCO_3^- above 28mm Hg, and high Pco_2 above 45mm Hg.
- Common causes of respiratory acidosis include:
  1. Respiratory depression
     a. Anesthetics
     b. Drugs (especially opioids and benzodiazepines)
     c. Brain injury
  2. Reduced alveolar-capillary diffusion
     a. Disease (emphysema, pneumonia, tuberculosis, fibrosis, or cancer)
     b. Pulmonary edema
     c. Atelectasis
     d. Pulmonary emboli
     e. Chest trauma
  3. Airway obstruction
     a. Foreign object in airway
     b. Disease (asthma, epiglottitis)
     c. Regional lymph node enlargement
  4. Inadequate chest expansion
     a. Skeletal deformities (kyphosis, scoliosis), trauma (flail chest, broken ribs), spinal cord injury
     b. Hemothorax or pneumothorax
     c. Respiratory muscle weakness
     d. Obesity
     e. Abdominal or thoracic masses

COMBINED METABOLIC AND RESPIRATORY ACIDOSIS

Metabolic and respiratory acidosis can occur at the same time. Uncorrected acute respiratory acidosis always leads to poor oxygenation and lactic acidosis (McCance, et al., 2014). For example, an adult who has diabetic ketoacidosis and chronic obstructive pulmonary disease has a combined metabolic and respiratory acidosis. Combined acidosis is more severe than either metabolic acidosis or respiratory acidosis alone.

INTERPROFESSIONAL COLLABORATIVE CARE
Assessment: Noticing
Signs and symptoms of acidosis are similar whether the cause is metabolic or respiratory (Chart 2-2). *Cognitive changes may be the*

| Chart 2-2 | Key Features of Acidosis |

Cardiovascular Signs and Symptoms
- Delayed electrical conduction
- Ranges from bradycardia to heart block
- Tall T waves
- Widened QRS complex
- Prolonged PR interval
- Hypotension
- Thready peripheral pulses

Central Nervous System Signs and Symptoms
- Depressed activity (lethargy, confusion, stupor, coma)

Neuromuscular Signs and Symptoms
- Hyporeflexia
- Skeletal muscle weakness
- Flaccid paralysis

Respiratory Signs and Symptoms
- Kussmaul respirations (in metabolic acidosis with respiratory compensation)
- Variable respirations (generally ineffective in respiratory acidosis)

Integumentary Signs and Symptoms
- Warm, flushed, dry skin in metabolic acidosis
- Pale to cyanotic and dry skin in respiratory acidosis

first signs of acidosis. Assess the patient's mental status for awareness of time, place, and person.

Laboratory Assessment

Arterial blood pH is the laboratory value used to confirm acidosis. Acidosis is present when arterial blood pH is less than 7.35. The serum potassium level is often high in acidosis as the body attempts to maintain electroneutrality during buffering.

METABOLIC ACIDOSIS
- The pH is low (<7.35) because buffering and respiratory compensation are not adequate to keep the amount of free hydrogen ions at a normal level.
- The bicarbonate level is low (<21 mEq/L [mmol/L]).

- The partial pressure of arterial oxygen (Pao_2) is normal because gas exchange is not impaired.
- The $Paco_2$ is normal or even slightly decreased because gas exchange is adequate and CO_2 retention is not a factor.

RESPIRATORY ACIDOSIS
- The pH is low (<7.35) because of the increased amount of free hydrogen ions in the blood.
- Bicarbonate level is normal or a little elevated (≥21 mEq/L [mmol/L]).
- The Pao_2 is low, less than 88mm Hg because gas exchange is impaired.
- The $Paco_2$ is high (>45mm Hg) because the pulmonary problem impairs gas exchange, causing poor oxygenation and CO_2 retention.
- *The hallmarks of respiratory acidosis are a decreasing Pao_2 coupled with a rising $Paco_2$.*

❗ NURSING SAFETY PRIORITY: Critical Rescue

Assess the cardiovascular system first in any patient at risk for acidosis because acidosis can lead to cardiac arrest from the accompanying hyperkalemia. If cardiac changes are present, respond by reporting these changes immediately to the primary health care provider.

Analysis: Interpreting
Patients experiencing acidosis have problems associated with the decreased function of excitable membranes.
- *For metabolic acidosis*, these problems include hypotension and decreased perfusion, impaired memory and cognition, and increased risk for falls.
- *For respiratory acidosis*, life-threatening problems are related to the cause of the respiratory impairment.

The priority patient problem for the patient experiencing respiratory acidosis is:
- Reduced GAS EXCHANGE resulting from underlying pulmonary disease

Planning and Implementation: Responding
Interventions for acidosis focus on correcting the underlying problem and monitoring for changes. Remember, acidosis is not a disease. It is a symptom of another health problem. To ensure appropriate interventions, first identify the specific type of acidosis present.

METABOLIC ACIDOSIS
- Administer IV fluids and maintain IV access.
- Monitor ABG and serum potassium results and report critical values to the primary health care provider.
- The cardiovascular system and the skeletal muscle system are sensitive to acidosis and are the most important systems to monitor.
- Carefully evaluate rate, rhythm, intervals, and other components of the electrocardiogram (ECG).
- Treat to control the cause. For example, if diabetic ketoacidosis is the cause, then insulin is given to correct the hyperglycemia and halt the production of ketone bodies.
- *Bicarbonate is administered only if serum bicarbonate levels are low and the pH is less than 7.2* (Ellis, 2015).

Considerations for Older Adults

- The older adult is at higher risk for respiratory acidosis in the presence of comorbidities of cardiac, respiratory, and kidney disease.
- The older adult is more likely to be taking drugs that interfere with acid-base balance, such as diuretics, nonsteroidal anti-inflammatories, laxatives, and antihypertensives.

RESPIRATORY ACIDOSIS
1. Promote adequate GAS EXCHANGE to restore acid-base balance by:
   a. Assessing the airway and breathing effectiveness
   b. Administering oxygen as prescribed; carefully monitor oxygen saturation levels
2. Positioning to provide maximal lung excursion
3. Administering drug therapy (as prescribed) that focuses on improving ventilation and GAS EXCHANGE rather than altering pH.
   a. Drug categories useful for respiratory acidosis include bronchodilators, corticosteroids, anti-inflammatories, and mucolytics
4. Administering naloxone (Narcan) if the cause of respiratory depression is anesthesia or opioid administration; this opioid reversal agent is short-acting and may need to be repeatedly administered if the respiratory-suppressing drug is long-acting.
5. Monitoring respiratory status at least every hour for response to therapy or worsening of breathing by assessing the following:
   a. Respiratory rate and depth

b. Oxygen saturation (Spo_2) and ABG values to maintain a normal range of oxygenation (Spo_2 greater than 90% to 92% and Pao_2 greater than 90mm Hg)

   c. Effort of breathing, including use of accessory muscles

   d. Breath sounds to determine if lung conditions are interfering with GAS EXCHANGE

   e. Color of nail beds and mucous membranes to avoid pallor or cyanosis

   f. Level of consciousness and mentation

Care Coordination and Transition Management

- Use fall precautions for any patient with a problem in ACID-BASE BALANCE.
- Do not discharge a patient from the acute care setting with a problem in ACID-BASE BALANCE unless the patient is transitioning to end-of-life care.

⊞ ACUTE CORONARY SYNDROMES: PERFUSION CONCEPT EXEMPLAR

OVERVIEW

- The term *acute coronary syndrome* (ACS) is used to describe patients who have either unstable angina or an acute myocardial infarction (MI or AMI). In ACS, it is believed that the atherosclerotic plaque in the coronary artery *ruptures,* resulting in platelet aggregation ("clumping"), thrombus (clot) formation, and vasoconstriction. The amount of disruption of the atherosclerotic plaque determines the degree of coronary artery obstruction (blockage) and the specific disease process.
- *Unstable angina* is chest pain or discomfort that occurs at rest or with exertion and causes severe activity limitation.
- *Myocardial infarction (MI)* occurs when myocardial tissue is abruptly and severely deprived of oxygen. When blood flow is quickly reduced by 80% to 90%, ischemia can lead to injury and necrosis of myocardial tissue if blood flow is not restored.
- There are two types of MI: non–ST-segment elevation MI (NSTEMI) and ST elevation MI (STEMI).
  1. NSTEMI: indicates myocardial ischemia
  2. STEMI: indicates myocardial necrosis. STEMI is attributable to rupture of the fibrous atherosclerotic plaque leading to platelet aggregation and thrombus formation at the site of rupture (Mc-Cance, et al., 2014). *The thrombus causes an abrupt 100% occlusion to the coronary artery, is a medical emergency, and requires immediate revascularization of the blocked coronary artery.*
- Infarction is a dynamic process that does not occur instantly. Rather, it evolves over a period of several hours.

INTERPROFESSIONAL COLLABORATIVE CARE

Assessment: Noticing

- If symptoms of coronary artery disease (CAD) are present, delay collecting historical data until interventions for symptom relief, vital sign instability, and dysrhythmias are started and the discomfort resolves.
- *Rapid assessment of the patient with chest pain or other presenting symptoms is crucial.*
- Assess for signs and symptoms of angina and MI.
  1. Quality, onset, duration, and alleviating and aggravating factors related to chest discomfort or presence and quality of atypical pain, including jaw pain, back pain, nausea and vomiting, palpitations, extreme fatigue, sudden and severe dyspnea, or diaphoresis dizziness, weakness
  2. VS, including heart rhythm and SpO_2
  3. Distal peripheral pulses and skin temperature
  4. Heart sounds, noting S_3 gallop or S_4
  5. Assess breath sounds for heart failure (HF is a serious complication of MI)
  6. Fear and anxiety, denial, or depression
  7. Elevated serum troponin levels
  8. 12-lead ECG changes:
     a. ST depression or elevation or T-wave inversion
     b. ST elevation or abnormal Q wave in two or more contiguous leads
  9. Results of echocardiography, exercise test (stress test), thallium scan, contrast-enhanced cardiovascular magnetic resonance (CMR), CT coronary angiography, and cardiac catheterization, if performed

Analysis: Interpreting

- The patient with CAD may have either stable angina or ACS. If ACS is suspected or cannot be completely ruled out, the patient is admitted to a telemetry unit for continuous monitoring or to a critical care unit if hemodynamically unstable.
- The priority collaborative problems for most patients with ACS include:
  1. Acute pain due to an imbalance between myocardial oxygen supply and demand
  2. Decreased myocardial tissue PERFUSION due to interruption of arterial blood flow
  3. Decreased functional ability due to fatigue caused by the imbalance between oxygen supply and demand
  4. Decreased ability to cope due to the effects of acute illness and major changes in lifestyle
  5. Potential for dysrhythmias
  6. Potential for heart failure

Planning and Implementation: Responding
MANAGE ACUTE PAIN

- Manage pain to improve oxygen supply to the myocardium and decrease myocardial oxygen demand.
  1. Nitroglycerin may be used to dilate peripheral veins, reducing oxygen demand.
  2. IV morphine relieves pain and dilates arteriole to improve oxygen supply in coronary arteries without complete blockage.
  3. Apply supplemental oxygen if SpO$_2$ is less than 92% to increase oxygen supply.

! NURSING SAFETY PRIORITY: Critical Rescue

If the patient is experiencing an MI, prepare him or her for transfer to a specialized unit where close monitoring and appropriate management can be provided. If the patient is at home or in the community, call 911 for transfer to the closest emergency department.

INCREASE MYOCARDIAL TISSUE PERFUSION

- Because MI is a dynamic process, restoring perfusion to the injured area (usually within 4 to 6 hours for NSTEMI and 60 to 90 minutes for STEMI) often limits the amount of extension and improves left ventricular function. Complete, sustained reperfusion of coronary arteries after an ACS has decreased mortality rates.
  1. Administer and monitor patient responses to drug therapy.
     a. Aspirin (325mg, chewed to hasten absorption) reduces platelet aggregation and prevents clot extension in coronary arteries.
     b. Glycoprotein (GP) IIb/IIIa inhibitors prevent fibrinogen from attaching to activated platelets at the site of the thrombus; abciximab (ReoPro), eptifibatide (Integrilin), or tirofiban (Aggrastat) may be administered IV when unstable angina or a NSTEMI is present.
     c. Antiplatelets such as clopidogrel (Plavix) or ticagrelor (Brilinta) may be given as an initial loading dose, with a daily dose for up to 12 months after diagnosis.

! NURSING SAFETY PRIORITY: Drug Alert

Dual antiplatelet therapy is suggested for all patients with ACS, incorporating aspirin and either clopidogrel (Plavix) or ticagrelor (Brilinta). The major side effect for *each* of these agents is bleeding. Observe for bleeding tendencies, such as nosebleeds or blood in the stool. Medications will need to be discontinued if evidence of bleeding occurs. Teach patients signs of bleeding.

d. A long-acting beta-blocker, usually metoprolol XL or carve-dilol CR, reduces HR and oxygen demand, decreases sympathetic stimulation of the compromised myocardium, and prevents life-threatening dysrhythmias.

! NURSING SAFETY PRIORITY: Drug Alert

Do not give beta-blockers if the pulse is below 55 or the systolic blood pressure (BP is below 100mm Hg without first checking with the primary health care provider. The beta-blocking agent may lead to persistent bradycardia or further reduction of systolic BP leading to poor peripheral and coronary perfusion.

e. Angiotensin-converting enzyme inhibitor (ACEI) or angiotensin receptor blocker may be given to prevent ventricular remodeling and development of HF especially if diabetes, hypertension, or early kidney disease is present.
f. For patients with angina, a calcium channel blocker may be prescribed to promote vasodilation and perfusion.
g. Statin therapy reduces the risk of developing recurrent MI, mortality, and stroke.
2. Support reperfusion therapy so that it occurs within 30 minutes of arrival to the hospital or emergency department.
a. Thrombolytic therapy using a fibrinolytic such as tissue plasminogen activator (t-PA, alteplase [Activase]) (IV or intracoronary), reteplase (Retavase) (IV or intracoronary), or Tenecteplase (TNK) (IV push [IVP]) dissolves thrombi in coronary arteries.

! NURSING SAFETY PRIORITY: Drug Alert

During and after thrombolytic administration, immediately report any indications of bleeding to the primary health care provider or Rapid Response Team. Observe for signs of bleeding by:
- Documenting the patient's neurologic status (in case of intracranial bleeding)
- Observing all IV sites for bleeding and patency
- Monitoring clotting studies
- Observing for signs of internal bleeding (monitor hemoglobin, hematocrit, HR, and BP)
- Testing stools, urine, and emesis for occult blood

b. Percutaneous coronary intervention (PCI) typically involves placement of a stent to open the clotted coronary artery.

(1) PCI, an invasive but technically nonsurgical technique, is performed to provide symptom reduction for patients with chest discomfort within 90 minutes of a diagnosis of AMI unless there are specific contraindications.

(2) Other nonsurgical techniques used to ensure patency of the vessel are stent placement, laser angioplasty, and atherectomy.

(3) Care after PCI includes:

- Monitoring for potential problems after the procedure, including acute closure of the vessel, reaction to the dye used in angiography, hypotension, hyperkalemia, and dysrhythmias
- Instructing the patient to report the development of chest pain immediately
- Frequently monitoring the insertion site for bleeding or vessel occlusion by palpating pulses, observing skin color and warmth of the limb, and marking the circumference of any hematoma where the catheter was inserted
  - Apply manual pressure if there is bleeding from the insertion site.
  - Report bleeding or changes in perfusion immediately to the physician.
- Maintaining limited backrest elevation and immobilization of the affected limb per institutional protocol
- Maintaining pressure dressing per institution protocol
- IV heparin and aspirin may be given after thrombolytic therapy to reduce additional clot formation; monitor activated partial thromboplastin time (aPTT).
- Apply manual pressure if there is bleeding from the insertion site and notify the physician if the bleeding is extensive or if oozing persists for longer than 15 minutes.

INCREASE FUNCTIONAL ABILITY

- Promote rest and provide assistance in ADLs to minimize oxygen demands during periods of angina.
- Progress patient mobility with supervision, starting with sitting at the edge of the bed and progressing to ambulation.
- Assess the patient's vital signs and level of fatigue with each higher level of activity.

- Notify the primary health care provider if there are indications of activity intolerance such as orthostatic hypotension, hypertension with activity, or complaints of dyspnea, chest pain, or dizziness.
- Monitor for indications of coronary artery reperfusion, including abrupt cessation of chest pain or discomfort, sudden onset of ventricular dysrhythmias, resolution of ST segment depression, and reduction of markers of myocardial damage over 12 hours.
- Facilitate referral to cardiac rehabilitation. Cardiac rehabilitation is divided into three phases:
  1. Phase 1 begins with acute illness and ends with discharge from the hospital.
  2. Phase 2 begins after discharge and continues through convalescence at home.
  3. Phase 3 involves long-term conditioning.

INCREASE ABILITY TO COPE

- Assess the patient's coping mechanisms (commonly denial, anger, and depression) and level of anxiety.
- Provide simple, repeated explanations of therapies, expectations, and surroundings.
- Help the patient identify the information that is most important to obtain.
- Denial that results in a patient's "acting out" and refusing to follow treatment regimen can be harmful.
  1. Remain calm and avoid confronting the patient.
  2. Clearly indicate when a behavior is not acceptable and is potentially harmful.
- Anger may be the result of a patient's attempt to regain control of his or her life.
  1. Encourage the patient to verbalize frustrations.
  2. Provide opportunities for decision-making and control.
- Depression may be a patient's response to grief.
  1. Listen to the patient, and do not offer false or general reassurances.
  2. Acknowledge depression and provide appropriate referral and follow-up.

IDENTIFY AND MANAGE DYSRHYTHMIAS (SEE DYSRHYTHMIAS, CARDIAC).

Dysrhythmias are the leading cause of prehospital death in most patients with ACS. Even in the early period of hospitalization, most patients with ACS experience some abnormal cardiac rhythm.
- Monitor ECG.
- Evaluate hemodynamic status with dysrhythmia onset.

MONITOR FOR AND MANAGE HEART FAILURE; SEE HEART FAILURE
- Decreased cardiac output due to heart failure is a relatively common complication after an MI resulting from left ventricular dysfunction, rupture of the intraventricular septum, papillary muscle rupture with valvular dysfunction, or right ventricular infarction.

Medical Management of Left Ventricular Failure
- Oxygen therapy (intubation and mechanical ventilation may be necessary)
- Diuretics, nitroglycerin, or nitroprusside to reduce preload
- IV morphine to decrease pulmonary congestion and relieve pain
- Invasive hemodynamic monitoring to titrate drug therapy

Medical Management of Right Ventricular Failure
- Enhance right ventricular function by administering fluids to maintain urine output >30 mL/kg/hour or right atrial pressure around 20mm Hg.
- Patients who do not respond to medical management of HF may require an intra-aortic balloon pump (IABP) or left ventricular assistive device to improve myocardial perfusion, reduce afterload, and facilitate perfusion.

Surgical Management
- Coronary artery bypass graft (CABG) surgery is indicated when other treatments are deemed unlikely to succeed or have been unsuccessful in managing CAD and ACS. This procedure is performed while the patient is under general anesthesia and undergoing cardiopulmonary bypass (CPB) surgery. A graft from the internal mammary or other blood vessel bypasses the occluded coronary vessel to restore blood supply to the myocardium. CABG can be done as a traditional open-heart technique or as a minimally invasive surgical (MIS) approach.
- Preoperative care includes:
  1. Familiarizing the patient and family with the cardiac surgical critical care environment if surgery is performed as an elective procedure
  2. Teaching the patient how to splint the chest incision, cough and deep breathe, perform arm and leg exercises, and what to expect during the postoperative period, including how pain will be managed
- CPB is used to provide oxygenation, circulation, and hypothermia intraoperatively during induced cardiac arrest. Blood is diverted from the heart to the bypass machine, where it is heparinized, oxygenated, and returned to the circulation through a cannula placed in the ascending aortic arch or femoral artery.
- Off-pump coronary artery bypass is performed without the use of CPB. It requires special surgeon training and is not yet common.

- Provide immediate postoperative care in a specialized unit.
  1. Maintain mechanical ventilation for 3 to 6 hours.
  2. Monitor chest tube output.
  3. Monitor pulmonary artery and arterial pressures.
  4. Frequently assess vital signs and cardiac rate and rhythm.
  5. Ensure that pain is appropriately managed.
  6. Treat symptomatic dysrhythmias according to unit protocols or primary health care provider's orders.
  7. Monitor for complications of open heart surgery, including:
     a. Fluid and electrolyte imbalances
     b. Hypotension and hypertension
     c. Hypothermia
     d. Bleeding
     e. Cardiac tamponade
     f. Neurologic defects that may include slowness to arouse, confusion, and stroke
- Provide continued postoperative care.
  1. Encourage deep breathing and coughing every 2 hours while awake and splinting the incision.
  2. Assist the patient in resuming activity and ambulation.
  3. Monitor for new onset chest pain and dysrhythmias, especially atrial fibrillation.
  4. Assess for wound or sternal infection (mediastinitis), such as fever (longer than 4 days), reddened sternum, purulent incisional drainage, and an elevated WBC count.
  5. Observe for indications of postpericardiotomy or post-CPB syndrome: pericardial and pleural pain, pericarditis, friction rub, elevated temperature and WBC count, and dysrhythmias; the problem may be self-limiting or may require treatment for pericarditis.

! NURSING SAFETY PRIORITY: Critical Rescue

Monitoring the ECG and using the bedside alarms to notify about changes in ST from baseline can provide an early warning of coronary artery occlusion after any of the radiologic or surgical interventions for CAD. Immediately notify the physician about new-onset dysrhythmias, ST elevation, and other changes in the ECG indicating ischemia, injury, or infarct.

Care Coordination and Transition Management

- Most patients are still recovering from their illness or surgery when discharged from the hospital; home health services may be required.

- Teach the patient and family about:
  1. The pathophysiology of CAD, angina, and MI
  2. Risk factor modification:
     a. Smoking cessation
     b. Dietary changes (limiting fat and sodium intake)
     c. BP control
     d. Blood glucose control
  3. Gradual increase in physical and sexual activity, according to cardiac rehabilitation protocol
  4. Cardiac drugs: dose effects, adverse effects, and rationale for use
  5. Occupational considerations, if any
  6. Complementary and alternative therapies such as progressive relaxation, guided imagery, music therapy, and pet therapy
- Teach patients to seek medical assistance if they experience:
  1. A pulse rate that remains 50 or less while awake
  2. Wheezing or difficulty breathing
  3. Weight gain of 3 pounds (6.6kg) in 1 week, or 1 to 2 pounds (2.2 to 4.4kg) overnight
  4. Slow or persistent increase in nitroglycerin use
  5. Dizziness, faintness, or shortness of breath with activity
- Patients should call for emergency transportation to the hospital if they experience the following:
  1. Chest discomfort that is not relieved with nitroglycerin
  2. Chest or epigastric discomfort with weakness, nausea, or fainting
  3. Other angina symptoms that are particular to the patient, such as fatigue, back pain, or palpitations
- Other important discharge plans include:
  1. Teaching for drug adherence and provider follow-up
  2. Referring the patient and caregiver for continued cardiac rehabilitation
- Referring the patient to cardiac rehabilitation as an outpatient for ongoing education and therapy related to nutrition, physical activity, strategies to adhere to drug regimen, pain management optimization, and best practices for self-management.

ACUTE RESPIRATORY DISTRESS SYNDROME

OVERVIEW

- Acute respiratory distress syndrome (ARDS) is acute respiratory failure with these features:
  1. Hypoxemia that persists even when 100% oxygen is given (refractory hypoxemia)
  2. Decreased pulmonary compliance
  3. Dyspnea

4. Noncardiac-associated bilateral pulmonary edema
5. Dense pulmonary infiltrates on x-ray (ground-glass appearance)

- ARDS can occur from both acute lung injury such as pneumonia, aspiration, or inhalation injury and nonpulmonary causes such as sepsis, shock, or acute pancreatitis and other inflammatory conditions.
- ARDS is typically the result of a systemic inflammatory response leading to injury at the alveolar-capillary membrane, causing protein-containing fluid to leak into alveoli. Fluid-filled alveoli cannot exchange oxygen and carbon dioxide.
- Fluid also leaks into the spaces between alveoli (interstitial edema), further compressing alveoli and reducing the capacity to exchange gases.
- ARDS also results in damage to the alveoli such that surfactant production is reduced, making the alveoli unstable and at risk for collapse, further impairing gas exchange.
- Lung volume and compliance are dramatically reduced with alveoli damage resulting in long-term consequences of prolonged illness and recovery.

⚕ Genetic/Genomic Considerations

An increased genetic risk is suspected in the development and progression of ARDS. Variations in the genes responsible for surfactant production appear to increase the predisposition to developing ARDS as does variation in the genes responsible for cytokine production during inflammatory events associated with sepsis. Ask about the patient's previous responses to infection or injury. If the patient has consistently had greater-than-expected inflammatory responses, he or she may be at increased risk for ARDS and should be monitored for manifestations of the disorder.

INTERPROFESSIONAL COLLABORATIVE CARE
Assessment: Noticing

- Assess breathing patterns. Assess for difficulty breathing (hyperpnea, noisy respirations, cyanosis, pallor, and retraction intercostally or substernally).
- *Abnormal lung sounds are **not** heard on auscultation because the edema occurs first in the interstitial spaces and not in the airways.*
- Assess vital signs at least hourly for hypotension, tachycardia, and dysrhythmias.
- The diagnosis of ARDS is established by a lowered partial pressure of arterial oxygen (Pao_2) value (decreased gas exchange and oxygenation), determined by arterial blood gas (ABG) measurements.

! NURSING SAFETY PRIORITY: Action Alert

Early identification of patients at high risk for ARDS can allow the nurse to plan interventions for prevention of this serious condition. Both aspiration and systemic infection increase ARDS risk. Use aspiration precautions and infection control measures to reduce risk in vulnerable patients.

- The course of ARDS and its management are divided into three phases:
  1. *Exudative phase:* This phase includes early changes of dyspnea and tachypnea resulting from the alveoli becoming fluid-filled and from pulmonary shunting and atelectasis. Early interventions focus on supporting the patient and providing oxygen.
  2. *Fibroproliferative phase:* Increased lung damage leads to pulmonary hypertension and fibrosis. The body attempts to repair the damage and increasing lung involvement reduces gas exchange and oxygenation. Multiple organ dysfunction syndrome can occur. Interventions focus on delivering adequate oxygen, preventing complications, and supporting the lungs.
  3. *Resolution phase:* Usually occurring after 14 days, resolution of the injury can occur; if not the patient either dies or has chronic disease. Fibrosis may or may not occur. Research indicates that patients surviving ARDS have neuropsychological deficits and poor quality-of-life scores.

Interventions: Responding
- Management includes:
  1. Endotracheal intubation and mechanical ventilation
  2. Antibiotics to manage identified infections
  3. Conservative IV fluid volume administration to prevent excess lung tissue fluid while managing hypotension and inadequate perfusion
  4. Enteral nutrition or parenteral nutrition as soon as possible to prevent malnutrition, loss of respiratory muscle function, and reduced immune response

! NURSING SAFETY PRIORITY: Critical Rescue

For the patient requiring emergency intubation and ventilation, bring the code (or "crash") cart, airway equipment box, and suction equipment (often already on the code cart) to the bedside. Maintain a patent airway through positioning (head tilt, chin lift) and the insertion of an oral or nasopharyngeal airway until the patient is intubated. Delivering manual breaths with a bag-valve-mask may also be required.

ADRENAL GLAND HYPOFUNCTION

OVERVIEW

- Adrenal insufficiency is the loss of cortisol and aldosterone.
  1. Low cortisol results in glucose dysregulation and hypoglycemia.
  2. Low aldosterone causes fluid and electrolyte imbalances, especially hyperkalemia, hyponatremia, and hypovolemia.
- Decreased production of these adrenocortical steroids occurs as a result of:
  1. Inadequate secretion of adrenocorticotropic hormone (ACTH) (hypopituitarism)
  2. Dysfunction of the hypothalamic-pituitary control mechanisms
     a. The most common cause of this type of dysfunction is the sudden cessation of long-term, high-dose corticosteroid (also called glucocorticoid) therapy.
     b. Other causes include cancer and severe, high acuity illness (sepsis, shock).
  3. Direct dysfunction of adrenal gland tissue that typically occurs gradually
     a. Causes include tuberculosis, autoimmune factors, HIV/AIDS, adrenal tumors, low perfusion states, and irradiation of the adrenal glands.
     b. Adrenalectomy with sudden loss of hormones is also an example of direct dysfunction.
- Acute adrenal insufficiency or *Addisonian crisis* is a life-threatening event in which the need for cortisol and aldosterone is greater than the available supply.
  1. It often occurs in response to a stressful event like surgery, trauma, and severe infection when the adrenal hormone output is already reduced.
  2. Death from hypoglycemia, shock, and hyperkalemia-associated cardiac problems can occur unless interventions are implemented rapidly.

INTERPROFESSIONAL COLLABORATIVE CARE
Assessment: Noticing

- Obtain patient information about:
  1. Change in activity level or lethargy and fatigue
  2. Increased salt craving or intake
  3. GI problems, such as anorexia, nausea and vomiting, diarrhea, and abdominal pain
  4. Unplanned weight loss
  5. History of radiation to the abdomen or head
  6. Past or current medical problems (e.g., tuberculosis, previous intracranial surgery)

7. Past and current drugs, especially steroids, anticoagulants, opioids, or cytotoxic drugs
- Assess for and document:
  1. Manifestations of hypoglycemia (low blood glucose level, sweating, headaches, tachycardia, and tremors)
  2. Manifestations of hypovolemia (e.g., postural hypotension, dehydration)
  3. Cardiac problems from hyperkalemia (e.g., dysrhythmias, T wave changes on ECG)
  4. Muscle weakness
  5. Electrolyte abnormalities (elevated serum potassium and low serum sodium levels)
  6. Areas of increased pigmentation, decreased pigmentation, or patchy pigmentation
  7. Decreased alertness, forgetfulness, confusion
- Diagnosis is based on clinical manifestations and:
  1. Laboratory findings of low serum cortisol, low fasting blood glucose, low sodium, and elevated potassium levels
  2. Altered plasma levels of ACTH and melanocyte-stimulating hormone (MSH)
  3. Low urinary 17-HYDROXYCORTICOSTEROID and 17-ketosteroid levels
  4. Magnetic resonance imaging (MRI) or CT scans of brain, abdomen, and pelvis
  5. ACTH stimulation testing

Interventions: Responding
- Cortisol and aldosterone deficiencies are corrected by hormone replacement therapy.
  1. For oral cortisol therapy divided doses are usually given, with two-thirds given in the morning and one-third in the late afternoon (or as prescribed). This divided dose mimics the normal release of this hormone.
- Nursing interventions to promote FLUID BALANCE, monitor for fluid deficit, and prevent hypoglycemia include:
  1. Weighing the patient daily and recording intake and output
  2. Assessing vital signs every 1 to 4 hours
  3. Checking for dysrhythmias or postural hypotension
  4. Monitoring glucose levels
  5. Monitoring laboratory values to identify hemoconcentration (e.g., increased hematocrit, blood urea nitrogen [BUN])
- Administer cortisol and aldosterone replacement therapy.
- Teach patients how to self-manage this replacement therapy, including the importance of daily drug use and potential need to alter dose during stressful physical conditions.

> **! NURSING SAFETY PRIORITY: Drug Alert**
>
> Prednisone and prednisolone are sound-alike drugs, and care is needed not to confuse them. Although they are both corticosteroids, they are not interchangeable because prednisolone is several times more potent than prednisone and dosages are not the same.

ALKALOSIS

OVERVIEW

In patients with alkalosis, the acid-base balance of the blood is disturbed and has an excess of bases, especially bicarbonate (HCO_3^-). The amount or strength of the bases is greater than normal compared with the amount of the acids. Alkalosis is a *decrease* in the free hydrogen ion level of the blood and is reflected by an arterial blood pH *above* 7.45.

- Alkalosis is not a disease; it is a condition caused by a metabolic problem, a respiratory problem, or both.
- Alkalosis can result from an actual or relative increase in the amount or strength (or both) of bases. In an actual base excess, alkalosis occurs when base (usually bicarbonate) is either overproduced or undereliminated.
- In *relative* alkalosis, the actual amount or strength of bases does not increase, but the amount of the acids decreases, creating an *acid deficit.*
- A relative base-excess alkalosis (actual acid deficit) results from an overelimination or underproduction of acids.
- Common causes of metabolic alkalosis include:
  1. Increase of base (especially bicarbonate)
     a. Excessive use of antacids or bicarbonate
     b. Milk-alkali syndrome
     c. Multiple transfusions of blood products
     d. IV administration of bicarbonate
     e. Total parenteral nutrition
  2. Acid loss
     a. Prolonged vomiting
     b. Continuous nasogastric suctioning
     c. Dehydration from excess diuretic use
     d. Hypercortisolism
     e. Hyperaldosteronism
- The hallmark of metabolic acidosis is an ABG result with an elevated pH and an elevated bicarbonate level, along with normal oxygen and carbon dioxide levels.

- Common causes of respiratory alkalosis include:
  1. Excessive loss of CO_2 though hyperventilation
     a. Hyperventilation can occur in response to anxiety, fear, or improper settings on mechanical ventilation. Hyperventilation can also occur from direct stimulation of the central respiratory centers because of fever, central nervous system lesions, and salicylates.
- The hallmark of respiratory alkalosis is an ABG result with an elevated pH coupled with a low carbon dioxide level. Usually the oxygen and bicarbonate levels are normal.

INTERPROFESSIONAL COLLABORATIVE CARE
Assessment: Noticing

Symptoms of problems with acid-base balance regulation are the same for metabolic and respiratory alkalosis. Many symptoms are the result of the low calcium levels (hypocalcemia) and low potassium levels (hypokalemia) that usually occur with alkalosis. These problems change the function of the nervous, neuromuscular, cardiac, and respiratory systems. See Chart 2-3 for key features of alkalosis.

Chart 2-3	Key Features of Alkalosis

Central Nervous System Signs and Symptoms
- Increased activity
- Anxiety, irritability, tetany, seizures
- Positive Chvostek sign
- Positive Trousseau sign
- Paresthesias

Neuromuscular Signs and Symptoms
- Hyperreflexia
- Muscle cramping and twitching
- Skeletal muscle weakness

Cardiovascular Signs and Symptoms
- Increased heart rate
- Normal or low BP
- Increased digitalis toxicity

Respiratory Signs and Symptoms
- Increased rate and depth of ventilation in respiratory alkalosis
- Decreased respiratory effort associated with skeletal muscle weakness in metabolic alkalosis

- Assessment findings include:
  1. CNS changes: caused by overexcitement of the nervous system
     a. Dizziness, agitation, confusion, and hyperreflexia, which can progress to seizures.
     b. Positive Chvostek sign and positive Trousseau sign
  2. Neuromuscular changes: related to hypocalcemia and hypokalemia
     a. Skeletal muscle weakness, muscle cramping and twitching, hyperreflexia, tetany
  3. Cardiovascular changes: occurs because alkalosis increases myocardial irritability, especially when combined with hypokalemia
     a. Thready pulse, increased heart rate, possible hypotension
  4. Respiratory changes, especially increases in the rate of breathing, are the main causes of respiratory alkalosis. Although the volume of air inhaled and exhaled with each breath is nearly normal, the total volume of air inhaled and exhaled each minute rises with the increased respiratory rate. The increased minute volume may be caused by anxiety or physiologic changes.

Interventions: Responding
- Management focuses on:
  1. Preventing further loss of hydrogen, potassium, calcium, and chloride ions
  2. Restoring fluid balance
  3. Monitoring changes in patient assessment
  4. Treating the cause of the alkalosis
  5. Providing patient safety
- Nursing care priority is prevention of injury from falls. The patient with alkalosis has hypotension and muscle weakness, which increase the risk for falls, especially among older adults.

ALLERGY AND ALLERGIC RESPONSES

OVERVIEW
- Allergy or hypersensitivity is an excessive IMMUNITY reaction with inflammation.
- Allergy occurs in response to the presence of an antigen (foreign protein or allergen) to which the patient usually has been previously exposed.
- Hypersensitivity reactions are classified into four basic types, determined by differences in timing, pathophysiology, and symptoms:
  1. Type I or immediate. It is also called atopic allergy.
     a. It results from the increased production of immunoglobulin E (IgE).
     b. Common conditions include allergies to pollen, bee venom, peanuts, shellfish, and many drugs.

A

    c. Symptoms can be life-threatening with angioedema, anaphylaxis, or relatively mild with rhinosinusitis.

2. Type II or cytotoxic
    a. It results from the reaction of immunoglobulin G (IgG) with host cell membrane or antigen adsorbed by host cell membrane.
    b. Common conditions include autoimmune hemolytic anemia, Goodpasture syndrome, and myasthenia gravis.

3. Type III or immune complex mediated
    a. It results from formation of immune complex of antigen and antibody, which deposits in walls of blood vessels and results in complement release and inflammation.
    b. Common conditions include serum sickness, vasculitis, systemic lupus erythematosus, and rheumatoid arthritis.

4. Type IV or delayed
    a. It results from reaction of sensitized T cells with antigen and release of lymphokines, which activates macrophages and induces inflammation.
    b. Common conditions include poison ivy, stem cell or solid organ rejections, positive tuberculosis (TB) skin test, and sarcoidosis.

 ALZHEIMER'S DISEASE: COGNITION EXEMPLAR

OVERVIEW

- Alzheimer's disease (AD) is a chronic, progressive, degenerative dementia that is characterized by memory loss and impaired cognition.
- AD is characterized by neurofibrillary tangles, amyloid-rich or neuritic plaques, and vascular degeneration.
- Age older than 65, gender (women), and genetics are important risk factors for the development of AD, although the exact cause of AD is not known.
- Other causes of dementia are stroke or cerebrovascular impairment, head injury, Parkinson's disease, Lewy body formation, human immune deficiency virus (HIV) infection, environmental toxins including metals, and chemical imbalances; repeated head trauma can also increase risk for AD.

Veteran's Health Considerations

Studies suggest that veterans of war who have a current or past history of post-traumatic stress disorder (PTSD) are at an increased risk of AD and other dementias (Sibener, et al., 2014). An additional factor that further increases the veteran's risk of AD is being a prisoner of war (POW) (Meziab, et al., 2014).

INTERPROFESSIONAL COLLABORATIVE CARE
Assessment: Noticing

- Assess and document abnormalities in cognition, including language, personality, and behavior:
  1. Onset, duration, progression of symptoms of impaired cognition
     a. Cognitive changes include decreased attention, concentration, judgment, perception, learning, and short-term memory.
     b. *One of the first symptoms of AD is short-term memory impairment.*
  2. Functional status and self-management skills
     a. Changes in self-management include requiring assistance in hygiene, dressing, following directions, or completing familiar activities.
  3. Oral and written communication skills
     a. Alterations in communication abilities, such as **apraxia** (inability to use words or objects correctly), **aphasia** (inability to speak or understand), **anomia** (inability to find words), and **agnosia** (loss of sensory comprehension), are due to dysfunction of the temporal and parietal lobes.
  4. Changes in mood, personality, or behavior
  5. Changes in behaviors and personality, such as aggressiveness, paranoia, inappropriate social interactions, rapid mood swings, and increased confusion at night or when fatigued
  6. Medical history including family history of AD, as well as history of head trauma, viral illness, or exposure to metal or toxic waste
  7. Available support systems (spouse, partner, adult children)
  8. Assess stage of dementia (Chart 2-4)

Chart 2-4	Key Features of Alzheimer's Disease

Early (Mild), or Stage I (first symptoms up to 4 years)
- Independent in ADLs
- Denies presence of symptoms
- Forgets names; misplaces household items
- Has short-term memory loss and difficulty recalling new information
- Shows subtle changes in personality and behavior
- Loses initiative and is less engaged in social relationships
- Has mild impaired COGNITION and problems with judgment
- Demonstrates decreased performance, especially when stressed

- Unable to travel alone to new destinations
- Often has decreased sense of smell

Middle (Moderate), or Stage II (2 to 3 years)
- Has impairment of all cognitive functions
- Demonstrates problems with handling or unable to handle money and finances
- Is disoriented to time, place, and event
- Possibly suffers from depression and/or agitated
- Increasingly dependent in ADLs
- Has visuospatial deficits: has difficulty driving and gets lost
- Has speech and language deficits: less talkative, decreased use of vocabulary, increasingly non-fluent, and eventually aphasic
- Incontinent
- Has episodes of wandering; trouble sleeping

Late (Severe), or Stage III
- Completely incapacitated; bedridden
- Totally dependent in ADLs
- Has loss of MOBILITY and verbal skills
- Has agnosia (loss of facial recognition)

LABORATORY AND IMAGING ASSESSMENT
- No laboratory test can confirm the diagnosis of AD. Definitive diagnosis is made on the basis of brain tissue examination at autopsy, which confirms the presence of neurofibrillary tangles and neuritic plaques.
- Genetic testing specifically for apolipoprotein E (apo-E) or amyloid beta protein precursor in the cerebrospinal fluid (CSF) may be helpful as a supportive test (not a predictive test) for the differential diagnosis of AD.
- A variety of laboratory or imaging tests are performed to rule out other treatable causes of dementia or delirium such as electrolyte derangements, metabolic derangements (glucose), and stroke.

Analysis: Interpreting
- The priority collaborative problems for patients with AD include:
  1. Decreased memory and COGNITION due to neuronal degeneration in the brain
  2. Potential for injury or accident due to wandering or inability to ambulate independently
  3. Potential for elder abuse by caregivers due to the patient's prolonged progression of disability and the patient's increasing care needs

Planning and Implementation: Responding

The priority for interprofessional care is safety! *Chronic confusion and physical deficits place the patient with AD at a high risk for injury, accidents, and elder abuse.*

MANAGING MEMORY AND COGNITIVE DYSFUNCTION

- Collaborate with the health care team to provide a structured and consistent environment.
  1. Provide a safe environment with adequate lighting, and remove items that can obstruct walking.
  2. Implement fall precautions in the acute care setting.
  3. Place the patient within easy view of the staff, preferably in a private room.
  4. Arrange the patient's schedule to provide as much uninterrupted sleep at night as possible. Fatigue increases confusion and behavioral problems such as agitation and aggression.
  5. Establish a daily routine, explaining changes in routine before they occur and again immediately before they take place.
  6. Place familiar objects, clocks, and single-date calendars in easy view of the patient. Encourage the family to provide pictures of family members and close friends that are labeled with the person's name on the picture.
  7. Use orientation and validation therapy; acknowledge the patient's feelings and concerns.
  8. Support use of cognitive stimulation and memory training.
  9. Collaborate with the physical and occupational therapists to assist the patient to maintain independence in ADLs as long as possible through the use of assistive devices (grab bars in the bathroom) and exercise programs.
  10. Develop an individualized bowel and bladder program for the patient.
  11. Attract the patient's attention before conversing, then use short, clear sentences.
  12. Allow sufficient time for the patient to respond and remind patient to complete one task at time.
  13. Keep environmental distractions and noise to a minimum.
  14. Provide drug therapy:
      a. Cholinesterase inhibitors are approved for symptomatic treatment of AD.

❗ NURSING SAFETY PRIORITY: Drug Alert

Teach the family to monitor the patient's heart rate and report dizziness or falls because these drugs can cause bradycardia. Therefore they are used cautiously for patients who have a history of heart disease.

b. N-methyl-D-aspartate (NMDA) receptor antagonist, memantine (Namenda), can slow the rate of damage to nerve cells.

c. Selective serotonin reuptake inhibitors like paroxetine (Paxil) and sertraline (Zoloft) are used to treat coexisting depression.

d. Psychotropic drugs, also called *antipsychotic* and *neuroleptic drugs*, should be reserved for a patient with emotional and behavioral health problems that may accompany dementia, such as hallucinations and delusions. Avoid using them for combativeness, agitation, or restlessness because they reduce mobility and self-management.

15. Use activities and recreation such as art, dance, and music in the long-term care setting to minimize agitation and support meaning and quality of life.

PREVENTING INJURIES OR ACCIDENTS

- The risk for injury can be related to falls, impaired mobility, wandering, or elder abuse.

1. Ensure that the patient always wears an identification bracelet or badge that cannot be removed by the patient. Devices that use global positioning system (GPS) can be embedded in the bracelet or badge to provide tracking abilities.

2. Ensure that alarms or other barriers to outside doors are working properly at all times.

3. Check on the patient often and provide a variety of structured activities such as walks, games, puzzles, music, or art to manage restlessness.

❗ NURSING SAFETY PRIORITY: Action Alert

In inpatient health care agencies, use the least restrictive physical restraints such as waist belts and geri-chairs with lapboards only as a last resort because they often increase patient restlessness and cause agitation. Federal regulations in long-term care facilities in the United States mandate that all residents have the right to be free of both physical and chemical restraints.

4. Assess for elder abuse; use state or facility guidelines.

5. Use calm, positive statements, and reassure the patient that he or she is safe, redirecting the patient as needed and using diversion.

6. Remove and secure all sharp objects and medications.

7. Implement seizure precautions if there is a history of seizures.

8. Keep an updated photograph of the patient that can be used if the patient wanders away.

9. Inform the patient's family about the Safe Return program, a national government-funded program of the Alzheimer's Association that assists in the identification and safe, timely return of individuals with AD and related dementias who wander off and become lost.

PREVENTING ELDER ABUSE AND MANAGING CAREGIVER ROLE STRAIN

- The following nursing planning and implementation steps are used to increase family coping and decrease caregiver role strain:
    1. Assess the family and other caregivers for signs of stress, such as anger, social withdrawal, anxiety, depression, and lack of concentration, sleepiness, irritability, and health problems; refer them to their primary health care provider.
    2. Encourage the family to maintain its own social network and to obtain respite care periodically.
    3. Assist the family to identify and develop strategies to cope with the long-term consequences of the disease, including recognition of the role of religion and spirituality in caregiving.
    4. Advise the family to seek legal counsel regarding the patient's competency and the need to obtain guardianship or durable power of attorney.
    5. Refer the family to a local support group affiliated with the Alzheimer's Association.

Care Coordination and Transition Management

- When possible, the patient should be assigned to a case manager who can assess the patient's need for health care resources and facilitate appropriate placement throughout the continuum of care.
- The patient is usually cared for in the home until late in the disease process. Therefore teach the patient and family:
    1. How to assist the patient with ADLs
    2. How to use adaptive equipment
    3. With dietary consultation, how to select and prepare food that the patient is able to chew and swallow
    4. How to prevent the patient from wandering
    5. What to do if the patient has a seizure
    6. How to protect the patient from injury
    7. Drug information (if drugs are prescribed) and how to secure drugs so the patient does not take them inappropriately
    8. How to implement validation and orientation therapy and use diversion, including activity or exercise
    9. How to obtain respite services
    10. Strategies that caregivers can use to reduce their stress, including:
        a. Maintaining realistic expectations for the person with AD

b. Trying to find positive aspects of each incident or situation

A

c. Using humor with the person who has AD
d. Setting aside time each day for rest or recreation, away from caregiving duties if possible
e. Seeking respite care periodically
f. Exploring alternative care settings early in the disease process for possible use later
g. Establishing advance directives early in the disease process with the person who has AD
h. Taking care of themselves by watching their diet, exercising, and getting plenty of rest
i. Being realistic about what they can do, and getting and accepting help from family, friends, and community resources
- Refer the patient, family, and significant others to the local chapter of the Alzheimer's Association for education and support.

Veterans Health Considerations

For veterans who have AD, help families locate the closest Veterans Administration (VA) for support and services. Services may include home-based primary care, homemaker and home health aides, respite care, adult day health care, outpatient clinics, inpatient hospital services, nursing home, or hospice care. Caregiver support is an essential part of all of these services.

ALLERGY, LATEX
OVERVIEW
- Latex allergy is a type I hypersensitivity reaction; the specific allergen is a protein found in processed natural latex rubber products. Patients may report an allergy or skin irritation to adhesive bandages and balloons.
- Allergic reactions to latex vary from contact dermatitis (mild) to anaphylaxis (severe).
- People at the greatest risk for latex allergy are those with a high-level exposure to natural latex products, such as patients with spina bifida or congenital urinary tract abnormalities and health care workers who use latex health care products (e.g., gloves, syringes, BP cuffs).
- Individuals with a latex allergy often have a history of other allergies, especially to specific foods (e.g., banana, avocado, some nuts).

! **NURSING SAFETY PRIORITY: Critical Rescue**

Use only latex-free products in the care of a patient with a known latex allergy.

INTERPROFESSIONAL COLLABORATIVE CARE

- Teach patients who are sensitive to latex to avoid products containing latex.
- When caring for a patient with a known latex allergy, the primary health care provider should:
  1. Remove any latex-containing product from his or her person (e.g., erasers, tourniquets, blood tubes)
  2. Use paper tape or other low-irritation adhesive products
  3. Check syringes, medication vials, and IV tubing for latex and use alternatives if latex is present
  4. Wash hands with soap and water (not alcohol-based rub) before entering the room or touching the patient to remove latex residue on the skin from health care products

 AMPUTATION: PERFUSION CONCEPT EXEMPLAR

OVERVIEW

- An **amputation** is the removal of a part of the body. Amputations may be elective or traumatic. Most are *elective* and are related to complications of peripheral vascular disease (PVD), arteriosclerosis, or numerous attempts to repair complex injuries. These complications result in impaired perfusion (ischemia) to distal areas of the lower extremity. Diabetes mellitus is often an underlying cause. *Traumatic* amputations most often result from accidents or war and are the primary cause of *upper extremity* amputation.

Veterans' Health Considerations

The number of traumatic amputations also increases during war as a result of hidden land mines (IEDs), bombs, and motor vehicle accidents (e.g., in Iraq and Afghanistan). Multiple limbs or parts of limbs may be amputated as a result of these devices. Thousands of veterans of war in the United States are amputees and have had to adjust to major changes in their lifestyles. Many veterans have multiple amputations that affect MOBILITY, ADL functional ability, and psychosocial health.

LEVELS OF AMPUTATION

- *Surgical amputations* are planned elective procedures performed for a variety of disorders and complications.

Lower Extremity (LE) Amputation

- Loss of the great toe is significant because it affects balance, gait, and push-off ability during walking.
- Midfoot amputations (e.g., Syme amputation) remove most of the foot but retain the intact ankle so that weight bearing can be

accomplished without the use of prosthesis and with reduced pain.

- Other lower extremity amputations are below-knee amputation (BKA), above-knee amputation (AKA), hip disarticulation, or removal of the hip joint, and hemipelvectomy (removal of half of the pelvis with the leg).
- The higher the level of amputation, the more energy is required for ambulation.

Upper Extremity (UE) Amputation

- Rare and more incapacitating than amputations of lower extremities.
- Early replacement with a prosthetic device is vital for the patient with UE amputation.
- Complications of elective or traumatic amputation include:
  1. Hemorrhage
  2. Infection
  3. Phantom limb pain
  4. Neuroma—a sensitive tumor consisting of damaged nerve cells
  5. Flexion contractures, especially of the hip or knee
  6. Psychological maladjustment

INTERPROFESSIONAL COLLABORATIVE CARE
Assessment: Noticing
- Assess:
  1. Neurovascular status of extremity to be amputated
     a. Examine skin color, temperature, sensation, capillary refill, and pulses
     b. Compare findings with those of the unaffected extremity
     c. Check and document the presence of discoloration, edema, ulcerations, hair distribution, and any necrosis
  2. Psychosocial responses
     a. Preparation for a planned amputation
     b. Presence of bitterness, hostility, or depression
     c. Expectations of how the loss of a body part may affect employment, social relationships, and recreational activities
     d. Current self-concept and self-image
     e. Willingness and motivation to withstand prolonged rehabilitation after the amputation
  3. Patient's and family's coping abilities
  4. Patient's religious, spiritual, and cultural beliefs
  5. Diagnostic assessment may include:
     a. Blood flow by Doppler ultrasonography or laser Doppler flowmetry or use of transcutaneous oxygen pressure ($TcPO_2$)

QSEN Safety

A high degree of teamwork is essential in the operating room (OR) to prevent mistakes. With the patient assisting, identify the limb or digit to be amputated preoperatively, and mark it with indelible ink. Follow time-out rules in the operating room, so that the correct patient and digit or limb is identified by at least two people.

Analysis: Interpreting
* The priority collaborative problems for patients with amputations include:
    1. Potential for decreased tissue perfusion in residual limb due to soft tissue damage, edema, and/or bleeding
    2. Acute and/or chronic pain related to soft-tissue damage, muscle spasm, and edema
    3. Decreased mobility due to pain, muscle spasm, soft-tissue damage, and/or lack of balance due to a missing body part
    4. Potential for infection related to a wound caused by surgery or trauma
    5. Decreased self-esteem due to one or more ADL deficits, disturbed self-concept, and/or lack of support systems

Planning and Implementation: Responding
MONITOR FOR DECREASED TISSUE PERFUSION
* Monitor for signs indicating that there is sufficient tissue perfusion:
    1. The skin at the end of the residual limb should be a normal skin color, have a brisk capillary refill, and be warm
    2. Perform neurovascular checks including assessing the closest proximal pulse for strength and compare it with that in the other extremity, mobility, and sensory perception

! NURSING SAFETY PRIORITY: Critical Rescue

If the patient has impaired perfusion, notify the surgeon immediately to communicate your assessment findings. If the patient's BP drops and the pulse increases, suspect covert (hidden) bleeding and notify the surgeon. To check for the presence of overt (obvious) bleeding, be sure to lift the residual limb and feel under the pressure dressing for dampness or drainage. If bleeding occurs, apply direct pressure and notify the Rapid Response Team or primary health care provider immediately. Continue to monitor the patient until help arrives.

❗ NURSING SAFETY PRIORITY: Critical Rescue

For prehospital care with any traumatic amputation:
- Call 911.
- Assess the patient for airway or breathing problems.
- Apply direct pressure to amputation site with layers of dry gauze or other cloth.
- Elevate the extremity above the patient's heart to decrease the bleeding.
- Wrap the completely severed digit or limb in a dry, sterile gauze or clean cloth.
- Put the digit or limb in a watertight, sealed plastic bag.
- Place the bag in ice water—never directly on ice. Use one part ice and three parts water.
- Be sure that the amputated part goes with the patient to the hospital.

MANAGE ACUTE AND/OR CHRONIC PAIN
- Pain management for surgical pain may start with opioids, then transition to nonsteroidal anti-inflammatory drugs (NSAIDs).
- Phantom limb pain (PLP) is managed with calcitonin, beta blocking agents, antidepressants, and antiepileptic drugs.
- Complementary and alternative therapies for pain following amputation are useful for many patients for both acute and chronic pain syndromes.

❗ NURSING SAFETY PRIORITY: Action Alert

If the patient reports PLP, recognize that the pain is real and should be managed promptly and completely.

PROMOTE MOBILITY
- Coordinate with the physical therapist to begin exercises as soon as possible after surgery.
- For patients with AKAs or BKAs, teach range-of-motion (ROM) exercises for prevention of flexion contractures, particularly of the hip and knee.
- Ensure that a trapeze and an overhead frame are used to aid in strengthening the upper extremities and allow the patient to move independently in bed.
- For patients with BKAs, teach how to push the residual limb down toward the bed while supporting it on a pillow.
- Follow primary health care provider and agency policy for elevation of a lower leg residual limb on a pillow while the patient is in a supine position.

- Coordinate with a certified prosthetist-orthotist (CPO) for appropriate postoperative planning.
- Instruct the patient being fitted for a leg prosthesis to bring a sturdy pair of shoes to the fitting.
- After surgery, apply the prescribed device, such as the Jobst air splint or elastic bandages, to shape and shrink the residual limb in preparation for the prosthesis. If elastic bandages are used, reapply the bandages in a figure-eight wrap every 4 to 6 hours or more often if they become loose.

PREVENT INFECTION

- Drug therapy with broad-spectrum prophylactic antibiotics may be used before, during, and after surgery.
- The surgeon usually removes the initial pressure dressing and drains 36 to 48 hours after surgery.
- Inspect the incision or wound for signs of infection. Record the appearance, amount, and odor of drainage, if present.
- The surgeon may want the incision open to air until staples or sutures are removed or may want the residual limb to have a continuous soft or rigid dressing made of fiberglass.
- A soft dressing is secured by an elastic bandage wrapped firmly around the residual limb.

PROMOTE SELF-ESTEEM

- If possible, arrange for the patient to meet with a rehabilitated amputee who is about the same age as him or her.
- Assess the patient's verbal and nonverbal references to the affected area and determine the patient preference for terminology (e.g., *stump*).
- Ask the patient to describe his or her feelings about changes in body image and self-esteem.
- Check whether the patient looks at the area during a dressing change.
- Document behavior that indicates acceptance or nonacceptance of the amputation.

Care Coordination and Transition Management

- Help the patient and family set realistic desired outcomes and take one day at a time.
- Teach the patient or family to care for the limb after it has healed by cleaning it each day with the rest of the body during bathing with soap and water.
- Teach the patient and family to inspect the limb every day for signs of inflammation or skin breakdown.
- Teach the patient and family how to care for the prosthesis if it is available.

- Collaborate with a social worker or vocational rehabilitation specialist to evaluate the skills of a patient who may need to change employment.
- If appropriate, refer the patient and family for professional assistance from a sex therapist, intimacy coach, or psychologist.
- Teach the patient and family about available resources and support from organizations such as the Amputee Coalition of America (ACA) (www.amputee-coalition.org) and the National Amputation Foundation (NAF) (www.nationalamputation.org).
- Refer to specialty veteran organizations and support groups if the individual has served in the military.

AMYOTROPHIC LATERAL SCLEROSIS
OVERVIEW

- Amyotrophic lateral sclerosis (ALS), also known as *Lou Gehrig's disease*, is a progressive degenerative disease involving the motor neurons of the brain, brain stem, and spinal cord.
- As motor neurons are lost, atrophy of muscles occurs, resulting in dysphagia, weakness of the extremities, spasticity, and dysarthria.
- As the disease progresses, flaccid quadriplegia develops. Increased risk for pneumonia and respiratory failure result from paralysis of breathing muscles, including the diaphragm.
- Treatment is symptomatic and directed toward the following: preventing complications of immobility, promoting comfort, providing ongoing support and counseling to the patient and family, and informing the patient about the need for advance directives such as a living will and durable power of attorney.
- The drug riluzole (Rilutek) is associated with increased survival time but there is no cure.

ANAL FISSURE
OVERVIEW

- An anal fissure is a tear in the anal lining.
- Diagnosis is made with inspection and palpation of the perianal area.
- Pain during and after defecation is the most common symptom; bleeding may also occur.
- Nonsurgical interventions include local symptomatic relief measures such as warm sitz baths, analgesics, and bulk-forming agents or osmotic laxatives.
- Surgical repair under local anesthesia may be necessary for chronic or recurrent fissures that do not respond to nonsurgical management.

ANAL FISTULA
OVERVIEW
- An anal fistula, is an abnormal tract leading from the anal canal to the perianal skin.
- Most anal fistulas result from anorectal abscesses, but they can be associated with tuberculosis, Crohn disease, or cancer.
- Symptoms include pruritus, purulent discharge, and tenderness or pain aggravated by bowel movements.
- Because fistulas do not heal spontaneously, surgery (fistulostomy) is necessary.
- Measures such as sitz baths, analgesics, and bulking products or stool softeners are used to reduce tissue trauma and discomfort.
- Hygiene is important; patients should be instructed to clean the anal area after each bowel movement.
- Patients should avoid constipation and straining with stool.

ANAPHYLAXIS
OVERVIEW
- Anaphylaxis is the most dramatic and life-threatening example of a type I hypersensitivity reaction.
- It occurs rapidly and systemically, affecting many organs within seconds to minutes of allergen exposure.
- Drugs and dyes are common allergens in acute care settings and food and insect bites/stings are common causes in community settings.
- Anaphylaxis episodes vary in severity and can be fatal. *The major factor in fatal outcomes for anaphylaxis is a delay in the administration of epinephrine* (Crawford & Harris, 2015a).

INTERPROFESSIONAL COLLABORATIVE CARE
Assessment: Noticing
- Assessment findings include:
  1. History of anaphylactic response and documentation of allergen
  2. Subjective feelings of uneasiness, apprehension, weakness, and impending doom
  3. Generalized itching, and urticaria (hives)
  4. Erythema and angioedema (diffuse swelling) of the eyes, lips, or tongue
  5. Bronchoconstriction, mucosal edema, and excess mucus production
  6. Crackles, wheezing, and reduced breath sounds on auscultation
  7. Laryngeal edema (hoarseness and stridor)
  8. Respiratory failure with hypoxemia

9. Rapid, weak, irregular pulse
10. Dysrhythmias
11. Increasing anxiety and confusion

A

! NURSING SAFETY PRIORITY: Critical Rescue

Closely monitor any patient receiving a drug that is associated with anaphylaxis to recognize symptoms early. If you suspect anaphylaxis, respond by immediately notifying the Rapid Response Team because most anaphylaxis deaths occur from a delay in treatment.

Interventions: Responding
* Emergency respiratory management
    1. Immediately assess the respiratory status, airway, and oxygen saturation of patients who show any symptoms of an anaphylactic reaction.
    2. If the airway is compromised in any way, call the Rapid Response Team and establish or stabilize the airway.
    3. Immediately discontinue the drugs of a patient having an anaphylactic reaction.
    4. Anticipate the following:
        a. Epinephrine (1:1000) 0.3 to 0.5 mL is the first-line drug for anaphylaxis. It is given IM or IV when symptoms appear.
        b. Antihistamines such as diphenhydramine (Benadryl, Allerdryl ✦) 25 to 100 mg are second-line drugs and are given IV or IM for angioedema and urticaria.
        c. Apply oxygen therapy using a high-flow, non-rebreather facemask at 90% to 100%.
        d. For bronchospasms, the patient may be given an inhaled beta-adrenergic agonist such as metaproterenol (Alupent) or albuterol (Proventil) via high flow nebulizer every 2 to 4 hours.
        e. Corticosteroids are added to emergency interventions, but they are not effective immediately. Oral steroids are continued (at lower doses) after the anaphylaxis is under control to prevent the late recurrence of symptoms.
    5. Document all drugs administered and observe patient responses to drugs.

! NURSING SAFETY PRIORITY: Critical Rescue

Administer epinephrine (1:1000) 0.3 to 0.5mL IM or IV as quickly as possible. Most deaths from anaphylaxis are related to delay in epinephrine administration. This drug constricts blood vessels, improves cardiac contraction, and dilates the bronchioles. The same dose may be repeated every 5 to 15 minutes if needed (Vacca & McMahon-Bowen, 2013).

- Supportive care
  1. Position the patient to maintain airway, breathing, and circulation. Elevate the backrest to 45 degrees unless hypotension is present.
  2. Raise the feet and legs to improve blood return to the heart.
  3. Monitor pulse oximetry and/or ABGs to determine oxygenation adequacy.
  4. Use suction to remove excess oral or nasal mucous secretions.
  5. Continually assess the patient's respiratory rate and depth.
  6. Reassure the patient that the appropriate interventions are being instituted.
  7. Observe the patient for fluid overload from the rapid drug and IV fluid infusions.
  8. Before discharge, instruct the patient to obtain and wear a medical alert bracelet or ID about the specific allergy.
  9. Teach the patient who carries an automatic epinephrine injector (EpiPen) how to care for, assemble, and use the device. Obtain a return demonstration.

ANEMIA

OVERVIEW

- Anemia is a reduction in the number of red blood cells (RBCs), the amount of hemoglobin, or the hematocrit (percentage of packed RBCs per deciliter of blood). *NOTE: A patient who is fluid overloaded may have reduced hematocrit and NOT be anemic. With correction of vascular fluid excess, the hematocrit returns to a normal value.*
- It is a clinical sign, not a specific disease, because it occurs with many health problems.
- Anemia can be caused by a deficiency in one of the components needed to make fully functional RBCs, increased destruction of RBCs, decreased RBC production, or blood loss.
  1. Examples of deficiency of components needed to make fully functional RBCs are:
     a. Iron-deficiency that can occur from a diet inadequate in iron intake, poor absorption of iron in the GI tract, and blood loss
     b. Vitamin B12 deficiency, from inadequate dietary intake (e.g., vegan or dairy-free diets), small bowel disease and

resection, chronic diarrhea or other malabsorption syndromes and a lack of intrinsic factor (a substance secreted by gastric mucosa to aid in B12 absorption)
   c. Folate (folic acid) deficiency from poor diet intake (especially a diet lacking green leafy vegetables and citrus fruits, beans, and nuts) or malabsorption syndromes and some drugs, including anticonvulsants
2. Examples of conditions that increase RBC destruction are:
   a. *Sickle cell disease,* an inherited disorder that results in defective hemoglobin synthesis
   b. *Glucose-6-Phosphate Dehydrogenase (G6PD) deficiency,* an X-linked recessive deficiency of an enzyme needed for RBC glucose metabolism
   c. *Autoimmune hemolytic anemia* occurs when antibodies attack and destroy one's own RBCs, including warm and cold antibody anemias
3. Examples of conditions that decrease RBC production are:
   a. Chronic liver disease
   b. Administration of chemotherapeutic agents to treat cancer
   c. Chronic kidney disease due to reduced synthesis of erythropoietin, a hormone produced in kidneys to stimulate bone marrow productions of RBCs
4. Examples of blood loss are:
   a. GI bleeding (the most common cause of anemia)
   b. Loss of blood during trauma, childbirth, or surgery

INTERPROFESSIONAL COLLABORATIVE CARE
Assessment: Noticing
- Assessment findings include:
  1. The complete blood count (CBC) shows reduced RBCs, hemoglobin, and hematocrit
  2. Weakness
  3. Color changes in skin and mucosa: pallor, petechiae, or ecchymosis
  4. Shortness of breath from reduced oxygen-carrying capacity
  5. Chest pain related to reduced oxygen-carrying capacity in the presence of cardiac disease
  6. Bone marrow biopsy may show abnormalities within this hematologic cell-forming organ

Interventions: Responding
- Management includes:
  1. Implementing diet therapy
     a. For iron deficiency, provide a scheduled iron supplement and instruct the patient to increase his or her oral intake of iron from food sources, such as red or organ meat, egg yolk, kidney beans, leafy vegetables, and raisins.

       (1) Teach the patient that oral iron supplements can change the color of stool to black and can promote constipation that can be treated with diet, stool softeners, osmotic laxatives, or bulk-forming agents.

    b. For vitamin B12 deficiency, teach the patient to eat foods high in vitamin B12, such as animal proteins, eggs, and dairy products. Provide vitamin B12 supplements.

       (1) For severe B12 deficiency (also known as pernicious anemia), administer vitamin B12 injections initially and anticipate ongoing and lifelong oral or parenteral supplementation.

    c. For folic acid deficiency, increase dietary intake of food sources of folic acid and provide scheduled folic acid replacement therapy.

2. Provide transfusion therapy when prescribed, using packed RBCs to maintain safe levels of oxygen-carrying hemoglobin to prevent disability, ischemia, and impaired perfusion.

❗ NURSING SAFETY PRIORITY: Action Alert

Problems in blood transfusion contribute to unintended mortality and morbidity. Use a consistent process to prevent problems in blood transfusion by identifying patients correctly *and* ensuring the correct blood product is administered.

- Ensure informed consent is obtained before non emergent transfusion of blood or blood products. Before the transfusion, the priority action is to determine that the blood component delivered is correct and that identification of the patient is correct. Check the primary health care provider's prescription, the patient's identity, and whether the identification band identifiers are identical to those on the blood component tag.
- The nurse who will be administering the blood products must be one of the two persons comparing the patient's identification with the information on the blood component bag.
- Be familiar with common and severe transfusion reactions. Monitor the patient closely during the first 15 minutes of transfusion therapy to detect adverse reactions.

3. Immunosuppressive therapy with drugs such as prednisone, antineoplastic, or immunomodulation drugs if increased destruction of RBCs is caused by an altered immune response

4. Splenectomy (removal of the spleen) when the immune system is implicated and the spleen is destroying normal RBCs or suppressing their development

5. Hematopoietic stem cell transplantation (bone marrow transplantation) to replace defective bone marrow

ANEURYSMS OF THE CENTRAL ARTERIES

OVERVIEW

* An aneurysm is a permanent, localized dilation of an artery that enlarges the artery to at least two times its normal diameter.
  1. It can be *fusiform* affecting the entire circumference of the artery or *saccular* affecting only a portion of the artery as an outpouching.
  2. *True* aneurysms are those caused by weakened medial arterial layer (stretching the inner and outer layers) from acquired or congenital problems while *false* aneurysms result from vessel injury or trauma to all three arterial layers.
  3. A *dissecting* aneurysm indicates that blood is accumulating within the layers (walls) of an artery. Blood loss can decrease blood flow distally and the enlarging accumulation of blood in the arterial wall can result in vessel rupture with abrupt and massive hemorrhage.
* Aneurysms tend to occur at curves, bifurcations, and where the arterial wall is not supported by muscle or bone.
* Aneurysms of the central vessels include abdominal aortic and thoracic aorta.
* Atherosclerosis is the most common cause of aneurysms with hypertension, hyperlipidemia, and cigarette smoking as modifiable contributing factors. Age, gender, genetics, or family history are nonmodifiable contributing factors.

INTERPROFESSIONAL COLLABORATIVE CARE
Assessment: Noticing
* Most patients with aortic aneurysm are asymptomatic.
* Assess for signs and symptoms of abdominal aortic aneurysms:
  1. Abdominal, flank, or back pain that is usually steady, with a gnawing quality, is unaffected by movement, and may last for hours or days
  2. Prominent pulsation in the upper abdomen (do not palpate)
  3. Abdominal or femoral bruit
* Assess for signs and symptoms of thoracic aneurysms:
  1. Back pain
  2. Shortness of breath
  3. Hoarseness
  4. Difficulty swallowing
* Assess for abdominal or thoracic aortic rupture:
  1. Pain that is described as tearing, ripping, and stabbing and located in the chest, back, and abdomen

2. Symptoms of hypovolemic hemorrhagic shock: hypotension, tachycardia, diaphoresis, absent or faint peripheral pulses, and decreased mentation
3. Nausea, vomiting, and apprehension

- Also assess for:
  1. Presence of a distorted aortic profile on thoracic or abdominal x-ray or CT scan
  2. Enlarged aortic profile by ultrasonography

Interventions: Responding

NONSURGICAL MANAGEMENT

- Antihypertensive drugs are prescribed to maintain normal BP and to decrease stress on an aortic aneurysm that is smaller than 2 or 3 inches (6cm) or when surgery is not feasible.
- Teach the patient the importance of keeping scheduled appointments to monitor the size of the aneurysm with ultrasound or CT.
- Review with the patient the clinical manifestations of dissecting the aneurysm and the need to use emergency transportation if symptoms occur.

SURGICAL MANAGEMENT

- Endovascular stent graft placement via an intra-aortic catheter is the procedure of choice to manage an aneurysm.
- Monitor the patient closely in the hospital and at home for the development of complications, such as bleeding, aneurysm rupture, peripheral embolization, and misdeployment of the stent graft. All of these complications require surgical intervention.
- Surgical removal of the aneurysm is used when the aneurysm ruptures or when endovascular graft placement is not possible. The excised portion of the aorta is replaced with a graft.
- Provide perioperative care:
  1. Maintain mean arterial pressure within prescribed ranges to promote tissue perfusion and avoid hypertension.
  2. Complete neurovascular checks: Assess all peripheral pulses, skin temperature, sensation, and movement with vital signs; mark where the pulse is felt or heard with bedside Doppler devices.
  3. Assess vital signs every hour to detect early signs of hypotension.
  4. Immediately report to the physician any signs of bleeding, leak, or occlusion at the surgical site or from a drain, such as pulse changes, severe pain, cool to cold extremities below the graft, white or blue extremities or flanks, abdominal distention and decreased urinary output, and decreased or absent motor movement or sensation below the aneurysm or graft site.

5. Abdominal aortic aneurysm repair can compromise the blood flow to the kidneys and spinal cord.

- Care of the patient undergoing thoracic aneurysm repair is similar to that for other thoracic surgeries. Additional postoperative care includes:
  1. Monitoring chest tube drainage for excess drainage such as more than 100mL for 2 hours
  2. Monitoring for cardiac dysrhythmias, paraplegia, acute kidney injury, and respiratory distress

! NURSING SAFETY PRIORITY: Critical Rescue

Report signs of hemorrhage or graft occlusion to the primary health care provider immediately.

Care Coordination and Transition Management

- Emphasize the importance of follow-up with ultrasound or CT scanning to monitor the size of the aneurysm in patients who have not had surgery.
- Emphasize the importance of controlling BP.

! NURSING SAFETY PRIORITY: Action Alert

Teach patient receiving treatment for hypertension about the importance of continuing to take prescribed drugs. Instruct them about the signs and symptoms that must promptly be reported to the primary health care provider, which include:
- Abdominal fullness or pain
- Chest or back pain
- Shortness of breath
- Difficulty swallowing or hoarseness
- Educate the patient and family with written and oral information

Teach the patient self-management activities, particularly during recovery from surgery to repair the aortic aneurysm:
- Avoiding lifting objects heavier than 15 to 20 pounds (6.8 to 9.1 kg) for 6 to 12 weeks postoperatively
- Providing wound care
- Providing pain management instruction
- Refer to home health nursing and other community agencies as needed.

ANEURYSMS OF THE PERIPHERAL ARTERIES
OVERVIEW

- An aneurysm is a permanent, localized dilation of an artery that enlarges the artery to at least two times its normal diameter. Refer to *Aneurysms of Central Arteries*.
- While uncommon, the typical peripheral arterial aneurysm is at the femoral or popliteal artery.
- Monitor patients for lower limb ischemia such a decreased pulse, cool skin, and pain.
- These aneurysms are managed with vascular surgery using a synthetic graft or autogenous saphenous vein graft repair (bypass).
- Report sudden development of pain or discoloration of the extremity immediately to the surgeon, it may indicate thromboembolism preprocedure or graft occlusion postprocedure.

ANGIOEDEMA: IMMUNITY CONCEPT EXEMPLAR
OVERVIEW

- Angioedema is a severe IMMUNITY reaction—a type I hypersensitivity reaction—that involves the blood vessels and all layers of the skin, mucous membranes, and subcutaneous tissues in the affected area.
- It is most often seen in the lips, face, tongue, larynx, and neck.
- Exposure to any ingested drug or chemical can cause the problem. The most common drugs associated with angioedema are angiotensin converting enzyme inhibitors (ACEIs) used for hypertension.

INTERPROFESSIONAL COLLABORATIVE CARE
Assessment: Noticing

- Ask the patient for a list of all drugs taken on a regular basis, especially drugs for BP control. Although it would be helpful to have more information, intervention is critically important because laryngeal edema can cause the patient to lose his or her airway.
- Airway and breathing
  1. Problems that indicate a need for immediate intervention are the inability to swallow, the feeling of a lump in the throat, or stridor.
  2. Anticipate that the patient will be anxious, particularly if he or she is hypoxic.
- Other signs and symptoms
  1. The patient with angioedema (with or without laryngeal edema) has deep, firm swelling of the face, lips, tongue, and neck. He or she may have difficulty speaking or drinking because the lips are so stiff from swelling. The face can be so

distorted that friends and relatives may not recognize the patient. Often nasal swelling interferes with breathing through the nose. When swelling occurs around the eyes and eyelids, the patient may not be able to see. Some patients may have urticaria (hives), but many do not.

Cultural and Spiritual Considerations

Patient-Centered Care

Black adults, especially African Americans, have a higher incidence of angioedema and laryngeal edema from ACEIs. In a large study of ACEI-induced angioedema, 55% of fatalities occurred among blacks. Any ACEI should be used cautiously in black patients. Be sure to observe the patient carefully for any signs and symptoms of angioedema and laryngeal edema after the first dose. Teach black patients taking a drug from this category about the signs and symptoms of angioedema and the importance of going to an emergency department or calling 911 immediately if symptoms appear.

Analysis: Interpreting

- The priority collaborative problems for patients with angioedema are:
  1. Potential for airway obstruction as a result of mucosal swelling
  2. Anxiety as a result of cerebral hypoxia and threat of death

Planning and Implementation: Responding

MAINTAIN A PATENT AIRWAY

- Administer oxygen to maintain gas exchange
- Establish intravenous access and administer drugs to interfere with the immune and inflammatory response including
  1. Antihistamine (H1 blocker)
  2. Corticosteroid
  3. Epinephrine

MINIMIZE ANXIETY

- Stay with the patient and reassure that proper treatment is occurring.
- Apply oxygen and monitor patient response to drug and oxygen therapy.
- Continually assess pulse oximetry, respiratory status, and the patient's ability to swallow.

Care Coordination and Transition Management

- With successful management, the patient is discharged to resume his or her usual activities.

- Determine the cause of the angioedema and teach the patient to avoid the offending agent.
- Ensure that he or she knows to seek emergency care as soon as any signs or symptoms of the problem occur.

APPENDICITIS

OVERVIEW

- Appendicitis is an acute inflammation of the vermiform appendix, the small finger-like pouch attached to the cecum of the colon.
- Inflammation of the appendix occurs when the lumen of the appendix is obstructed.
- Inflammation leads to infection as bacteria invade the wall of the appendix.
- Appendicitis is the most common cause of pain in the right lower abdominal quadrant.

Considerations for Older Adults

Appendicitis is relatively rare at extremes in age. However, perforation is more common in older people, causing a higher mortality rate. The diagnosis of appendicitis is difficult to establish in older adults because symptoms of pain and tenderness may not be as pronounced in older adults. This difference results in treatment delay and an increased risk for perforation, peritonitis, and death.

INTERPROFESSIONAL COLLABORATIVE CARE

Assessment: Noticing

- Assessment findings include:
  1. Abdominal pain in the right lower quadrant (McBurney's point); although pain can be anywhere in the abdomen or flank
  2. Abdominal pain that increases with cough or movement and is relieved by flexion of the right hip or knees suggests a perforated appendix with peritonitis
  3. Nausea and vomiting
  4. Abdominal muscle rigidity or rebound tenderness may indicate perforation and peritonitis
  5. Normal or slightly elevated temperature, tachycardia, hypo- or hypertension
  6. Increased WBC count with neutrophilia, increased segmented neutrophils
  7. Ultrasound or CT scan showing an enlarged appendix

Interventions: Responding

- Provide routine preoperative care; withhold oral fluids 2 to 4 hours preoperatively to surgical appendectomy (removal of the appendix).
- Administer opioid analgesics and antibiotics.
- Keep the patient in a semi-Fowler's position so that any abdominal drainage can be contained in the lower abdomen.
- An appendectomy may be performed as a traditional procedure through external skin incision (laparoscopy or open procedure) or via endoscopy.
- Provide routine postoperative care with an anticipated length of stay of less than 24 hours for uncomplicated procedures and 3 to 5 days when perforation or peritonitis is present.
- Administer analgesics and antibiotics to patients with a complicated appendicitis presentation and surgery.

ARTERIOSCLEROSIS AND ATHEROSCLEROSIS

OVERVIEW

- Arteriosclerosis is a thickening or hardening of the arterial wall often associated with aging.
- Atherosclerosis, a type of arteriosclerosis, involves the formation of a plaque within the arterial wall and is the leading cardiovascular disease.
- The exact pathophysiologic mechanism of atherosclerosis is unknown but is thought to occur with inflammation of the vessel.
- After the vessel becomes inflamed, a fatty streak appears on the intimal surface of an artery and, over time, develops into a fibrous plaque that obstructs the blood flow of the artery.
- When plaque ruptures, the exposed underlying tissue causes platelet adhesion and rapid thrombus formation. The thrombus may suddenly block a blood vessel, resulting in ischemia and infarction (e.g., MI, ischemic stroke, arterial occlusion).
- The rate of progression of plaque formation and rupture is thought to be influenced by genetic factors, diabetes and other chronic conditions, and lifestyle (e.g., smoking, dietary intake of fat, sedentary habits).

INTERPROFESSIONAL COLLABORATIVE CARE
Assessment: Noticing

- Assess:
  1. Risk for cardiovascular disease, using history and standard tools
  2. BP in both arms and note any differences
  3. Pulses at all major sites and note any bruits and diminishment or absence

4. Presence of prolonged capillary refill or cool extremities
5. Serum cholesterol (total, low-density lipoprotein [LDL], protective high-density lipoprotein [HDL]) and triglyceride levels

Interventions: Responding

- Interventions include:
  1. Teaching the patient to adopt dietary habits to reduce risk, including limiting saturated fat to 5% to 6% of calories and emphasizing the intake of vegetables, fruit, and whole grains. DASH or Mediterranean diets are examples of guideline diets.
  2. Developing and reinforcing the plan for regular activity with at least 40 minutes 3 to 4 times weekly that is moderate-to-vigorous (Eckel, et al., 2014)
  3. Administering drug therapy as prescribed:
     a. Cholesterol-lowering drugs, usually a statin
  4. Using best practices to assist patients to stop smoking and informing nonsmokers to avoid secondhand smoke
  5. Planning for follow-up and ongoing care with primary care provider at least annually

 ARTHRITIS, RHEUMATOID: IMMUNITY CONCEPT EXEMPLAR

OVERVIEW

- Rheumatoid arthritis (RA) is a condition of altered IMMUNITY that occurs when transformed autoantibodies (rheumatoid factors [RFs]) cause inflammation.
- RA is a chronic, progressive, systemic inflammatory autoimmune disease process that damages and destroys synovial joints and other body tissues; inflammatory responses may occur in any organ or body system in which connective tissue is prevalent.
  1. Affected body systems include cardiovascular (e.g., vasculitis, myocarditis, pericarditis), lung (e.g., pleurisy, pneumonitis), eyes, and skin.
  2. Inflammatory factors also contribute to anorexia, weight loss, and nutritional derangements.
- Onset may be acute and severe or slow and insidious, and the pattern of illness progression includes remissions and exacerbations.
- Permanent joint changes may be avoided or mitigated when RA is diagnosed early. Early aggressive treatment to suppress synovitis may lead to a remission.
- Genes, typically associated with human leukocyte antigen (HLA)-DR proteins, are thought to combine with environmental conditions to trigger RA.

INTERPROFESSIONAL COLLABORATIVE CARE

A

Assessment: Noticing

- Assess for early disease manifestations, including:
  1. Joint stiffness, swelling, pain (especially of the upper extremities); usually bilateral (affecting both sides) and symmetric (same joints) symptoms
  2. Fatigue, generalized weakness
  3. Anorexia, weight loss
  4. Persistent, low-grade fever
  5. Joint dislocation or infection (one hot, swollen joint; pain out of proportion to other joints)

! NURSING SAFETY PRIORITY: Critical Rescue

Cervical RA may result in subluxation (partial joint dislocation), especially of the first and second vertebrae. This complication may be life-threatening because branches of the phrenic nerve that supply the diaphragm are restricted and respiratory function may be compromised. The patient is also in danger of becoming quadriparetic (weak in all extremities) or quadriplegic (paralyzed in all extremities). If cervical pain (may radiate down one arm) or loss of range of motion is present in the cervical spine, keep the neck straight in a neutral position to prevent permanent damage to the spinal cord or spinal nerves. *Notify the primary health care provider immediately about these neurologic changes.*

- Assess for late disease manifestations:
  1. Affected joints become deformed
  2. Muscles atrophy above and below affected joints
  3. ROM decreases and can cause pain (e.g., carpal tunnel syndrome)
  4. Subcutaneous nodules along muscles or tendons and Baker's cysts (enlarged popliteal bursae behind the knee)
  5. Tendonitis or tendon rupture (especially the Achilles tendon)
  6. Exacerbations, often called *flares*, manifested by increased joint swelling and tenderness and moderate to severe weight loss, fever, and extreme fatigue
  7. Infection in affected joints and skin
  8. Systemic complications:
     a. Vasculitis or inflammation of blood vessels, particularly of small- to medium-sized vessels
     b. Cardiac inflammation such as myocarditis or pericarditis
     c. Lung inflammation such as pleurisy, pneumonitis, diffuse interstitial fibrosis, and pulmonary hypertension

    d. Skin inflammation including
      (1) Ischemic skin and nail lesions that appear in small groups as small, brownish spots
      (2) Larger skin lesions that appear on the lower extremities and may lead to ulceration, and that heal slowly as a result of vascular changes leading to poor peripheral circulation
    e. Peripheral neuropathy, causing footdrop and paresthesias
    f. Carpel tunnel syndrome or complications around wrist mobility with pain
    g. Ocular involvement, such as iritis or scleritis
    h. Sjögren syndrome (eye, mouth, and vaginal dryness)
    i. Felty syndrome (splenomegaly with neutropenia, leukopenia, thrombocytosis)

- Assess for psychosocial issues
  1. Fear of becoming disabled and dependent, uncertainty about the disease process, altered body image, devaluation of self, frustration, and depression are common.
  2. Extreme fatigue and impaired comfort may result in a reluctance to socialize.
  3. Body changes may cause poor self-esteem and body image.
  4. The patient may grieve, experience degrees of depression, or have feelings of helplessness caused by a loss of control over a disease that can "consume" the body.
- Assess laboratory data
  1. Laboratory tests help support a diagnosis of RA, but no single test or group of tests can confirm diagnosis.
- Other diagnostic assessments
  1. Joint x-rays
  2. Bone scan or joint scan
  3. Arthrocentesis, a procedure to aspirate a sample of the synovial fluid to relieve pressure and analyze the fluid for inflammatory cells and immune complexes, including RF

Analysis: Interpreting
- The priority collaborative problems for patients with RA include:
  1. Chronic inflammation and pain due to systemic autoimmune disease process
  2. Potential for decreased mobility related to joint deformity, muscle atrophy, and fatigue
  3. Potential for decreased self-esteem image related to joint deformity

Planning and Implementation: Responding
Patients who have RA are managed in the community under the supervision of a qualified primary health care provider. The goal of management is that the disease goes into remission and its progression

slows to decrease pain, prevent joint destruction, and increase mobility. When patients with RA are admitted to the inpatient acute care or long-term care facility, it is usually for health problems other than for complications of arthritis.

MANAGE CHRONIC INFLAMMATION PAIN

1. Synovectomy: removal of inflamed synovium may be needed for joints such as the knee or elbow.
2. Total joint arthroplasty (TJA) may be indicated when other measures fail to relieve pain.
3. Drug therapy used to treat RA:
   a. **NSAIDs** are sometimes used for RA to help promote comfort and decrease inflammation.
   b. **First-Line Disease-Modifying Antirheumatic Drugs (DMARDs)** are used to slow the progression of RA:
      (1) Methotrexate (MTX)(Rheumatrex), an immunosuppressive medication, in a low, once-a-week dose (generally 25 mg or less per week orally) is the mainstay of therapy for RA because it is effective and relatively inexpensive.
      (2) Leflunomide (Arava)
      (3) Hydroxychloroquine (Plaquenil)
   c. Biological response modifiers (BRMs), sometimes called biologics, are one of the newest classes of DMARDs.
      (1) Most BRMs neutralize the biologic activity of tumor necrosis factor–alpha (TNFA) by inhibiting its binding with TNF receptors. Any one of the BRMs may be tried.
      (2) Common examples include etanercept (Enbrel), infliximab (Remicade), adalimumab (Humira), and certolizumab (Cimzia).
         i. Do not give BRMs if patient has a serious infection, TB, or MS because they may exacerbate these health problems.
         ii. Teach patients taking BRMs to avoid getting live vaccines.
         iii. Teach patients to avoid crowds and people with infections because serious infections, especially respiratory infections, can lead to hospitalization or cause death.
   d. Glucocorticoids (steroids)—usually prednisone (Deltasone)—are given for their fast-acting anti-inflammatory and immunosuppressive effects.

Nonpharmacologic Management

1. Nonpharmacologic pain-relief measures: rest, positioning, ice, and heat

2. Plasmapheresis (or plasma exchange) to remove the antibodies causing the disease
3. Complementary and integrative therapy to relief pain such as hypnosis, acupuncture, magnet therapy, imagery, or music therapy
4. Stress management to reduce pain perception
5. Nutrition to meet caloric and protein goals

PROMOTE MOBILITY

1. Identify assistive devices to allow the patient as much independence as possible.
2. Help the patients acquire household items with handles.
3. Teach the patient to use larger muscle groups to perform tasks usually performed by fine muscle groups (e.g., use the flat of the hand to squeeze toothpaste tubes instead of the fingers).
4. Refer the patient to an occupational or physical therapist or the Arthritis Foundation for special assistive and adaptive devices.
5. Collaborate with the health care team to alleviate or manage factors that contribute to fatigue and immobility:
   a. Anemia
      (1) Administer iron, folic acid, vitamin supplements, or a combination of these.
      (2) Assess the patient for drug-related GI bleeding, such as that caused by NSAID therapy, by testing the stool for occult blood.
   b. Muscle atrophy
      (1) Collaborate with a physical therapist to develop and help the patient implement a personalized daily exercise program.
      (2) Encourage patient to maintain independence in ADLs and set priorities in care or assistance in care.
   c. Inadequate rest
      (1) Arrange for a quiet environment.
      (2) Encourage the patient to develop a bedtime routine for sleep hygiene, such as drinking a warm beverage before bedtime.
6. Teach principles of energy conservation.
   a. Pacing activities
   b. Setting priorities
   c. Planning rest periods

ENHANCE SELF-ESTEEM

1. Identify factors to enhance self-esteem when dysfunction or joint deformity occurs.
2. Determine the patient's perception of role and social changes and identify sources of support for role changes and to avoid isolation.

3. Communicate acceptance of the patient; establish a trusting relationship.

Care Coordination and Transition Management

1. Remind patients to avoid crowds and other possible sources of infection when they are taking drugs that decrease immunity.
2. Assist the patient and family to identify structural changes needed in the home before discharge.
3. Instruct patients with arthritic pain to use multiple modalities for pain relief, including ice/heat, rest, positioning, complementary and alternative therapies, and medications as prescribed.
4. Reinforce information about drug therapy.
5. Teach the patient to consult with the primary health care provider before trying any over-the-counter (OTC) or home remedies.
6. Teach joint protection measures related to splinting, positioning, and function.
7. Review energy conservation measures.
8. Review the prescribed exercise program.
9. Encourage patients with arthritis and connective tissue diseases to discuss their chronic illness and identify coping strategies that have previously been successful.
10. Refer the patient to the nutritionist, counselor, home health nurse, rehabilitation therapist, financial counselor, and local and state support groups as needed.

ASTHMA

OVERVIEW

- Asthma is chronic disease with intermittent and reversible airflow obstruction affecting only the airways, not the alveoli.
- Airway obstruction occurs in two ways:
  1. Inflammation, obstructing the lumen (the inside) of airways, occurs in response to the presence of specific allergens; general irritants such as cold air, dry air, or fine airborne particles; microorganisms; and aspirin.
  2. Airway tissue sensitivity (hyperresponsiveness), obstructing airways by constricting bronchial smooth muscle and causing a narrowing of the airway from the outside, can occur with exercise, an upper respiratory illness, and for unknown reasons.
- Severe airway obstruction from acute asthma can be fatal.
- Although asthma may be classified into different types based on the events known to trigger the attacks, the pathophysiology is similar for all types of asthma regardless of the triggering event.

- Asthma can occur at any age. About half of adults with asthma also had the disease in childhood. Asthma is more common in urban settings than in rural settings.

Considerations for Older Adults

Asthma occurs as a new disorder in about 3% of people older than 55 years. Another 3% of people older than 60 years have asthma as a continuing chronic disorder. Lung and airway changes as a part of aging make any breathing problem more serious in the older adult. One problem related to aging is a change in the sensitivity of beta-adrenergic receptors. When stimulated, these receptors relax smooth muscle and cause bronchodilation. As these receptors become less sensitive, they no longer respond as quickly or as strongly to agonists (e.g., epinephrine, dopamine) and beta-adrenergic drugs, which are often used as rescue therapy during an acute asthma attack. Teaching older patients how to avoid asthma attacks and to use preventive drug therapy correctly are nursing priorities.

Gender Health Considerations

The incidence of asthma is about 35% higher among women than men, and the asthma death rates are also higher among women. Obesity and hormonal fluctuations around the menstrual cycle are thought to contribute to the difference in incidence, and undertreatment of the disease is thought to be a factor in the higher death rate. Teaching women how to be a partner in asthma management and the correct use of preventive and rescue drugs remains a nursing priority in improving the outcomes of the disease.

INTERPROFESSIONAL COLLABORATIVE CARE
Assessment: Noticing
- Obtain the patient's personal history.
  1. Episodes of dyspnea, chest tightness, coughing, wheezing, and increased mucus production
  2. Specific patterns of dyspnea appearance (at night, with exercise, seasonally, or in association with other specific activities or environments)
  3. Other allergic symptoms such as rhinitis, skin rash, or pruritus, and whether other family members have asthma or respiratory problems

- Signs and symptoms during an attack include:
  1. Audible wheeze (at first, louder on exhalation)
  2. Increased respiratory rate
  3. Coughing
  4. Inability to complete a sentence of more than five words
  5. Decreased oxygen saturation
  6. Pallor or cyanosis of oral mucous membranes and nail beds
  7. Tachycardia
  8. Changes in level of consciousness
  9. Use of accessory muscles (muscle retraction at the sternum, the suprasternal notch, and between the ribs)
- Physical changes from frequent asthma attacks include:
  1. Increased anteroposterior (AP) chest diameter
  2. Increased space between the ribs
- Laboratory assessment data changes during an asthma attack:
  1. Decreased PaO_2
  2. Decreased $PaCO_2$ (early in attack)
  3. Elevated $PaCO_2$ (later in attack)
- Laboratory assessment data changes from allergic asthma:
  1. Elevated serum eosinophil count
  2. Elevated immunoglobulin E (IgE) levels
  3. Sputum-containing eosinophils, mucous plugs, and shed epithelial cells (Curschmann spirals)
- Diagnostic assessment:
  1. Pulmonary function tests (PFTs) measured using spirometry, especially:
     a. Forced vital capacity (FVC) (volume of air exhaled from full inhalation to full exhalation)
     b. Forced expiratory volume in the first second (FEV_1) (volume of air blown out as hard and fast as possible during the first second of the most forceful exhalation after the greatest full inhalation)
     c. Peak expiratory flow (PEF) (fastest airflow rate reached at any time during exhalation)
  2. Chest x-ray

Interventions: Responding

- The goals of asthma therapy are to improve airflow, relieve symptoms, and prevent episodes by making the patient an active partner in the management plan.
- Priority patient education focuses on:
  1. Teaching the patient to assess asthma severity at least once daily with a peak flowmeter and adjust drugs to manage inflammation and bronchospasms to prevent or relieve symptoms

2. Assisting the patient to establish a "personal best" PEF by measuring his or her PEF twice daily for 2 to 3 weeks when asthma is well controlled and using this value to compare against all other readings
3. Instructing the patient to evaluate when to use a rescue inhaler ("yellow zone" or PEF is between 50% and 80% of personal best) and when to seek emergency assistance ("red zone" or PEF is below 50% of personal best)

❗ NURSING SAFETY PRIORITY: Critical Rescue

Teach the patients that if a "red zone" reading occurs when using the peak flowmeter to immediately use the fast-acting bronchodilating drugs and seek emergency help.

4. Teaching the patient to keep a symptom and intervention diary to learn his or her triggers of asthma symptoms, early cues for impending attacks, and personal response to drugs
5. Stressing the importance of proper use of the asthma action plan for any severity of asthma
- Drug therapy focuses on prevention of asthma attacks (preventive therapy) and stopping attacks that have already started (rescue therapy).
- Many preventive and rescue drugs are delivered as dry powder inhalers (DPIs) or as aerosol metered dose inhalers (MDIs). Teach patients the proper ways to use and store these inhalers.
- Preventive therapy drugs are those used to change airway responsiveness to prevent asthma attacks from occurring. They are used every day, regardless of symptoms.
  1. Bronchodilators cause bronchiolar smooth muscle relaxation and include beta$_2$ agonists, cholinergic antagonists, and methylxanthines.
     a. Short-acting bronchodilators provide rapid but short-term relief. They're most useful when administered as an asthma attack begins. One example is albuterol.
     b. Long-acting beta$_2$ agonists (LABAs) are delivered by inhaler directly to the site of action, the bronchioles. They need time to build up an effect, but the effects are longer lasting. Examples include formoterol (Perforomist) and salmeterol (Serevent).
     c. Combination drugs with a LABA and inhaled corticosteroid; the use of LABAs is recommended for co-administration with inhaled steroids.

! **NURSING SAFETY PRIORITY: Drug Alert**   A

These drugs are useful in preventing an asthma attack but have no value during an acute attack. Teach patients *not* to use LABAs to rescue them during an attack or when wheezing is getting worse.

> d. Cholinergic antagonists (anticholinergic drugs) are similar to atropine and block the parasympathetic nervous system, causing bronchodilation and decreased pulmonary secretions. Most are used by inhaler.
>> (1) Ipratropium (Atrovent)
>> (2) Tiotropium (Spiriva)
> e. Xanthines are used when other types of management are ineffective:
>> (1) Theophylline (Theo-Dur)
>> (2) Aminophylline (Truphylline)
2. Anti-inflammatory drugs alter the immune and inflammatory responses in the airways. Some are given systemically and have more side effects. Others are used as inhalants and have few systemic side effects.
> a. Inhaled corticosteroids (ICSs):
>> (1) Fluticasone (Ellipta, Flovent)
>> (2) Budesonide (Pulmicort)
> b. Cromones:
>> (1) Nedocromil (Tilade)
> c. Leukotriene antagonists:
>> (1) Montelukast (Singulair)

! **NURSING SAFETY PRIORITY: Critical Rescue**

Teach the patient to always carry the rescue short-acting beta agonist drug inhaler with him or her and to ensure that there is enough drug remaining in the inhaler to provide a quick dose when needed.

- Regular exercise, including aerobic exercise, is a recommended part of asthma therapy.
  1. Teach patients to examine the conditions that trigger an attack and adjust the exercise routine as needed.
  2. Some patients may need to premedicate with inhaled SABAs before beginning activity.
- Supplemental oxygen with a high flow rate or high concentration is often used during an acute asthma attack. Oxygen is delivered by mask, nasal cannula, or endotracheal tube.

- Heliox, a mixture of helium and oxygen (often 50% helium and 50% oxygen) can help improve oxygen delivery to the alveoli.
- *Status asthmaticus* is a severe, life-threatening acute episode of airway obstruction that intensifies once it begins and often does not respond to usual therapy.
  1. Assess for manifestations, including:
     a. Extremely labored breathing and wheezing
     b. Use of accessory muscles
     c. Distention of neck veins
     d. PEF below 50% of expected for patient's age, size, and gender
     e. Oxygen saturation less than 80%
  2. Apply oxygen.
  3. Anticipate administration of immediate therapy, including:
     a. IV fluids
     b. Repeated doses of inhaled bronchodilators
     c. IV steroids
  4. Prepare for emergency intubation.

 ## ATRIAL FIBRILLATION: PERFUSION CONCEPT EXEMPLAR

OVERVIEW
- Atrial fibrillation (AF) is a common dysrhythmia that can lead to impaired perfusion.
- This alteration in cardiac function allows for blood to pool placing the patient at risk at risk for clotting concerns such as DVT or PE.
- As AF progresses, cardiac output decreases by as much as 20% to 30%.
- AF is frequently associated with cardiovascular disease.

INTERPROFESSIONAL COLLABORATIVE CARE
Assessment: Noticing
- Determine history of cardiovascular disease such as hypertension, heart failure, or acute coronary syndrome.
- Determine characteristics of the heart rate and rhythm.
  1. Multiple rapid impulses from many atrial foci depolarize the atria in a totally disorganized manner at a rate of 350 to 600 times per minute; ventricular response is usually 120 to 200 beats per minute.
  2. The electrocardiogram shows a chaotic rhythm with no clear P waves, and an irregular ventricular response.
- Assess for poor perfusion:
  1. Fatigue or weakness
  2. Shortness of breath

3. Dizziness
4. Anxiety
5. Syncope
6. Palpitations
7. Chest discomfort or pain
8. Hypotension
- Definitive diagnosis occurs with a 12 lead ECG.

Analysis: Interpreting

- The priority collaborative problems for most patients with atrial fibrillation are:
  1. Potential for embolus formation due to irregular cardiac rhythm
  2. Potential for heart failure due to altered conduction pattern

Planning and Implementation: Responding

Interventions for AF depend on the severity of the problem and the patient's response. Be sure to individualize care based on the patient's values and preferences, your clinical expertise, and best current evidence.

PREVENT EMBOLUS FORMATION

Reduce potential for embolus formation related to irregular cardiac rhythm by slowing the ventricular rate to 60 to 90 beats per minute and, if possible restoring the rhythm to sinus rhythm

---

❗ NURSING SAFETY PRIORITY: Action Alert

The loss of coordinated atrial contractions in AF can lead to pooling of blood resulting in CLOTTING. *The patient is at high risk for pulmonary embolism!* Thrombi may form within the right atrium and then move through the right ventricle to the lungs. If pulmonary embolism is suspected remain with the patient and monitor for shortness of breath, chest pain, and/or hypotension. Initiate the rapid response team and notify the provider.

In addition, the patient is at risk for systemic emboli, particularly an embolic stroke, which may cause severe neurologic impairment or death. Monitor patients carefully for signs of stroke. Initiate rapid response team if stroke is suspected to facilitate timely diagnosis.

Patients with AF who have valvular disease are particularly at risk for venous thromboembolism (VTE). In VTE, the patient may complain of lower extremity pain and swelling. Anticipate ultrasound of vasculature and initiation of systemic anticoagulation.

- Administer drugs to slow conduction:
  1. Calcium channel blockers like diltiazem (Cardizem)
  2. Amiodarone (Cordarone)
  3. Dronedarone (Multaq); avoid this drug in patients with heart failure because it can cause an exacerbation of cardiac symptoms; with permanent AF, it increases the risk of stroke, myocardial infarction or cardiovascular death.
  4. Beta blockers, such as metoprolol (Toprol, Betaloc ♣) and esmolol (Brevibloc)
  5. Digoxin (Lanoxin, Toloxin ♣) for patients with heart failure and AF.
- If AF is new and NOT permanent, administer drugs to control rhythm, such as:
  1. Flecainide (Tambocor)
  2. Dofetilide (Tikosyn)
  3. Propafenone (Rythmol)
  4. Ibutilide (Corvert)
- Anticipate continuous cardiac monitoring and frequent 12 lead ECGs with new onset AF.
- Administer anticoagulation therapy:
  1. Warfarin
  2. Novel oral anticoagulants (NOACs) such as dabigatran (Pradaxa), rivaroxaban (Xarelto), apixaban (Eliquis), or edoxaban (Savaysa) may be given on a long-term basis to prevent strokes associated with nonvalvular AF. Because these drugs achieve a steady state, there is no need for laboratory test monitoring.
- Monitor for bleeding with anticoagulation therapy
  1. Warfarin is monitored with international normalized ratio (INR) to achieve a goal of two to three times normal; these values increase bleeding risk.
  2. NOACs do not require serum monitoring. The only NOAC with a reversal agent is dabigatran (Pradaxa). Idarucizumab (Praxbind), an intravenous monoclonal antibody, binds to dabigatran, thereby preventing dabigatran from inhibiting thrombin.

❗ NURSING SAFETY PRIORITY: Drug Alert

Teach patients taking any type of anticoagulant drug to report bruising, bleeding nose or gums, and other signs of bleeding to their primary health care provider immediately.

PREVENT HEART FAILURE
- Promote cardiac output by restoration of normal conduction or achieving a ventricular rate of 60 to 90 beats per minute.

1. Nonsurgical interventions
   a. Antidysrhythmic drugs described earlier
   b. Electrical cardioversion, a synchronized countershock delivered in a monitored setting with experts to provide advanced cardiac life support
   c. Biventricular pacemaker/defibrillator placement
2. Surgical interventions
   a. Left atrial appendage closure to reduce the area for clot formation and subsequent emboli when the patient is not able to safely take anticoagulants
   b. Radiofrequency catheter ablation (RCA), an invasive procedure that may be used to destroy an irritable focus in atrial or ventricular conduction

Care Coordination and Transition Management

- Teach self-management of drug therapy, including antidysrhythmic and anticoagulant agents.
- Provide emotional support; it is common for patients with AF to experience anxiety.
- Evaluate the need for home health care or care coordination to promote ongoing access to services, including laboratory testing of INR or pacemaker testing.
- Remind patients to report any signs of a change in heart rhythm, such as a significant decrease in pulse rate, a rate more than 100 beats/min, or increased rhythm irregularity.

B

BLINDNESS

See *Visual Impairment (Reduced Vision)*.

BREAST CONDITION, FIBROCYSTIC

OVERVIEW

- The two main features of fibrocystic breast condition (FBC) are fibrosis and cysts in lobules, ducts, and stromal tissue of the breast.
- This condition occurs in almost half of women during their life span, most commonly in premenopausal women between ages 20 and 50 years of age.
- FBC is thought to be caused by an imbalance in the normal estrogen-to-progesterone ratio.
- Typical symptoms include breast pain and tender lumps or areas of thickening in the breasts. The lumps are rubbery, ill-defined, and commonly found in the upper outer quadrant of the breast.

INTERPROFESSIONAL COLLABORATIVE CARE

- Management of FBC focuses on the symptoms of the condition:
  1. Supportive measures such as the use of mild analgesics or limiting salt intake before menses can help decrease swelling.
  2. Wearing a supportive bra can reduce pain by decreasing tension on the ligaments, although some women find that not wearing a bra is more comfortable.
  3. Local application of ice or heat may provide temporary relief of pain.
  4. If drug therapy is indicated, oral contraceptives may be prescribed to suppress oversecretion of estrogen, and progestins may be used to correct luteal insufficiency.

! NURSING SAFETY PRIORITY: Drug Alert

Explain to women the benefits and risks associated with hormonal drug therapy for FBC, such as stroke, liver disease, and increased intracranial pressure. Teach them to seek medical attention immediately if any signs and symptoms of these complications occur.

  5. Vitamins C, E, and B complex may reduce cyst formation.
  6. Diuretics may be prescribed to decrease premenstrual breast engorgement.
  7. Reduction of dietary fat and caffeine has been suggested, although the role of caffeine and fat in FBC is unclear.
  8. Teach patients to follow guidelines for breast self-examination, obtain breast examinations by a health care provider regularly, and undergo mammographic or magnetic resonance imaging (MRI) diagnostic testing.

BURNS

OVERVIEW

- A burn is a complex injury with loss of TISSUE INTEGRITY that results from exposure to temperature extremes, mechanical abrasion, chemical abrasion, radiation, and electrical currents.
- Local and systemic problems resulting from burns include fluid and electrolyte imbalances, protein losses, sepsis, and changes in metabolic, endocrine, respiratory, cardiac, hematologic, immune, and psychological function.
- The priorities in care are prevention of infection and closure of the burn wound because a lack of or delay in wound healing is a

key factor for all systemic problems and a major cause of disability and death among patients who are burned.

- Burn severity is determined by the extent to which skin and the underlying tissue is damaged (wound depth) and by how much of the body surface area is involved. Wound depth in burns has four classifications and two classes have subcategories:

1. *Superficial-thickness wounds* have the least damage because only the epidermis is damaged. The epithelial cells and basement membrane, needed for total regrowth, remain. Common causes of superficial-thickness wounds are prolonged exposure to low-intensity heat (e.g., sunburn) or short (flash) exposure to high-intensity heat. Redness with mild edema, pain, and increased sensitivity to heat occur as a result. Desquamation (peeling of dead skin) occurs 2 to 3 days after the burn with healing occurring in 3 to 6 days without a scar or other complication.

2. *Partial-thickness wounds* involve the entire epidermis and various depths of the dermis. Depending on the amount of dermal tissue damaged, partial-thickness wounds are further subdivided into superficial partial-thickness and deep partial-thickness injuries.

   a. *Superficial partial-thickness wounds* are caused by injury to the upper third of the dermis, leaving a good blood supply. Wounds are pink, moist, and blanch (whiten) when pressure is applied. Blisters often form. Nerve endings are exposed, and any stimulation (touch or temperature change) causes intense pain. With care, these burns heal in 10 to 21 days with no permanent scar, but some minor pigment changes may occur.

   b. *Deep partial-thickness wounds* extend deeper into the skin dermis and fewer healthy cells remain. The wound surface is red and dry, with white areas in deeper parts; blisters do not form. Edema is moderate and reduced blood flow can result in a deeper injury. Pain may be less compared with more superficial burns because more nerve endings have been destroyed. Healing occurs over 3 to 6 weeks with scar formation.

3. *Full-thickness wounds* occur with destruction of the entire epidermis and dermis, leaving no skin cells to repopulate. The wounded tissue does not regrow and the wound will require grafting. The wound has a hard, dry, leathery eschar that must slough off or be removed from the burn wound before healing can occur. The wound may be waxy white, deep red, yellow, brown, or black. Sensation is reduced or absent in these areas because of nerve ending destruction. Edema is severe under the eschar in a full-thickness wound.

   a. When the injury is circumferential (completely surrounds an extremity or the chest), blood flow and chest movement for breathing may be reduced by tight eschar.

    b. *Escharotomies* (incisions through the eschar) or *fasciotomies* (incisions through eschar and fascia) may be needed to relieve pressure and allow normal blood flow and breathing.

  4. *Deep full-thickness wounds* extend beyond the skin into underlying fascia and tissues. Muscle, bone, and tendons are damaged and exposed. The wound is blackened and depressed, and sensation is completely absent. Healing takes weeks to months.

- Mechanisms of burn injury and emergency interventions to limit injury
  1. *Dry heat injuries* result from open flames. The patient should stop, drop, and roll to smother the flames.
  2. *Moist heat (scald) injuries* are caused by contact with hot liquids or steam. Clothes that are saturated with hot liquids should be removed immediately.
  3. *Contact burns* occur when hot metal, tar, or grease contact the skin, often leading to a full-thickness injury. Removal of the hot substance limits the injury.
  4. *Chemical burns* occur as a result of accidents in the home or workplace. The severity of the injury depends on the duration of contact, the concentration of the chemical, the amount of tissue exposed, and the action of the chemical. Dry chemicals should be brushed off the skin and clothing. Wet clothing is removed. Depending on the specific agent, the skin may be flushed with water or covered with mineral oil.
  5. *Electrical injury burns* occur when an electrical current enters the body. These injuries have been called the "grand masquerader" of burn injuries because the surface injuries may look small but the associated internal injuries can be huge. The longer the electricity is in contact with the body, the greater the damage. The patient should be removed from the source of the electricity in such a way that the care provider does not place himself or herself in danger (use a wooden pole, rather than a metal one, to separate the person from the electrical source). *The person must not be touched directly while he or she is in contact with the electrical source.*
  6. *Radiation injuries* occur when people are exposed to large doses of radioactive material. The most common type of tissue injury from radiation exposure occurs with therapeutic radiation. More serious injury occurs in industrial settings where radioactive energy is produced or radioactive isotopes are used. Removal of the patient from the source of radiation limits the injury.
- Physiologic responses to a burn injury
  1. Circulation to burned skin is disrupted immediately.
     a. Macrophages from damaged tissue release chemicals that cause vasoconstriction.

b. Thrombosis may occur, causing decreased perfusion, tissue necrosis, and additional injury.

c. Vasoconstriction is followed by vasodilation and subsequent fluid shift from blood vessels into interstitial spaces (also known as third spacing or capillary leak syndrome).

   (1) Extensive edema occurs when tissue exudate is large or severe.

   (2) Fluid shifts can cause pulmonary edema and lung injury.

   (3) Fluid shift and low perfusion to the GI tract can contribute to a paralytic ileus or GI ulcer formation.

2. Fluid and electrolyte shifts along with loss of plasma proteins can decrease intravascular volume and blood pressure, leading to indirect injury from low perfusion to essential organs like brain, heart, and kidney.

   a. Tachycardia and increased cardiac output occur to compensate for hypotension.

   b. Fluid shifts can cause pulmonary edema and lung injury.

3. The endocrine system responds to a burn with stress hormones, releasing catecholamines and cortisol.

   a. This stress response alters caloric and protein metabolism, increases nutritional needs, and raises the core body temperature.

   b. Hypermetabolism puts the burned patient at risk for hypoglycemic episodes and further tissue damage.

4. Disrupted skin integrity increase risk for infection and the inflammatory response to burn injury alters immune function and healing.

- Health promotion and maintenance

  1. Teach everyone to check water temperature before immersion and to set hot water tanks at <140°F (60°C).

  2. Stress the importance of never adding a flammable substance to an open flame.

  3. Teach all family members to plan escape routes and leave a burning building and to use smoke and carbon monoxide detectors.

RESUSCITATION PHASE OF BURN INJURY

OVERVIEW

The resuscitation phase is the first phase of a burn injury. It begins at the onset of injury and continues for about 24 to 48 hours. During this phase the injury is evaluated and the immediate problems of fluid loss, edema, and reduced blood flow are assessed. Events within these first hours after the burn are critical and can make the difference between life and death for the patient with a burn injury.

INTERPROFESSIONAL COLLABORATIVE CARE

Assessment: Noticing

- Obtain the following personal patient information:
  1. Age to determine risk for complications; complications are more common in ages >50 years
  2. Height and weight (to calculate fluid replacement and energy requirements)
  3. Medical history (especially cardiac or kidney disease, alcoholism, substance abuse, diabetes mellitus)
  4. Use of prescribed, over-the-counter (OTC), or street drugs within the past 24 hours
  5. Smoking history
  6. Level of pain
  7. Allergies
  8. Immunization status (especially tetanus)
- Assess for:
  1. Airway and inhalation injury
     a. Changes in the appearance or function of the mouth, nose, or throat
     b. Facial burns; singed hair on the head, eyebrows, eyelids, or nose
     c. Blisters or soot on the lips, on oral mucosa, or in sputum
     d. "Smoky" smell of the breath
     e. Progressive hoarseness, wheezing, crowing, stridor
     f. Decreased oxygen saturation
     g. Drooling (inability to swallow oral secretions)
     h. Respiratory pattern, rate, and effort

❗ NURSING SAFETY PRIORITY: Critical Rescue

Monitor the patient's respiratory efforts closely. For a burn patient in the resuscitation phase who is hoarse, has a brassy cough, drools, has difficulty swallowing, or produces an audible breath sound on exhalation, respond by immediately applying oxygen and notifying the Rapid Response Team.

  2. Carbon monoxide poisoning
     a. Headache
     b. Decreased cognitive functioning, confusion, coma
     c. Tinnitus
     d. Nausea
     e. Absence of cyanosis or pallor (lips and mucous membranes may appear bright red)
     f. Elevated carboxyhemoglobin levels
  3. Smoke poisoning/inhalation
     a. Atelectasis, pulmonary edema
     b. Hemorrhagic bronchitis (6 to 72 hours after injury)

4. Thermal injury from aspiration of scalding liquid
   a. Heat damage to pharynx, oropharynx, and nasopharynx can cause edema and upper airway obstruction and requires early intubation.
   b. Observe for hoarseness, stridor, or shortness of breath.
   c. Pulmonary fluid overload:
      (1) Dyspnea
      (2) Hypoxia
      (3) Respiratory crackles
5. Cardiovascular changes
   a. Hypovolemic and cardiogenic shock
   b. Circulatory overload with heart failure
   c. Rapid, thready pulse
   d. Hypotension
   e. Reduced peripheral pulses
   f. Slow or absent capillary refill
   g. Generalized edema
   h. Weight gain
   i. Baseline and continuous electrocardiographic tracings
6. Renal or urinary changes
   a. Decreased (less than 0.5 to 1mL/kg/hr) or absent urine output
   b. High urine specific gravity
   c. Proteinuria
7. Skin changes
   a. Depth of injury
   b. Size of injury by the total body surface area (TBSA)
   c. Color and appearance
8. Gastrointestinal changes
   a. Decreased or absent bowel sounds
   b. Nausea, vomiting
   c. Abdominal distention
   d. Gastritis, GI ulcer formation
   e. Gross or occult blood in vomitus, GI secretions, or stool
- Laboratory assessment
   1. Increased white blood cells (WBCs), with the differential reporting increased neutrophils
   2. Electrolytes
   3. Liver enzyme studies
   4. Clotting studies

🌐 Cultural Considerations

For black individuals with an African heritage, a serum laboratory assay called a sickle cell preparation may be appropriate if sickle status is unknown. The trauma of a burn injury can trigger a sickle cell crisis in patients who have the disease and in those who carry the trait.

Analysis: Interpreting

- The priority problems for the patient with burn injuries in the resuscitation phase who have sustained a burn injury greater than 25% of the TBSA are:
    1. Potential for decreased oxygenation due to upper airway edema, pulmonary edema, airway obstruction, or pneumonia
    2. Potential for shock due to increase in capillary permeability, active fluid volume loss, electrolyte imbalance, and inadequate fluid resuscitation
    3. Pain (acute and chronic) due to tissue injury, damaged or exposed nerve endings, débridement, dressing changes, invasive procedures, and donor sites
    4. Potential for acute respiratory distress syndrome (ARDS) due to inhalation injury

Planning and Implementation: Responding

SUPPORTING OXYGENATION

Nonsurgical Management

- Interventions include airway maintenance, promotion of ventilation, monitoring gas exchange, oxygen therapy, drug therapy, positioning, and deep breathing.
- Assess hourly for fluid overload (e.g., presence of lung crackles, distended neck veins, decreased cognition, decreased oxygen saturation, fluid intake greater than urine output).
- Keep emergency airway equipment at the bedside during the resuscitation phase of care.
    1. Arterial oxygenation < 60mm Hg is an indication for intubation and mechanical ventilation.
    2. Assess and document the patient's response to interventions such as positioning or coughing and deep breathing to improve respiration and responses to changes in oxygen therapy.
        a. Monitor oxygen saturation continuously; communicate decrements greater than 5% or values less than 92% immediately to prescribing health care provider and anticipate oxygen supplementation interventions.
        b. Evaluate ABG levels for pH (acidemia indicates poor perfusion); low oxygenation (Pao_2 less than 90mm Hg) or hypercarbia ($Paco_2$ greater than 46mm Hg).

❗ NURSING SAFETY PRIORITY: Critical Rescue

Immediately report any signs of respiratory distress or concerning change in respiratory patterns to the health care team and the respiratory therapist.

Surgical Management
- A tracheotomy may be needed when long-term intubation is expected. This procedure increases the risk for infection in burn patients. Emergency tracheotomies are performed when an airway becomes occluded and oral or nasal intubation cannot be achieved.

PREVENTING HYPOVOLEMIC SHOCK
- Interventions are aimed at increasing blood fluid volume, supporting compensatory mechanisms, and preventing complications. Nonsurgical management is often sufficient for achieving these aims. Surgical management is required most often for full-thickness burns.

Nonsurgical Management
- Fluid volume and tissue blood flow are restored through IV fluid therapy (rapid IV therapy is called *fluid resuscitation* and is guided by a well-established formula based on the size and depth of burn injury) and drug therapy. Priority nursing interventions are carrying out fluid resuscitation and monitoring for indications of effectiveness or complications.
  1. Fluid replacement formulas are calculated from the time of injury, not the time of arrival to the hospital.
  2. Fluids are infused rapidly or gradually to achieve a typical goal of urine output at 0.5 mL/kg/hour.

Considerations for Older Adults

In older patients, especially those with cardiac disease, a complicating factor in fluid resuscitation may be acute exacerbation of heart failure or concurrent myocardial infarction. Drugs that increase cardiac output (e.g., dopamine [Intropin]) or that strengthen the force of myocardial contraction may be used along with fluid therapy.

Surgical Management
- An escharotomy may be needed when tight eschar impairs tissue perfusion.
- A fasciotomy (a deeper incision extending through the fascia) may be needed to relieve constriction from fluid buildup when a burn completely surrounds an extremity.

MANAGING PAIN AND ALTERATIONS IN COMFORT
- Pain associated with burns is both acute and chronic when burns are extensive or deep. Pain management is tailored to the patient's tolerance for pain, coping mechanisms, and physical status. The priority nursing actions include continually assessing the patient's

pain level, using appropriate pain-reducing strategies, and preventing complications.

Nonsurgical Management

- Interventions for the patient having pain include drug therapy opioid and nonopioid analgesics, complementary therapy measures, and environmental manipulation.
- Assess the patient's pain level hourly until pain is well controlled, then every 2 to 4 hours.
- For the alert patient, consider using patient-controlled analgesia.

> **❗ NURSING SAFETY PRIORITY: Critical Rescue**
>
> Give opioid drugs for pain only by the intravenous route during the resuscitation phase. Absorption through the GI tract, subcutaneous, or muscle tissues may be delayed. Later, as circulation recovers in these tissues, doses can be rapidly absorbed resulting in lethal blood levels of analgesics.

- Provide a quiet environment to promote rest and sleep.
- Coordinate with all members of the health care team to ensure that most procedures are performed during the patient's waking hours.
- Use alternative and complementary pain management techniques, including relaxation techniques, meditative breathing, guided imagery, music therapy, massage, and healing or therapeutic touch.

Surgical Management

- Surgical management for pain involves early surgical excision of the burn wound.

PREVENTING ACUTE RESPIRATORY DISTRESS SYNDROME

- The goal of care is to provide balanced fluid intake, avoiding fluid overload, and preventing lung tissue damage from high tidal volumes during mechanical ventilation. (See ARDS later in chapter.)

ACUTE PHASE OF BURN INJURY

OVERVIEW

- The acute phase of burn injury begins 36 to 48 hours after injury when fluid shift resolves and lasts until wound closure is complete.
- Interprofessional team care is directed toward continued assessment and maintenance of the cardiovascular, respiratory, neuroendocrine, immune, musculoskeletal, and GI systems; providing nutrition, burn wound care, and pain control; and implementing psychosocial support.

- Complications of this phase include pneumonia, malnutrition, loss of musculoskeletal function, infection, and sepsis.

INTERPROFESSIONAL COLLABORATIVE CARE

Assessment: Noticing
- Assess for:
  1. Cardiopulmonary dysfunction
     a. Pneumonia
     b. Respiratory failure
  2. Neuroendocrine dysfunction
     a. Hypothermia
     b. Weight loss, negative nitrogen balance, malnutrition
  3. Immune system dysfunction
     a. Wound appearance
     b. Systemic infection and sepsis
  4. Musculoskeletal dysfunction
     a. Muscle atrophy
     b. Contracture formation manifested by decreased range of motion (ROM)
     c. Immobilization and immobility
  5. Pain
  6. Maladaptive psychosocial responses

Analysis: Interpreting
- Priority nursing problems for patients with burn injuries greater than 25% TBSA in the acute phase of recovery are:
  1. Wound care management due to impaired tissue integrity associated with burn injury and skin grafting procedures
  2. Potential for infection of open burn wounds due to the presence of multiple invasive catheters, reduced immune function, and poor nutrition
  3. Weight loss due to increased metabolic rate, reduced calorie intake, and increased urinary nitrogen losses
  4. Decreased mobility due to open burn wounds, pain, scars, and contractures
  5. Decreased self-esteem due to trauma, changes in physical appearance and lifestyle, and alterations in sensory and motor function

Planning and Implementation: Responding
MANAGING WOUND CARE
Nonsurgical Management
- Assess all burn wounds at least daily for:
  1. Adequacy of circulation
  2. Size and depth of injury
  3. Presence of infection

4. Evidence of healing: granulation, re-epithelialization, scar tissue formation, decreased wound size

• Participate in wound débridement procedures to remove eschar and other cellular debris from the burn wound.

1. *Mechanical débridement* can be performed one or two times daily with hydrotherapy. Hydrotherapy is performed by showering the patient on a special shower table or washing only small areas of the wound at the bedside. Burn areas are washed thoroughly and gently with mild soap or detergent and water; nurses and skilled technicians use forceps and scissors to remove loose, dead tissue.

2. *Enzymatic débridement* can occur naturally by autolysis or, more commonly, artificially by the application of exogenous agents. A topical agent is applied directly to the burn wound in once-daily dressing changes. The enzymes digest collagen in necrotic tissues.

3. Dress the burn wound using standard wound dressings, biologic dressings, synthetic dressings, or artificial skin after cleaning and débridement.

   a. *Standard wound dressings* are multiple layers of roller-type gauze over a topical agents. The number of gauze layers depends on the depth of the injury, amount of drainage expected, area injured, patient's mobility, and frequency of dressing changes. Dressings are changed every 12 to 24 hours.

   b. *Biologic dressings* are skin or membranes obtained from human tissue donors or animals. When applied over open wounds, a biologic dressing rapidly adheres and promotes healing or prepares the wound for permanent skin graft coverage. Types of biologic dressings include:

      (1) *Homografts (allografts)* are human skin obtained from a cadaver and provided through a skin bank.

      (2) *Heterografts (xenografts)* are skin obtained from another species. Pig skin is the most common heterograft and is compatible with human skin.

      (3) *Cultured skin* can be grown from a small specimen of epidermal cells from an unburned area of the patient's body. Cells are grown in a laboratory to produce cell sheets that can be grafted on the patient to generate a permanent skin surface.

      (4) *Artificial skin* is an alternative approach to closure of the burn wound. This substance has two layers: a Silastic epidermis and a porous dermis made from beef collagen and shark cartilage.

   c. *Biosynthetic wound dressings* are a combination of a nylon fabric that is partially embedded into a silicone film. Collagen is incorporated into both the silicone and nylon components. The nylon fabric forms an adherent bond with the wound surface until epithelialization has occurred. The porous silicone film allows exudates to pass through.

   d. *Synthetic dressings* are made of solid silicone and plastic membranes (e.g., polyvinyl chloride, polyurethane). They are applied directly to the surface of a clean or surgically prepared wound and remain in place until they fall off or are removed. These dressing are typically transparent and used at graft donor sites.

Surgical Management

- Surgical management of burn wounds focuses on excision and grafting for wound closure. Surgical excision is performed early in the post burn period. Grafting may be performed throughout the acute phase as burn wounds are made ready and donor sites are available. Early grafting reduces the time patients are at risk for infection and sepsis. Wound covering by autografting involves taking healthy skin from an area of the patient's intact skin and transplanting it to an excised burn wound.

MINIMIZING POTENTIAL FOR INFECTION

- Burn wound infection can occur through *auto-contamination,* in which the patient's own normal flora overgrows and invades other body areas, and *cross-contamination,* in which organisms from other people or environments are transferred to the patient.

Nonsurgical Management

- Use infection control interventions to prevent transmission, provide a safe environment, and monitor for early detection of infection.
- Drug therapy for infection prevention
  1. Tetanus toxoid, an IM vaccine, is routinely given when the patient is admitted to the hospital. Additional administration of tetanus immune globulin (human) (Hyper-Tet) is recommended when the patient's history of tetanus immunization is not known.
  2. Topical antimicrobial drugs are used to prevent infection in burn wounds. The goal of this therapy is to reduce bacterial growth in the wound and prevent systemic sepsis. Common topical agents are bacitracin, silver sulfadiazine, and mafenide (Sulfamylon). Other products with antimicrobials such as Acticoat, Mepilex Ag, and Aquacel Ag release antimicrobials over several days and can be left in place for up to 7 days, reducing dressing changes.
- Drug therapy for treatment of infection
  1. Systemic broad-spectrum antibiotics are used when burn patients have symptoms of an infection, including sepsis. After results of blood cultures and sensitivity status are available,

specific drugs may be changed to those that are effective against the specific organisms causing the infection.

- Providing a safe environment
  1. Use strict aseptic technique when caring for patients who have open burn wounds to prevent infection.
     a. Monitor vital signs (VS) at least every 8 hours for indications of wound infection or sepsis (tachycardia, hypotension, fever); monitor more frequently with patients who have more than 25% TBSAs.
     b. Do not share equipment among patients.
     c. Use disposable items as much as possible.
     d. Ensure daily cleaning of patient's room and bathroom.
  2. Do not keep plants or flowers in the patient's room; they are a source of microbes.
  3. Restrict visitors to healthy adults.
  4. Consider infection control isolation measures to prevent cross contamination.
- Monitoring for early recognition of infection by assessing the burn wounds at each dressing change for:
  1. Pervasive odor
  2. Color changes: focal, dark red, brown discoloration in the eschar
  3. Change in texture
  4. Purulent drainage
  5. Exudate
  6. Sloughing grafts
  7. Redness at the wound edges extending to nonburned skin

  Surgical Management
- Infected burn wounds with colony counts of or near 10^5 colonies per gram of tissue are life-threatening and may require surgical excision to control these infections.

MINIMIZING WEIGHT LOSS
- Coordinate with the dietitian to calculate the patient's caloric and protein goals.
- Nutritional requirements for a patient with a large burn area can exceed 5000 kcal/day and include a diet high in protein for wound healing.
- Nasoduodenal tube feedings are often started within 4 hours of beginning fluid resuscitation to prevent nutritional deficit.
- Encourage patients who can eat solid foods to ingest as many calories as possible.
- Take the patient's preferences into consideration for diet planning and food selection.
- Encourage patients to request food whenever they feel they can eat, not just according to the hospital's standard meal schedule.

- Offer frequent high-calorie, high-protein supplemental feedings.
- Keep an accurate calorie count for foods and beverages that are ingested by the patient.

MAINTAINING MOBILITY

Nonsurgical Management

1. Maintain the patient in a neutral body position with minimal flexion to prevent contractures.
2. Use splints and other devices on the joints of the hands, elbows, knees, neck, and axillae to prevent contractures.
3. Use ROM exercises at least three times daily. ROM can be active (performed by the patient) or passive (performed by the clinician).
4. For burned hands, urge the patient to perform active ROM exercises for the hand, thumb, and fingers every hour while awake.
5. Start ambulation as soon as possible after the fluid shifts have resolved and perform two to three times daily.
6. Apply pressure dressings after grafts heal to help prevent contractures and tight hypertrophic scars; pressure dressings are worn at least 23 hours every day until the scar tissue is mature (at 12 to 24 months).

Surgical Management

- Surgical management can be used to restore mobility from contractures. Surgical release of joints and tendons is most commonly performed in the neck, axilla, elbow flexion areas, and hand.

SUPPORT POSITIVE SELF-ESTEEM

Nonsurgical Management

- Assess which stage of grief the patient is experiencing and help interpret his or her behavior.
- Reassure the patient that feelings of grief, loss, anxiety, anger, fear, and guilt are normal.
- Coordinate with other health care team members (e.g., psychologist, psychiatrist, social worker, clergy or religious leader) in addressing these problems.
- Accept the physical and psychological features of the patient.
- Present patients and families with realistic expected outcomes regarding the patient's functional capacity and physical appearance.
- Plan and encourage the patient's active participation in self-care activities.
- Urge families to include the patient in family decision making to the same degree that he or she participated in this process before the injury.

- Provide information sessions and counseling for the family to help identify effective patterns of support.
- Facilitate the patient's use of established support systems and the development of new support resources.
- Make referrals to support groups.
  Surgical Management
- Reconstructive and cosmetic surgery can restore function and improve the patient's appearance, often increasing his or her feelings of self-worth and promoting a positive body image. Teach the patient and family about expected cosmetic outcomes.

REHABILITATIVE PHASE OF BURN INJURY

OVERVIEW
- The technical rehabilitative phase begins with wound closure and ends when the patient returns to the highest possible level of functioning.
- The emphasis during this phase is the psychosocial adjustment of the patient, the prevention of scars and contractures, and the resumption of preburn activity, including resuming work, family, and social roles.
- This phase may take years or even last a lifetime as patients adjust to permanent limitations that may not be apparent until long after the initial injury.

INTERPROFESSIONAL COLLABORATIVE CARE
- Explore the patient's feelings about the burn injury.
- Ask the patient or a family member whether there is a history of psychological problems.
- Assess and document the type of coping mechanisms the patient has used successfully during times of stress to assist with a future plan of care.
- Assess the patient's family unit and the family members' history of interaction.
- Identify cultural and ethnic factors, and take these into consideration when planning psychosocial interventions.

Care Coordination and Transition Management
- Discharge planning for the patient with a burn injury begins at the time of admission to the hospital or burn center.
- Help the patient adjust to the reaction of others to the sight of healing wounds and disfiguring scars.
- Teach the patient and family:
  1. How to perform dressing changes
  2. Signs and symptoms of infection
  3. Drug regimens

4. Proper use of prosthetic and positioning devices
5. Correct application and care of pressure garments
6. Comfort measures to reduce pruritus
7. Dates for follow-up appointments
- Additional common discharge needs of the patient with burns include:
  1. Financial assessment
  2. Evaluation of family resources with possible home assessment (on-site visit)
  3. Psychological referral
  4. Determination of disposition: home, home with home care services, rehabilitation, long-term care, or other setting
  5. Medical equipment or prosthetic training
  6. Referral to community resources
  7. Re-entry programs for school or work environment

C

CANCER

OVERVIEW

- Cancer is abnormal cellular regulation.
- *Cancer cells,* also called *malignant cells,* are abnormal, serve no useful function, and invade and destroy normal body tissues. Without treatment, cancer leads to loss of function in tissues and organs and, ultimately, death of the individual with cancer.
- *Carcinogens* are substances that can damage normal cell deoxyribonucleic acid (DNA) and change the activity of genes. Carcinogens may be chemicals, physical agents, or viruses.
- *Neoplasia* is any new or continued cell growth not needed for normal development or replacement of dead and damaged tissues. This new growth may be benign or malignant.
- *Benign tumor cells* are normal cells growing in the wrong place or at the wrong time. They are not needed for normal growth and development. Although benign tumors do not invade other tissues, depending on their location, they can damage normal tissue and may need to be removed.
- A *primary tumor* is the original tumor, identified by the normal tissue from which it arose.
- A *metastatic tumor* is one that has spread from the original site, usually through the blood or lymph, into other tissues and organs, where it can establish metastatic or secondary tumors that grow and cause more damage and dysfunction.

- *Grading* of a tumor classifies cellular aspects of the cancer and ranks cancers for the degree of malignancy based on cancer cell appearance, growth rates, and aggressiveness compared with the normal tissues from which they arose. A low grade is less malignant.
- *Staging* describes the extent or severity of a person's cancer. The TNM staging system is based on the size of the primary tumor (T), whether cancer cells have spread to nearby lymph nodes (N), and whether metastasis (M) or spread of cancer to other parts of the body has occurred. Staging is important because for most cancers the smaller the cancer is at diagnosis, the fewer the lymph nodes that are involved; and the less it has spread, the greater the chances are that treatment will result in a cure. Staging also influences selection of therapy.
- Advanced cancers often affect:
  1. Immunity and other blood-producing functions
  2. Gastrointestinal (GI) function
  3. Peripheral nerve function
  4. Central motor and sensory function
  5. Respiratory and cardiac function
  6. Comfort

PERSONAL FACTORS AND CANCER DEVELOPMENT

Personal factors, including immunity, age, and genetic risk, also affect whether an adult is likely to develop cancer.

- Immunity protects the body from foreign invaders. Cancer incidence increased among patients with reduced immunity such as:
  1. Adults older than age 60: *Advancing age* is the single most important risk factor for cancer (ACS, 2017).
  2. Organ transplant recipients.
  3. Patients with AIDS.
- Genetic testing for cancer predisposition is available to confirm or rule out an adult's genetic risk for some specific cancer types.
  1. These tests do not diagnose the presence of cancer; they only provide risk information.
  2. When a patient tests positive for a known cancer-causing gene mutation, his or her risk for cancer development is greatly increased; however, the cancer still may never develop.

🧬 Genetic/Genomic Considerations: Patient-Centered Care

Genetic risk for cancer occurs only in a small percent of the population; however, adults who have a genetic predisposition are at very high risk for cancer development. Mutations in suppressor genes or oncogenes can be inherited when they occur in sperm and ova and are then passed on to one's children, in whom all cells contain the inherited mutations. Thus for some adults, tight CELLULAR REGULATION is lost as a result of a mutation in a suppressor gene, which reduces or halts its function and allows oncogene overexpression. In other adults, the suppressor genes are normal, and the oncogene is mutated and does not respond to suppressor gene signals, thus reducing cellular regulation and increasing the risk for cancer development. Be sure to include questions about any genetic condition in the family when performing a family history.

C

CANCER PREVENTION

- Primary Prevention: The use of strategies to prevent the actual occurrence of cancer.
  1. *Avoidance of known or potential carcinogens* is an effective prevention strategy when a cause of cancer is known and avoidance is easily accomplished.
     a. For example, teach adults to use skin protection during sun exposure to avoid skin cancer. Most lung cancer can be avoided by not using tobacco and eliminating exposure to loose asbestos particles.
  2. *Modifying associated factors* appears to help reduce cancer risk.
     a. Absolute causes are not known for many cancers, but some conditions appear to increase risk. Examples are the increased incidence of cancer among adults who consume alcohol; the association of a diet high in fat and low in fiber with colon cancer, breast cancer, and ovarian cancer; and a greater incidence of cervical cancer among women who have multiple sexual partners (ACS, 2017).
  3. *Removal of "at-risk" tissues* reduces cancer risk for an adult who has a known high risk for developing a specific type of cancer.
  4. *Vaccination* is a newer method of primary cancer prevention. Currently, the only vaccines approved for prevention of cancer are related to prevention of infection from several forms of the human papilloma virus (HPV). These vaccines are Gardasil and Cervarix.
  5. *Chemoprevention* is a strategy that uses drugs, chemicals, natural nutrients, or other substances to disrupt one or more steps important to cancer development.

Veterans' Health Considerations

The incidence of tobacco-related cancers is high among military veterans. One reason is that, at one time, cigarette smoking was considered "manly" among military personnel. The cost of cigarettes was low in stores on military installations (no state taxes were applied). In addition, military field meals such as "C-rations" or "K-rations" included free cigarettes. Ask patients about their military service and whether cigarette smoking started, continued, or increased during that time.

- Secondary Prevention: The use of screening strategies to detect cancer early, at a time when cure or control is more likely.
  1. Regular screening for cancer does not reduce cancer incidence but can greatly reduce some types of cancer deaths.
  2. Examples of recommended screenings include (ACS, 2017):
     a. The choice of annual mammography for women 40 to 44 years of age, annual mammography for women 45 to 54 years of age, and annual or biennial mammography for women older than 55 years of age
     b. Annual clinical breast examination for women older than 40 years; every 3 years for women age 20 to 39 years
     c. Colonoscopy at age 50 years and then every 10 years
     d. Annual fecal occult blood for adults of all ages
     e. Digital rectal examination (DRE) for men older than 50 years

INTERPROFESSIONAL COLLABORATIVE CARE
Assessment: Noticing
Impact of Cancer on Physical Function:
- **Impaired Immunity and Clotting:** Impaired immunity and blood-producing functions can occur when cancer starts in or invades the bone marrow, where blood cells are formed.
- **Altered GI Function:** Tumors of the GI tract increase the metabolic rate and the need for nutrients; however, many patients suffer from disease- and treatment-related appetite loss, and alterations in taste that have a negative impact on nutrition, leading to weight loss.
- **Altered Peripheral Nerve Function:** Although tumors in the spine can change peripheral nerve function, the more common cause is chemotherapy. Neurotoxic chemotherapy agents injure peripheral nerves, leading to peripheral neuropathy with reduced sensory perception.
- **Motor and Sensory Deficits:** Motor and sensory perception deficits occur when cancers invade bone or the brain or compress nerves. In patients with bone metastasis, the primary cancer started in another organ (e.g., lung, prostate, breast).
- **Cancer Pain:** The patient with cancer may have pain, especially chronic pain. Pain does not always accompany cancer, but it can be a major problem.

- **Altered Respiratory and Cardiac Function:** Cancer can disrupt respiratory function, capacity, and gas exchange and may result in death. Tumors that grow in the airways cause obstruction. If lung tissue is involved, lung capacity is decreased, leading to dyspnea and hypoxemia. Cancer cells thicken the alveolar membrane and damage lung blood vessels, both of which impair gas exchange.

Interventions: Responding

Therapies for cancer include surgery, radiation therapy, cytotoxic agents, biological and immunomodulation drugs, hormonal manipulation, and photodynamic therapy.

NONSURGICAL MANAGEMENT

Radiation Therapy: Radiation therapy (radiotherapy) uses high-energy radiation from gamma rays, radionuclides, or ionizing radiation beams to kill cancer cells, provide disease control, or relieve symptoms.

- *External beam* or *teletherapy* is radiation delivered from a source outside of the patient. *Because the source is external, the patient is not radioactive and there is no hazard to others.* Usually, the total dosage is delivered in one to five separate treatment sessions.
- *Brachytherapy,* also known as internal radiotherapy, means "short" (close) therapy. The radiation source comes into direct, continuous contact with the tumor for a specific time period. *With all types of brachytherapy, the radiation source is within the patient. Therefore the patient emits radiation for a period of time and is a potential hazard to others.*

Chart 2-5	Best Practice for Patient Safety and Quality Care

Care of the Patient with Sealed Implants of Radioactive Sources

- Assign the patient to a private room with a private bath.
- Place a "Caution: Radioactive Material" sign on the door of the patient's room.
- If portable lead shields are used, place them between the patient and the door.
- Keep the door to the patient's room closed as much as possible.
- Wear a dosimeter film badge at all times while caring for patients with radioactive implants. The badge offers no protection but measures a person's exposure to radiation. Each person caring for the patient should have a separate dosimeter to calculate his or her specific radiation exposure.

- Wear a lead apron while providing care. Always keep the front of the apron facing the source of radiation (do not turn your back toward the patient).
- If you are attempting to conceive, do not perform direct patient care regardless of whether you are male or female.
- Pregnant nurses should not care for these patients; do not allow pregnant women or children younger than 16 years to visit.
- Limit each visitor to one-half hour per day. Be sure visitors stay at least 6 feet from the source.
- Never touch the radioactive source with bare hands. In the rare instance that it is dislodged, use a long-handled forceps to retrieve it. Deposit the radioactive source in the lead container kept in the patient's room.
- Save all dressings and bed linens in the patient's room until after the radioactive source is removed. After the source is removed, dispose of dressings and linens in the usual manner. Other equipment can be removed from the room at any time without special precautions and does not pose a hazard to other people.

- Radiation therapy has both short- and long-term effects, depending upon the area(s) radiated.
  1. Short-term effects include radiodermatitis or redness and desquamation of skin, hair loss, altered taste, fatigue, and bone marrow suppression.
  2. Long-term effects include tissue and organ scarring and fibrosis at the site of radiation, development of new cancer long after treatment, sterility (if radiation occurs near reproductive organs), and acceleration of atherosclerosis and cardiovascular disease.
  3. Germ cells (ova and sperm) are exquisitely sensitive to damage from radiation. Reproductive organs are shielded. Counseling about reproductive choices is a part of informed consent for cancer treatments.

Cytotoxic Systemic Therapy: Cytotoxic systemic therapy refers to the use of antineoplastic (chemotherapy) drugs that are used to kill cancer cells and disrupt their CELLULAR REGULATION.

Genetic/Genomic Considerations

Patient-Centered Care

It is now possible to check the patient's genetic profile to determine the likelihood of experiencing dangerous side effects from some cytotoxic agents. Genomic profiling, known as *pharmacogenomics*, allows a more individualized approach to chemotherapy selection and side effect management. In addition, checking the genetic profile of the tumor can determine its sensitivity to various chemotherapy and targeted therapy agents. This practice individualizes cancer therapy and improves therapy outcomes. Expected future outcomes include an economic advantage for cancer care as decisions for treatment can be based on likelihood of effectiveness for a given patient rather than on a tumor type or stag disease. Remind patients that assessing genetic sensitivity can result in a selection of therapy that differs from that of other adults with the same cancer type.

- *Chemotherapy*: The treatment of cancer with chemical agents, is used to kill cancer cells and increase survival time. This killing effect on cancer cells is related to the ability of chemotherapy to damage DNA and interfere with cell division. The chemotherapy drug categories are:
  1. *Alkylating agents* prevent proper DNA and ribonucleic acid (RNA) synthesis thereby inhibiting cell division.
  2. *Antimetabolites* are used by cells in place of essential chemicals in cellular reactions. Because antimetabolites cannot function in reactions, their presence impairs cell division.
  3. *Antimitotic agents* interfere with the formation and actions of microtubules so cells cannot complete mitosis during cell division.
  4. *Antitumor antibiotics* damage the cell's DNA and interrupt DNA or RNA synthesis.
  5. *Topoisomerase inhibitors* disrupt an enzyme (topoisomerase) essential for DNA synthesis and cell division causing cell death.
  6. *Miscellaneous* chemotherapy drugs are those with mechanisms of action that are either unknown or do not fit those of other drug categories.
  7. *Combination chemotherapy* is common; more than one specific anticancer drug is administered in a timed manner.

Temporary and permanent damage can occur to normal tissues from chemotherapy because it is systemic and exerts its effects on all cells. These adverse effects include:
  1. Irritation and damage at the site of administration. Most chemotherapeutic agents are given intravenously.
  2. Bone marrow suppression: anemia, reduced immunity (reduced white blood cells [WBCs] and low neutrophils [neutropenia]), and thrombocytopenia with associated fatigue, immunosuppression, and bleeding and clotting abnormalities

! NURSING SAFETY PRIORITY: Action Alert

The priority interventions for the patient with neutropenia are protecting him or her from infection within the health care system and teaching the patient and family how to reduce infection risk in the home. Total patient assessment, including a review of common symptoms associated with infection (e.g., fever, sore throat, urinary frequency or discomfort, purulent drainage), skin and mucous membrane inspection, lung sounds, mouth assessment, and inspection of venous access device insertion sites, must be performed every 8 hours by a registered nurse for hospitalized patients.

Considerations for Older Adults
Patient-Centered Care
Older adults are at even greater risk for chemotherapy-induced neutropenia because of age-related changes in bone marrow function. Using growth factors, such as filgrastim (Neupogen) and pegfilgrastim (Neulasta), before neutropenia occurs rather than later, can reduce the severity of neutropenia and the risk for infectious complications. Use frequent hand washing during times of immunosuppression. Be extra vigilant in assessing older adults for early indicators of infection.

3. Chemotherapy-induced nausea and vomiting (CIN); antiemetics are available to relieve nausea and vomiting
4. Mucositis (sores in mucus membranes) and stomatitis (sores in the oral cavity)
5. Alopecia (hair loss)
6. Changes in cognitive function that are usually temporary and resolve but may persist with permanent anatomic changes to the brain
7. Chemotherapy-induced peripheral neuropathy (loss of sensory perception or motor function of peripheral nerves)

! NURSING SAFETY PRIORITY: Critical Rescue

Monitor patients with reduced IMMUNITY to recognize signs of infection. When any temperature elevation (>100°F or 37.8°C) is present, respond by reporting this to the primary health care provider immediately and implement standard infection protocols. When IV anti-infective drugs are started, the neutropenic patient is admitted to the hospital. The patient with neutropenia but no other symptoms of communicable disease is NOT an infection hazard to other people; however, other people can be an infection hazard to the patient.

Immunotherapy: Biologic or Targeted Therapy
- *Biological response modifiers (BRMs)* enhance or alter an adult's biologic responses to cancer cells.
- As antineoplastic agents, these therapies include monoclonal antibodies and small molecule drugs that interfere with interleukin and interferon that influence attacks on cancer cells by macrophages, natural killer (NK) cells, or other immune cells.
    1. Monoclonal antibody therapy uses human and/or mouse proteins to form antibodies against given targets known to be present in or on certain types of cancer cells.
    2. Small molecule targeted therapies generally block the growth and spread of cancer by interfering with cellular growth pathways or molecules involved in the growth and progression of cancer cells (e.g., tyrosine kinase, hormone blocking agents, angiogenesis inhibitors, epidermal growth factor blockers).
- As supportive therapy, BRMs induce rapid recovery of bone marrow cells after suppression by radiation or chemotherapy and include colony-stimulating factors or "growth factors."
- Patients receiving interleukins have generalized, severe inflammatory reactions because these drugs are proteins and can stimulate a hypersensitivity response.

Hormonal Manipulation
- *Hormonal manipulation* involves changing the body's usual hormone responses.
- Hormonal manipulation may include the use of corticosteroids, steroid analogues, and enzyme inhibitors (aromatase inhibitors [AIs], gonadotropin-releasing hormone analogues, antiandrogens, and antiestrogens).
- These agents are used to block receptors and thus affect CELLULAR REGULATION by preventing the cancer cells from receiving normal hormonal growth stimulation.

Photodynamic Therapy
- *Photodynamic therapy (PDT)* is the selective destruction of cancer cells through a chemical reaction triggered by high-energy laser light.
    1. An agent that sensitizes cells to light is injected IV along with a dye to achieve cell death with exposure to specific wavelengths of laser light administered later.
    2. The application of PDT is contraindicated in patients with known tumor involvement of a major blood vessel, due to the triggering of a severe or fatal episode of bleeding.

- PDT is used most often for non-melanoma skin cancers, ocular tumors, GI tumors, and cancers located in the upper airways.

SURGICAL

- Surgery for cancer involves the removal of diseased tissue and may be used for prophylaxis, diagnosis, cure, control, palliation, determination of therapy effectiveness, and reconstruction.

Oncological Emergencies

- **Sepsis and Disseminated Intravascular Coagulation (DIC):** *Sepsis,* or *septicemia,* is a condition in which organisms enter the bloodstream (bloodstream infection [BSI]) and can result in septic shock, a life-threatening condition. Adults with cancer who have low WBCs (neutropenia) and impaired immunity from cancer therapy are at risk for infection and sepsis.
  1. Often a low-grade fever (100.4°F or 38°C) is the only sign of infection.
  2. Extensive, abnormal clotting occurs throughout the small blood vessels of patients with DIC. This widespread clotting depletes circulating clotting factors and platelets. As this happens, extensive bleeding occurs. Bleeding from many sites is the most common problem and ranges from oozing to fatal hemorrhage.
- **Syndrome of Inappropriate Antidiuretic Hormone:** In healthy adults, antidiuretic hormone (ADH) is secreted by the posterior pituitary gland only when more fluid (water) is needed in the body, such as when plasma volume is decreased. Certain conditions induce ADH secretion when not needed by the body, which leads to syndrome of inappropriate antidiuretic hormone (SIADH). Cancer is a common cause of SIADH, especially small cell lung cancer (SCLC). SIADH also may occur with other cancers, including head and neck, melanoma, GI, prostate, and hematologic malignancies, especially when metastatic tumors are present in the brain.

! NURSING SAFETY PRIORITY: Critical Rescue

Monitor patients at least every 2 hours to recognize signs and symptoms of increasing fluid overload (bounding pulse, increasing neck vein distention [jugular venous distention (JVD)], presence of crackles in lungs, increasing peripheral edema, reduced urine output) because pulmonary edema can occur very quickly and lead to death. When symptoms indicate that the fluid overload from SIADH either is not responding to therapy or is becoming worse, respond by notifying the primary health care provider immediately.

- **Spinal Cord Compression:** Spinal cord compression (SCC) is an oncologic emergency that requires immediate intervention to relieve pain and prevent neurologic damage. Damage from SCC occurs either when a tumor directly enters the spinal cord or spinal column, or when the vertebrae collapse from tumor degradation of the bone. Tumors metastasizing from the lung, prostate, breast, and colon account for most SCC.
    1. The symptoms of SCC can vary depending on the severity and location of the compression. Back pain is a common first symptom and occurs before other problems or nerve deficits. Other symptoms include weakness, loss of sensation, urinary retention, and constipation.
- **Hypercalcemia:** Hypercalcemia (increased serum calcium level) occurs in up to one-third of patients with cancer. It is a metabolic emergency and can lead to death. Breast, lung, and renal cell carcinomas; multiple myeloma; and adult T-cell leukemia and lymphoma are the most common causes among cancer patients. These cancers can secrete parathyroid hormone, causing bone to release calcium.
    1. Early symptoms of hypercalcemia are nonspecific. Common symptoms include skeletal pain, kidney stones, abdominal discomfort, and altered cognition that can range from lethargy to coma.
- **Superior Vena Cava Syndrome:** The superior vena cava (SVC), which returns all blood from the head, neck, and upper extremities to the heart, has thin walls, and compression or obstruction by tumor growth or by clots in the vessel leads to congestion of the blood. This is known as *superior vena cava syndrome (SVCS)* and can occur quickly or develop gradually over time. Compression of the SVC is painful and can be life-threatening.
    1. Early signs and symptoms include edema of the face, especially around the eyes (periorbital edema) on arising in the morning, and tightness of the collar. As the compression worsens, the patient develops engorged blood vessels and erythema of the upper body, edema in the arms and hands, and dyspnea. The development of stridor (a high-pitched crowing sound) indicates narrowing of the pharynx or larynx and is an alarming sign of rapid SVCS progression. Symptoms are more apparent when the patient is in the supine position.
- Tumor lysis syndrome: In tumor lysis syndrome (TLS), large numbers of tumor cells are destroyed rapidly. The intracellular contents of damaged cancer cells, including potassium and purines (DNA components), are released into the bloodstream faster than the body can eliminate them. Unlike other oncologic emergencies, TLS is a positive sign that cancer treatment is

effective in destroying cancer cells. Severe or untreated TLS can cause tissue damage, acute kidney injury (AKI), and death (Wang et al., 2015).

Care Coordination and Transition Management

- Teach patients to reduce risk for cancer and cancer recurrence by:
  1. Wearing sunscreen and avoiding sunburn
  2. Stopping or never starting cigarette smoking
  3. Eating a diet with five or more servings of fruit and vegetables daily
  4. Identifying environmental or occupational carcinogens and wearing protective gear to reduce exposure
- Offer fertility-protective approaches such as harvest and storage of ova or sperm before cancer treatment, particularly if sterility is a risk from treatment.
- Teach all adults the benefits of participating in specific routine screening techniques such as Papanicolaou (Pap) test, mammogram, and colonoscopy as part of health maintenance.
- Teach everyone to recognize the warning signs for cancer so that it can be diagnosed and treated in early stages. Use the acronym *CAUTION*:
  1. **C**hanges in bowel or bladder habits
  2. **A** sore that does not heal
  3. **U**nusual bleeding or discharge
  4. **T**hickening or lump in the breast or elsewhere
  5. **I**ndigestion or difficulty swallowing
  6. **O**bvious change in a wart or mole
  7. **N**agging cough or hoarseness
- For patients undergoing surgical management of cancer or solid tumors, provide postoperative care and advise to follow-up with the oncologist.
- For patients undergoing chemotherapy or radiation therapy, teach the signs of infection and the urgency of follow-up even with mild infection if in an immunosuppressed state.
- Teach the warning signs of cancer and cancer recurrence.
- Assess the patient's and family's ability to cope with the uncertainty of cancer and its treatment and with the changes in body image and role.
- Coordinate with the health care team to provide ongoing health, financial, spiritual, and psychosocial support for the patient and family.
- Encourage the patient and family to express their feelings and concerns.
- When cancer or cancer surgery is disfiguring, encourage the patient to look at the surgical site, touch it, and participate in any dressing changes or incisional care required.

- Provide information about support groups, such as those sponsored by the American Cancer Society or specialty cancer organizations.
- Discuss with the patient the idea of having a person who has coped with the same issues come for a visit.
- Teach the patient about the importance of performing and progressing the intensity of any prescribed exercises to regain as much function as possible and prevent complications.
- Coordinate with the physical therapist, occupational therapist, and family members to plan strategies individualized to each patient to regain or maintain optimal function.

C

Common Cancer Sites	Nursing Considerations

BONE	• The most common symptoms are pain and swelling at the site of the bone tumor.
	• Fragility from the deterioration in the bone matrix can result in spontaneous and debilitating fractures.
	• Treatment includes:
	  1. Pain management
	  2. Bracing to reduce pain and prevent fracture
	  3. Chemotherapy alone or in combination with radiation therapy to shrink the tumor
	  4. Surgery to remove the tumor or the limb with the diseased bone (amputation)
	  5. Rehabilitation and psychosocial support for the person with extensive surgery to remove cancerous bone

BREAST	• Breast cancer is a common problem of impaired CELLULAR REGULATION. (See Ignatavicius, Workman, & Rebar, 9e for fully processed Breast Cancer Exemplar)
	  1. Breast cancer is divided into two broad categories: noninvasive and invasive.
	    a. *Noninvasive cancers* remain within the breast ducts and make up 20% of breast cancers.
	    b. *Invasive cancers* penetrate the tissue surrounding the ducts and make up 80% of all breast cancers.
	      (1) The most common invasive breast cancer is *infiltrating ductal carcinoma,* originating in mammary ducts and invading surrounding tissue.

Continued

Common Cancer Sites	Nursing Considerations

The priority collaborative problems for patients with breast cancer include:

1. Potential for metastasis of cancer to other parts of the body due to lack of treatment or inadequate treatment response
   a. Teach the patient to follow-up with radiation, chemotherapy, hormone therapy, or targeted therapy.
   b. For those who cannot have surgery or whose cancer is too advanced, these therapies are used to promote comfort (palliation).
2. Potential for decreased ability to cope due to unanticipated breast cancer diagnosis and its treatment
   a. Teach women ways to minimize surgical area deformity and enhance body image, such as the use of breast prosthesis or the option of breast reconstruction.
   b. Address the reactions of family and significant others to the diagnosis of breast cancer; provide support and education.

Promote a return to normal cellular regulation with surgical removal of the tumor and adjunctive drug or radiation therapy.

- Reinforce information about the type of surgery planned, which may be a lumpectomy, partial, modified, or complete mastectomy.
- Breast reconstruction is common for women without complications from the cancer surgery and may be performed during the cancer surgery or at a later time.
- Radiation therapy is administered after breast-conserving surgery to kill remaining breast cancer cells.
- Chemotherapy for breast cancer is delivered intravenously when breast cancer is invasive.

Common Cancer Sites	Nursing Considerations
	1. A common chemotherapy regimen for breast cancer treatment is doxorubicin (Adriamycin, Caelyx~), cyclophosphamide (Cytoxan), and paclitaxel (Taxol), which, in the US, is also known as AC-T (Burchum & Rosenthal, 2016). Administered over 3 to 6 months in cycles of 2 to 3 weeks each month.
	• Targeted therapy for breast cancer involves the use of drugs that target specific features of cancer cells, such as a protein, an enzyme, or the formation of new blood vessels. The advantage of targeted therapy over traditional chemotherapy is that it is less likely to harm normal, healthy cells and has fewer side effects. One of the first targeted therapies developed for breast cancer is the monoclonal antibody trastuzumab (Herceptin).
	• Hormonal therapy is used to reduce the estrogen available to breast tumors to stop or prevent their growth.

Genetic/Genomic Considerations

Mutations in several genes, such as *BRCA1* and *BRCA2,* are related to hereditary breast cancer. People who have specific mutations in either one of these genes are at a high risk for developing breast cancer and ovarian cancer. However, only 5% to 10% of all breast cancers are hereditary. Only women with a strong family history and a reasonable suspicion that a mutation is present have genetic testing for *BRCA* mutations. Encourage women to talk with a genetics counselor to carefully consider the benefits and potential harmful consequences of genetic testing before these tests are done.

CERVICAL	• Risk factors include:
	1. Infection with human papillomavirus (HPV)
	2. History of sexually transmitted disease
	3. Multiple sex partners

Continued

Common Cancer Sites	Nursing Considerations

4. Younger than 18 years of age at first intercourse
5. Multiparity (multiple pregnancies)
6. Smoking
7. Oral contraceptive use
8. Obesity, poor diet

The HPV vaccine protects against the high-risk HPV strains that are responsible for most cervical (and penile) cancer.

- Cervical cancer can be detected at early stages, when cure is most likely, through a periodic pelvic examination and Pap test. Diagnosis is made by cytological examination of the Pap smear.
- Ask the patient about vaginal bleeding. Cervical cancer may manifest as spotting between menstrual periods or after sexual intercourse or douching.
  - The classic symptom of invasive cancer is painless vaginal bleeding. As the cancer grows, bleeding increases in frequency, duration, and amount, and it may become continuous.
- Surgical management for small, early-stage cervical cancer includes electrosurgical excision, laser therapy, and cryosurgery.
- Surgical management at the microinvasive stage depends on the patient's health, desire for future childbearing, tumor size, stage, cancer cell type, and preferences.
- A *conization,* in which a cone-shaped area of cervix is removed surgically, can remove the affected tissue while preserving fertility.
- Radiation therapy is reserved for invasive cervical cancer.
- Chemotherapy may be used with radiation for invasive cervical cancer.

COLORECTAL
- Colorectal cancer (CRC), or cancer of the colon or rectum, is a common malignancy or impaired CELLULAR REGULATION. (See Ignatavicius, Workman, & Rebar, 9e for fully processed Colorectal Cancer Exemplar.)

Common Cancer Sites	Nursing Considerations

- Most CRCs are adenocarcinomas arising from the glandular epithelial tissue of the colon and developing as a multi-step process.
- Complications include bowel perforation with peritonitis, abscess or fistula formation, frank hemorrhage, and complete intestinal obstruction.
- Risk factors include:
  1. Age older than 50 years
  2. Genetic predisposition
     a. People with a first-degree relative (sister, sibling, or child) diagnosed with CRC have three to four times the risk of developing the disease.
  3. Personal or family history of cancer or diseases that predispose to cancer (e.g., familial adenomatous polyposis [FAP], hereditary nonpolyposis colorectal cancer [HNPCC])
  4. Crohn's disease or ulcerative colitis
- Assess for:
  1. Rectal bleeding (the most common symptom) and stool characteristics
  2. Anemia (low hemoglobin level and hematocrit; stool positive for occult blood)
  3. Cachexia (late sign)
  4. Abdominal distension or mass (late sign)
- Diagnostic assessment includes:
  1. Fecal occult blood test (FOBT)
  2. Carcinoembryonic antigen (CEA) blood test
  3. Colonoscopy
  4. CT or MRI of the abdomen with additional views for evaluation of metastasis (pelvis, thorax, and brain)
- Surgical management with tumor removal is the primary approach to treatment. Nonsurgical management reduces the potential for cancer recurrence and metastasis and provides symptom management and psychosocial support.
  1. Radiation to reduce tumor size and as a palliative measure to reduce pain, hemorrhage, bowel obstruction, or metastasis.

Continued

Common Cancer Sites	Nursing Considerations

2. *Chemotherapy* is used after surgery to interrupt cancer cell division and improve survival.
3. *Targeted biotherapy* for advanced CRC may also be used.
4. Symptom relief for pain (opioids) and emesis (antiemetics)

- In a colon resection, the bowel segment containing the tumor is removed along with several inches of bowel beyond the tumor margin and regional lymph nodes followed by an end-to-end anastomosis. This surgical procedure may be the traditional open method or a laparoscopy (minimally invasive approach).
- A colectomy (colon removal) with temporary or permanent colostomy may be needed.
- In an abdominal peritoneal (A-P) resection, the sigmoid colon and rectum are removed, the anus is closed, and a permanent colostomy is formed.
  1. Managing the colostomy, if present:
     a. If an ostomy pouch is not in place, cover the stoma with petroleum gauze to keep it moist, followed by a dry, sterile dressing
     b. Collaborate with the enterostomal therapist
     c. Observe the stoma for color, discharge, and intactness of surrounding skin
     d. Anticipate colostomy functioning 2 to 4 days after surgery; stool is liquid immediately after surgery but becomes more solid
     e. Empty the pouch when excess gas has collected or when it is one-third to one-half full of stool

Common Cancer Sites	Nursing Considerations

! NURSING SAFETY PRIORITY: Action Alert

Report any of these problems related to the colostomy to the surgeon:
- Signs of ischemia and necrosis (dark red, purplish, or black color; dry, firm, or flaccid)
- Unusual or excessive bleeding
- Mucocutaneous separation (breakdown of the suture line securing the stoma to the abdominal wall)

- Teach the patient and family colostomy care, including:
  1. Normal appearance of a stoma, including size and how to measure size
  2. Signs and symptoms of complications
  3. The choice, use, care, and application of the appropriate appliance to cover the stoma
  4. How to protect the skin adjacent to the stoma
  5. Dietary measures to control gas and odor

ENDOMETRIAL (UTERINE)
- Endometrial cancer (cancer of the inner lining of the uterus) is the most common gynecologic cancer.
- Adenocarcinoma is the most common type, accounting for 80% of all cases.
  1. It is slow growing with initial growth in the uterine cavity, followed by extension into the myometrium and cervix.
- Risk factors associated with endometrial cancer include:
  1. Prolonged exposure to estrogen without the protective effects of progesterone
  2. Women in reproductive years
  3. Family history of endometrial cancer
  4. Diabetes mellitus
  5. Hypertension
  6. Obesity
  7. Uterine polyps
  8. Late menopause
  9. Nulliparity (no childbirths)

Continued

Common Cancer Sites	Nursing Considerations

10. Smoking
11. Tamoxifen (Nolvadex) given for breast cancer

- The primary symptom is postmenopausal bleeding as well as low back, abdominal, or pelvic pain.
- *Transvaginal ultrasound* and *endometrial biopsy* are the gold standard tests for the presence of endometrial thickening and cancer.
- Surgical removal and cancer staging of the tumor is first-line therapy. Typically, a total hysterectomy is done (see *Uterine Fibroids [Leiomyomas], Surgical Management, Hysterectomy*).
- Radiation therapy and chemotherapy are used postoperatively and depend on the surgical staging.

HEAD AND NECK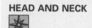

- Head and neck cancers begin as a loss of CELLULAR REGULATION and occur in structures within the larynx, trachea, throat, oral cavity, or on the tongue. (See Ignatavicius, Workman & Rebar, 9e, for fully processed Head and Neck Cancer Exemplar.)
- Other origins of head and neck cancers include the salivary glands, thyroid, and other structures.
- Head and neck cancers are usually squamous cell carcinomas or slow growing tumors that are curable when diagnosed and treated at an early stage.
- The cause of head and neck cancers is unknown, but the two greatest risk factors are tobacco and alcohol use, especially in combination.
- Assess for signs and symptoms:
  1. Malnutrition or weight loss
  2. Hoarseness
  3. Lumps on the head or in the neck
  4. Mouth sores
- The goal of treatment is to remove or eradicate the cancer while preserving as much normal function as possible. The specific treatment depends on the extent and location of the lesion.

Common Cancer Sites	Nursing Considerations

- Radiation therapy is used alone or in combination with chemotherapy or surgery. Because radiation therapy slows tissue healing, it may not be performed before surgery.
  1. Complications of radiation therapy for head and neck cancer include increased hoarseness, dysphagia, skin problems, and dry mouth (leading to halitosis, taste changes, increased risk for dental caries and dental infection).
  2. Dry mouth (xerostomia) is a long-term complication and may be permanent. Interventions to improve comfort are:
     a. Providing fluid intake and room or oxygen humidification
     b. Administering artificial saliva, moisturizing gels, or saliva stimulants (e.g., Salagen, cevimeline)
- Chemotherapy can be used alone or in addition to surgery or radiation for head and neck cancer.
  1. Specific treatment regimens and drug combinations vary, but the most commonly used agent for head and neck cancer include cisplatin (Platinol).
  2. Targeted therapy (biotherapy) for advanced head and neck cancers may include cetuximab (Erbitux) to inhibit growth factors.
- Tumor size and location (according to tumor-nodes-metastasis [TNM] classification) determines the type of surgery needed for the specific head and neck cancer.
- Very small, early-stage tumors may be removed by laser therapy or photodynamic therapy, but few head and neck tumors are found at this stage, and most require extensive traditional surgery.
- Traditional surgical procedures for head and neck cancers include:
  1. *Laryngectomy* (total and partial): removal of the larynx.
  2. *Tracheotomy:* creation of a new artificial airway by opening the wall of the trachea.

Continued

C

Common Cancer Sites	Nursing Considerations

3. *Oropharyngeal cancer resections*
4. *Cordectomy:* vocal cord removal.
5. *Radical neck dissection,* which is removal of the primary tumor along with lymph node dissection; it may involve removing skin, muscle, bone, and other structures.
6. *Composite resections* are a combination of surgical procedures, including partial or total glossectomy, partial mandibulectomy, and, if needed, nodal neck dissection.

! NURSING SAFETY PRIORITY: Critical Rescue

If a carotid artery leak is suspected, call the Rapid Response Team, and do not touch the area because additional pressure could cause an immediate rupture. When the carotid artery ruptures, large amounts of bright red blood spurt quickly. If the carotid artery ruptures because of drying or infection, immediately place constant pressure over the site and secure the airway. Maintain direct manual continuous pressure on the carotid artery and immediately transport the patient to the operating room for carotid resection. Do not leave the patient. Carotid artery rupture has a high risk of stroke and death. Nursing response can save the patient's life.

- Observe the patient who has had a subtotal, vertical, or supraglottic laryngectomy for aspiration.
- Evaluate the stoma following a laryngectomy and all grafts and flaps every 1 to 2 hours for the first 72 hours.
- Monitor pain, pulse/perfusion, capillary refill, color, and drainage at the surgical site.
- Position the patient so that the side of the head and neck with the flaps is not dependent.
- Observe for carotid artery leakage or rupture.
  1. Rupture results in large amounts of bright red blood spurting quickly.
  2. Leakage shows as oozing of bright red blood.

Common Cancer Sites	Nursing Considerations
	• Acute surgical pain is typically managed by patient-controlled analgesic pumps intravenously initially then transitioned to an enteral nonsteroidal anti-inflammatory drug (NSAID).
	1. Chronic pain from nerve root involvement or from radiation treatment is managed with nonopioids like NSAIDs or tricyclic antidepressants.
	• Teach the patient and family about:
	1. Stoma, tracheostomy, or laryngectomy and incision care
	2. Communication methods and wearing a medical alert bracelet to inform the reader about emergency airway/communication challenges
	3. Smoking cessation
LUNG	• Lung cancers arise as a result of failure of CELLULAR REGULATION in bronchial epithelium and are classified as small cell lung cancer (SCLC) or non–small cell lung cancer (NSCLC).
	• The overall 5-year survival rate for all patients with lung cancer is only 16% because most lung cancers are diagnosed at a late stage when metastasis is present.
	• Risk factors for lung cancer:
	• Cigarette smoking is the major risk factor and is responsible for 85% of all lung cancer deaths.
	• Nonsmokers exposed to passive, or secondhand, smoke have a greater risk for lung cancer than nonsmokers.
	• Environmental exposure such as asbestos, coal distillates, mustard gas, and radiation
	• Common signs and symptoms of lung cancer are associated with respiratory problems and include dyspnea, pallor or cyanosis, tachycardia, bloody sputum, and cough.
	• Pain is common when lymph nodes are enlarged and press on nerves.

C

Continued

Common Cancer Sites	Nursing Considerations

Interprofessional Collaborative Care
- Assess for pulmonary manifestations
  1. Dyspnea
  2. Hoarseness
  3. Abnormal breath sounds: wheezing, decreased or absent breath sounds
  4. Breathing pattern abnormalities
  5. Areas of tenderness or masses palpated on the chest wall
  6. Tracheal deviation
  7. Pleural friction rub
  8. Asymmetry of diaphragm movement
  9. Use of accessory muscles manifested by retraction between ribs or at sternal notch
- Assess for nonpulmonary manifestations
  1. Weight loss, anorexia, dysphagia
  2. Fatigue
  3. Muffled heart sounds
  4. Dysrhythmias
  5. Bone pain
  6. Fever/chills related to pneumonitis, bronchitis, and pneumonia
  7. Paraneoplastic endocrine syndromes caused by hormones secreted by tumor cells, such as SIADH
- Diagnosis of lung cancer is made on the basis of:
  1. Chest x-ray
  2. CT scan
  3. Fiberoptic bronchoscopy
  4. Thoracoscopy or thoracentesis to view and biopsy lung tissue

Nonsurgical Management
- Chemotherapy is often the treatment of choice for lung cancers, and it may be used alone or as adjuvant therapy In combination with surgery.
- *Targeted therapy* drugs include:
  1. Erlotinib (Tarceva), an oral drug
  2. Bevacizumab (Avastin), given IV
  3. Crizotinib (Xalkori), an oral drug

Common Cancer Sites	Nursing Considerations

- *Radiation therapy* may be used for locally advanced lung cancers confined to the chest. It is typically used in addition to surgery or chemotherapy.
- Common side effects of radiation therapy for lung cancer are:
  1. Chest skin irritation and peeling
  2. Fatigue, nausea, and weight loss
  3. Wheezing from inflamed airways
  4. Esophagitis and changes in taste
- *Photo dynamic therapy* (PDT) may be used to remove small bronchial tumors when they are accessible by bronchoscopy.
- Surgery is the main treatment for stage I and stage II NSCLC. Total removal of a non–small cell primary lung cancer is undertaken in hope of achieving a cure. If complete removal is not possible, the surgeon removes the bulk of the tumor.
- The specific surgery depends on the stage of the cancer and the patient's overall health and functional status. Surgeries include:
  1. Wedge resection or removal of the peripheral portion of small areas of tumor and surrounding tissue
  2. Removal of a lung segment (segmental resection)
  3. Removal of a lobe (lobectomy)
  4. Removal of an entire lung (pneumonectomy)
- Refer to the peri operative care section

Postoperative care specific to lung cancer:
1. Maintain closed-chest (chest tube) drainage system to remove air and blood from the pleural space and re-expand the lung.
2. Respiratory management
   a. Maintain a patent airway.
   b. Assess respiratory status at least every 2 hours for the first 12 to 24 hours.
   c. Perform oral suctioning as necessary.

Continued

Common Cancer Sites	Nursing Considerations

    d. Provide oxygen therapy or mechanical ventilation as prescribed.

    e. Assist the patient to a semi-Fowler's position or to sit up in a chair as soon as possible.

    f. For a patient with spontaneous respirations, encourage the patient to use the incentive spirometer every hour while awake.

    g. If coughing is permitted, help the patient cough by splinting any incision and ensuring that the chest tube does not pull with movement.

3. Manage acute surgical pain, typically with patient-controlled analgesia (PCA) and a nerve or epidural block.

! NURSING SAFETY PRIORITY: Action Alert

For a water seal chest tube drainage system, 2 cm of water is the minimum needed in the water seal to prevent air from flowing backward into the patient. Check the water level every shift, and add sterile water to this chamber to the level marked on the indicator (specified by the manufacturer of the drainage system).

- Palliative treatment may focus on symptom management, rather than cure.
- Dyspnea management is a priority. Dyspnea is reduced with oxygen, drug therapy, radiation, management of pleural effusion, pain relief, and positioning for comfort. For example, the patient with severe dyspnea may be most comfortable sitting in a lounge chair or reclining chair.

OVARIAN
- Most ovarian cancers are epithelial tumors that form on the surface of the ovaries.
- These tumors grow rapidly, spread quickly, and are often bilateral.

Common Cancer Sites	Nursing Considerations

- Ovarian cancers are often detected at late stages when metastasis has occurred by direct extension into nearby organs and through blood and lymph circulation to distant sites. Free-floating cancer cells also spread through the abdomen.
- Women who have a mutation in the BRCA1 or BRCA2 genes are at high risk for developing ovarian cancer over their lifetime, although the actual number of women with these genes is relatively small.

Interprofessional Collaborative Care
- Assess for risks factors and signs and symptoms of ovarian cancer:
  1. Abdominal pain, swelling, or bloating
  2. Vague GI disturbances such as dyspepsia (indigestion) and gas
  3. Urinary frequency or incontinence
  4. Unexpected weight loss
  5. Vaginal bleeding
- Diagnosis and staging are performed by surgical exploration and biopsy analysis.
- Nursing care of the patient with ovarian cancer is similar to that for endometrial or cervical cancer.
- Treatment options depend on the extent of the cancer and usually include surgery first, followed by chemotherapy. Radiation therapy is used for more widespread cancers.
- Total abdominal hysterectomy and bilateral salpingo-oophorectomy (BSO) are the surgical procedures for all stages of ovarian cancer.
- When cancer has spread to other abdominal organs or lymph nodes, the tumors can be removed during the surgery.
- After surgery, nursing care is similar to that of the patient undergoing a hysterectomy for uterine leiomyomas or care for the postoperative abdominal surgery patient.
- For all stages of ovarian cancer, chemotherapy drugs may be used. Drugs may include cisplatin (Platinol), carboplatin, and paclitaxel (Taxol). They may be given IV or intraperitoneally.

Continued

Common Cancer Sites	Nursing Considerations
PANCREATIC	• Pancreatic tumors are highly malignant and originate in the epithelial cells (adenocarcinoma) of the pancreatic ductal system.
	• These cancers grow rapidly and spread to surrounding organs (stomach, duodenum, gallbladder, and intestine) by direct extension and invasion of the lymphatic and vascular system.
	• Pancreatic cancer may also result from metastasis from cancer of the lung, breast, thyroid, or kidney or from skin melanoma.
	• Most pancreatic cancers are not diagnosed until the disease is advanced, and the overall survival rate is low.

Interprofessional Collaborative Care
- Assess for signs and symptoms:
  1. Jaundice and pruritus
  2. Clay-colored stool and dark, frothy urine
  3. Abdominal pain described as a vague, constant dullness in the upper abdomen and nonspecific in nature; pain related to eating or activity; or back pain
  4. Weight loss (unplanned)
  5. Anorexia accompanied by early satiety, nausea, flatulence, and vomiting
  6. High blood glucose levels
  7. Splenomegaly
  8. GI bleeding
  9. Leg or calf pain (from thrombophlebitis)
  10. Fatigue and weakness
  11. Dull sound on abdominal percussion indicating ascites
- Diagnostic assessment may include:
  1. Elevated levels of serum amylase, serum lipase, alkaline phosphatase, and bilirubin
  2. Elevated level of CEA
  3. Elevated levels of serum markers: CA-19-9 and CA-242
  4. Abdominal ultrasound or CT
  5. Endoscopic retrograde cholangiopancreatography (ERCP)
  6. Aspiration of pancreatic ascitic fluid

Common Cancer Sites	Nursing Considerations

- Management of the patient with pancreatic cancer is geared toward preventing tumor spread and decreasing pain. These measures are palliative, not curative.
- Pancreatic cancer is often metastatic and recurs despite treatment.

Nonsurgical Management
- Drug therapy includes:
  1. High doses of opioid analgesia; dependency is not a consideration because of the poor prognosis
  2. Chemotherapy with drug combinations
  3. Targeted therapies that inhibit growth factors, angioneogenesis, and tyrosine kinase, an enzyme used in cancer cells
- *External beam radiation therapy* to shrink pancreatic tumor cells, alleviating obstruction and improving food absorption, may provide pain relief but has not increased survival rates.
- Implantation of radon seeds in combination with systemic or intra-arterial administration of floxuridine (FUDR) has also been used.
- Biliary stents may be inserted to relieve biliary obstruction.

Surgical Management
- Surgery consists of complete or partial pancreatectomy.
- The classic surgery, the Whipple procedure, entails extensive surgical manipulation, including resection of the proximal head of the pancreas, the duodenum, a portion of the jejunum, the stomach (partial or total gastrectomy), and the gallbladder, with anastomosis of the pancreatic duct (pancreatojejunostomy), the common bile duct (choledochojejunostomy), and the stomach (gastrojejunostomy) to the jejunum. The spleen may also be removed (splenectomy). This surgery may be performed by the traditional open abdominal method or by laparoscopic minimally invasive surgery (in select cancers).

Continued

Common Cancer Sites	Nursing Considerations

- Palliative measures to relieve obstruction, such as cholecystojejunostomy, may be performed.
- Refer to the peri operative care section
- Postoperative care specific to pancreatic cancer includes:
  1. Monitoring the drainage tubes and their patency to remove drainage and secretions from the area and to prevent stress on the anastomosis site
  2. Monitoring drainage for color, consistency, and amount
  3. Observing for fistula formation and excoriation (drainage of pancreatic fluids is corrosive and irritating to the skin, internal leakage causes peritonitis)
  4. Placing the patient in a semi-Fowler's position to reduce stress on the incision and anastomosis and to optimize lung expansion
  5. Assessing blood glucose levels for transient hyperglycemia or hypoglycemia resulting from surgical manipulation of the pancreas
  6. Monitoring the patient for pitting edema of the extremities and dependent edema in the sacrum and back

PROSTATE

- Prostate cancer is another exemplar of impaired CELLULAR REGULATION and the second most common type of cancer in men, most commonly affecting men older than 65 years. (See Ignatavicius, Workman & Rebar, 9e, for fully processed Prostate Cancer Exemplar)
- Most prostate tumors are adenocarcinomas arising from epithelial cells located in the posterior lobe or outer portion of the gland, and most are androgen-sensitive (need testosterone to grow).
- Of all malignancies, prostate cancer is one of the slowest growing, and it metastasizes (spreads) in a predictable pattern. Common sites of metastasis are the nearby lymph nodes, bones, lungs, and liver.

Common Cancer Sites	Nursing Considerations

Interprofessional Collaborative Care
- Assess for signs and symptoms:
  1. Urine quality and characteristics, including force of stream
  2. Pain in the pelvis, spine, hips, or rib
  3. Swollen lymph nodes, especially in the groin areas
  4. Psychosocial issues
- Diagnostic assessment for cancer and metastasis may include:
  1. Digital rectal examination (DRE): prostate that is found to be stony hard and have palpable irregularities or indurations is suspected to be malignant.
  2. Elevated levels of prostate-specific antigen (PSA), greater than 2.5 ng/mL
  3. Elevated *early prostate cancer antigen (EPCA-2)*
  4. Elevated levels of serum acid phosphatase in advanced disease
  5. Elevated serum alkaline phosphatase may indicate bone metastases
  6. Transrectal ultrasound (TRUS) of the prostate (may be paired with prostate biopsy)
  7. Prostate tissue biopsy
  8. Lymph node biopsy
  9. CT scan of the pelvis and abdomen
  10. MRI

! NURSING SAFETY PRIORITY: Action Alert

After a *transrectal ultrasound with biopsy,* instruct the patient about possible complications, although rare, including hematuria with clots, signs of infection, and perineal pain. Teach him to report fever, chills, bloody urine, and any difficulty voiding. Advise him to avoid strenuous physical activity and to drink plenty of fluids, especially in the first 24 hours after the procedure. Teach him that a small amount of bleeding turning the urine pink is expected during this time. However, bright red bleeding should be reported to the health care provider immediately.

Continued

Common Cancer Sites	Nursing Considerations

- Goals of care include preventing metastasis from impaired cellular regulation and supporting the patient with psychosocial interventions.
- Because prostate cancer is slow growing with late metastasis, older men who are asymptomatic may choose observation without immediate active treatment, an option known as *active surveillance (AS)*.
  1. The average time from diagnosis to start of treatment is up to 10 years.
  2. During AS, men are monitored at regular intervals through DRE and PSA testing.
  3. If obstruction occurs, a transurethral resection of the prostate (TURP) may be done.
  4. Factors that are considered in choosing AS include potential side effects of treatment (e.g., urinary incontinence, ED), estimated life expectancy, and the risk for increased morbidity and mortality from not seeking active treatment.
- Active treatment occurs when symptoms become bothersome or when the cancer is more aggressive with concerning changes between surveillance periods.
  1. *Surgery is the most common intervention for a cure*. Minimally invasive approaches are usually performed.
     a. The most common procedure is the *laparoscopic radical prostatectomy (LRP)* with robotic assistance.
     b. A newer procedure is *transrectal high-intensity focused ultrasound* (HIFU) and cryosurgery with smaller incisions and fewer complications.
     c. Less common is an open surgical technique for radical prostatectomy (prostate removal).
     d. A bilateral orchiectomy (removal of both testicles) is another palliative surgery that slows the spread of cancer by removing the main source of testosterone.

Common Cancer Sites	Nursing Considerations

2. Postoperative care interventions include the typical care for a surgical patient with emphasis on maintaining hydration, caring for wound drains (open procedure), managing pain, and preventing pulmonary complications.

- Nonsurgical management is usually an adjunct to surgery but may be done as an alternative intervention if the cancer is widespread or the patient's condition or age prevents surgery.
- External or internal radiation therapy may be used in the treatment of prostate cancer or for palliation of late-stage symptoms.
  1. *External beam radiation therapy* (EBRT) comes from a source outside the body. Patients are usually treated 5 days each week for 6 to 9 weeks.
  2. *Internal radiation therapy (brachytherapy)* can be delivered by implanting low-dose radiation seeds directly into and around the prostate gland.
- Drug therapy
  1. Hormone therapy
     a. *LH-RH agonists* such as leuprolide (Lupron), goserelin (Zoladex), and triptorelin (Trelstar). These drugs stimulate the pituitary gland to release the luteinizing hormone (LH); once LH is depleted, testosterone production in testes decreases.
     b. *Anti-androgen drugs,* also known as *androgen deprivation therapy (ADT),* block the body's and tumor's ability to use the available androgens. Examples include flutamide (Eulexin, Euflex), bicalutamide (Casodex), and nilutamide (Nilandron).
  2. Chemotherapy may be an option for patients whose cancer has spread and for whom other therapies have not worked.
     a. Docetaxel (Taxotere) plus prednisone or a combination of cisplatin (Platinol) and etoposide (VP-16, VePesid) may be used.

Continued

Common Cancer Sites	Nursing Considerations
	• Home care management of the patient after a radical prostatectomy includes:
	1. Collaborating with the case manager to coordinate the efforts of various primary health care providers and possibly a home care nurse
	2. Health teaching about:
	a. Indwelling urinary catheter care if recovering from an open procedure
	b. Restriction for activity or weight lifting; these may be as brief as 2 to 3 days for minimally invasive procedures and as long as 6 weeks for open surgical procedures
	c. Perineal exercises (Kegal) may reduce the severity of urinary incontinence after radical prostatectomy; teach the patient to contract and relax the perineal and gluteal muscles
	d. Teach the patient to avoid straining at defecation until surgical sites have healed
	• Refer patients with ED or urinary incontinence to a urologist or other specialist.

🌐 Cultural and Spiritual Considerations: Patient-Centered Care

Race is the second-most common risk factor for prostate cancer because the disease affects African Americans more often than other ethnic/racial groups, followed by Caucasians (Euro-Americans) and Hispanic-American men.

SKIN	• Overexposure to sunlight is the major cause of skin cancer. Genetic predisposition and the presence of precancerous lesions are also associated with skin cancers. There are four common skin cancers:
	1. Actinic keratosis (premalignant): small macules or papule with rough, adherent flaking

Common Cancer Sites	Nursing Considerations

2. Squamous cell carcinoma: firm, nodular lesions topped with a crust; larger tumors can result in metastases
3. Basel cell carcinoma: pearly papule with a central crater on sun-exposed areas of skin; often with dilated blood vessels (telangiectasia)
4. Melanoma: irregularly shaped pigmented papule that is highly invasive and has great morbidity and mortality

Interprofessional Collaborative Care
- Biopsy of the lesion is a typical first step to diagnosis and staging.
- Surgical management to excise the lesion is often necessary.
- Cryosurgery or cell destruction by local application of liquid nitrogen can be used for some premalignant lesions.
- Topical chemotherapy can be used for actinic dermatosis and widespread basal cell treatment.
- Drug therapy for melanoma can include targeted biological therapy to manage cellular regulation and systemic chemotherapy to destroy cancer cells.

Care Coordination and Transition Management
- Prepare patients for self-management by teaching steps to avoid skin cancer, particularly avoiding exposure to sun and examining one's body for changes in spots, moles, scars and other lesions.
- Advise patients to seek medical advice if you note changes in skin, particularly changes in color, rapid growth, swelling around a lesion, or new bleeding or draining near a lesion.

UROTHELIAL (BLADDER)
- Urothelial cancers are malignant tumors of the urothelium, the lining of transitional cells in the kidney, renal pelvis, ureters, urinary bladder, and urethra.

Continued

Common Cancer Sites	Nursing Considerations

- Most urothelial cancers occur in the bladder; the term *bladder cancer* is the general term used to describe this condition.
- Most urinary tract cancers occur in the transitional cell layer and are treated with surgical excision.
- Chemotherapy and radiation therapy are also used. When chemotherapy is instilled into the bladder additional teaching and processes for safe urine disposal are needed.
- When the bladder is removed, surgical techniques are used to divert urine flow, including construction of a neobladder.
- If the cancer is untreated, the tumor cells invade surrounding tissues, the cancer spreads to distant sites (liver, lung, and bone), and the condition ultimately leads to death.
- Causes of urothelial cancers include tobacco use; exposure to toxic chemicals used in fuels, hair dye, rubber, paint, electric cable, and textile industries; *Schistosoma haematobium* (a parasite) infection; excessive use of drugs containing phenacetin; and long-term use of cyclophosphamide (Cytoxan, Procytox ♣).

Interprofessional Collaborative Care
Assessment
- Assess signs and symptoms:
  1. Description of change in color, frequency, amount of urine
  2. Presence of any abdominal discomfort
  3. Presence of dysuria, frequency, or urgency
  4. Overall appearance of the patient, especially skin color and general nutritional status
  5. Abdomen for asymmetry, tenderness, and bladder distention
  6. Urine for color, clarity, presence of blood (first sign of bladder cancer), cells, and sediment

Common Cancer Sites	Nursing Considerations

- Diagnostic assessment includes:
  1. Urinalysis
  2. Bladder wash specimens and bladder biopsy
  3. CT scan or MRI for deep, invasive tumors

Nonsurgical Management
- Intravesical instillation of Bacille Calmette-Guérin (BCG), a live virus is used to prevent recurrence of superficial bladder cancers.
- Multiagent chemotherapy or radiation therapy may prolong life after metastasis has occurred but rarely results in a cure.

Surgical Management
- The type of surgery for bladder cancer depends on the type and stage of the cancer and the patient's general health.
- Transurethral resection of the bladder tumor (TURBT) or partial cystectomy is performed for small, early, superficial tumors, and only a portion of the bladder is removed.
- Complete bladder removal (cystectomy) with additional removal of surrounding muscle and tissue offers the best chance of a cure for large, invasive bladder cancers.
- The common types of urinary drainage following a cystectomy are ileal conduit, continent pouch, bladder reconstruction (also known as *neobladder*), and ureterosigmoidostomy.
  1. *Ileal conduit* results in the ureters surgically placed in the ileum, which is brought to the skin surface as a stoma. Urine is collected in a pouch on the skin around the stoma.
  2. *Continent pouch* (e.g., Kock's pouch) are internal pouches constructed from an ileal segment. Although these pouches open to the outside of the abdomen, a fold prevents urine leakage. Urine is drained with intermittent catheterization, and an external pouch is not needed.

Continued

Common Cancer Sites	Nursing Considerations

3. *Neobladder* is reconstruction of the bladder from bowel tissue and connecting it to the urethra. Many patients learn to control voiding from the neobladder and neither external pouching nor intermittent catheterization is needed.

4. *Ureterosigmoidostomy* results in the ureters surgically placed into a specially constructed segment of the sigmoid colon. No external pouching is needed.

- Refer to the peri operative care section.
- Postoperative care specific to bladder cancer includes:

  1. Ensure education about the specific urinary diversion and postoperative care requirements for self-care practices, methods of pouching, control of urine drainage, and management of odor

  2. Coordinate with an ET for wound, skin, stoma, and pouch care

  3. Monitor urine output and urine characteristics

  4. Manage the drain and catheter for patients who have had construction of a continent reservoir

  5. Perform initial irrigation and intermittent catheterization of the neobladder

  6. Teach the patient with a neobladder how to use new cues to know when to void, such as voiding at prescribed times or noticing a feeling of neobladder pressure

- Patients who have a neobladder created often have extreme weight loss during the first few weeks after surgery. Collaborate with a dietitian to develop a diet plan specific to the patient to meet his or her caloric needs.

- Teach patients who come into contact with chemicals in their workplaces or with leisure-time activities to avoid direct skin and mucous membrane contact with these chemicals.

- Provide health teaching to the patient and family about:

Common Cancer Sites	Nursing Considerations
	1. Drugs, diet, and fluid therapy; the use of external pouching systems; and the technique for catheterizing a continent reservoir
	2. Avoiding foods that are known to produce gas if the urinary diversion uses the intestinal tract
	• Assist the patient to prepare for the impact of urinary diversion on self-image, body image, sexual functioning, and self-esteem.
	• Refer patients and families to community support.

CARDIAC TAMPONADE

OVERVIEW

- Acute cardiac tamponade may occur when small volumes (20 to 30 mL) of fluid accumulate in the pericardium.
- It is a medical emergency and requires prompt confirmation with an echocardiogram and primary health care provider intervention.

INTERPROFESSIONAL COLLABORATIVE CARE

- Signs and symptoms of cardiac tamponade include:
  1. Paradoxical pulse (*pulsus paradoxus*) with the systolic BP 10 mm Hg or more on exhalation compared with inhalation
  2. Hypotension
  3. Jugular venous distension
  4. Decreased HR
  5. Muffled heart sounds
  6. Dyspnea, anxiety, and fatigue
- Anticipate emergent interventions of IV fluid administration and *pericardiocentesis* or insertion of a long, large bore needle into the pericardium to remove fluid by the provider.

CARDIOMYOPATHY

OVERVIEW

- Cardiomyopathy is a subacute or chronic heart muscle disease.
- Cardiomyopathy is divided into four categories on the basis of abnormalities in structure and function.
  1. *Dilated cardiomyopathy* (DCM), the most common type, involves extensive damage to the myofibrils and interference with

myocardial metabolism; both ventricles are dilated and systolic function is impaired.

2. *Hypertrophic cardiomyopathy* (HCM) is characterized by asymmetric ventricular hypertrophy and disarray of the myocardial fibers resulting in a stiff left ventricle and diastolic filling abnormalities. In about 50% of patients, HCM is transmitted as a single-gene autosomal dominant trait.

3. *Restrictive cardiomyopathy* (RCM), the rarest of the four cardiomyopathies, is caused by ventricles that restrict filling during diastole. The disease can be primary or caused by endocardial or myocardial disease such as sarcoidosis or amyloidosis.

4. *Arrhythmogenic right ventricular* (ARV) *cardiomyopathy* (dysplasia) results from replacement of myocardial tissue with fibrous and fatty tissue, usually as a familial condition and can affect both the right and left ventricles despite the name.

INTERPROFESSIONAL COLLABORATIVE CARE
Assessment: Noticing
- Assess for signs and symptoms of cardiomyopathy.
  1. Signs of reduced cardiac output, manifested by dyspnea on exertion, decreased exercise capacity, fatigue, and palpitations
  2. Dizziness or syncope
  3. Irregular pulse and abnormal or irregular heart rhythms, especially atrial fibrillation and ventricular dysrhythmias
  4. Some patients die without any symptoms; this is one type of sudden cardiac death
  5. Left or biventricular heart failure
  6. Enlarged heart on CXR and echocardiography
  7. Nonsurgical management

Interventions: Responding
- Care of the patient with cardiomyopathy is similar to that for patients with heart failure (see *Heart Failure*) and dysrhythmias.
- Nonsurgical management includes:
  1. Administering diuretics, vasodilating agents, and cardiac glycosides to increase cardiac output
  2. Administering antidysrhythmics and agents to slow HR
  3. Providing an implantable defibrillator or defibrillator-pacemaker to control dysrhythmias

SURGICAL MANAGEMENT
- The type of surgery performed depends on the type of cardiomyopathy.
  1. Ventriculomyomectomy is the excision of a portion of the hypertrophied ventricular septum to create a widened outflow

tract. This is the most common surgical treatment for obstructive HCM.
2. Percutaneous alcohol septal ablation to improve forward flow of ventricular blood into the aorta.
3. Heart transplantation is the treatment of choice for patients with severe DCM; a donor heart from a person of comparable body weight and ABO compatibility is transplanted into a recipient within 6 hours of procurement.
- For the patient who receives a heart transplant, provide postoperative care similar to patients who have open heart surgery and organ transplantation.

C

❗ NURSING SAFETY PRIORITY: Critical Rescue

After cardiac transplant surgery, perform frequent comprehensive cardiovascular and respiratory assessments according to agency or heart transplant surgical protocol. *Report any of these manifestations to the surgeon immediately: shortness of breath, fluid gain (edema, pulmonary crackles, abdominal bloating), new bradycardia, hypotension, atrial fibrillation or flutter, and fatigue or decreased activity tolerance.* To detect rejection, the surgeon performs right endomyocardial biopsies at regularly scheduled intervals and whenever heart failure-like symptoms occur.

CARDITIS, RHEUMATIC (RHEUMATIC ENDOCARDITIS)

OVERVIEW

- *Rheumatic carditis (rheumatic endocarditis)* develops after an infection with group A beta-hemolytic streptococci in some individuals.
- Inflammation is evident in all layers of the heart and results in impaired contractile function of the myocardium, thickening of the pericardium, and inflamed endocardium, leading to inflammation of valve leaflets and valvular damage.

INTERPROFESSIONAL COLLABORATIVE CARE

- Common signs and symptoms include:
  1. Evidence of an existing streptococcal infection: fever, sore throat, tachycardia, and elevated serum findings of antideoxyribonuclease B titer, antistreptolysin O titer, complement assay, and C-reactive protein
  2. New-onset murmur, pericardial friction rub, precordial pain, and/or extreme fatigue

- Management includes antibiotic therapy to manage streptococcal infection and follow-up care to manage heart valve or heart damage (see *Valvular Heart Disease* and *Cardiomyopathy*).

CARPAL TUNNEL SYNDROME
OVERVIEW
- Carpal tunnel syndrome (CTS) is a condition in which the median nerve in the wrist becomes compressed, causing pain and numbness.
- Risk factors include common repetitive strain injury (RSI), synovitis, excessive hand exercise, edema or hemorrhage into the carpal tunnel, thrombosis of the median artery, Colles' fracture of the wrist, and hand burns. CTS is also a common complication of certain metabolic and connective tissue diseases.

INTERPROFESSIONAL COLLABORATIVE CARE
- Common signs and symptoms include:
  1. Positive results for the Phalen maneuver, producing paresthesia in the palmar side of the thumb, index, and middle finger and radial half of the ring finger within 60 seconds; the patient is asked to relax the wrist into flexion or place the back of the hands together with both wrists simultaneously
  2. Positive results for the Tinel sign, which is the same response as for the Phalen maneuver, elicited by tapping lightly over the area of the median nerve in the wrist
  3. Weak pinch, clumsiness, and difficulty with fine movements that progresses to muscle weakness progressing to muscle wasting in the affected hand
  4. Wrist swelling and autonomic changes such as skin discoloration, nail brittleness, and increased or decreased palmar sweating
- Diagnostic assessment may include any of these: standard x-rays, electromyography (EMG), MRI, and ultrasonography.

NONSURGICAL MANAGEMENT INCLUDES:
- Drug therapy with NSAIDs
- Wrist immobilization with a splint or brace to place the wrist in a neutral position or slight extension during the day, during the night, or both

SURGICAL MANAGEMENT
- Surgery is performed to relieve the pressure on the median nerve by cutting or laser.
  Postoperative Care:
  1. See *Peri Operative Care*
  2. Check the dressing for drainage and tightness and the hand and fingers for neurovascular status

3. Explain to the patient that hand movements may be restricted for 6 to 8 weeks and discomfort can last that long or longer
• Multiple surgeries may be needed to fully decompress the median nerve

 CATARACTS

OVERVIEW
• A cataract is a lens opacity that distorts the image projected onto the retina, reducing visual sensory perception.
• Cataracts can occur at any age, and may be caused by trauma or exposure to toxic agents, or result from comorbidities like diabetes, and occurring with aging.

INTERPROFESSIONAL COLLABORATIVE CARE
Assessment: Noticing
1. Family history for cataracts and exposure to lens-damaging drugs or toxins
2. Visual acuity
3. Assess concerns about reduced vision
• Improve vision
1. Surgery is the only cure for cataracts. However, patients often live with reduced vision for years before the cataract is removed. Driving privileges may be restricted or withheld during this period of reduced vision.
   a. The most common surgical procedure is removal of the lens by phacoemulsification and replacement with a clear plastic lens for specific vision correction.
   b. Stress that care after surgery requires the instillation of different types of eye drops several times each day for 2 to 4 weeks.
   c. Instruct the patient on the importance of following the prescribed regimen for eye drops after surgery.
   d. Instruct the patient to notify the ophthalmologist if there is significant swelling or bruising around the eye; pain occurring with nausea or vomiting; increasing redness of the eye, a change in visual acuity, tears, and photophobia; and yellow or green drainage.

! NURSING SAFETY PRIORITY: Critical Rescue

Teach the patient to report any reduction in vision immediately to the ophthalmologist.

Care Coordination and Transition Management

1. Help the patient and family plan the eye drop schedule and daily home eye examination.
2. Review these indications of complications after cataract surgery with the patient and family:
   a. Sharp, sudden pain in the eye
   b. Bleeding or increased discharge
   c. Green or yellow, thick drainage
   d. Lid swelling
   e. Reappearance of a bloodshot sclera after the initial appearance has cleared
   f. Decreased vision
   g. Flashes of light or floating shapes
3. Teach the patient about activity restrictions such as avoiding heavy lifting or vacuuming.

CELIAC DISEASE

OVERVIEW

- Celiac disease is a multi-system autoimmune disease that has cycles of remission and exacerbation characterized by inflammation of small intestinal mucosa leading to malabsorption syndrome.
- Like other autoimmune inflammatory conditions it is thought to be caused by a combination of genetic, immunologic, and environmental factors.
- Symptoms include anorexia; diarrhea and/or constipation; steatorrhea (fatty stools); abdominal pain, distension, and bloating; and weight loss.
- Malnutrition symptoms occur over time when nutrients cannot be absorbed (malabsorption syndrome). Patients may have malnutrition-related muscle weakness, anemia, osteoporosis, PN, infertility, weight loss, fluid retention, and easy bruising.

INTERPROFESIONAL COLLABORATIVE CARE

- Dietary management with a gluten-free diet promotes disease remission.

CHLAMYDIAL INFECTION

OVERVIEW

- *Chlamydial trachomatis* is an intracellular bacterium that causes genital chlamydial infection, which is the most common sexually transmitted disease (STD) in the United States.
- The incubation period ranges from 1 to 3 weeks, but the pathogen may be present in the genital tract for months without producing symptoms. Many infected persons are asymptomatic.

- The main symptom in men is urethritis with dysuria, frequent urination, and a watery, mucoid discharge. Complications include epididymitis, prostatitis, infertility, and reactive arthritis (also known as Reiter syndrome).
- Women may have a mucopurulent cervicitis that occurs with a change in vaginal discharge, easily induced cervical bleeding, urinary frequency, and abdominal discomfort or pain. Complications include salpingitis, PID, ectopic pregnancy, and infertility.
- Chlamydia infections are reportable to the local health department.

INTERPROFESSIONAL COLLABORATIVE CARE

- The primary treatment is antibiotic therapy with azithromycin (Zithromax) or doxycycline; other agents can be used.
- Test and treat sexual partners.
- Educate patients about:
  1. The mode of disease transmission and incubation period
  2. Manifestation, including the possibility of asymptomatic infections
  3. Essential elements of treatment with antibiotic
  4. The need for abstinence from sexual intercourse until the patient and partner have completed treatment
  5. No test of cure is required, but all women should be re-screened 3 to 4 months after treatment because of the high risk for PID if re-infection occurs
  6. The need for the patient and partner to return for evaluation if symptoms recur or new symptoms develop

CHOLECYSTITIS: NUTRITION CONCEPT EXEMPLAR

OVERVIEW

- Cholecystitis is an inflammation of the gallbladder that can occur as an acute or chronic process and results in and alters NUTRITION.
- Acute calculous cholecystitis usually develops in association with cholelithiasis (gallstones). About one-half of the adult population in the United States has asymptomatic gallstones.
  1. Gallstones are composed of substances normally found in bile, such as cholesterol, bilirubin, bile salts, calcium, and various proteins.
  2. Gallstones are classified as either cholesterol stones or pigment stones.
- Acalculous cholecystitis occurs in the absence of gallstones and is associated with biliary stasis caused by any condition that affects the regular filling or emptying of the gallbladder, such as decreased blood flow to the gallbladder, or anatomic problems, such as kinking of the gallbladder neck or cystic duct that can result in pancreatic enzyme reflux into the gallbladder.

- Chronic cholecystitis results when repeated episodes of cystic duct obstruction result in chronic inflammation, and the gallbladder becomes fibrotic and contracted, resulting in decreased motility and deficient absorption.
- Complications of cholecystitis include pancreatitis and cholangitis (inflammation and infection of the common bile ducts).
- Cholangitis is usually associated with choledocholithiasis (common bile duct stones).
- Jaundice (yellow discoloration of body tissues) and icterus (yellow discoloration of the sclera) can occur in acute disease but are most commonly seen in the chronic phase of cholecystitis. Jaundice results from increased bilirubin in the body that collects in the skin and sclera. Itching and a burning sensation result.

INTERPROFESSIONAL COLLABORATIVE CARE
Assessment: Noticing
- Record patient information:
  1. Height and weight, body mass index, and waist circumference
  2. Gender, age, race, and ethnic group
  3. Fatty food intolerances and related GI symptoms, including flatulence, dyspepsia (indigestion), eructation (belching), anorexia, nausea, vomiting, and abdominal pain in relation to fatty food intake
  4. Family history of gallbladder disease
  5. In women, history of estrogen replacement therapy

⚮ Gender Health Considerations: Patient-Centered Care

Women between 20 and 60 years of age are twice as likely to develop gallstones as men. Obesity is a major risk factor for gallstone formation, especially in women. Pregnancy and drugs such as hormone replacements and birth control pills alter hormone levels and delay muscular contraction of the gallbladder, decreasing the rate of bile emptying. The incidence is higher in women who have had multiple pregnancies. Combinations of causative factors increase the incidence of stone formation, especially in women.

- Assess for signs and syptoms:
  1. Abdominal pain of varying intensity in the right upper abdominal quadrant, including radiation to the right upper shoulder; ask the patient to describe the intensity, duration, precipitating factors, and relief measures

! NURSING SAFETY PRIORITY: Critical Rescue

Biliary colic may be so severe that it occurs with tachycardia, pallor, diaphoresis, and prostration (extreme exhaustion). Assess the patient for possible shock caused by biliary colic. Notify the primary health care provider or Rapid Response Team if these symptoms occur. Stay with the patient, and keep the head of the bed flat.

2. Other GI symptoms, including nausea, vomiting, dyspepsia, flatulence, eructation, and feelings of abdominal heaviness, guarding, rigidity, rebound tenderness (Blumberg sign)
3. Late signs and symptoms of chronic cholecystitis:
   a. Jaundice, clay-colored stools, and dark urine
   b. Steatorrhea (fatty stools)
   c. Elevated temperature with tachycardia and dehydration from fever and vomiting
   d. Results of serum liver enzyme and bilirubin tests (may be elevated); amylase (may be elevated if pancreas is involved)
   e. Increased WBC count

Analysis: Interpreting

The priority collaborative problems for patients with cholecystitis include:

1. Weight loss due to decreased intake because of pain, nausea, and inflammation
2. Acute pain due to cholecystitis

Planning and Implementation: Responding

NONSURGICAL MANAGEMENT

Promote nutrition

1. Provide small-volume, low-fat meals
2. Administer fat-soluble vitamins and bile salts
3. Weigh patient to assess for concerning weight loss
4. Monitor nutrition parameters such as blood urea nitrogen (BUN) and serum prealbumin, albumin, and total protein

Manage acute pain

1. Withhold food and oral fluids during nausea and vomiting episodes; to avoid airway compromise, nasogastric (NG) decompression is initiated for severe vomiting.
2. Drug therapy includes:
   a. Opioid analgesics to relieve pain and reduce spasm; all opioids may cause some sphincter of Oddi spasm, worsening pain
   b. Ketorolac (Toradol) may be used for mild-to-moderate pain
   c. Antiemetics to provide relief from nausea and vomiting
   d. Oral bile acid dissolution or gallstone stabilizing agents such as ursodiol (Actigall) and chenodiol (Chenodal) may be given for up to 2 years to dissolve or stabilize gallstones

3. *Extracorporeal shock wave lithotripsy (ESWL)* may be used to break up small stones or for those who are not good surgical candidates.
4. Insertion of a percutaneous transhepatic biliary catheter (drain) using CT or ultrasound guidance to open the blocked duct(s) so that bile can flow (cholecystostomy) may be used.

SURGICAL MANAGEMENT

- Cholecystectomy is the surgical removal of the gallbladder and may be done laparoscopically (minimally invasive surgical approach) or, less often, in a traditional open abdominal approach.
- Preoperative care is similar to other patients having surgery.
- Provide postoperative care for patients with laparoscopic cholecystectomy by:
  1. Promoting nutrition in collaboration with the surgeon and dietitian, generally starting with clear liquids and advancing to solid food within 24 to 48 hours following surgery
  2. Teaching the patient the importance of early ambulation to absorb the carbon dioxide that is retained in the abdomen after a laparoscopic procedure
  3. Inform the patient that shoulder pain is both expected and common; the pain decreases as the gases expanding the abdomen are dissipated.
  4. Inform the patient that he or she can return to usual activities 1 to 3 weeks after the procedure.

! NURSING SAFETY PRIORITY: Action Alert

After a laparoscopic cholecystectomy, assess the patient's oxygen saturation level frequently until the effects of the anesthesia have passed. Remind the patient to perform deep-breathing exercises every hour.

- Use of the open surgical approach (abdominal laparotomy) has greatly declined during the past several decades. Patients who have this type of surgery usually have severe biliary obstruction and the ducts are explored to ensure patency.
- Provide postoperative care for traditional surgery patients:
  1. Postoperative incisional pain after a traditional cholecystectomy is controlled with opioids using a patient-controlled analgesia (PCA) pump.
  2. Advance the diet from clear liquids to solid foods, as tolerated by the patient.
  3. Maintain the patient's surgical drain (Jackson-Pratt drain).
     a. This tube is placed in the gallbladder bed to prevent fluid accumulation. The drainage is usually serosanguineous

(serous fluid mixed with blood) and is stained with bile in the first 24 hours after surgery. Antibiotic therapy is given to prevent infection.

4. Assist the patient with early ambulation.

Care Coordination and Transition Management

- Education needs to be started as soon as a patient has an initial experience with cholecystitis and has been provided with appropriate pain relief.
- Assess the patient's and family's knowledge of the disease and provide teaching as needed.
- The desired outcomes for discharge planning and education are to avoid further episodes of cholecystitis.
- Key teaching points include reminding the patient to avoid fatty, fried, and "fast" foods, and to report any signs of postoperative complications to the primary health care provider immediately.

CHRONIC OBSTRUCTIVE PULMONARY DISEASE: GAS EXCHANGE CONCEPT EXEMPLAR

OVERVIEW

- Chronic obstructive pulmonary disease (COPD) interferes with airflow and GAS EXCHANGE.
- Cigarette smoking is the greatest risk factor for COPD; other contributing factors include chronic exposure to inhaled particles, fuels, and a history of asthma.
- Two common conditions that lead to COPD are emphysema and chronic bronchitis.
- *Emphysema* is a chronic irreversible condition characterized by:
  1. Loss of lung elasticity
  2. Hyperinflation of the lung (air trapping)
- Emphysema is associated with higher-than-normal levels of protease enzymes used to destroy and eliminate inhaled particulate matter. Over time, proteases damage alveoli and small airways. Smoking triggers increase synthesis of proteases.
- Emphysema is classified as panlobular, centrilobular, or paraseptal, depending on the pattern of destruction and dilation of the gas-exchanging units (acini). Each type can occur alone or in combination in the same lung. Most are associated with smoking or chronic exposure to other inhalation irritants.

 Genetic/Genomic Considerations

The gene for alpha-1 antitrypsin (AAT) has many known variations, and some increase the risk for emphysema. Different variations result in different levels of AAT deficiency, which is why the disease is more severe for some adults than for others (OMIM, 2016b). The most serious variation for emphysema risk is the Z mutation, although others also increase the risk but to a lesser degree. Urge patients who have any AAT deficiency to avoid smoking and other environmental pollutants.

- *Bronchitis* is an inflammation of the bronchi and bronchioles characterized by:
  1. Increased number and size of mucous glands in airways that produce large amounts of thick mucus
  2. Thickening of bronchial walls that impairs airflow
- Complications of COPD include hypoxemia, hypercarbia, respiratory infections, heart failure, dysrhythmias, and respiratory failure.
- Respiratory infection can cause an acute exacerbation (worsening) in COPD symptoms.

INTERPROFESSIONAL COLLABORATIVE CARE
Assessment: Noticing
- Obtain and record patient information and history:
  1. Age, occupational history, and family history
  2. Smoking history, including the length of time the patient has smoked and the number of packs smoked daily
  3. Occupational or environmental exposure to lung irritants
  4. History of asthma
  5. Current breathing problems:
     a. Does the patient have difficulty breathing while talking? Can he or she speak in complete sentences, or is it necessary to take a breath between every one or two words?
     b. Ask about the presence, duration, or worsening of wheezing, coughing, and shortness of breath, and what activities trigger these problems.
     c. If the cough is productive, what is the sputum color and amount, and has the amount increased or decreased?
     d. What is the relationship between activity tolerance and dyspnea? How is the patient's activity level and shortness of breath now compared with a month earlier and a year earlier? Is he or she having any difficulty with eating, sleeping, or performing activities of daily living (ADLs)?
  6. How are the patient's weight and general appearance? The patient with severe COPD is thin with loss of muscle mass in the extremities, has enlarged neck muscles and a barrel-shaped chest, and is slow moving and slightly stooped.

- Assess for signs and symptoms
  1. Respiratory changes
     a. Subjective report of dyspnea using a standard approach such as a Visual Analog Dyspnea Scale
     b. Rapid, shallow respirations, paradoxical respirations, or use of accessory muscles
     c. Limited diaphragmatic movement (excursion)
     d. Abnormal lung sounds
     e. Increased anterior-posterior chest diameter
     f. Cough with or without sputum production
  2. Cardiovascular changes
     a. Tachycardia and dysrhythmias
     b. Swelling of feet and ankles
     c. Cyanosis, or blue-tinged, dusky appearance
     d. Clubbing of the fingers
  3. Psychosocial issues
     a. Social isolation due to decreased mobility and energy
     b. Anxiety and fear related to dyspnea that may reduce the patient's ability to participate in a full life
     c. Patient's and family's concerns of their feelings about COPD progression to a life-limiting disorder
     d. Patient's and family's awareness and use of support groups and services
  4. Diagnostic and laboratory tests
     a. Serial arterial blood gas (ABG) values for hypoxemia and hypercarbia
     b. Oxygen saturation by pulse oximetry
     c. Sputum cultures
     d. Hematocrit and hemoglobin to evaluate polycythemia, a compensation for chronic hypoxia
     e. Serum electrolyte levels that support respiratory effort because low phosphate, potassium, calcium, or magnesium levels can reduce (breathing) muscle strength
     f. Serum AAT levels in patients with a family history of COPD
     g. Chest x-ray
     h. Pulmonary function test (PFT)
     i. Peak expiratory flow rates
     j. Carbon monoxide diffusion test

Analysis: Interpreting

- The priority collaborative problems for patients with COPD include:
  1. Decreased gas exchange due to alveolar-capillary membrane changes, reduced airway size, ventilatory muscle fatigue, excessive mucus production, airway obstruction, diaphragm flattening, fatigue, and decreased energy

2. Weight loss due to dyspnea, excessive secretions, anorexia, and fatigue
3. Anxiety due to a change in health status, and situational crisis
4. Decreased endurance due to fatigue, dyspnea, and an imbalance between oxygen supply and demand
5. Potential for pneumonia or other respiratory infections

Planning and Implementation: Responding

IMPROVE GAS EXCHANGE AND REDUCE CARBON DIOXIDE RETENTION

- Most patients with COPD use nonsurgical management to improve or maintain gas exchange.
  - *Nonsurgical Management*
- Maintain a patent airway.
- Assessing breathing rate, rhythm, use of accessory muscles, breath sounds, SpO_2, and dyspnea as part of physical assessment and before and after interventions.
- Position to provide lung expansion with positioning, including Fowler/high backrest elevation.
- Monitoring for changes in respiratory status in the hospitalized patient with COPD at least every 2 hours.
- Determining whether any factors are contributing to increased work of breathing, such as respiratory infection.
- Teaching breathing techniques:
  1. Diaphragmatic or abdominal breathing
  2. Pursed-lip breathing
- Enhancing coughing effectiveness:
  1. Assist the patient to a sitting position with shoulders turned inward, head bent slightly downward, and a pillow hugged to the stomach.
  2. Teach the patient to take a few breaths, exhaling more fully each time, and after three to five breaths take a deeper breath and bend forward slowly while coughing two or three times ("mini-coughs"). Repeat this procedure at least twice.
- Providing oxygen therapy to maintain a peripheral oxygenation (SpO_2) of 88% to 92%.
- Ensuring that there are no open flames or other combustion hazards in rooms where oxygen is in use.
- Suctioning only when needed can remove sputum and mucus.
- Develop intake goals as hydration may thin sticky secretions.
- Vibratory positive expiratory pressure device (a handheld plastic pip and bowl) can help patients remove secretions.
- Vibratory chest vest devices can also help move secretions from distal to proximal airways for removal.
- Drug therapy includes:
  1. Inhaled bronchodilator drugs, such as albuterol (Proventil, Ventolin), ipratropium (Atrovent, Apo-Ipravent♥), tiotropium

(Spiriva), and theophylline (Elixophyllin, Theo-Dur, Uniphyl, Theolair), and many others.

2. Inhaled or systemic corticosteroids to reduce inflammation, such as fluticasone (Flovent) and prednisone (Deltasone ✤, Medrol)

3. Mucolytic drugs, such as acetylcysteine (Mucosil, Mucomyst ✤) or dornase alfa (Pulmozyme)

- Teach patients and family members the correct techniques for using inhalers and how to care for them properly.
- Teach patients about value of exercise conditioning or pulmonary rehabilitation to prevent general and pulmonary muscle deconditioning.
  1. Collaborate with the physical therapist and patient to plan an individualized exercise program.
  2. Remind the patient to perform planned exercises at least two or three times each week.

Surgical Management

- Lung transplantation may be performed for select patients with end-stage COPD.
- Lung reduction surgery can improve gas exchange through removal of the hyperinflated lung tissue areas that are useless for gas exchange.
- Preoperative care includes routine preoperative care described in Part One and:
  1. Pulmonary rehabilitation to maximize lung and muscle function
  2. Testing with pulmonary plethysmography, gas dilution, or perfusion scans to determine the location of greatest lung hyperinflation and poorest lung blood flow
- Postoperative care includes routine postoperative care and:
  1. Close monitoring for respiratory problems
  2. Chest tube management
  3. Maintenance of bronchodilator and mucolytic therapy
  4. Collaboration with the respiratory therapist to administer inhaled drugs and adjust oxygen therapy before activity
- Preventing weight loss.
- Weight loss occurs in patients with COPD as a result of food intolerance, nausea, early satiety, poor appetite, and meal-related dyspnea.
- The increased work of breathing raises calorie and protein needs.
- Malnourished patients lose muscle mass and strength, lung elasticity, and alveolar-capillary surface area that contribute to poor gas exchange.
- Collaborate with the dietician to provide sufficient protein and calories to support the work of breathing.

- Monitor patient weight and other indicators of nutrition, such as skin condition and serum prealbumin levels.
- Manage eating to avoid dyspnea and shortness of breath.
  1. Urge the patient to rest before meals.
  2. Teach the patient to plan the biggest meal of the day for the time when he or she is most hungry and well rested. Four to six small meals each day may be preferred to three larger ones.
  3. Suggest the use of a bronchodilator 30 minutes before the meal.
- Encourage the patient to select food that is appealing, easy to chew, and not gas forming.
  1. Suggest dietary supplements, such as Pulmocare, that provide nutrition with reduced carbon dioxide production.
  2. If early satiety is a problem, advise the patient to minimize drinking fluids before and during meals.

MINIMIZE ANXIETY

- Anxiety can be related to dyspnea, a change in health status, and situational crisis.
- Patients with COPD often have increased anxiety during acute dyspnea episodes, especially if they feel as though they are choking on excessive secretions. Anxiety has been shown to cause dyspnea.
- Help the patient develop a written plan that states exactly what to do if symptoms flare.
- Stress the use of pursed-lip and diaphragmatic breathing techniques during periods of anxiety or panic.
- Recommend professional counseling, if needed, as a positive suggestion. Stress that talking with a counselor can help identify techniques to maintain control over the dyspnea and feelings of panic.
- Explore other approaches to control dyspnea episodes and panic attacks, such as progressive relaxation, hypnosis therapy, and biofeedback.

IMPROVE ACTIVITY TOLERANCE

- Activity intolerance is related to fatigue, dyspnea, and an imbalance between oxygen supply and demand.
- Teach energy conservation techniques to plan and pace activities for maximal tolerance and minimal discomfort.
  1. Work with the patient to develop a personal daily schedule for activities and rest periods.
  2. Teach about the use of adaptive tools for housework, such as long-handled dustpans, sponges, and dusters, to reduce bending and reaching.
  3. Suggest how to organize workspaces so that items used most often are within easy reach.

  4. Teach the patient not to talk when engaged in other activities that require energy, such as walking.
  5. Teach him or her to avoid breath holding while performing any activity.
- Assist with ADLs of eating, bathing, and grooming based on assessment of the patient's needs and fatigue level.
- Assess the patient's response to activity by noting skin color changes, pulse rate and regularity, BP, and work of breathing.
- Suggest the use of supplemental oxygen during periods of high-energy use, such as bathing or walking.

PREVENT RESPIRATORY INFECTION
- Patients with COPD who have excessive secretions or who have artificial airways are at increased risk for respiratory tract infections.
- Teach patients to avoid large crowds and anyone who is ill.
- Stress the importance of receiving a pneumonia vaccination and a yearly influenza vaccination.

Care Coordination and Transition Management
- Coordinate with all members of the health care team to individualize plans for the patient to be discharged to home.
- Determine what equipment and assistance will be needed in the home setting.
- Teach the patient and family about:
  1. The disease and its course
  2. Drug therapy
  3. Manifestations of infection, especially pneumonia
  4. Avoidance of respiratory irritants, including smoking cessation
  5. Nutrition therapy regimen
  6. Stress and anxiety management
  7. Breathing and coughing techniques
  8. Energy conservation measures while maintaining self-care activities
- Collaborate with the care manager and social worker to obtain needed home services:
  1. Oxygen and nebulizer
  2. Hospital-type bed
  3. Home health nurse or aide
  4. Financial assistance
- Provide appropriate referrals, as needed:
  1. Home care visits
  2. Housekeeping assistance and meal preparation
  3. Support groups
  4. Smoking cessation programs

CIRRHOSIS: CELLULAR REGULATION CONCEPT EXEMPLAR

OVERVIEW

- Cirrhosis is characterized by widespread fibrotic (scarred) bands of connective tissue that change the liver's normal makeup and its associated cellular regulation.
- The most common causes for cirrhosis in the United States are chronic alcoholism, chronic viral hepatitis, nonalcoholic steatohepatitis (NASH), bile duct disease, and genetic diseases.
- Cirrhosis of the liver can be divided into several common types, depending on the cause of the disease.
  1. *Postnecrotic cirrhosis* is caused by viral hepatitis, especially hepatitis C, and certain drugs or other toxins.
  2. *Laennec* cirrhosis, or *alcoholic cirrhosis,* is caused by chronic alcoholism.
  3. *Biliary cirrhosis,* also called *cholestatic cirrhosis,* is caused by chronic biliary obstruction or autoimmune disease.
- Complications of cirrhosis include:
  1. *Portal hypertension:* A persistent increase in pressure within the portal vein develops as a result of increased resistance or obstruction to flow. Blood flow backs into the spleen, causing splenomegaly. Veins in the esophagus, stomach, intestines, abdomen, and rectum become dilated. Dilated vessels develop weakened walls, leading to plasma leak and hemorrhage.
  2. *Ascites:* Free fluid accumulates within the peritoneal cavity. Increased hydrostatic pressure from portal hypertension results in venous congestion of the hepatic capillaries, causing plasma to leak directly from the liver surface and portal vein. Other contributing factors include reduced circulating plasma protein and increased hepatic lymphatic formation. Massive ascites can cause abdominal compartment syndrome.
  3. *Gastroesophageal varices:* Thin-walled, distended esophageal veins result from increased portal hypertension. Varices occur most often in the lower esophagus, stomach, and rectum. Fragile varices can rupture, resulting in gastrointestinal bleeding.
  4. *Splenomegaly* (enlarged spleen) results from the pressure of portal hypertension. The enlarged spleen destroys platelets (thrombocytopenia), adding to the increased risk for bleeding.
  5. *Reduced bile production,* preventing the absorption of fat-soluble vitamins and decreased synthesis of clotting factors depending on vitamin K leading to coagulopathy manifested by bruising and bleeding.
  6. *Jaundice* caused by ineffective excretion of bile from hepatic (hepatocellular disease) or bile duct tracts from scarring

(intrahepatic obstruction). Patients with jaundice often report pruritus (itching).

7. *Hepatic encephalopathy* (also called *portal-systemic encephalopathy* [PSE]): This is a complex, neurologic syndrome. It is associated with elevated serum ammonia levels. Early symptoms include sleep disturbance, mood disturbance, mental status changes, and speech problems. Later, altered level of consciousness, impaired thinking processes, and neuromuscular disturbances (e.g., "liver flap") are common symptoms.

8. *Hepatorenal syndrome:* Progressive, oliguric kidney failure is associated with hepatic failure, resulting in functional impairment of kidneys with normal anatomic and morphologic features. It is manifested by a sudden decrease in urinary output and elevated serum urea nitrogen and creatinine levels, with abnormally decreased urine sodium excretion and increased urine osmolality.

9. *Spontaneous bacterial peritonitis* from translocation of bowel bacteria to ascitic fluid.

INTERPROFESSIONAL COLLABORATIVE CARE
Assessment: Noticing
- Document patient information and history:
  1. Age, gender, and race
  2. Employment history, including working conditions exposing the patient to toxins
  3. History of individual and family liver disease
  4. Medical conditions, including viral hepatitis (especially B, C, and D), systemic viral infections, biliary tract disorders, autoimmune disorders, heart failure, respiratory disorders, and liver injury. Blood transfusions and blood borne infections from tattoos may be associated with hepatitis.
  5. Sexual history
  6. History of or present alcohol or substance use

☒ Gender Health Considerations: Patient-Centered Care

The amount of alcohol necessary to cause cirrhosis varies widely from individual to individual, and there are gender differences. In women, it may take as few as two or three drinks per day over a minimum of 10 years. In men, perhaps six drinks per day over the same time period may be needed to cause disease. However, a smaller amount of alcohol over a long period of time can increase memory loss from alcohol toxicity of the cerebral cortex. Binge drinking can increase risk for hepatitis and fatty liver.

- Because cirrhosis has a slow onset, many of the *early* signs and symptoms are vague and nonspecific. Assess for:
  1. Generalized weakness, fatigue
  2. Weight changes (loss or gain)
  3. GI symptoms, such as anorexia and vomiting
  4. Abdominal distension, pain, or tenderness
  5. Jaundice of the skin and sclera
  6. Dry skin, rashes, or pruritus
  7. Petechiae and bruising or excessive bleeding from minor injury
  8. Palmar erythema
  9. Spider angiomas on the nose, cheeks, upper thorax, and shoulders
  10. Hepatomegaly palpated in the right upper quadrant, confirmed by palpation, ultrasound, or radiographic imaging
  11. Ascites revealed by bulging flanks and dullness on percussion of the abdomen
  12. Protruding umbilicus
  13. Hematemesis or melena
  14. Fetor hepaticus (the fruity, musty breath odor of chronic liver disease)
  15. Amenorrhea in women
  16. Testicular atrophy, gynecomastia, and impotence in men
  17. Changes in mentation and personality
  18. Asterixis (a coarse tremor characterized by rapid, nonrhythmic extension and flexion in the wrist and fingers)
  19. Elevated serum liver enzymes (aspartate aminotransferase [AST], alanine aminotransferase [ALT], and lactate dehydrogenase [LDH]), biliary biomarkers (alkaline phosphatase, gamma-glutamyl transpeptidase [GGT]), and serum bilirubin levels
  20. Decreased hemoglobin, total serum protein, and albumin levels
  21. Positive hepatitis A, B, C, or D panel
  22. Altered coagulation factors, prolonged bleeding times
  23. Elevated serum ammonia level
  24. Ultrasound, followed by CT or MRI to determine the hepatomegaly or the cause of cirrhosis
  25. Esophagogastroduodenoscopy (EGD) to visualize the upper GI tract and detect complications of cirrhosis

Analysis: Interpreting
- The priority collaborative problems for patients with cirrhosis include:
  1. Fluid overload due to third spacing of abdominal and peripheral fluid

2. Potential for hemorrhage due to portal hypertension
3. Potential for hepatic encephalopathy due to shunting of portal venous blood and/or increased serum ammonia levels

Planning and Implementation

- The goals of care are to manage the underlying cause of hepatitis (infection, alcohol abuse) and reduce complications of impaired CELLULAR REGULATION leading to excess fluid volume, bleeding, and hepatic encephalopathy.

MANAGE FLUID VOLUME

- Monitor respiratory status to avoid complications from pulmonary edema.
    1. Monitor Spo_2 with vital signs.
    2. Elevate the head of the bed to minimize shortness of breath and position for comfort.
- Provide nutrition therapy
    1. Provide a low-sodium diet initially, restricting sodium to 1 to 2 g/day.
    2. Suggest alternatives to salt, such as lemon, vinegar, parsley, oregano, and pepper.
    3. Collaborate with the dietitian to explain the purpose of diet and meal planning; suggest elimination of table salt, salty foods, canned and frozen vegetables, and salted butter and margarine.
    4. Supplement vitamin intake with thiamine, folate, and multivitamin preparations.
    5. Record the patient's daily weight.
- Provide drug therapy
    1. Give diuretics to reduce intravascular fluid and to prevent cardiac and respiratory impairment.
    2. Monitor intake and output carefully with daily weight.
    3. Monitor serum electrolytes.
- Paracentesis may be indicated if dietary restrictions and drug administration fail to control ascites.
    1. Explain the procedure and verify informed consent obtained.
    2. Obtain vital signs and weight, and check allergies.
    3. Assist the patient to an upright position at the side of the bed.
    4. Monitor vital signs every 15 minutes during the procedure; rapid, drastic removal of ascitic fluid leads to decreased abdominal pressure, which may contribute to vasodilation and shock.
    5. Measure and record drainage; send samples to laboratory if ordered.
    6. Position the patient in a semi-Fowler's position in bed, and maintain bed rest until vital signs are stable.
    7. Assess the patient's lung sounds.

PREVENT OR MANAGE HEMORRHAGE

- All patients with cirrhosis should be screened for esophageal varices by endoscopy to detect them early *before they bleed.* If patients have varices, they are placed on preventive therapy. If acute bleeding occurs, early interventions are used to manage it. *Because massive esophageal bleeding can cause rapid blood loss, emergency interventions are needed.*
  1. Prevent hypertension by determining systemic and mean arterial BP goals. Decreasing systemic BP reduces hepatic pressures and portal vessel leak.
  2. Institute frequent monitoring and communicate observations about bleeding immediately to the provider. Coagulopathy and high BP can place the patient at significant risk for hemorrhage.
  3. Provide protection from gastric acid-related damage with a proton pump inhibitor or H_2 histamine blocker.
  4. Support the patient during endoscopic therapy to reduce bleeding from varicies.
     a. Endoscopic variceal banding decreases the blood supply to the varicies.
     b. Endoscopic sclerotherapy allows varicies to be injected with a sclerosing agent to decrease bleeding.
     c. Vasoconstrictive drug therapy with octreotide (Sandostatin) or vasopressin are used emergently to decrease bleeding.
  5. Initiate rescue therapy with esophagogastric balloon tamponade to compress bleeding vessels.
     a. The large esophageal balloon compresses the esophagus; a smaller gastric balloon helps anchor the tube and exerts pressure against bleeding varices at the distal esophagus and the stomach. A third lumen terminates in the stomach and is connected to suction, allowing the aspiration of gastric contents and blood.
     b. Keep tube taped and secure and place scissors at the bedside for emergent situations from a migrating tamponade tube blocking the airway.
     c. Monitor the patient for respiratory distress caused by obstruction from the esophageal balloon or aspiration; if distress occurs, cut both balloon ports to allow for rapid balloon deflation and tube removal.
  6. Provide procedural-related care:.
     a. An ERCP uses the endoscope to inject contrast material via the sphincter of Oddi to view the biliary tract and allow for stone removals, sphincterotomies, biopsies, and stent placements if required.
     b. EGD is used to directly visualize the upper GI tract and to detect the presence of bleeding or oozing esophageal varices,

stomach irritation and ulceration, or duodenal ulceration and bleeding. EGD is performed by introducing a flexible fiberoptic endoscope into the mouth, esophagus, and stomach while the patient is under moderate sedation. A camera attached to the scope permits direct visualization of the mucosal lining of the upper GI tract.

   c. *Transjugular intrahepatic portal-systemic shunting (TIPS)* is a nonsurgical procedure whereby the physician implants a shunt between the portal vein and the hepatic vein to reduce portal venous pressure and control bleeding.

7. Administer blood products (red blood cells [RBCs] and fresh-frozen plasma) and IV fluids to sustain circulation and perfusion during episodes of bleeding.

8. Give vasopressin to promote coagulation.

! NURSING SAFETY PRIORITY: Action Alert

Avoid placing or manipulating the nasogastric or orogastric tube in a patient who is at high risk for or diagnosed with esophageal varices because tube movement can injure a fragile, dilated vessel, causing it to rupture and bleed.

PREVENT OR MANAGE HEPATIC ENCEPHALOPATHY

• Provide a safe environment

1. Altered mentation places the patient at risk for falls, aspiration, and pressure ulcer formation from prolonged immobility. Institutional interventions should be put in place to avoid these adverse events.

2. Administer lactulose to promote fecal excretion of ammonia.

3. Administer a nonabsorbable oral antibiotic to destroy bowel flora and diminish protein breakdown and ammonia formation.

• Provide nutrition therapy

1. Patients with chronic cirrhosis have altered nutritional requirements for vitamins, minerals, carbohydrates, and protein; collaborate with the dietitian and gastroenterologist or hepatologist to set dietary goals and identify restrictions.

2. Patients with acute cirrhosis or encephalopathy have protein intake limited in the diet to reduce intestinal bacteria formation of ammonia.

3. Be aware of decreased metabolism of many drugs, especially opioids, sedatives, and other central nervous system (CNS) agents due to impaired liver cell functions.

Care Coordination and Transition Management

• Health teaching is individualized for the patient, depending on the cause of the disease.

- Identify if the patient needs a family member or friend to help with drugs, or needs a home health care nurse or aide.
- Teach the patient and family to:
  1. Follow the prescribed diet.
  2. Restrict sodium intake if ascites occur.
  3. Obtain and record daily weights and report increase of 5 pounds or more over any 3-day period.
  4. Restrict protein intake if the patient is susceptible to encephalopathy.
  5. Take diuretics as prescribed, report symptoms of hypokalemia, and consume foods high in potassium.
  6. Take H_2 receptor antagonist agent or proton pump inhibitor.
  7. Avoid all nonprescription drugs.
  8. Avoid alcohol (refer to Alcoholics Anonymous if patient is addicted to alcohol).
  9. Recognize signs and symptoms of PSE.
  10. Notify the patient's health care provider immediately in case of GI bleeding or PSE.
  11. Keep follow-up visits with the physicians.
  12. Address end-of-life concerns with patients who experience progressive cirrhotic disease; include preferences and values about transplantation in this discussion.

✴ COLITIS, ULCERATIVE: ELIMINATION CONCEPT EXEMPLAR

OVERVIEW

- Ulcerative colitis (UC) creates widespread inflammation of the rectum and rectosigmoid colon but can extend to the entire colon, affecting ELIMINATION.
- UC is characterized by hyperemic intestinal mucosa (increased blood flow) with resultant edema. In more severe inflammation, the lining can bleed and small ulcers occur.
- Abscesses can form in ulcerative areas and result in tissue necrosis, perforation, and peritonitis.
- Edema and mucosal thickening can lead to a narrowed colon and bowel obstruction.
- Complications of the disease include fistula formation, toxic megacolon, hemorrhage, increased risk for colon cancer, and malabsorption.
- Extraintestinal clinical manifestations include polyarthritis, oral and skin lesions, iritis, and hepatic and biliary disease.
- The patient's stool typically contains blood and mucus. Patients report tenesmus (an unpleasant and urgent sensation to defecate) and lower abdominal colicky pain relieved with defecation.

Malaise, anorexia, anemia, dehydration, fever, and weight loss are common.

INTERPROFESSIONAL COLLABORATIVE CARE
Assessment: Noticing
- Document patient information and history:
  1. Family history of inflammatory bowel disease
  2. Previous and current therapy for illnesses, including surgeries
  3. Diet history, including usual patterns and intolerances of food
  4. History of weight changes
  5. Presence of abdominal pain, cramping, urgency, and diarrhea
  6. Bowel elimination patterns; color, consistency, and character of stools; and the presence or absence of blood
  7. Relationship between the occurrence of diarrhea and the timing of meals, pain, emotional distress, and activity
  8. Extraintestinal symptoms such as arthritis, mouth sores, vision problems, and skin disorders
- Assess signs and symptoms:
  1. Abdominal cramping, pain, and distention
  2. Bloody diarrhea, tenesmus
  3. Fever, tachycardia
  4. Patient's understanding of the disease process
  5. Psychosocial impact of the disease; the inability to control symptoms, especially diarrhea, can be disruptive and stress producing
  6. Abnormal laboratory values: hematocrit, hemoglobin, WBC count, erythrocyte sedimentation rate, C-reactive protein, and electrolytes
  7. Results from most recent colonoscopy or magnetic resonance enterography

Analysis: Interpreting
- The priority collaborative problems for patients with ulcerative colitis include:
  1. Diarrhea due to inflammation of the bowel mucosa
  2. Acute pain or chronic non-cancer pain due to inflammation and ulceration of the bowel mucosa and skin irritation
  3. Potential for lower GI bleeding and resulting anemia due to UC

Planning and Implementation: Responding
- Management of UC is aimed at relieving the symptoms and reducing intestinal motility, decreasing inflammation, and promoting intestinal healing.

DECREASE DIARRHEA
Nonsurgical Management
  1. Record patient responses to interventions, noting changes in the color, volume, frequency, and consistency of stools.

2. Monitor the skin in the perianal area for irritation and ulceration resulting from loose, frequent stools.
3. Monitor immune function and results of stool or other cultures.

- Drug therapy
  1. Aminosalicylates are used to reduce inflammation.
  2. Corticosteroids (also called glucocorticoids) are used during exacerbations of the illness.
  3. Antidiarrheal drugs are given to provide symptomatic management of diarrhea; they are given cautiously because they can precipitate colonic dilation and toxic megacolon.
  4. Immunomodulators to alter (modulate) the immune response are most effective when given with corticosteroids. Examples include infliximab (Remicade) and adalimumab (Humira).
- Nutrition therapy may include:
  1. NPO status with total parenteral nutrition (TPN) for the patient with severe symptoms
  2. Elemental formulas, which are absorbed in the small intestine, minimizing bowel stimulation
  3. Avoiding caffeine, alcohol, or foods that cause symptoms
- Ensure that the patient has easy access to the bedside commode or bathroom.
- Explore psychosocial concerns such as body image, fear, and anxiety.
- Complementary and alternative therapies may include flaxseed, selenium, vitamin C, biofeedback, yoga, acupuncture, and Ayurveda (combination of diet, herbs, and breathing exercises).

Surgical Management
- The need for surgery is based on the patient's response to medical interventions.
- Surgical procedures include:
  1. A temporary or permanent *ileostomy*
     a. An ileostomy is a procedure in which a loop of the ileum is placed through an opening in the abdominal wall (stoma) for drainage of fecal material.
     b. Initial output from the ileostomy is a loose, dark green liquid; over time, the volume decreases, becomes thicker, and turns yellow-green or yellow-brown.
     c. A foul or unpleasant odor may be a symptom of some underlying problem (blockage or infection).
  2. Restorative proctocolectomy with ileo pouch–anal anastomosis (RPC-IPAA) has become the gold standard for patients with UC. This a two-stage procedure.
     a. First the surgeon removes the colon and most of the rectum, leaving the anus and anal sphincter remain intact. The surgeon creates an internal pouch (reservoir) using a portion of

the small intestine. The pouch, sometimes called a *J-pouch,* *S-pouch,* or *pelvic pouch,* is then connected to the anus. A temporary ileostomy through the abdominal skin is created to allow healing of the internal pouch.
  b. In the *second* surgical stage, the loop ileostomy is closed and elimination returns through the anus.

❗ NURSING SAFETY PRIORITY: Critical Rescue

The ileostomy stoma is usually placed in the right lower quadrant of the abdomen below the belt line. It should not be prolapsed or retract into the abdominal wall. Assess the stoma frequently. It should be pinkish to cherry red to ensure an adequate blood supply. *If the stoma looks pale, bluish, or dark, report these findings to the health care provider immediately.*

MINIMIZE PAIN
- Assess the patient for changes in pain intensity that may indicate disease or surgical complications, such as increased inflammation, obstruction, hemorrhage, or peritonitis.
- Assess for pain, including its character, pattern of occurrence (e.g., before or after meals, during the night, before or after bowel movements), and duration.
- Assist the patient to reduce or eliminate factors that increase the pain.
- Take measures to relieve irritated skin caused by contact with diarrheal stool or ileostomy drainage.
- Assist the patient to use other pain relief measures such as biofeedback and music therapy.

MONITOR FOR LOWER GASTROINTESTINAL BLEEDING
- Monitor the patient for bright red or black and tarry stools and symptoms of GI bleeding.
- Notify the health care provider immediately of GI bleeding because blood transfusion or surgical interventions may be necessary.

❗ NURSING SAFETY PRIORITY: Critical Rescue

Recognize that it is important to monitor stools for blood loss for the patient with UC. The blood may be bright red (frank bleeding) or black and tarry (melena). Monitor hematocrit, hemoglobin, and electrolyte values, and assess vital signs. Prolonged slow bleeding can lead to anemia. Observe for fever, tachycardia, and signs of fluid volume depletion. Changes in mental status may occur, especially among older adults, and may be the first indication of dehydration or anemia.

If symptoms of GI bleeding begin, respond by notifying the health care provider immediately. Blood products are often prescribed for patients with severe anemia. Prepare for the blood transfusion by inserting a large-bore IV catheter if it is not already in place.

Care Coordination and Transition Management
- Health teaching includes the following:
  1. Provide information on the nature of the disease, including acute episodes, remissions, and symptom management
  2. Self-management strategies to reduce or control pain, promote adequate nutrition, manage clinical manifestations, and monitor for complications
  3. Provide additional information for the patient with an ostomy regarding:
     a. Ostomy or pouch care
     b. Skin care, including anal and peristomal skin
     c. Special issues related to drugs (e.g., to avoid taking enteric-coated drugs and capsule drugs); the patient should inform health care providers and the pharmacist that he or she has an ostomy
     d. Symptoms indicating a need to contact the provider such as increased or no drainage, stomal swelling, or discoloration of the stoma
     e. Activity limitations, including avoidance of heavy lifting
     f. The importance of adequate fluid intake, especially during periods of high ostomy output
- Refer the patient to home health care ostomy or outpatient clinics.
- Refer the patient to support groups for ostomy recipients and organizations that provide education and support for individuals with inflammatory bowel disease.

COMPARTMENT SYNDROME

OVERVIEW
- Compartment syndrome occurs when tissue pressure within a confined body space becomes elevated and restricts blood flow.
  1. Compartments are areas in the body where muscles, blood vessels, and nerves are contained within fascia.
  2. Fascia is an inelastic tissue that surrounds groups of muscles, blood vessels, and nerves in the body.
- It is usually a complication of musculoskeletal trauma in the lower leg and forearm, but it can be seen with severe burns, extensive insect bites, acute arterial occlusion (thrombosis or embolism), massive infiltration of IV fluids, and with abdominal swelling (ascites).

- Pressure to the compartment can also occur from an external source, such as tight, bulky dressings and casts.
- If the condition is not treated, cyanosis, tingling, numbness, pain, paresis, and permanent tissue damage can occur.
- Complications of compartment syndrome can include infection, persistent motor weakness in the affected extremity, contracture, and myoglobinuric renal failure.
- In extreme cases, amputation or opening the abdomen becomes necessary.

INTERPROFESSIONAL COLLABORATIVE CARE

- Nursing care includes:
  1. Identifying patients who may be at risk
  2. Monitoring for early signs of compartment syndrome by assessing for the "six Ps" of ischemia:
     a. Pain
     b. Pressure
     c. Paralysis
     d. Paresthesia
     e. Pallor
     f. Pulselessness
  3. Invasive monitoring of compartment pressure in patients at especially high risk for compartment syndrome using a hand-held device with a digital display or a pressure monitor such as that used for abdominal compartment syndrome evaluation
  4. When external conditions are causing the syndrome, implementing interventions to relieve the pressure:
     a. Loosening dressings or tape
     b. Following agency protocol about cutting a tight cast

! NURSING SAFETY PRIORITY: Critical Rescue

When manifestations indicate compartment syndrome, notify the surgeon immediately because irreversible damage can occur within a few hours.

- Surgical intervention is a fasciotomy (opening in the fascia) made by incising through the skin and subcutaneous tissues into the fascia of the affected compartment to relieve the pressure and restore circulation to the affected area.
- After fasciotomy, the open wound is packed and dressed on a regular basis until swelling resolves.
- Débridement and skin grafting may be required to manage or close the fasciotomy.

CORNEAL ABRASION, INFECTION, AND ULCERATION
OVERVIEW

* A *corneal abrasion* is a painful scrape or scratch of the cornea that disrupts the integrity of this structure, most commonly caused by the presence of a small foreign body, trauma, and contact lens use.
* The abrasion provides a portal of entry for organisms, leading to *corneal infection.*
* *Corneal ulceration* is a deeper disruption of the corneal epithelium, often occurring with bacterial, fungal, or viral infection. *This problem is an emergency and can lead to permanently impaired vision.*

INTERPROFESSIONAL COLLABORATIVE CARE

* Assess for these problems in the affected eye:
  1. Pain
  2. Reduced vision
  3. Photophobia
  4. Eye secretions with cloudy or purulent fluid on eyelids or eyelashes
  5. Hazy, cloudy cornea with a patchy area of ulceration
  6. Damaged areas appear green with fluorescein stain
* Drug therapy delivered as eye drops
  1. Antibiotics, antifungals, and antivirals are prescribed to reduce or eliminate the organisms. Usually, a broad-spectrum antibiotic is prescribed first, and it may be changed when culture results are known.
  2. Usually the anti-infective therapy involves instilling eye drops every hour for the first 24 hours.
  3. Corticosteroids may be used with antibiotics to reduce the inflammatory response in the eye.
  4. Anesthetic drops can be used to decrease pain.
* Educate the patient for self-management
  1. Teach the patient how to apply the eye drops correctly.
  2. Teach the patient to wash hands after touching the affected eye.
  3. If both eyes are infected, separate bottles of antibiotics are prescribed; label each bottle right or left and treat each eye separately, washing hands between care for each eye.
  4. Teach the patient to not wear contact lenses during the entire time that these drugs are being used.

❗ NURSING SAFETY PRIORITY: Action Alert

Stress the importance of applying the drug as often as prescribed, even at night, and to complete the entire course of antibiotic therapy. Stopping the infection at this stage can save the vision in the infected eye. Instruct the patient to make and keep all follow-up appointments; usually the patient is seen again in 24 hours or less.

CORNEAL OPACITIES AND KERATOCONUS
OVERVIEW
- The cornea can permanently lose its shape, become scarred or cloudy, or become thinner, reducing useful visual sensory perception.
- *Keratoconus* is the degeneration of the corneal tissue resulting in an abnormal corneal shape that can occur with trauma or may occur as part of an inherited disorder.

INTERPROFESSIONAL COLLABORATIVE CARE
- *Keratoplasty* is the surgical removal of diseased corneal tissue and replacement with tissue from a human donor cornea (corneal transplant). For a misshaped cornea that is still clear, surgical management involves a corneal implant that adjusts the shape of the cornea.
- Provide preoperative care as outlined in Part One and:
  1. Assess the patient's knowledge of the surgery and of expected care before and after surgery
  2. Inform the patient that local anesthesia commonly is used
- Provide postoperative care and:
  1. Maintain the eye protective shield and dressing care as prescribed by the surgeon.
  2. Educate the patient or caregiver about eye drop instillation, typically antibiotics.
  3. Teach the patient and caregiver to examine the eye daily for the presence of infection, graft rejection, and reduced visual acuity.
     a. Report immediately to the surgeon the presence of purulent discharge, a continuous leak of clear fluid from around the graft site (not tears), or excessive bleeding.
  4. Instruct the patient to avoid activities that promote rapid or jerky head motions or increase intraocular pressure for several weeks after surgery.

CORONARY ARTERY DISEASE
See Acute Coronary Syndrome

CROHN'S DISEASE
OVERVIEW
- Crohn's disease is a chronic inflammatory disease of the small intestine (most often), colon, or both segments of the GI tract.

- "Skip lesions" with thickened intestinal walls, alternating with healthy tissue, can result in deep fissures and ulcerations predisposing the patient to development of bowel fistulas.
- Narrowing of the bowel lumen (strictures) contributes to GI symptoms and complications.
- Complications of Crohn's disease include malabsorption, fistulas, hemorrhage, abscess formation, and intestinal obstruction. Severe malnutrition and debilitation over time can occur with reduced intestinal absorption of nutrients.

INTERPROFESSIONAL COLLABORATIVE CARE

- Assess for:
  1. Abdominal pain, distension, or masses
  2. Frequency and consistency of stools; presence of blood or fat (steatorrhea) in the stool
  3. Weight loss (indicates serious nutritional deficiencies)
  4. Diet history or nutritional intake
  5. Family history of the disease
  6. Distention, masses, or visible peristalsis
  7. Ulcerations or fissures of the perianal area
  8. Bowel sounds may be diminished or absent in the presence of severe inflammation; high-pitched over narrowed bowel loops
  9. Results of diagnostic imaging tests that show narrowing, ulcerations, strictures, and fistulas consistent with Crohn's disease
  10. Results of laboratory studies, especially CBC and electrolytes
      a. Low hemoglobin and hematocrit (anemia) may indicate GI bleeding, malnutrition, or both.
      b. Elevated WBC levels may indicate exacerbation or complications (fistula formation, perforation, or peritonitis).

! NURSING SAFETY PRIORITY: Action Alert

For the patient with Crohn's disease, be especially alert for manifestations of peritonitis, hemorrhage, intestinal obstruction, nutritional deficits, and fluid imbalances. Early detection of a change in the patient's status helps reduce these potentially life-threatening complications.

- The care of the patient with Crohn's disease is similar to care for the patient with UC (*see Colitis, Ulcerative*).

! NURSING SAFETY PRIORITY: Action Alert

Adequate nutrition and fluid and electrolyte balance are priorities in the care of the patient with a fistula. GI secretions are high in volume and rich in electrolytes and enzymes. The patient is at high risk for malnutrition, dehydration, and electrolyte imbalance, particularly hypokalemia. Assess for these conditions and collaborate with the health care team to manage them. Decreases in urinary output and daily weights indicate possible dehydration and thus should be monitored.

- Malnutrition can result in poor fistula and wound healing, loss of lean muscle mass, decreased immune system response, and increased morbidity and mortality.
  1. Consult with the dietitian to individualize diet and monitor tolerance to nutritional intake.
  2. Assist the patient to select high-caloric, high protein, high-vitamin, low-fiber meals.
  3. Offer oral supplements such as Ensure and Vivonex.
  4. Record food intake and accurate calorie count.
  5. TPN may be needed for severe exacerbations while the patient is NPO.
- Electrolyte therapy includes:
  1. Fluid and electrolyte replacement by oral liquids and nutrients, as well as IV fluids
  2. Cautious use of antidiarrheal agents to decrease fluid loss
  3. Monitoring of intake, output, and daily weights
- Impaired skin integrity results from fistula formation. The degree of associated problems is related to the location of the fistula, the patient's general health status, and the character and amount of fistula drainage.
  1. In collaboration with the wound enterostomal therapist, apply a pouch or drain to the fistula to prevent skin irritation and to measure the drainage. Negative pressure wound therapy may promote healing when the fistula is large.
  2. Provide skin barriers to prevent skin irritation and excoriation.
  3. Protect the adjacent skin and keep it clean and dry.
  4. Observe for subtle signs of infection or sepsis such as fever, abdominal pain, or change in mental status.
- Some patients with Crohn's disease require surgery such as a bowel resection and anastomosis with or without a colon resection to improve the quality of life.
- Strictureplasty may be performed for bowel strictures.

CYSTIC FIBROSIS

OVERVIEW

- Cystic fibrosis (CF) is a genetic disease that affects many organs and lethally impairs lung function.
- The underlying problem of CF is blocked chloride transport in cell membranes, causing the formation of thick and sticky mucus.

- This mucus plugs up glands in the lungs, pancreas, liver, salivary glands, and testes, causing atrophy and organ dysfunction.
- Nonpulmonary problems include pancreatic insufficiency with malnutrition and intestinal obstruction, poor growth, male sterility, diabetes, and cirrhosis of the liver.
- The primary cause of death in the patient with CF is respiratory failure.
- The disorder is most common among white individuals, and about 4% are carriers. It is very rare among African Americans or Asians. Males and females are affected equally.

Genetic/Genomic Consideration

Interprofessional Care

CF is an autosomal recessive disorder in which both gene alleles must be mutated for the disease to be expressed. The CF gene (CTFR cystic fibrosis transmembrane conductance regulator) produces a protein that controls chloride movement across cell membranes. The severity of CF varies greatly; however, life expectancy is always considerably reduced, with an average of 40 years. Adults with one mutated allele are carriers and have few or no symptoms of CF but can pass the abnormal allele on to their children. More than 1700 different mutations have been identified. The inheritance of different mutations is responsible for variation in disease severity. Help patients understand why their symptoms may be more or less severe than others with the disease, even within the same family.

INTERPROFESSIONAL COLLABORATIVE CARE

- The major diagnostic test is sweat chloride analysis, and additional genetic testing can be performed to determine which specific mutation a person may have.
- Assess for these nonpulmonary manifestations: abdominal distention, gastroesophageal reflux, rectal prolapse, foul-smelling stools, steatorrhea (excessive fat in stools), small stature, and underweight for height.
- Assess for these common pulmonary manifestations: frequent or chronic respiratory infections, chest congestion, limited exercise tolerance, cough, sputum production, use of accessory muscles, and decreased pulmonary function (especially forced vital capacity and forced exhalation volume over 1 second [FEV_1]).

Interventions

- Nutrition management focuses on weight maintenance, vitamin supplementation, diabetes management, and pancreatic enzyme replacement (enzymes must be taken with food).

- Pulmonary management is focused on preventive maintenance and management of pulmonary exacerbation.
  1. Preventive or maintenance therapy involves the use of a regimen of chest physiotherapy, positive expiratory pressure, active cycle breathing technique, and an individualized regular exercise program. Drug therapy includes bronchodilators, anti-inflammatory agents, mucolytics, and antibiotics.
  2. Exacerbation therapy is needed when the patient with CF has a change in manifestations from baseline. Management focuses on mucus clearance, oxygenation, and, if infection is present, antibiotic therapy. Additional therapies are:
     a. Heliox delivery of 70% oxygen and 30% helium
     b. Airway clearance techniques (ACTs) four times each day
     c. Intensified bronchodilator and mucolytic therapies, corticosteroids
  3. *Gene therapy* for CF is available for use in patients with specific gene mutations. These drugs target the CFR channel so the transporter can move chloride across the cell membrane, reducing sodium and fluid absorption so that mucus is less thick and sticky.
     a. The drug ivacaftor (Kalydeco) has been found to be of value to patients with CF who have specific mutations in the *CFTR* gene.
     b. The combination drug lumacaftor/ivacaftor (Orkami) is effective for patients whose CF is caused by the F508del mutation, the most common mutation involved in CF.
  4. Teach patients about protecting themselves by avoiding direct contact of bodily fluids such as saliva and sputum. Teach them not to routinely shake hands or kiss people in social settings. Hand washing is critical because the organism also can be acquired indirectly from contaminated surfaces such as sinks and tissues.
- The surgical management of the patient with CF involves lung transplantation.
  1. Anti-rejection drug regimens must be started immediately after surgery. The drugs generally are used long-term to prevent rejection after organ transplantation. Anti-rejection drugs are immunosuppressive and increase the risk for serious infection.

CYSTITIS (URINARY TRACT INFECTION)
OVERVIEW
- *Cystitis* is an inflammation or infection of the urinary bladder.
- Infectious causes are bacteria, viruses, fungi, and parasites.
  1. Cystitis with infection is a "urinary tract infection"(UTI).
     a. A UTI is further categorized as *uncomplicated* or *complicated*.

(1) Uncomplicated UTI is an acute invasion of pathogenic microbes (typically *Escherichia coli*) and can be treated without concern for pre-existing conditions or anatomic complexity.

(2) Complicated UTI is characterized by an anatomic or functional abnormality of the urinary tract or a condition that increases the risk for treatment failure (i.e., unresolved infection after treatment) such as the presence of a multidrug resistant organism (MDRO), pregnancy, male gender, obstruction, diabetes, neurogenic bladder, urologic disease, chronic kidney disease, and immunosuppression.

- Noninfectious inflammation causes include chemical exposure, radiation therapy, and immunologic responses in chronic inflammatory disease.
  1. *Interstitial cystitis* is a chronic inflammation of the lower urinary tract (bladder, urethra, and adjacent pelvic muscles).
  2. Cystitis may sometimes occur as a complication of other disorders, such as gynecologic cancers, PIDs, endometriosis, Crohn's disease, diverticulitis, lupus, or tuberculosis.

Teamwork and Collaboration: Informatics

The urinary tract is the infection source of severe sepsis or septic shock in about 10% to 30% of cases. The spread of the infection from the urinary tract to the bloodstream is termed bacteremia or **urosepsis**. Urosepsis is associated with a mortality rate of 30% Timely reporting of abnormal CBC results (especially an elevated WBC count), abnormal urinalysis results (especially positive nitrogen and leukocyte esterase), and positive urine culture reports are essential to initiating and evaluating effective antibiotic treatment.

INTERPROFESSIONAL COLLABORATIVE CARE
Assessment: Noticing
- Assess for:
  1. Increased frequency or urgency in voiding
  2. Urgency and pain or discomfort on urination
  3. Change in urine color, clarity, or odor; presence of pus (WBCs) or blood (RBCs)
  4. Presence of nitrogen or leukocyte esterase with urinalysis
  5. Positive urine culture
  6. Elevated plasma WBCs
  7. Abdominal or back pain
  8. Bladder distention
  9. Feelings of incomplete bladder emptying

10. Voiding in small amounts or inability to urinate
11. Difficulty in initiating urination
12. Urinary meatus inflammation
13. Prostate gland changes or tenderness

Considerations for Older Adults

- The symptoms of UTI may be as vague as increasing mental confusion or unexplained falls.
- Sudden onset of or worsening of incontinence may be an early symptom.
- Fever, tachycardia, tachypnea, and hypotension even without any urinary symptoms may be signs of urosepsis.
- Loss of appetite, nocturia, and dysuria are common symptoms.

Interventions: Responding
- Drug therapy includes:
  1. Antibiotics: In uncomplicated UTIs (also called acute bacterial cystitis), a 3-day course of oral antibiotic treatment is recommended. A 7- to 14-day course of oral or parenteral antibiotics may be needed for complicated UTIs and for urosepsis.
  2. Analgesics or antipyretics may be used to promote comfort.
  3. Antispasmodics may be used to decrease bladder spasm and promote complete bladder emptying in certain chronic conditions or with recurrent UTI.
  4. Antifungal agents such as amphotericin B in daily bladder instillations and ketoconazole (Nizoral) in oral form may be used if the infecting microbe is fungal.
- Diet therapy includes:
  1. Ensure sufficient fluid intake to maintain clear or light yellow urine (2.2 to 3 L/day), unless contraindicated in a chronic condition.
  2. Cranberry juice or tablets taken daily may reduce the frequency of recurrent UTIs but should be avoided with interstitial cystitis.
- Other therapy includes providing warm sitz baths to relieve perineal discomfort.
- Surgical interventions for management of noninfectious cystitis include urologic procedures for structural abnormalities or endourologic procedures to manipulate or pulverize kidney stones if these conditions are associated with cystitis.
- Teach the patient to:
  1. Self-administer drugs and complete all of the prescribed antibiotic or antimicrobial agent.

2. Expect changes in color of urine with some treatments.
3. Use appropriate techniques to prevent discomfort with sexual activities and how to prevent postcoital infections.
4. Consume liberal fluid intake to maintain urine color as clear or light yellow.
5. Clean the perineum after urination.
6. Empty the bladder as soon as the urge is felt.
7. Avoid known irritants such as caffeine, carbonated beverages, tomato products, chemicals in bath water (e.g., bubble baths), vaginal washes, and scented toilet tissue.
8. Seek prompt medical care if symptoms recur.
- Pregnant women with cystitis require prompt and aggressive antibiotic treatment because this infection can lead to preterm labor and premature birth.

CYSTOCELE

OVERVIEW

- A cystocele is a protrusion of the bladder through the vaginal wall resulting from weakened pelvic structures.
- Causes include obesity, advanced age, childbearing, or genetic predisposition.

INTERPROFESSIONAL COLLABORATIVE CARE

- Assess for:
  1. Difficulty in emptying the bladder
  2. Urinary frequency and urgency or other symptoms of UTI
  3. Stress urinary incontinence
  4. Bulging of the anterior vaginal wall, especially when the woman is asked to bear down during a pelvic examination
- Diagnostic tests may include cystography, measurement of residual urine, IV urography (IVU), voiding cystourethrography (VCUG), cystometrography, and uroflowmetry.
- Management of patients with mild symptoms is conservative and may include:
  1. Use of a pessary for bladder support
  2. Application of intravaginal estrogen to prevent atrophy and weakening of vaginal walls
  3. Kegel exercises to strengthen perineal muscles
- Surgical intervention for severe symptoms is usually a vaginal sling or an anterior colporrhaphy (anterior repair) to tighten the pelvic muscles for better bladder support (see *Prolapse, Pelvic Organ*).

DEHYDRATION: FLUID AND ELECTROLYTE CONCEPT EXEMPLAR

OVERVIEW

- Dehydration is a condition of impaired FLUID AND ELECTROLYTE BALANCE resulting in fluid volume deficit.
- Fluid intake or fluid retention is less than what is needed to meet the body's fluid needs.
- It may be an *actual* decrease in total body water caused by either too little intake of fluid or too great a loss of fluid; or it can occur as a *relative* deficit, without an actual loss of total body water, such as when water shifts from the plasma into the interstitial space.

Considerations for Older Adults

Older adults are at high risk for dehydration because they have less total body water than younger adults. In addition, many older adults have decreased thirst sensation and may have difficulty with walking or other motor skills needed for obtaining fluids. They also may take drugs such as diuretics, antihypertensives, and laxatives that increase fluid excretion. Assess the fluid and electrolyte balance status of all older adults in any setting.

- *Isotonic dehydration* is the most common type of fluid volume deficit, in which fluid is lost from the extracellular fluid (ECF) space, including both the plasma and the interstitial spaces. See chart 2-6 for common causes of dehydration.

Chart 2-6	Common Causes of Fluid Imbalances: Dehydration

- Hemorrhage
- Vomiting
- Diarrhea
- Profuse salivation
- Fistulas
- Ileostomy
- Profuse diaphoresis
- Burns
- Severe wounds
- Long-term NPO status

- Diuretic therapy
- GI suction
- Hyperventilation
- Diabetes insipidus
- Difficulty swallowing
- Impaired thirst
- Unconsciousness
- Fever
- Impaired motor function

INTERPROFESSIONAL COLLABORATIVE CARE

Assessment: Noticing

- Obtain and record patient information:
  1. Nutritional history
  2. Fluid history
     a. Intake and output volumes
     b. Weight (a weight change of 1 pound corresponds to fluid volume change of about 500 mL)
  3. Presence of excessive sweating, diarrhea
  4. Drug therapy (especially diuretics and laxatives)
  5. Medical history
     a. Diabetes
     b. Kidney disease
  6. Level of consciousness and functional status
  7. Amount of strenuous physical activity
  8. Exposure to high environmental temperatures
  9. Dizziness or light headedness when standing
- Physical assessment/signs and symptoms
  1. Vital signs, including orthostatic heart rate (HR) and blood pressure (BP) if patient is able to sit or stand
  2. Cardiovascular changes
     a. Tachycardia at rest
     b. Weak peripheral pulses
     c. Low systolic or mean arterial BP
     d. Decreased pulse pressure
     e. Flat neck and hand veins in dependent position
  3. Respiratory changes
     a. Increased respiratory rate
     b. Increased respiratory depth
  4. Skin changes
     a. Dry mucous membranes
     b. Tongue has a paste-like coating or fissures
     c. Dry, flaky skin
     d. Poor skin turgor (skin "tents" when pinched)

Considerations for Older Adults

Assess skin turgor in an older adult by pinching the skin over the sternum or on the forehead, rather than the back of the hand, because these areas more reliably indicate hydration. As a person ages, the skin loses elasticity and tents on hands and arms even when the person is well hydrated.

5. Neurologic changes
   a. Alterations of mental status (especially confusion)
   b. Fever
6. Kidney function
   a. Urine output less than 0.5 to 1 mL/kg/hour for 2 or more hours or less than 500 mL/day
   b. Increased urine concentration (specific gravity greater than 1.030, dark amber, strong odor)

D

❗ NURSING SAFETY PRIORITY: Critical Rescue

Urine output below 500 mL/day for any patient without kidney disease is cause for concern and should be reported to the primary health care provider.

- Diagnostic assessment: No single laboratory test result confirms or rules out dehydration. Instead, it is determined by laboratory findings along with clinical manifestations. Common laboratory findings for dehydration include:
  1. Elevated levels of hemoglobin and hematocrit
  2. Increased serum osmolality, glucose, protein, blood urea nitrogen, and various electrolytes

❗ NURSING SAFETY PRIORITY: Action Alert

Hemoconcentration is not present when dehydration is from hemorrhage. Therefore do not rely only on laboratory values to identify dehydration.

Analysis: Interpreting
- The priority problems for the patient who has dehydration are:
  1. Dehydration due to excess fluid loss or inadequate fluid intake
  2. Potential for injury due to blood pressure changes and muscle weakness

Planning and Implementation: Responding
- Goals of care for the patient with dehydration are to prevent further fluid loss, increase fluid volumes to normal, and prevent injury.

RESTORE FLUID BALANCE
  1. Monitor vital signs, especially HR and BP to anticipate a return to normal ranges.
     a. Monitor the cardiac and pulmonary status at least every hour when patients with dehydration are receiving intravenous (IV) fluid replacement therapy to avoid overtreatment.

  b. Use daily weights to determine fluid gains or losses (1 L = 1 kg = 2.2 pounds).

 2. Replace fluids.

  a. Oral fluid replacement is used for correction of mild to moderate dehydration if the patient is alert enough to swallow and can tolerate oral fluids.

  b. IV fluid replacement is used when dehydration is severe and when the patient cannot safely swallow or cannot tolerate oral fluids.

   (1) Crystalloids are IV fluids that contain water, minerals (electrolytes), and sometimes other water-soluble substances such as glucose.

   (2) Colloids are IV fluids that contain larger nonwater-soluble molecules that increase the osmotic pressure in the plasma volume.

 3. Measure intake and output.

  a. Evaluate for a daily urine output within 500 mL of daily fluid intake.

  b. Evaluate urine output for an average of 30 mL/hour or 0.5 to 1 ml/kg/hour.

 4. Drug therapy may correct some causes of the dehydration:

  a. Antidiarrheal drugs

  b. Antiemetics

  c. Antipyretics

PREVENT INJURY

 1. Assess muscle strength, gait stability, and level of alertness.

  a. Implement fall precautions for safety.

  b. Instruct the patient to get up slowly from a lying or sitting position and to immediately sit down if he or she feels light-headed.

 2. Evaluate for a return to normal skin turgor.

Care Coordination and Transition Management

• Because dehydration is a symptom or complication of another health problem or drug therapy, even severe dehydration is resolved before patients return home or to residential care.

 1. Educate the patient and family to prevent recurrence by:

  a. Reviewing signs and symptoms for a change in fluid and electrolyte balance including a sudden change in cognition and HR

  b. Maintaining fluid intake of at least 1500 mL or intake of 500 mL greater than output unless another condition requires restricted fluid intake

  c. Instructing patients at risk for fluid imbalance to weigh themselves on the same scale daily, close to the same time each day, and with about the same amount of clothing on each time and to monitor these daily weights for changes or trends

d. Instructing caregivers of older adults who have cognitive impairments or mobility problems to schedule offerings of fluids at regular intervals throughout the day

DEMENTIA

See *Alzheimer's Disease*

DIABETES INSIPIDUS

OVERVIEW

- Diabetes insipidus (DI) is a disorder of the posterior pituitary gland in which water loss is caused by either an antidiuretic hormone (ADH) deficiency or an inability of the kidneys to respond to ADH.
- The result of DI is the excretion of large volumes of dilute urine.
- DI is classified into types, depending on whether the problem is caused by too little ADH or an inability of the kidneys to respond to ADH.

INTERPROFESSIONAL COLLABORATIVE CARE

Assessment: Noticing

- Most symptoms of DI are related to dehydration.
    1. Poor skin turgor, dry mucous membranes, weight loss, or thirst

Interventions: Responding

NONSURGICAL MANAGEMENT

Management Focuses on Controlling Symptoms with Drug Therapy

- Drug therapy may include:
    1. Desmopressin acetate (DDAVP), a synthetic form of vasopressin given intranasally in a metered spray or as an oral tablet; frequency of dosing depends on the patient's response

> **! NURSING SAFETY PRIORITY: Drug Alert**
>
> The parenteral form of desmopressin is 10 times stronger than the oral form, and the dosage must be reduced.

- Nursing interventions include:
    1. Replacing fluids by encouraging the patient to drink fluids equal to the amount of urinary output (if the patient is unable to do so, provide IV, as prescribed)

> **! NURSING SAFETY PRIORITY: Critical Rescue**
>
> Patients with DI are at risk for severe dehydration and hypovolemic shock because they cannot reduce urine output even in the presence of low oral fluid intake. Provide ongoing access to oral or IV fluids and monitor patient response to intake and output every 4 hours around the clock.

2. Monitoring intake and output with daily weights and communicating imbalances in a timely manner; a loss of 1 kg is equivalent to losing 1 L of fluid
3. Monitoring for vital sign changes indicating poor tissue perfusion (e.g., low BP; rapid, thready pulse; decreased consciousness)
4. Monitoring for indications of dehydration, including dry skin, poor skin turgor, and dry or cracked mucous membranes
5. Monitoring serum and urine laboratory results for effectiveness of therapy

- Self-management education and skills includes:
  1. Assisting the patient to drink fluids in an amount equal to urine output and teaching the patient that polyuria and thirst are signals for the need for another drug dose
  2. Teaching the patient to use daily weights and symptoms of dehydration to adjust medication accordingly. Signs of dehydration indicate the need for additional DDAVP and symptoms of overhydration or water intoxication indicate a need to reduce drug dose.
  3. Encouraging the patient with chronic DI to wear a medical alert bracelet or necklace at all times

✳ DIABETES MELLITUS: GLUCOSE REGULATION CONCEPT EXEMPLAR

OVERVIEW

- Diabetes mellitus (DM) is a chronic endocrine disorder of impaired glucose regulation that affects the function of all cells and tissues.
- Glucose regulation is the result of a complex cascade of insulin and other hormones.
- Movement of glucose into many cells requires the presence of glucose transporters and insulin. Insulin is needed for metabolism of carbohydrates, proteins, and fats.
- Acute manifestations of DM are hyperglycemia (elevated blood glucose levels), polyuria (excessive urination), polydipsia (excessive thirst and drinking), and polyphagia (hunger).
- DM is classified according to the cause of the disease and the severity of insulin lack. The three most common types of DM are type 1, type 2, and gestational diabetes.
  1. *Type 1 diabetes* (T1D) is an autoimmune disorder in which beta cells of the pancreas are destroyed and no insulin is produced. T1D:
     a. Is abrupt in onset

b. Requires insulin injections to prevent hyperglycemia and ketosis and to sustain health
c. Represents fewer than 10% of all people who have diabetes
d. Occurs primarily in childhood and adolescence but can occur at any age
e. May follow viral infection; viral infection can trigger auto-immune destructive actions

2. *Type 2 diabetes* (T2D) is a problem resulting from a reduction in the ability of most cells to respond to insulin (insulin resistance), poor control of liver glucose output, and decreased beta cell function. T2D:

a. Is generally slow in onset and may be present for years before it is diagnosed
b. May require oral drug therapy or insulin to correct hyperglycemia
c. Is usually found in middle-aged and older adults but may occur in younger people
d. May be part of metabolic syndrome or obesity
e. Is usually not associated with ketoacidosis
f. Represents about 90% of all people who have diabetes

3. Gestational diabetes mellitus (GDM):

a. Occurs during pregnancy and is confirmed by an oral glucose tolerance test
b. Is associated with large birth weight (baby weighs more than 9 pounds)
c. Is associated with increased risk for T2D in the woman diagnosed with GDM long after pregnancy

Acute complications of DM

1. Diabetic ketoacidosis (DKA) is caused by the absence of insulin and generation of ketoacids.
2. Hyperglycemic-hyperosmolar state (HHS) is caused by insulin deficiency and profound dehydration.

Considerations for Older Adults

Older adults with DM are at the greatest risk for dehydration and subsequent HHS. The onset of HHS is slow and may not be recognized. The older patient often seeks medical attention later and is sicker than younger patients. The mortality rate for HHS in older adults is as high as 40% to 70%.

! NURSING SAFETY PRIORITY: Action Alert

HHS does not occur in people who are adequately hydrated. Take steps to avoid dehydration in susceptible patients.

3. Hypoglycemia is caused by too much insulin or too little glucose.

Chronic Complications of DM

- DM can lead to organ complications and early death because of changes in large blood vessels (*macrovascular*) and small blood vessels (*microvascular*) in tissues and organs. These blood vessel changes lead to complications from poor tissue PERFUSION and cell ischemia.
  1. Macrovascular complications
     a. Coronary heart disease
     b. Cerebrovascular disease
     c. Peripheral vascular disease
  2. Microvascular complications
     a. Nephropathy
     b. Neuropathy
     c. Retinopathy
- Although no intervention prevents all complications, complications can be slowed significantly by maintaining serum glucose between 60 and 150 mg/dL ("tight control") and:
  1. Managing lipids to prevent hyperlipidemia, usually through drug therapy (statins)
  2. Ensuring BP is maintained below 140/90 or, in younger patients, below 130/80, usually through drug therapy to manage *hypertension*
  3. Promoting a healthy lifestyle of smoking cessation, balanced diet, and regular activity or exercise
  4. Adding low dose daily aspirin to prevent clotting in coronary arteries associated with *acute coronary syndrome*s

🌐 Cultural and Spiritual Considerations

Racial and ethnic minorities have a higher prevalence and greater burden of DM compared with non-Hispanic whites, and some minority groups also have higher rates of complications. The rate of DM is 13% among African Americans and 12.8% in the Hispanic population compared with non-Hispanic white Americans. At nearly 16.1%, American Indians and Alaska Indians have the highest age-adjusted prevalence of DM among US racial and ethnic groups (CDC, 2015). *The increase in obesity and sedentary lifestyles in the North American population intensifies this growing problem.*

The outcomes for minority patients with diabetes are worse than for non-Hispanic whites with DM. Factors for these outcome differences include lack of access to health care, lifestyle issues, mistrust of the health care system, reduced financial resources, and lack of knowledge about GLUCOSE REGULATION and complications. Be alert to the risk for DM whenever you are interviewing or assessing adults who belong to these higher risk groups.

INTERPROFESSIONAL COLLABORATIVE CARE

Assessment: Noticing

D

- Ask about and record patient history:
  1. Age and weight
  2. Birth weight of children or diagnosis of GDM or glucose intolerance during pregnancy
  3. History of recent illness, infection, or extreme stress
  4. Omission of insulin or oral diabetic drugs if the patient is known to have DM
  5. Change in eating habits
  6. Change in exercise schedule or activity level
  7. Presence and duration of polyuria, polydipsia, polyphagia, and loss of energy
  8. Presence of cardiovascular disease such as hyperlipidemia, hypertension, heart failure, or stroke
- Laboratory assessment:
  1. Elevated blood glucose
     a. Fasting blood glucose level higher than 126 mg/dL on two occasions
     b. Oral glucose tolerance test (2 hour post-load test) with glucose greater than 200 mg/dL
     c. Glycosylated hemoglobin assay (HbA1c) results greater than 6.5%
     d. A random blood glucose greater than 200 mg/dL with concurrent polyuria, polydipsia, or unexplained weight loss
  2. Islet cell autoantibodies (ICAs), autoantibodies to insulin, and autoantibodies to glutamic acid decarboxylase (GAD65) with new onset of T1D
  3. Positive results for urinary ketones; presence of albumin and glucose in the urine
  4. Serum levels of lipids (cholesterol)
  5. Dehydration (e.g., poor skin turgor, dry mucous membranes, hemoconcentration with elevated hematocrit and hemoglobin levels, decreased urine output, dark and strong-smelling urine)
  6. Serum levels of kidney disease such as elevated blood urea nitrogen, creatinine, electrolyte abnormalities
  7. Symptoms of infection including elevated WBCs, fever, or unexplained pain in skin, bones, and visceral organs

Analysis: Interpreting

- The priority collaborative problems for patients with diabetes DM include:
  1. Potential for injury due to hyperglycemia
  2. Potential for impaired wound healing due to endocrine and vascular effects of diabetes
  3. Potential for injury due to diabetic neuropathy
  4. Pain due to diabetic neuropathy
  5. Potential for injury due to diabetic retinopathy-induced reduced vision
  6. Potential for kidney disease due to impaired kidney circulation
  7. Potential for hypoglycemia
  8. Potential for diabetic ketoacidosis
  9. Potential for hyperglycemic-hyperosmolar state and coma

Planning and Implementation: Responding

PREVENT INJURY FROM HYPERGLYCEMIA

- Glucose monitoring
- Nutrition intervention
- Planned exercise
- Drug therapy

NONSURGICAL MANAGEMENT

Glucose Monitoring

- The patient needs to know how to perform all aspects of self-monitoring of blood glucose (SMBG).
  1. Help the patient select a meter based on the cost of the meter and strips, ease of use, and the availability of repair and servicing.
  2. Results are influenced by many factors including: the amount of blood on the strip; environmental conditions of altitude, temperature, and moisture; and patient-specific conditions of hematocrit, triglyceride level, and presence of hypotension.
  3. Teach the patient how to clean the equipment to prevent infection.
  4. *Continuous blood glucose monitoring* (CGM) systems monitor glucose levels in interstitial fluid to provide real-time glucose information to the user. The system consists of three parts: a disposable sensor that measures glucose levels, a transmitter that is attached to the sensor, and a receiver that displays and stores glucose information.
     a. After an initiation or warm-up period, the sensor gives glucose values every 1 to 5 minutes. Sensors may be used for 3 to 7 days, depending on the manufacturer.
     b. CGM provides information about the current blood glucose level, provides short-term feedback about results of

treatment, and provides warnings when glucose readings become dangerously high or low.

Nutrition Therapy

1. Use interprofessional collaboration to formulate an individualized meal plan for the patient based on overall glycemic control, blood lipids, and weight management goals.

    a. Carbohydrate intake is advised to be 45% of daily calories, with a minimum of 130 g/day.

    b. A protein intake of 15% to 20% of total daily calories is appropriate for patients with normal kidney function.

    c. Limit total fat intake to 20% to 30% of daily calories. Choose mono- and poly-unsaturated fats over unsaturated and avoid all *trans* fats.

    d. Fiber intake improves carbohydrate metabolism and lowers cholesterol levels. Advise a goal of 25 g of fiber daily.

    e. Warn the patient that fat "substitutes" or replacements may increase carbohydrate content in foods.

2. Day-to-day consistency in the timing and amount of food eaten helps control blood glucose. Patients taking insulin or oral drugs associated with hypoglycemia need to eat at consistent times that are coordinated with the timed action of the drug.

3. Explain and reinforce how to read food labels.

4. Reinforce dietary teaching such as how to follow the exchange system for meal planning and how to perform carbohydrate counting.

5. Support and reinforce information provided by the dietician regarding how to make adjustments in nutritional intake during illness, planned exercises, and social occasions.

6. Socioeconomic factors may affect a patient's ability to prepare the proper foods; collaborate with the case manager, diabetic educator, and social worker to identify sources of healthy food choices

Considerations for Older Adults

A realistic approach to NUTRITION therapy is essential for the older patient with DM. Changing the eating habits of 60 to 70 years is very difficult. The nurse, dietitian, and patient assess the patient's usual eating patterns. Teach the older patient taking diabetic drugs the importance of eating meals and snacks at the same time every day, eating the same amount of food from day to day, and eating all food allowed on the diet.

Planned Exercise
- Collaborate with the patient and rehabilitation specialist to develop an exercise program that includes at least 150 min/week of moderate-to-intensive (50% to 70% maximum HR) aerobic physical activity divided into 3 days, or 75 min/week of vigorous aerobic physical activity or an equivalent combination of the two.

! NURSING SAFETY PRIORITY: Action Alert

Teach patients with type 1 DM to perform vigorous exercise only when blood glucose levels are 100 to 250 mg/dL (5.6 to 13.8 mmol/L) and no ketones are present in the urine.

- Instruct the patient to have a complete physical examination before starting an exercise program.
- Instruct the patient to wear proper footwear with good traction and cushioning and to examine the feet after exercise.
- Discourage exercise in extreme heat or cold or during periods of poor glucose control.
- Advise the patient to stay hydrated.
- Patients with DM should evaluate serum glucose before and after vigorous exercise and follow advice about carbohydrate intake to prevent hypoglycemia with exercise.

Drug Therapy
Drug therapy is indicated when a patient with type 2 DM does not achieve blood glucose control with diet changes, regular exercise, and stress management. Several categories of drugs are available to lower blood glucose levels. Patients with type 1 DM require insulin therapy for blood glucose control. Drug therapy is used to achieve blood glucose control of A1C at 7.0% or below. Chart 2-7 reviews common examples of antidiabetic drugs.

Chart 2-7 Common Examples of Antidiabetic Drugs

Drug Class	

• Sulfonylureas
  Glipizide (Glucotrol)
  Glimepiride (Amaryl)
	• Oral drug that triggers release of insulin from pancreatic cells. Hypoglycemia is the most serious complication.

| Chart 2-7 | Common Examples of Antidiabetic Drugs—cont'd |

Drug Class

• Meglitinide Analogs Repaglinide (Prandin) Nateglinide (Starlix)	• Oral drugs that trigger insulin release. • Short-acting and given at meal time. • Associated with hypoglycemia.
• Biguanides Metformin (Glucophage)	• Metformin (Glucophage) is an oral drug that does not increase insulin secretion. It decreases liver glucose production and decreases intestinal absorption of glucose. It also improves insulin sensitivity by increasing peripheral glucose uptake and utilization.
• Thiazolidinediones Rosiglitazone (Avandia) Pioglitazone (Actos)	• These oral drugs work by increasing the sensitivity of insulin receptors, which promotes the use of glucose in peripheral tissues. • These drugs are associated with cardiac complications and carry a **Black Box Warning**.
• Alpha-glucosidase inhibitors Acarbose (Precose) Miglitol (Glyset)	• These oral drugs reduce hyperglycemia after meals by slowing digestion within the intestine. • Drugs in this class do not cause hypoglycemia.
• Incretin mimetics Albiglutide (Tanzeum) Dulaglutide (Trulicity) Exenatide (Byetta) Exenatide extended release (Bydureon) Liraglutide (Victoza)	• These drugs given by injection act like natural "gut" hormones that work with insulin to lower plasma glucose levels. • These drugs may be used with insulin to manage T1 DM or with oral agents to manage T2D.

D

Continued

Chart 2-7 Common Examples of Antidiabetic Drugs—cont'd

Drug Class

• DPP-4 inhibitors Sitagliptin (Januvia) Saxagliptin (Onglyza) Linagliptin (Tradjenta) Alogliptin (Nesina)	• DPP-4 is an enzyme that breaks down the natural gut hormones. By reducing the inactivation of the incretin hormones, these oral DDP-4 inhibitors control hyperglycemia after meals.
• Amylin analog Pramlintide (Symlin)	• This injectable drug is similar to amylin, a naturally occurring hormone. • Amylin levels are deficient in patients with type 1 DM who are also deficient in insulin. • Pramlintide (Symlin) works by delayed gastric emptying; reducing after-meal blood glucose levels; and triggering satiety (in the brain).
• Sodium-glucose cotransport inhibitors Canagliflozin (Invokana) Dapagliflozin (Farxiga) Empagliflozin (Jardiance)	• These oral drugs prevent kidney reabsorption of glucose that was filtered from the blood into the urine. • The filtered glucose is excreted in the urine rather than moving back into the blood.
• Combination agents	• Combination agents combine drugs with different mechanisms of action. Glucovance, for example, combines glyburide with metformin. Combining drugs with different mechanisms of action may be highly effective in maintaining desired blood glucose control.

❗ NURSING SAFETY PRIORITY: Drug Alert

DPP-4 inhibitors and the incretin mimetics may be associated with an increased risk for pancreatitis. Warn patients taking these drugs to immediately report signs of jaundice; sudden onset of intense abdominal pain that radiates to the back, left flank, or left shoulder; and gray-blue discoloration of the abdomen or periumbilical area to the primary health care provider.

! NURSING SAFETY PRIORITY: Drug Alert

Metformin can cause lactic acidosis in patients with kidney impairment and should not be used by anyone with kidney disease. To prevent lactic acidosis and acute kidney injury, the drug is withheld before and after using contrast medium or any surgical procedure requiring anesthesia until adequate kidney function is established.

Insulin Therapy
- Insulin therapy is required for type 1 DM and may be used for type 2 DM.
  1. Insulin is available in rapid-, short-, intermediate-, and long-acting forms. Some insulins can be mixed, while others will need to be administered separately.
  2. The Institute for Safe Medication Practices (ISMP) and The Joint Commission's National Patient Safety Goals identify insulin as a *High-Alert* drug. High-Alert drugs are those that have an increased risk for causing patient harm if given in error. The ISMP cautions that digital displays on some of the newer insulin pens can be misread. If the pen is held upside down, as a left-handed person might do, a dose of 52 units actually appears to be a dose of 25 units, and a dose of 12 units looks like a dose of 21 units.
  3. Insulin regimens try to duplicate the normal release pattern of insulin from the pancreas such that a long-acting insulin is used for basic, ongoing metabolism and a short- or rapid-acting insulin is used at meal time.

! NURSING SAFETY PRIORITY: Drug Alert

Do not mix any other insulin type with insulin glargine, insulin detemir, or with any of the premixed insulin formulations, such as Humalog Mix 75/25.

  4. Teach the patient that insulin type, injection techniques, site of injection, and individual response can all affect absorption, onset, degree, and duration of insulin activity, and reinforce that changing insulin may affect blood glucose control.
  5. Complications of insulin therapy include:
     a. Hypoglycemia
     b. *Dawn phenomenon,* a fasting hyperglycemia thought to result from the nocturnal release of growth hormone secretion that may cause blood glucose elevations around 5:00 to 6:00 AM, is managed or prevented by providing more insulin for the overnight period.

c. *Somogyi* phenomenon, a morning hyperglycemia resulting from an effective counterregulatory response to nighttime hypoglycemia, is managed or prevented by ensuring adequate dietary intake at bedtime and evaluating the insulin dose and exercise program.

d. *Hypertrophic lipodystrophy,* a spongy swelling at or around injection sites

e. *Lipoatrophy,* a loss of subcutaneous fat in areas of repeated injection, is treated by injection of human insulin at the edges of the atrophied area.

6. Insulin may be administered by:

a. A syringe and subcutaneous technique, based on intermittent testing of glucose; some patients may use a prefilled "pen," cartridge, or syringe

b. External insulin pump containing a syringe and reservoir with rapid- or short-acting insulin connected to the patient by an infusion set; the patient can adjust dosing based on glucose testing

c. Internal insulin pumps implanted into the peritoneal cavity where insulin can be absorbed in a more physiologic manner

7. Teach the patient about storage, dose preparation, injection procedures, and complications associated with drug therapy.

8. Instruct the patient to always buy the same type of syringes and use the same gauge and needle length; short needles are not used for an obese patient.

SURGICAL MANAGEMENT

• Surgical interventions for diabetes include islet cell or pancreas transplantation. When successful, this procedure eliminates the need for insulin injections, blood glucose monitoring, and many dietary restrictions.

1. Immunosuppressive therapy is needed for life to prevent rejection of the transplanted pancreas.

2. Complications include venous thrombosis, rejection, and infection.

• Provide preoperative care as described in Part One and:

1. Monitor hydration and IV fluids and urine output

2. Monitor blood glucose results and administer insulin to maintain serum glucose at less than 180 mg/dL

• Provide postoperative care as described including:

1. Send scheduled glucose evaluation; physical stress from surgery, anesthesia, or hypothermia may cause hyperglycemia

2. Monitor fluid and electrolyte balance; hyperglycemia and kidney conditions may contribute to problems with fluid and electrolyte balance

3. Maintain tight glycemic control throughout the postoperative phase
4. Monitor for postoperative complications, including:
   a. MI
   b. Hypoglycemia and hyperglycemia; monitor at least four times daily
   c. Hyperkalemia or hypokalemia
   d. Impaired wound healing or wound infection; an unanticipated episode of hyperglycemia may indicate a new infection
   e. Acute kidney injury or progression of chronic kidney disease

D

PREVENT INJURY FROM PERIPHERAL NEUROPATHY
- Patients with DM need intensive teaching about foot care because foot injury is a common complication. Once a failure of TISSUE INTEGRITY has occurred and an ulcer has developed, there is an increased risk for wound progression that may eventually lead to amputation.
- Promote wound healing when diabetic ulcers occur.
  1. Nonhealing foot wounds cause more inpatient hospital days than any other complication of diabetes.
  2. Loss of pain, pressure, and temperature sensation in the foot increases the risk for injury and ulceration.
  3. Foot deformities common in diabetic neuropathy may lead to callus formation, ulceration, and increased areas of pressure.
  4. Foot care education includes:
     a. Teaching preventive foot care to the patient; sensory neuropathy, ischemia, and infection are the leading causes of foot disease
     b. Recommending that the patient have shoes fitted by an experienced shoe fitter such as a certified podiatrist, and instructing the patient to change shoes at midday and in the evening and to wear socks or stockings with shoes
     c. Instructing the patient on how to care for wounds
  5. Refer the patient to a specialist for orthotic devices to eliminate pressure on infected or open wounds of the foot.
  6. Topical application of growth factors may be used to accelerate tissue healing for long-standing foot ulcers.
  7. Wound care for diabetic ulcers includes a moist wound environment, débridement of necrotic tissue, and offloading or elimination of pressure.

MANAGE PAIN RELATED TO NEUROPATHY
- Drug therapy and adjunctive therapy to manage peripheral neuropathic pain may include:
  1. Anticonvulsants such as gabapentin (Neurontin)
  2. Tricyclic antidepressants, particularly amitriptyline (Elavil, Levate ♣), nortriptyline (Pamelor), or selective serotonin

and norepinephrine reuptake inhibitors, such as duloxetine (Cymbalta)
3. Capsaicin cream, 0.075% (e.g., Zostrix-HP, Axsain ✿)
4. Distraction, positioning, and orthotics

PREVENT INJURY FROM REDUCED VISION
- Encourage all patients to have a baseline ophthalmic examination and yearly follow-up examinations.
- Advise the patient to seek a retinal specialist if problems are present.
- Collaborate with the rehabilitation specialist to recommend strategies to improve the patient's visual abilities; strategies include improving lighting, placing dark equipment against a white background, coding objects such as insulin vials with bright colors or felt-tip markers, and using large-type books and newspapers.
- Various stages of diabetic retinopathy can be treated with laser therapy or surgery.
- Teach the patient with limited vision the following strategies for using adaptive devices to self-administer insulin:
  1. Ensuring proper placement of the device on the syringe
  2. Holding the insulin bottle upright when measuring insulin
  3. Avoiding air bubbles in the syringe by pulling a small amount of insulin into the syringe, moving the plunger in and out three times, and measuring insulin on the fourth draw

REDUCE THE RISK FOR KIDNEY DISEASE
- Aggressive control of blood glucose and hypertension in patients without albuminuria can avoid nephropathy. Once albuminuria develops, management focuses on controlling blood pressure and blood glucose and avoiding nephrotoxic agents.
- Screen urine annually to quantify urine albumin; persistent albuminuria in the range of 30 to 299 mg/24 hours (formerly called microalbuminuria) is the earliest stage of nephropathy in type 1 DM and a marker for the development of nephropathy in type 2 DM.
- Teach the patient to avoid nephrotoxins including NSAIDs and some contrast dyes.
- Teach the patient to limit protein to 0.8 g/kg of body weight per day if he or she has overt nephropathy.
- Teach the patient about the signs and symptoms of urinary tract infection (UTI).

PREVENT HYPOGLYCEMIA
- Monitor glucose levels before administering hypoglycemic agents, before meals, at bedtime, and when the patient is symptomatic.
- Treat the patient with mild hypoglycemia (hungry, irritable, shaky, weak, headache, fully conscious, blood glucose less than

70 mg/dL [3.4 mmol/L]) and who is able to swallow with 15 to 20 g of glucose, such as *one* of these:
1. 2 or 3 glucose tablets
2. 4 oz. of fruit drink
3. 8 oz. of skim milk
4. 6 saltines
5. 3 graham crackers
6. 6 to 10 hard candies
7. 4 cubes or 2 teaspoons of sugar
- The blood glucose level should be tested after 15 minutes.
- Treat the patient with moderate hypoglycemia (cold and clammy skin, pale, rapid pulse, rapid shallow respirations, marked changes in mood, drowsiness, blood glucose less than 40 mg/dL [2.2 mmol/L]) with 15 to 30 g of rapidly absorbed carbohydrates and additional food such as low-fat milk or cheese after 10 to 15 minutes.

D

! NURSING SAFETY PRIORITY: Critical Rescue

Assess patients to recognize the presence and severity of hypoglycemia. For the patient with *severe* hypoglycemia (unable to swallow, unconscious or convulsing, blood glucose usually less than 20 mg/dL [1.0 mmol/L]), respond by:
1. Giving glucagon 1 mg subcutaneously or IM
2. Repeating the dose in 10 minutes if the patient remains unconscious
3. Notifying the primary health care provider immediately, and following instructions

---

PREVENT DIABETIC KETOACIDOSIS
- DKA occurs in people with T1D and is often precipitated by illness, especially infection.
- DKA is a condition of metabolic acidosis and severe dehydration with electrolyte derangements.
- Laboratory diagnosis is based on serum glucose level equal to or greater than 300 mg/dL (16.7 mmol/L), arterial pH less than 7.35, arterial bicarbonate level less than 15 mEq/L, blood urea nitrogen level greater than 30 mg/dL, creatinine level greater than 1.5 mg/dL, and ketonuria.
- Clinical manifestations of dehydration and acidosis include decreased skin turgor, dry mucous membranes, hypotension, tachycardia, tachypnea, Kussmaul respirations, abdominal pain, nausea, and vomiting. Central nervous system depression results in changes in consciousness varying from lethargy to coma.

- Death occurs in 1% to 10% of these cases even with appropriate treatment. Mortality is highest for older patients who also have infection, stroke, myocardial infarction, vascular thrombosis, intestinal obstruction, or pneumonia.
- Monitor the patient for signs and symptoms of DKA: hyperglycemia, metabolic acidosis, and urinary ketones. Classic symptoms are polyuria, polydipsia, polyphagia, a rotting citrus fruit odor to the breath, vomiting, abdominal pain, dehydration, weakness, confusion, shock, and coma. Mental status can vary from total alertness to profound coma.
- If ketoacidosis occurs, interventions include the following:
  1. Give insulin bolus as indicated, followed by a continuous drip
  2. Check the patient's BP, pulse, and respirations every 15 minutes until stable
  3. Replace both fluid volume and ongoing losses, monitoring for heart failure symptoms and pulmonary edema if large volume of IV fluid is administered
  4. Record urine output, temperature, and mental status every hour
  5. Assess the patient's level of consciousness and blood glucose levels every hour until stable; once stable, assess every 4 hours
  6. Monitor the patient for dehydration and hypokalemia (symptoms are muscle weakness, abdominal distention or paralytic ileus, hypotension, and weak pulse); before administering potassium, ensure that the patient's urine output is at least 30 mL/hr
- Instruct the patient about how to prevent future episodes of DKA by contacting the primary health care provider when the blood glucose is greater than 250 mg/dL, when ketonuria is present for longer than 24 hours, when he or she is unable to take food or fluids, and when illness persists for longer than 1 to 2 days.

PREVENT HYPERGLYCEMIC-HYPEROSMOLAR STATE

- HHS, is a hyperosmolar (increased blood osmolarity) state caused by hyperglycemia. Both HHS and DKA are caused by hyperglycemia and dehydration. HHS differs from DKA in that ketone levels are absent or low and blood glucose levels are much higher (Chart 2-8). Blood glucose levels may exceed 600 mg/dL (33.3 mmol/L), and blood osmolarity may exceed 320 mOsm/L.
  1. Administer IV fluids and insulin as indicated, and monitor and assess the patient's response to therapy.
  2. Assess for signs of cerebral edema and immediately report to the physician a change in the level of consciousness; change in pupil size, shape, or reaction to light; or seizure activity.

Chart 2-8	Differences Between DKA and HHS

	Diabetic Ketoacidosis (Dka)	Hyperglycemic-Hyperosmolar State (Hhs)
Onset	Sudden	Gradual
Precipitating factors	Infection	Infection
	Other stressors	Other stressors
	Inadequate Insulin dose	Poor fluid intake
Symptoms	Ketosis: Kussmaul respiration, "rotting fruit" breath, nausea, abdominal pain	Altered central nervous system function with neurologic symptoms
	Dehydration or electrolyte loss: polyuria, polydipsia, weight loss, dry skin, sunken eyes, soft eyeballs, lethargy, coma	Dehydration or electrolyte loss: same as for DKA

D

Care Coordination and Transition Management

- Discharge planning includes:
  1. Ensuring that the patient understands the significance, symptoms, causes, and treatment of hypoglycemia and hyperglycemia
  2. Assisting the patient to identify the items needed for the administration of insulin and for glucose monitoring
  3. Teaching the patient how to monitor blood sugar level
  4. Teaching the patient how to administer drugs and prevent hypoglycemia
  5. In collaboration with the dietician, teaching the patient the skills associated with food choices and meal planning
  6. Referring the patient to a diabetes educator for the necessary instruction
  7. Helping the patient adapt to DM, including teaching stress management techniques and identifying coping mechanisms
  8. Referring the patient to the American Diabetes Association and its resources
  9. Providing information about community resources, such as diabetic education programs

DIVERTICULA, ESOPHAGEAL
OVERVIEW
- Diverticula are sacs resulting from the herniation of esophageal mucosa and submucosa into surrounding tissue.
- Patients with esophageal diverticula are at risk for esophageal perforation.
- The most common form of esophageal diverticula is *Zenker's* diverticula, usually located near the hypopharynx and occurs most often in older adults.

INTERPROFESSIONAL COLLABORATIVE CARE
Assessment: Noticing
- Assessment findings include:
  1. Dysphagia
  2. Regurgitation
  3. Feelings of fullness or pressure
  4. Halitosis
  5. Nocturnal cough

Interventions: Responding
- Diet therapy and positioning are the primary interventions for controlling symptoms.
  1. Collaborate with the dietitian to determine the size and frequency of meals and the texture and consistency that can best be tolerated by the patient.
  2. Elevate the head of the bed for sleep to avoid reflux of gastric contents onto diverticula.
  3. Teach the patient to avoid the recumbent position and vigorous exercise for at least 2 hours after eating to prevent reflux.
  4. Teach the patient to avoid restrictive clothing at the abdomen and thorax and to minimize stooping or bending to reduce reflux.
- Surgical management is aimed at excision of the diverticula.
- Postoperative care
  1. Monitor for bleeding and perforation.
  2. Do not irrigate the nasogastric (NG) tube used for decompression unless specifically ordered by the primary health care provider.
  3. Maintain hydration and nutrition through IV fluids and enteral feedings until oral intake is permitted; NPO status may be several days' duration to allow esophageal healing.
  4. Manage the patient's postoperative pain.
  5. Teach the patient to observe for complications such as infection or poor wound healing.

DIVERTICULAR DISEASE

OVERVIEW

- Diverticular disease includes diverticulosis and diverticulitis.
  1. *Diverticula* are pouch-like herniations of the mucosa through the muscular wall of any portion of the gut.
  2. *Diverticulosis* can occur in any segment of the gut but it most commonly refers to diverticula of the colon. High intraluminal pressure forces the formation of a pouch in the weakened area of the mucosa, commonly near blood vessels.
  3. *Diverticulitis,* or inflammation of one or more diverticula, results when the diverticulum retains undigested food that compromises the blood supply to that area and facilitates bacterial invasion of the diverticular sac.
  4. Complications of diverticula and diverticulitis are abscess formation and perforation followed by peritonitis.

INTERPROFESSIONAL COLLABORATIVE CARE

Assessment: Noticing

- Patients with diverticulosis are usually asymptomatic; a minor history of left quadrant pain or constipation may be reported.
- Diverticula are identified by colonoscopy; a screening abdominal ultrasound may reveal thickened bowel wall
- Assess for signs and symptoms of diverticulitis:
  1. Abdominal pain that may begin as intermittent and may progress to continuous; pain may be localized to the left lower quadrant and increase with coughing, straining, or lifting
  2. Fever
  3. Nausea and vomiting
  4. Abdominal distention
  5. Blood in the stool (microscopic to larger amounts)
  6. Elevated WBCs; reduced hematocrit and hemoglobin if bleeding occurs
  7. Hypotension and dehydration occur if bleeding occurs (see *Shock*)
  8. Signs of septic shock occur if peritonitis has occurred
  9. Intake and output, including NG tube (amount, color, and quality) if used for gastric decompression or to manage vomiting

Interventions: Responding

- Drug therapy is used to treat infection and inflammation from diverticulitis.
  1. Administer broad-spectrum antibiotics such as metronidazole (Flagyl) plus trimethoprim/sulfamethoxazole (Bactrim, Septra), or ciprofloxacin (Cipro).
  2. Implement management for mild or moderate pain; if pain is severe, use opioids.

3. Laxatives and enemas are not given because they increase intestinal motility.

- An NG tube is inserted if nausea, vomiting, or abdominal distention is severe. Report the appearance of output.
- Diet therapy:
  1. Provide IV fluids for hydration during the acute phase of the disease or when the patient is NPO.
  2. Consult with a dietitian to promote healthy food choices.

SURGICAL MANAGEMENT

- Patients with diverticulitis need emergent surgery if any of the following occurs:
  1. Rupture of the diverticulum with subsequent peritonitis
  2. Abdominal or pelvic abscess
  3. Bowel obstruction
  4. Fistula
  5. Uncontrolled bleeding
- Surgical management includes a colon resection with an end-to-end anastomosis or temporary or permanent colostomy.
- Preoperative care is provided as described in Part One and includes:
  1. Reinforcing physician teaching about the possible need for a temporary or permanent colostomy
  2. Administering IV fluids, antibiotics, and pain medications, as prescribed
- Postoperative care includes:
  1. Maintaining a drainage system at the abdominal incision site
  2. If a colostomy was created, monitoring colostomy stoma for color and integrity, anticipating that a gray or black color or separation between the mucous membranes and skin is indicative of poor healing and requires immediate communication with the surgeon
  3. Providing the patient with an opportunity to express feelings about the colostomy
  4. Consulting with the wound or ostomy specialist
  5. Providing written postoperative instructions on:
     a. Wound care
     b. Avoidance of activities that increase intra-abdominal pressure, including straining at stool, bending, lifting heavy objects, and wearing restrictive clothing
     c. Pain management, including prescriptions
- Teach the patient and family to:
  1. Follow dietary considerations for diverticulosis, which include consultation with the dietitian. Keep a food diary to note food associations with symptoms and to implement the following:
     a. Eat a diet high in cellulose and hemicellulose, which are found in wheat bran, whole-grain breads, cereals, fresh fruit, and vegetables

   b. Use a bulk-forming laxative such as psyllium (Metamucil) to increase fecal size and consistency if recommended fiber intake of 25 to 35 g daily is not tolerated

   c. Encourage fluids to prevent bloating that may accompany a high-fiber diet

   d. Avoid alcohol, which has an irritant effect on the bowel

   e. Do not exceed a fat intake of 30% of the total daily caloric intake

2. Avoid all fiber when symptoms of diverticulitis are present because high-fiber foods are then irritating. As inflammation resolves, gradually add fiber back into the diet.

3. Monitor for signs and symptoms of diverticulitis (e.g., fever, abdominal pain, bloody stools).

4. Avoid enemas and irritant or stimulant laxatives.

DUMPING SYNDROME

OVERVIEW

- Dumping syndrome is a group of vasomotor symptoms that occurs after eating following recovery from surgical procedures that reduce the size of the stomach such as a partial or full gastrectomy (for cancer or perforation from peptic ulcer disease) or bariatric surgery (to reduce complications from morbid obesity).
- This syndrome is believed to occur as a result of the rapid emptying of food contents into the small intestine that shifts fluid into the gut, causing abdominal distention.
- *Early dumping syndrome* typically occurs within 30 minutes of eating. Symptoms include vertigo, tachycardia, syncope, sweating, pallor, palpitations, and the desire to lie down. Report these manifestations to the surgeon in the postoperative recovery period, and encourage the patient to lie down.
- *Late dumping syndrome*, which occurs 90 minutes to 3 hours after eating, is caused by a release of an excessive amount of insulin. The insulin release follows a rapid rise in the blood glucose level that results from the rapid entry of high-carbohydrate food into the jejunum. Observe for manifestations, including dizziness, light-headedness, palpitations, diaphoresis, and confusion and encourage the patient to lie down and reconsider dietary choices.

INTERPROFESSIONAL COLLABORATIVE CARE

- Dumping syndrome is managed by nutrition changes that include decreasing the amount of food taken at one time and eliminating liquids ingested with meals. In collaboration with the dietitian, teach the patient to eat a high-protein, high-fat, low- to moderate-carbohydrate diet.

DUCTAL ECTASIA
OVERVIEW
- Ductal ectasia is a benign breast problem characterized by breast duct dilation and thickened wall, particularly in women approaching menopause.
- The ducts become blocked, distended, and filled with cellular debris, activating an inflammatory response.
- Manifestations are a hard and tender mass with irregular borders, greenish brown nipple discharge, enlarged axillary nodes, and redness and edema over the mass.
- Ductal ectasia does not increase breast cancer risk, but the mass may be difficult to distinguish from breast cancer. Nipple discharge is examined microscopically for any atypical or malignant cells.

INTERPROFESSIONAL COLLABORATIVE CARE
- Warm compresses and antibiotics may be helpful in relieving symptoms and improving drainage. The affected area may be excised.
- Nursing interventions focus on reducing the anxiety and providing support through the diagnostic and treatment procedures.

DYSRHYTHMIAS
OVERVIEW
- Cardiac dysrhythmias are abnormal rhythms of the heart's electrical system that can affect its ability to effectively pump oxygenated blood throughout the body.
- Some dysrhythmias are life threatening, and others are not. They are the result of disturbances in cardiac electrical impulse formation, conduction, or both.
- Any disorder of the heartbeat is called a dysrhythmia.

NORMAL SINUS RHYTHM
- Originates from the sinoatrial (SA) node (dominant pacemaker) that meets these ECG criteria:
  1. Rate: atrial and ventricular rates of 60-100 beats/min
  2. Rhythm: atrial and ventricular rhythms are regular
  3. P waves: present, consistent configuration, one P wave before each QRS complex
  4. PR interval: 0.12 to 0.20 second and constant
  5. QRS duration: 0.04 to 0.10 second and constant

SINUS ARRHYTHMIA
- Sinus arrhythmia has all the characteristics of normal sinus rhythm (NSR) except for its irregularity. The PP and RR intervals

vary, with the difference between the shortest and the longest intervals being greater than 0.12 second.

COMMON DYSRHYTHMIAS
Premature Complexes
- *Premature complexes* are early complexes that occur when a cardiac cell or group of cells other than the SA node becomes irritable and fires an impulse before the next sinus impulse is generated.
  1. *Bigeminy* occurs when normal complexes and premature complexes occur alternately in a repetitive two-beat pattern, with a pause occurring after each premature complex so that complexes occur in pairs.
  2. *Trigeminy* is a repetitive three-beat pattern, usually occurring as two sequential normal complexes followed by a premature complex and a pause, with the same pattern repeating itself in triplets.
  3. *Quadrigeminy* is a repetitive four-beat pattern, usually occurring as three sequential normal complexes followed by a premature complex and a pause, with the same pattern repeating itself in a four-beat pattern.

Bradydysrhythmias
- *Bradydysrhythmias* are characterized by a HR less than 60 beats/min.
  1. The patient may tolerate a low HR if BP is adequate.
  2. Symptomatic bradydysrhythmias lead to hypotension, myocardial ischemia or infarction, other dysrhythmias, and heart failure.

Tachydysrhythmias
- *Tachydysrhythmias* are HRs greater than 100 beats/min.
  1. Signs and symptoms include palpitations; chest discomfort; pressure or pain from myocardial ischemia or infarction; restlessness; anxiety; pale, cool skin; and syncope from hypotension.
  2. They may cause heart failure as indicated by dyspnea, orthopnea, pulmonary crackles, distended neck veins, fatigue, and weakness.
- Dysrhythmias are further classified according to their site of origin.

Sinus Dysrhythmias
  1. Sinus tachycardia, which occurs when the SA node discharge exceeds 100 beats/min. Treatment is based on identifying the underlying cause (e.g., angina, fever, hypovolemia, pain); beta-adrenergic blocking agents may be prescribed.
  2. Sinus bradycardia, a decreased rate of SA node discharge of less than 60 beats/min. If the patient is symptomatic, treatment

includes atropine, a pacemaker, and avoidance of parasympathetic stimulations such as prolonged suctioning.

Atrial Dysrhythmias

1. *Premature atrial complex* (PAC) occurs when atrial tissue becomes irritable. This ectopic focus fires an impulse before the next sinus impulse is due.
   a. No intervention is generally needed except to treat the cause, such as heart failure or valvular disease.
2. *Supraventricular tachycardia* (SVT) involves the rapid stimulation of atrial tissue at a rate of 100 to 280 beats/min.
   a. Drug therapy is prescribed for some patients to convert SVT to an NSR. Adenosine (Adenocard) is used to terminate the acute episode and is given rapidly (over several seconds) followed by a normal saline bolus.
   b. Oxygen therapy, antidysrhythmic drugs, vagal maneuvers by the provider, or synchronized cardioversion may be needed.
   c. Sustained SVT may need to be treated with radiofrequency catheter ablation.

> **! NURSING SAFETY PRIORITY: Drug Alert**
>
> Side effects of adenosine include significant bradycardia with pauses, nausea, and vomiting. When administering adenosine, be sure to have emergency equipment readily available!

3. *Atrial fibrillation* (AF) is characterized by chaotic depolarization of the atria decreasing cardiac output and PERFUSION. It is considered uncontrolled when the ventricular rate is 120-200 beats/min. See Atrial Fibrillation Exemplar.
   a. Drug treatment is used to prevent embolus formation related to irregular cardiac rhythm and to slow cardiac rate from altered conduction pattern or to return the rhythm to normal.
4. *Atrial flutter* is a rapid atrial depolarization occurring at a rate of 250 to 350 times/min with flutter rather than P waves mapped on ECG; ventricular response is considered uncontrolled with rates of 120 to 200 beats/min.
   a. Treatment is the same as for AF.
   b. Atrial flutter often deteriorates in AF.

Ventricular Dysrhythmias

- Ventricular dysrhythmias are potentially more life threatening than atrial dysrhythmias because the left ventricle pumps oxygenated blood throughout the body to perfuse vital organs and other tissues.

1. *Premature ventricular complexes* (PVCs) (also called premature ventricular contractions) result from irritability of ventricular cells.

   a. They may need no treatment or treatment may focus on underlying causes such as electrolyte derangements(s), low oxygenation, caffeine, stress, and acute coronary syndrome.

   b. When PVCs cause symptoms of low cardiac output, the condition is treated with the drugs that manage ventricular tachycardia.

2. *Ventricular tachycardia* (VT), sometimes referred to as *V tach*, occurs with repetitive firing of an irritable ventricular ectopic focus, usually at a rate of 140 to 180 beats/min or more. VT may result from increased automaticity or a re-entry mechanism. It may be intermittent (nonsustained VT) or sustained, lasting longer than 15 to 30 seconds. The rapid rate and loss of atrial volume results in decreased cardiac output.

   a. Patients are at risk for VT during acute coronary syndromes, following surgical manipulation of the heart or pericardium, or with electrolyte imbalances.

! NURSING SAFETY PRIORITY: Critical Rescue

In many patients, VT causes cardiac arrest. Assess the patient's circulation, airway, breathing, level of consciousness, and oxygenation level. For the *stable* patient with sustained VT, administer oxygen and confirm the rhythm via a 12-lead ECG. Amiodarone (Cordarone), lidocaine, or magnesium sulfate may be given.

   b. Current Advanced Cardiac Life Support (ACLS) guidelines state that elective cardioversion is highly recommended for stable VT.

   c. Common drugs to manage VT include mexiletine (Mexitil) or sotalol (Betapace, Rylosol), to prevent further occurrences.

3. *Ventricular fibrillation* (VF) sometimes called *V fib*, is the result of electrical chaos in the ventricles and is *life threatening!* Impulses from many irritable foci fire in a totally disorganized manner so ventricular contraction cannot occur. *There is no cardiac output or pulse and therefore no cerebral, myocardial, or systemic perfusion. This rhythm is rapidly fatal if not successfully ended within 3 to 5 minutes.*

    a. *The priority is to defibrillate the patient immediately according to ACLS protocol.*

    b. If a defibrillator is not readily available, high-quality cardiopulmonary resuscitation (CPR), also known as Basic Cardiac Life Support (BCLS), must be initiated and continued until the defibrillator arrives. An automated external defibrillator (AED) is frequently used because it is simple for both medical and lay personnel.

    c. Antidysrhythmic drugs may be used after return of an organized rhythm; the most common drug used in amiodarone (Cordarone).

4. Ventricular asystole, sometimes called *ventricular standstill,* is the complete absence of any ventricular rhythm. There are no electrical impulses in the ventricles and therefore *no* ventricular depolarization, no QRS complex, no contraction, no cardiac output, and no perfusion to the rest of the body.

    a. CPR must be initiated immediately when asystole occurs.

- When finding an unresponsive patient, confirm unresponsiveness and call 911 (in community or long-term care setting) or the emergency response team (in the hospital). Gather the AED or defibrillator *before initiating CPR.* Guidelines for CPR have changed from an ABC (airway-breathing-compressions) approach to the initial priorities of CAB (compressions-airway-breathing) (AHA, 2015).

! NURSING SAFETY PRIORITY: Critical Rescue

Early defibrillation is critical in resolving pulseless VT or VF. It must not be delayed for any reason after the equipment and skilled personnel are present. The earlier defibrillation is performed, the greater the chance of survival! *Do not defibrillate ventricular asystole.* The purpose of defibrillation is disruption of the chaotic rhythm allowing the SA node signals to restart. In ventricular asystole, no electoral impulses are present to disrupt.

Before defibrillation, loudly and clearly command all personnel to clear contact with the patient and the bed and check to see they are clear before the shock is delivered. Deliver shock and immediately resume CPR for 5 cycles or about 2 minutes. Reassess the rhythm every 2 minutes and, if indicated, charge the defibrillator to deliver an additional shock at the same energy level previously used. During the 2-minute intervals while high-quality CPR is being delivered, the ACLS team administers medications and performs interventions to try and restore an organized cardiac rhythm. *Discussion of ACLS protocol is beyond the scope of this text.*

INTERPROFESSIONAL COLLABORATIVE CARE

- Assess patients with dysrhythmias for a decrease in cardiac output resulting in inadequate oxygenation and perfusion to vital organs: VS, pulses, and level of consciousness unless the monitored rhythm is VF. If VF, initiate rapid response team and begin CPR.
- Interpret common dysrhythmias, especially bradycardia, tachycardia, AF, VT, VF, PVCs, and asystole, using the steps of ECG analysis. Respond with immediate communication to the primary health care provider when a patient has a new abnormal rhythm.
- Identify and intervene in life-threatening situations by providing CPR, electrical therapy (cardioversion or defibrillation), or drug administration.
- Anticipate blood collection for evaluation of serum electrolytes and possibly serum levels of antidysrhythmic drugs if these type of drugs have been prescribed.
- Anticipate the need for IV access and fluids and place a peripheral catheter if one is not present and functioning.
- If sinus rhythm or spontaneous circulation returns during treatment, transport the patient to the ICU and use best practices to hand off the patient (SBAR or agency format).
- Some institutions allow or encourage family members to be present at resuscitation event; contact the chaplain or social worker to provide family members with support and debriefing if they witness urgent care around a dysrhythmia.

Care Coordination and Transition Management

- If an implantable defibrillator or pacemaker is newly placed for treatment, teach the patient about incisional care and safe practice, including avoiding strong magnets or microwave transmission.
- Teach patients with dysrhythmias the correct drug, dose, route, time, and side effects of prescribed drugs, and teach them to notify their primary care provider if adverse effects occur.
- Teach patients taking anticoagulant therapy to report any signs of bruising or unusual bleeding immediately to their primary health care provider.
- Teach family members where to learn CPR to decrease their anxiety while living with a patient with dysrhythmias or ICD/pacemaker.

E

ECTASIA, DUCTAL

OVERVIEW

- Ductal ectasia is a benign breast problem in women approaching menopause, caused by thickening and dilation of breast ducts.
- The ducts are blocked, becoming distended and filled with cellular debris, which activates an inflammatory response.
- Manifestations are a hard and tender mass with irregular borders; greenish brown nipple discharge; enlarged axillary nodes; and redness and edema over the mass.
- Ductal ectasia does not increase breast cancer risk, but the mass may be difficult to distinguish from breast cancer. Because the risk for breast cancer is increased among women in the menopause age group, accurate diagnosis is vital.
- Nipple discharge is examined microscopically for any atypical or malignant cells.

INTERPROFESSIONAL COLLABORATIVE CARE

- Warm compresses and antibiotics may be helpful in relieving symptoms and improving drainage. The affected area may be excised.
- Nursing interventions focus on reducing the anxiety and providing support through the diagnostic and treatment procedures.

ENCEPHALITIS

OVERVIEW

- Encephalitis, an inflammation of the brain parenchyma (brain tissue) and often the meninges, is most often caused by infective organisms.
- Encephalitis can be life-threatening or lead to persistent neurologic problems such as learning disabilities, epilepsy, memory, or fine motor deficits.

INTERPROFESSIONAL COLLABORATIVE CARE

Assessment: Noticing

- Assessment findings include:
  1. Fever
  2. Nausea and vomiting
  3. Stiff neck; nuchal rigidity
  4. Decreased level of consciousness and impaired cognition
  5. Motor dysfunction
  6. Focal neurologic deficits
  7. Symptoms of increased intracranial pressure
  8. Ocular palsies
  9. Facial weakness

10. Abnormal cerebrospinal fluid analysis
11. Elevated white blood cell (WBC) count

! NURSING SAFETY PRIORITY: Critical Rescue

Level of consciousness is the most sensitive indicator of neurologic status. Inform the health care provider of worsening cognition or decreased arousal because this may mean worsening of acute neurologic disease.

Interventions: Responding
- The treatment for encephalitis is similar to that for meningitis.
  1. Maintain a patent airway; avoid aspiration.
  2. Encourage and assist the patient to reposition, and deep breathe frequently; suction if respiratory status is compromised.
  3. Monitor vital signs and neurologic signs, such as level of consciousness, orientation, pupil responses, and motor movement.
  4. Elevate the head of the bed 30 to 45 degrees.
  5. Administer acyclovir (Zovirax) for herpes encephalitis as prescribed; no specific drug therapy is available for infection by arboviruses or enteroviruses.
  6. If there are neurologic disabilities, the patient is discharged to a rehabilitation setting or a long-term care facility.

ENDOCARDITIS, INFECTIVE
OVERVIEW
- Infective endocarditis (previously called bacterial endocarditis) refers to a microbial infection (virus, bacterium, fungus) involving the endocardium.
- Infective endocarditis occurs primarily in patients who are IV drug abusers, have had cardiac valve replacements, have experienced systemic infection, or have structural cardiac defects.
- Portals of entry for infecting organisms include:
  1. Oral cavity, especially if dental procedures have been performed
  2. Skin rashes, lesions, or abscesses
  3. Infections (cutaneous, genitourinary or gastrointestinal (GI), systemic)
  4. Surgical or invasive procedures, including IV line placement

INTERPROFESSIONAL COLLABORATIVE CARE
Assessment: Noticing
- Assessment findings include:
  1. Signs of infection, including fever, chills, malaise, night sweats, and fatigue
     a. Older adults may remain afebrile.

2. Heart murmurs: Almost all patients with infective endocarditis develop murmurs.
3. *Heart failure is the most common complication of infective endocarditis*
   Right-sided heart failure, evidenced by:
   a. Peripheral edema
   b. Weight gain
   c. Anorexia
   Left-sided heart failure, evidenced by:
   a. Fatigue
   b. Shortness of breath
   c. Crackles
4. Evidence of arterial embolization from fragments of vegetation on valve leaflets, which may travel to other organs and compromise function. Manifestations of acute embolization include:
   a. Splenic emboli: sudden abdominal pain and radiation to the left shoulder
   b. Kidney infarction: flank pain that radiates to the groin and is accompanied by hematuria or pyuria
   c. Mesenteric emboli: diffuse abdominal pain, often after eating and abdominal distention
   d. Brain emboli: signs of stroke, confusion, reduced concentration, and difficulty speaking
   e. Pulmonary emboli: pleuritic chest pain, dyspnea, and cough
5. Petechiae of the neck, shoulders, wrists, ankles, mucous membranes, or conjunctivae
6. Splinter hemorrhages, black longitudinal lines, or small red streaks in the nail bed
7. Osler's nodes (reddish, tender lesions with a white center on the pads of the fingers, hands, and toes)
8. Janeway's lesion (nontender hemorrhagic lesion found on the fingers, toes, nose, and earlobes)
9. Positive blood culture
10. Low hemoglobin level and hematocrit
11. Abnormal transesophageal echocardiography

Interventions: Responding

- Interventions include:
  1. Administering IV antimicrobial therapy as prescribed
  2. Monitoring the patient's tolerance to activity
  3. Protecting the patient from contact with potentially infective organisms
  4. Informing the Rapid Response Team of symptoms of embolization; collaborating and communicating to prevent complications from embolization, particularly decreased oxygenation, brain injury, and acute coronary syndrome

- Surgical intervention includes removal of the infected valve, repair or removal of congenital shunts, repair of injured valves and chordae tendineae, and draining abscesses in the heart or elsewhere.
- Preoperative and postoperative care for the patient having surgery involving the valves is similar to that described for patients undergoing a coronary artery bypass grafting or valve replacement.

Care Coordination and Transition Management

- Teach the patient and family:
  1. Information on the cause of the disease and its course, drug regimens, signs and symptoms of infection, and practices to prevent future infections
  2. How to administer IV antibiotic and care for the IV or peripherally inserted central catheter (PICC) site, ensuring that all supplies are available to the patient discharged to home
  3. The importance of good personal and oral hygiene, such as using a soft toothbrush, brushing the teeth twice each day, and rinsing the mouth with water after brushing
  4. To avoid the use of dental irrigation devices and dental floss
  5. To inform health care providers and dentists about the history of endocarditis so that prophylactic antibiotics are given before treatment

ENDOMETRIOSIS

OVERVIEW

- Endometriosis occurs when the endometrial (inner uterine) tissue implants *outside* the uterine cavity, most commonly on the ovaries and the cul-de-sac (posterior rectovaginal wall) and less commonly on other pelvic organs and structures.
- This tissue responds to cyclic hormonal stimulation just as if it were in the uterus.
- Monthly cyclic bleeding occurs at the site of implantation, where it is trapped, causing pain, irritation, scarring, and adhesion formation in the surrounding tissue.
- When endometriosis is on an ovary, a *chocolate cyst* (endometrioma) can form.
- The cause of endometriosis is unknown.
- The disorder is most often found in women during their reproductive years and can lead to infertility.

INTERPROFESSIONAL COLLABORATIVE CARE

Assessment: Noticing

- Obtain patient information about:
  1. Menstrual history, sexual history, and bleeding characteristics
  2. Pain, which is the most common symptom of endometriosis

3. Dyspareunia (painful sexual intercourse)
4. Painful defecation
5. Low backache
6. Infertility
7. GI disturbances
- Assess for and document:
  1. Pelvic tenderness
  2. Tender nodules in the posterior vagina and limited movement of the uterus
  3. Anxiety because of uncertainty about the diagnosis and potential infertility
- Diagnostic studies may include tests to rule out other diagnoses such as:
  1. Pelvic inflammatory disease (PID) caused by chlamydia or gonorrhea
  2. Ovarian cancer detected by serum cancer antigen CA 125
  3. Pelvic masses detected by transvaginal ultrasound
  4. Laparoscopy and biopsy to determine endometrial tissue typing

Interventions: Responding
NONSURGICAL MANAGEMENT
- Hormonal contraceptives for cycle control
- Heatpacks, relaxation techniques, yoga, and biofeedback to improve blood flow to painful areas
- Calcium and magnesium may relieve muscle cramping for some patients.

SURGICAL MANAGEMENT
- Surgical management of endometriosis with laser therapy through laparoscopy removes the implants and adhesions, allowing the woman to remain fertile.
- In women with intractable pain, severing a pelvic nerve may provide relief.
- If the patient does not wish to have children, the uterus and ovaries may be removed.
- Nursing care is similar to that for a woman undergoing a vaginal hysterectomy (see *Surgical Management* under *Leiomyomas, Uterine*).

 END-OF-LIFE CARE: COMFORT CONCEPT EXEMPLAR

OVERVIEW
- Although dying is part of the normal life cycle, it is often feared as a time of pain and suffering.
- **Palliative care** is a philosophy of care for people with life-threatening disease that assists patients and families in identifying their outcomes for care, assists them with informed decision making, and facilitates quality symptom management.
  1. Palliation is the relief or management of symptoms, particularly symptoms that are distressing to the patient or caregivers.

2. Palliative care is associated with positive patient outcomes of restored function, high patient satisfaction, cost reductions in health care, and slowing the progression of disease.
- **End-of-life care** is often used synonymously with **hospice** care.
  1. Hospice care implies a prognosis of 6 months or less; end-of-life care implies weeks to days of life.
  2. Hospice care uses a coordinated, interprofessional approach to focus on quality of life among patients at the end of life and their families. This approach neither hastens nor postpones death; hospice staff provides interventions to meet the needs of a dying patient.
     a. Hospice is considered the model for quality, compassionate care for people facing a life-limiting illness or injury.
     b. Hospice provides expert medical care, pain management, and emotional and spiritual support expressly tailored to the person's needs and wishes.
     c. Support is also provided to the person's loved ones.
- Euthanasia is a term that has been used to describe the process of ending one's life and is intimately tied to ethics.
  1. *Active euthanasia* implies that health care providers take action (e.g., give medication or treatment) that purposefully and directly causes the patient's death. *Active euthanasia, even with the patient's permission, is not supported by most health professional organizations in the United States, including the American Nurses Association.*
  2. *Physician-assisted suicide (PAS),* sometimes referred to as assisted dying, is gaining world-wide public support. PAS is now legally approved in Oregon, Washington, Vermont, Montana, and New Mexico in the U.S. In 2015, Canada's Supreme Court recently overturned a ban on PAS.
  3. *Withdrawing or withholding life-sustaining therapy,* formerly called *passive euthanasia,* involves discontinuing one or more therapies that might prolong the life of a person who cannot be cured by the therapy.
  4. A newer concept as the legal alternative method for death in all 50 states is *voluntary stopping of eating and drinking (VSED),* also called *terminal dehydration* (Lachman, 2015). In all cases, the principles of informed consent must be met: the patient is competent, the death is voluntary, and the patient understands the benefit, burden, and consequences of the death.
- *Death* is the cessation of integrated tissue and organ function, manifested by lack of heartbeat, absence of spontaneous respirations, or irreversible brain dysfunction.
- A *good death* is one that is free from avoidable distress and suffering for patients, families, and caregivers, in agreement with

patients' and families' wishes, and consistent with clinical practice standards.

- *Advance directives* are legal documents that detail preferences for health care, including care at the end of life.
    1. Advance directives are instructional "living wills" which identify what one would (or would not) want if the individual is near death.
    2. Some states also have directives referred to as *POLST* (physician orders for life-sustaining treatment), which document additional instructions in case of cardiac or pulmonary arrest.
    3. Advance directives also refer to durable power of attorney for health care documents that establish proxy decision makers when a patient does not have decisional capacity.
    4. The Patient Self-Determination Act of 1990 requires that all patients admitted to any health care agency be asked if they have advance directives.

INTERPROFESSIONAL COLLABORATIVE CARE
Assessment: Noticing
1. Assess distressing symptom(s) by intensity, frequency, duration, quality, and exacerbating (worsening) and relieving factors.
2. Use a consistent method for rating the intensity of symptoms to facilitate ongoing assessments and evaluate treatment response.
3. Assess and document the effects of an intervention on distress and comfort.

Interventions: Responding
- The desired outcomes for a patient with distressing symptoms are that the patient will have:
    1. Needs and preferences met
    2. Control of symptoms of distress
    3. Meaningful interactions with family or friends
    4. A peaceful death

MANAGING SYMPTOMS OF DISTRESS
Manage Pain
1. Assess distressing symptom(s) by intensity, frequency, duration, quality, and exacerbating (worsening) and relieving factors.
2. Use a consistent method for rating the intensity of symptoms to facilitate ongoing assessments and evaluate treatment response.
3. Both nonopioid and opioid analgesics play a role in pain management.
4. Complementary and integrative health concepts are often integrated into the pain management plan.
    a. Massage
    b. Music therapy
    c. Therapeutic touch

   d. Aromatherapy with lavender, capsicum, bergamot, chamomile, rose, ginger, rosemary, lemongrass, sage, and camphor

Manage Weakness
1. For palliation, collaborate with physical and occupational therapists to reduce energy expenditure and maintain muscle strength and integrity.
2. For patients at end-of-life, consider bed rest to avoid falls and injuries.
3. Weakness combined with decreased neurologic function may impair the ability to swallow (dysphagia).
4. For palliative care, consult with speech-language pathologist to improve swallowing ability.
5. For end-of-life care, limit oral intake and teach families about the risk for aspiration; with great sensitivity, reinforce that having no appetite or desire for food or fluids is expected.

E

! NURSING SAFETY PRIORITY: Patient-Centered Care

Dysphagia near death presents a problem for oral drug therapy. Although some tablets may be crushed, drugs such as sustained-release capsules should not be taken apart. Reassess the need for each medication. Collaborate with the prescriber about discontinuing drugs that are not needed to control pain, dyspnea, agitation, nausea, vomiting, cardiac workload, or seizures. In collaboration with a pharmacist experienced in palliation, identify alternative routes and/or alternative drugs to promote COMFORT and maintain control of symptoms. Choose the least invasive route such as oral, buccal mucosa (inside cheek), transdermal (via the skin), or rectal. Some oral drugs can be given rectally. Depending on the patient needs, the subcutaneous or IV routes may be used if access is available. The intramuscular route is almost never used at the end of life because it is considered painful and drug distribution varies among patients.

Manage Breathlessness/Dyspnea
1. Perform a thorough assessment of the patient's dyspnea.
   a. Include onset, severity (e.g., 0-to-10 scale), and precipitating factors.
   b. Precipitating factors may include time of day, position, anxiety, pain, cough, or emotional distress.
2. Providing oxygen therapy may relieve dyspnea, especially with activity. Collaborate with the respiratory therapist to determine the need for home oxygen when Spo_2 is consistently less than 90%.

3. Administer drug therapy including:
   a. *Bronchodilators,* such as albuterol (Proventil) or ipratropium bromide (Atrovent, Apo-Ipravent) via a metered dose inhaler (MDI) or nebulizer, may be given for symptoms of bronchospasm (heard as wheezes).
   b. *Corticosteroids,* such as prednisone (Deltasone, Winpred), may be given for bronchospasm and inflammatory problems.
   c. *Diuretics,* such as furosemide (Lasix, Uritol) may be given to decrease blood volume, reduce vascular congestion, and reduce the workload of the heart for dyspnea from heart failure.
   d. *Antibiotics* may be indicated for dyspnea related to a respiratory infection.
   e. *Opioids such as morphine sulfate are the standard treatment for dyspnea near death.* They work by:
      1. Altering the perception of air hunger by reducing anxiety and associated oxygen consumption
      2. Reducing pulmonary congestion.
   g. Loud, wet respirations (referred to as **death rattle**) are disturbing to family and caregivers even when they do not seem to cause dyspnea. They managed with *anticholinergics,* such as atropine (ophthalmic) solution 1% given sublingually every 4 hours as needed or hyoscyamine (Levsin) every 6 hours, are commonly given to dry up secretions.
4. Provide nonpharmacologic interventions including:
   a. Limiting exertion to avoid exertional dyspnea
   b. Insertion of a long-term urinary (Foley) catheter to avoid dyspnea on exertion
   c. Positioning the patient with the head of the bed up either in a hospital bed or a reclining chair to increase chest expansion
   d. Applying wet cloths to the patient's face
   e. Encouraging imagery and deep breathing

Manage Nausea and Vomiting
1. Assess for bowel obstruction and constipation.
   a. If constipation is identified as the cause of nausea and vomiting, give the patient a biphosphate enema (e.g., Fleet) to remove stool quickly.
2. Administer antiemetic agents such as ondansetron (Zofran), dexamethasone (Decadron, Deronil, Dexasone), or metoclopramide (Reglan, Maxeran).
3. Aromatherapy using chamomile, camphor, fennel, lavender, peppermint, and rose may reduce or relieve vomiting. Some patients, however, may have worse nausea with aroma. Ask the patient and family about preferences.

Manage Agitation and Delirium

1. Asses for pain or urinary retention, constipation, or another reversible cause.
2. Administer an antipsychotic to calm the agitated patient; stop the drug as soon as possible.

❗ NURSING SAFETY PRIORITY: Drug Alert

Do not give the patient more than one antipsychotic drug at a time because of the risk for adverse drug events (ADEs). A neuroleptic drug such as a low dose of haloperidol (Haldol, Peridol) 0.5 to 2 mg orally, IV, subcutaneously, or rectally may be used for agitated, hyperactive delirium to prevent self- or caregiver harm.

3. Music therapy may produce relaxation by quieting the mind and promoting a restful state.
4. Aromatherapy with chamomile may also help overcome anxiety, anger, tension, stress, and insomnia.

Manage Seizures

1. Assess risk for or occurrence of seizure at end of life; seizure may occur in patients with brain tumors, advanced AIDS, and pre-existing seizure disorders.
2. Benzodiazepines, such as diazepam (Valium) and lorazepam (Ativan), are the drugs of choice and can be given as a rectal gel or sublingual solution.

Manage Refractory Symptoms of Distress at End of Life

1. Drug therapy for symptoms of distress at end of life is guided by protocols, using medications believed to be safe, with the intent of alleviating suffering.
2. *There is no evidence that administering medications for symptoms of distress using established protocols hastens deaths.*
3. The ethical responsibility of the nurse in caring for patients near death is to follow guidelines for drug use to manage symptoms and to facilitate prompt and effective symptom management until death.

MEET PSYCHOSOCIAL NEEDS

1. Use a spiritual assessment tool to identify sources of strength and support. One strategy is to use the classic HOPE mnemonic as a guide:

   H: Sources of hope and strength
   O: Organized religion (if any) and role that it plays in one's life
   P: Personal spirituality, rituals, and practices
   E: Effects of religion and spirituality on care and end-of-life decisions

2. Regardless of whether a person has had an affiliation with a religion or a belief in God or other Supreme Being, he or she can experience what is referred to as *spiritual* or *existential distress.*
   a. Existential distress is brought about by the actual or perceived threat to one's continued existence.
3. Acknowledge the patient's spiritual pain, and encourage verbalization.
4. Provide opportunity for uninterrupted time with family members, friends, and other individuals who support the patient's health.
5. Establish and review patient preferences and values regarding quality of life and treatment options.

🌐 Cultural and Spiritual Considerations

Patient-Centered Care

Spirituality is whatever or whoever gives ultimate meaning and purpose in one's life that invites particular ways of being in the world in relation to others, oneself, and the universe. A person's spirituality may or may not include belief in God. **Religions** are formal belief systems that provide a framework for making sense of life, death, and suffering and responding to universal spiritual questions. Religions often have beliefs, rituals, texts, and other practices that are shared by a community. Spirituality and religion can help some patients cope with the thought of death, contributing to quality of life during the dying process.

ASSIST WITH GRIEVING

- Interventions to assist patients and families in grieving and mourning are based on cultural beliefs, values, and practices. Some patients and their families express their grief openly and loudly, whereas others are quiet and reserved.
  1. Provide appropriate emotional support to allow patients and their families to verbalize their fears and concerns.
     a. *Intervene with those grieving an impending death by "being with" as opposed to "being there."* "Being with" implies you are physically and psychologically with the grieving patient, empathizing to provide emotional support. Listening and acknowledging the legitimacy of the patient's and/or family's impending loss are often more therapeutic than speaking; this concept is often referred to as **presence.**
     b. *Do not minimize a patient's or family member's reaction to an impending loss/death.* An example of therapeutic communication might be "This must be very difficult for you" or "I'm sorry this is happening."

    c. *Storytelling through reminiscence and life review can be an important activity for patients who are dying.* **Life review** is a structured process of reflecting on what one has done through their life. This is often facilitated by an interviewer. **Reminiscence** is the process of randomly reflecting on memories of events in one's life.

2. Assess coping ability of the patient and family or other caregiver. Some basic beliefs about dying, death, and afterlife for some of the major religions are described below under the heading *Cultural Considerations*.

- Prepare the family for the patient's death:
  1. Physical manifestations of approaching death
     a. Cold, mottled, discolored extremities
     b. Increased sleeping
     c. Food and fluid decrease
     d. Incontinence
     e. Congestion and gurgling
     f. Breathing pattern change
     g. Disorientation
     h. Restlessness
  2. Emotional manifestations of approaching death
     a. Withdrawal
     b. Vision-like experiences
     c. Letting go
     d. Saying goodbye
  3. Vital signs: anticipate hypotension; slow, fast, or irregular heartbeat; and fast, shallow, or irregular respiratory rate
  4. Signs that death has occurred
     a. Breathing stops
     b. Heart stops beating
     c. Pupils become fixed and dilated
     d. Body color becomes pale and waxen
     e. Body temperature drops
     f. Muscles and sphincters relax
     g. Urine and stool may be released
     h. Eyes may remain open and there is no blinking
     i. Jaw may fall open
     j. Trickling of fluids internally may be heard

🌐 Cultural Considerations

- Death-related beliefs and practices vary by ethnicity, religion, and race.
1. Christianity
   a. There are many Christian denominations, which have variations in beliefs regarding medical care near the end of life.

   b. Roman Catholic tradition encourages individuals to receive the Sacrament of the Sick, administered by a priest at any point during an illness. This sacrament may be administered more than once. Not receiving this sacrament will *not* prohibit them from entering heaven after death.

   c. People may be baptized as Roman Catholics in an emergency situation (e.g., the person is dying) by a layperson. Otherwise, they are baptized by a priest.

   d. Christians believe in an afterlife of heaven or hell once the soul has left the body after death.

2. Judaism

   a. The dying person is encouraged to recite the confessional or the affirmation of faith, called the *Shma*.

   b. According to Jewish law, a person who is extremely ill and dying should not be left alone.

   c. The body, which was the vessel and vehicle to the soul, deserves reverence and respect.

   d. The body should not be left unattended until the funeral, which should take place as soon as possible (preferably within 24 hours).

   e. Orthodox Judaism does not allow autopsies except under special circumstances.

   f. The body should not be embalmed, displayed, or cremated.

3. Islam

   a. Islam is based on belief in one God, Allah, and his prophet, Muhammad. The Qur'an is the scripture of Islam, composed of Muhammad's revelations of the Word of God (Allah).

   b. Death is seen as the beginning of a new and better life.

   c. God has prescribed an appointed time of death for everyone.

   d. The Qur'an encourages humans to seek treatment and not to refuse treatment. The belief is that only Allah cures, but that Allah cures through the work of humans.

   e. Upon death, the eyelids are to be closed and the body should be covered. Before moving and handling the body, contact someone from the person's mosque to perform rituals of bathing and wrapping body in cloth.

🌐 Considerations for Older Adults

Pain relief is often the priority need of older adults and is often underreported and undertreated. Do not withhold opioid drugs from older adults. Instead, reduce starting doses, make dose increases slowly, and monitor for changes in mental status or excessive sedation.

- Provide for the care of the patient after death.
  1. Provide all care with respect to communicate that the person was important and valued.
  2. Notify mortality services and the local organ procurement agency if this step is hospital or agency policy.
  3. Ask the family or significant others if they wish to help wash the patient, comb his or her hair, or otherwise prepare the body.
     a. If no autopsy is planned, remove or cut all tubes and lines according to agency policy.
     b. Determine whether any organs will be donated after death (e.g., bone, corneas, or body for research or education).
     c. Close the patient's eyes.
     d. Insert dentures if the patient wore them.
     e. Straighten the patient and lower the bed to a flat position.
     f. Place waterproof pads under the patient's hips and around the perineum to absorb any excrement.
  4. Allow the family or significant others to see the patient in private and to perform any religious or cultural customs they wish (e.g., prayer).
  5. Ensure that the nurse or physician has completed and signed the death certificate.
  6. Prepare the patient for transfer to either a morgue or funeral home; wrap the patient in a shroud and attach identification tags per agency policy.

EPIDIDYMITIS

OVERVIEW

- *Epididymitis* is an inflammation of the epididymis, which may result from an infectious (most common) or noninfectious source such as trauma.
- Main manifestations include pain along the inguinal canal and along the vas deferens, followed by pain and swelling in the scrotum and the groin.
- It can be a complication of a sexually transmitted disease (STD), such as gonorrhea or chlamydia.
- If untreated, the infection can spread and an abscess may form, requiring an orchiectomy (removal of one or both testes). If both testes are affected, sterility may result.
- Less often, it can be a complication of long-term use of an indwelling urinary catheter, prostatic surgery, or a cystoscopic examination.

INTERPROFESSIONAL COLLABORATIVE CARE

- Obtain patient information about:
  1. Pain along the inguinal canal
  2. Pain and swelling of the scrotum and groin

- Assess for and document:
  1. Pyuria, bacteria
  2. Regional lymph node swelling
  3. Signs of infection such as fever, chills, and elevated WBCs
- Diagnosis is made on the basis of manifestations and a smear or culture of the urine or prostate secretions to identify the causative organism.
- Interventions include:
  1. Drug therapy
     a. Antibiotics
     b. Nonsteroidal anti-inflammatory drugs (NSAIDs) to decrease inflammation and promote comfort
  2. Comfort measures, including:
     a. Elevating or supporting the swollen scrotum (use a jock strap)
     b. Applying cold compresses or ice to the scrotum intermittently
     c. Taking sitz baths
     d. Avoiding lifting, straining, or sexual activity until the infection is under control (which may take as long as 4 weeks)
- The sexual partner should be treated if the infection is caused by a sexually transmitted infection (STI).
- An epididymectomy (excision of the epididymis from the testicle) may be needed if the problem is recurrent or chronic.
- An ultrasound study can rule out an abscess or tumor.

ERECTILE DYSFUNCTION

OVERVIEW

- *Erectile dysfunction* (ED) is the inability to achieve or maintain an erection for sexual intercourse. There are two major types: organic and functional.
- *Organic ED* is a gradual deterioration of function. The man first notices diminishing firmness and a decrease in frequency of erections. Causes include:
  1. Inflammation of the prostate, urethra, or seminal vesicles
  2. Surgical procedures such as prostatectomy
  3. Pelvic fractures
  4. Lumbosacral injuries
  5. Vascular disease, including hypertension
  6. Chronic neurologic conditions, such as Parkinson's disease or multiple sclerosis
  7. Endocrine disorders, such as diabetes mellitus or thyroid disorders
  8. Smoking and alcohol consumption
  9. Drugs
  10. Poor overall health that prevents sexual intercourse

- *Functional ED* usually has a psychological cause. Men with functional ED have normal nocturnal (nighttime) and morning erections. Onset is usually sudden and proceeded by a period of high stress.

INTERPROFESSIONAL COLLABORATIVE CARE

- Assess the medical, social, and sexual history to help determine the cause of ED.
- Hormone testing is used for patients who have a poor libido, small testicles, or sparse beard growth.
- Duplex Doppler ultrasonography may be performed to determine the adequacy of arterial and venous blood flow to the penis.

Nonsurgical Management

- Functional ED is managed by sexual counseling and drugs that increase penile blood flow.
- Nonsurgical management of organic ED may include:
  1. Drug therapy to improve penile blood flow, phosphodiesterace-5 (PDE-5) inhibitors such as:
     a. Sildenafil (Viagra)
     b. Vardenafil (Levitra)
     c. Tadalafil (Cialis)

! NURSING SAFETY PRIORITY: Drug Alert

Instruct patients taking PDE-5 inhibitors to abstain from alcohol before sexual intercourse because it may impair the ability to have an erection. Common side effects of these drugs include dyspepsia (heartburn), headaches, facial flushing, and stuffy nose. If more than one pill a day is being taken, leg and back cramps, nausea, and vomiting also may occur. *Teach men who take nitrates to avoid these drugs because the vasodilation effects can cause a profound hypotension and reduce blood flow to vital organs.* For patients who cannot take these drugs or do not respond to them, other methods are available to achieve an erection.

  2. Vacuum devices
     a. A vacuum device is a cylinder that fits over the penis, and a vacuum is created with a pump. The vacuum draws blood into the penis to maintain an erection.
     b. The advantage of this procedure is that the device is easy and safe to use regardless of what drugs the patient may be taking.
  3. Intracorporal injections
     a. Vasoconstrictive drugs can be injected directly into the penis to reduce blood outflow and make the penis erect.

b. Common agents are papaverine, phentolamine (Regitine), and alprostadil.
c. Adverse effects include priapism (prolonged erection), penile scarring, fibrosis, bleeding, bruising at the injection site, pain, infection, and vasovagal responses.

Surgical Management

- Penile implants can be surgically placed when other modalities fail. Devices include semirigid, malleable, or hydraulic inflatable and multicomponent or one-piece instruments.
- Advantages include the man's ability to control his erections.
- The major disadvantages include device failure and infection.

ESOPHAGEAL TUMORS: NUTRITION CONCEPT EXEMPLAR

OVERVIEW

- Esophageal tumors can be benign but most are malignant (cancerous).
- Esophageal tumors grow rapidly because there is no serosal layer to limit their extension. Because the esophageal mucosa is richly supplied with lymph tissue, there is early spread of tumors to lymph nodes.
- Risk factors for development of esophageal tumors are smoking, obesity, excessive alcohol intake, and untreated gastrointestinal reflux disease (GERD) leading to Barrett's esophagus, a condition of cell dysplasia (abnormal cell growth) from exposure to acid and pepsin.

INTERPROFESSIONAL COLLABORATIVE CARE

Assessment: Noticing

- Assess for risk factors related to the development of esophageal tumors
  1. Primary risk factors associated with the development of esophageal cancer are smoking and obesity.
- Assess for signs and symptoms, including:
  1. Dysphagia (difficulty swallowing)
  2. Odynophagia (painful swallowing)
  3. Regurgitation or vomiting
  4. Halitosis (foul breath) and chronic hiccups
  5. Chronic cough, increased oropharyngeal or respiratory secretions
  6. Hoarseness when tumors in the upper esophagus involve the larynx
- Psychosocial concerns around choking (anxiety) and other distressing symptoms, including decreased pleasure and social support around meal time when eating is not easy or possible
- Consider the results of common diagnostic tests, including:
  1. Barium swallow study with fluoroscopy
  2. Esophageal ultrasound (EUS) with fine needle aspiration to examine the tumor tissue

3. Esophagogastroduodenoscopy (EGD) may be performed to inspect the esophagus and obtain tissue specimens for cell studies and disease staging.

Analysis: Interpreting

- The most specific common problem for patients with esophageal cancer is potential for compromised nutrition due to impaired swallowing and possible metastasis.

Planning and Implementation: Responding

PROMOTE NUTRITION

- Interventions to maintain or improve nutrition status focus on treatments that remove or shrink the obstructive tumor. Methods to reduce the effects of treatment that can impact nutrition are also a priority. Surgery is the most definitive intervention for esophageal cancer.

NONSURGICAL MANAGEMENT

- Promote nutrition to maintain weight, caloric, and protein goals in collaboration with the dietician
- Provide semisoft and thickened liquids because they are easier to swallow
- Consult with speech-language pathologist (SLP) for swallowing therapy
- Consult with the occupational therapist for feeding therapy

❗ NURSING SAFETY PRIORITY: Critical Rescue

When the patient with an esophageal tumor is eating or drinking, recognize that you must monitor for signs and symptoms of aspiration, such as choking or coughing. Food aspiration can cause airway obstruction, pneumonia, or both, especially in older adults. In coordination with the SLP, teach family members and caregivers how to feed the patient, if needed. Teach them how to monitor for aspiration and how to respond quickly to implement appropriate measures if choking occurs.

- Anticipate that chemotherapy, targeted therapy, or radiation will be used to shrink the tumor. These treatments are further described under *Cancer*, in this section.
- Photodynamic therapy (PDT) is used as a palliative treatment for patients with advanced esophageal cancer who are not candidates for surgery.
- Esophageal dilation may be performed as necessary throughout the course of the disease to achieve temporary but immediate relief of dysphagia.

SURGICAL MANAGEMENT

- The purposes of surgical resection vary from palliation to cure.
- Esophagectomy is the removal of all or part of the esophagus.

- Esophagogastrostomy involves the removal of part of the esophagus and proximal stomach.
- A jejunostomy tube may be placed for postoperative enteral feeding.
- Preoperative nursing care focuses on teaching and on psychological support regarding the surgical procedure and preoperative and postoperative instructions.
- The patient requires intensive postoperative care and is at risk for multiple serious complications.
  1. Keep the postoperative patient in a semi-Fowler's or high-Fowler's position to support ventilation and prevent reflux.
  2. Monitor for symptoms of fluid overload and dehydration.
  3. Monitor for atrial fibrillation that results from irritation of the vagus nerve during surgery.
  4. Monitor for wound healing and anastomotic leak for as long as 10 days after surgery.

! NURSING SAFETY PRIORITY: Action Alert

Respiratory care is the highest postoperative priority for patients having an esophagectomy. For those who had traditional surgery, intubation with mechanical ventilation is needed for at least the first 16 to 24 hours. Pulmonary complications include atelectasis and pneumonia. The risk for postoperative pulmonary complications is increased in the patient who has received preoperative radiation. Once the patient is extubated, begin deep breathing, turning, and coughing every 1 to 2 hours. Assess the patient for decreased breath sounds and shortness of breath every 1 to 2 hours. Provide incisional support and adequate analgesia for effective coughing.

Care Coordination and Transition Management
- Treatment for esophageal tumors can have long-lasting fatigue and weakness; help the patient to plan for sequencing activities of daily living to reflect reduced energy.
- Assess resources for follow-up care such as transportation for radiation and chemotherapy.
- Consider home health services to promote ongoing respiratory care if the patient is at high risk for aspiration.
- Teach the patient or family to immediately report to the health care provider the presence of fever and a swollen, painful neck incision.
- Discuss strategies for ongoing nutrition support, including weight monitoring.

F

FATIGUE SYNDROME, CHRONIC
OVERVIEW
Chronic fatigue syndrome (CFS), also known as *chronic fatigue and immune dysfunction syndrome* (CFIDS), is characterized by severe fatigue for 6 months or longer, usually following flu-like symptoms.
* For a diagnosis of CFS, four or more of the following criteria must be met:
  1. Sore throat
  2. Substantial impairment in short-term memory or concentration
  3. Tender lymph nodes
  4. Muscle pain
  5. Multiple joint pain with redness or swelling
  6. Headaches of a new type, pattern, or severity (not familiar to the patient)
  7. Unrefreshing sleep
  8. Postexertional malaise lasting more than 24 hours
* There is no test to confirm the disorder, and the cause is unknown.

INTERPROFESSIONAL COLLABORATIVE CARE
* Management is supportive and focuses on alleviation or reduction of symptoms.
  1. Nonsteroidal anti-inflammatory drugs (NSAIDs) for body aches and pain
  2. Low-dose antidepressants for alleviating symptoms and promoting sleep
  3. Teaching the patient to follow healthy practices
     a. Adequate sleep
     b. Proper nutrition
     c. Regular exercise (but not excessive enough to increase fatigue)
     d. Stress management
     e. Energy conservation
     f. Use of complementary and alternative therapies that include acupuncture, tai chi, massage, and herbal supplements
* Refer the patient to support groups and reputable Internet sites for information and web-based support.

FIBROMYALGIA SYNDROME
OVERVIEW
* Fibromyalgia syndrome (FMS) is a chronic pain syndrome not an inflammatory disease.

- Pain, stiffness, and tenderness can be accompanied by numbness, tingling, severe fatigue, and sleep disturbances.
- Pain and tenderness (called trigger points) are located at specific sites at the back of the neck, upper chest, trunk, low back, and extremities and can be palpated to elicit pain in a predictable, reproducible pattern.
- Secondary FMS can accompany any connective tissue disease, particularly lupus and rheumatoid disease.
- Other signs symptoms include:
  1. Gastrointestinal (GI) disturbances, including abdominal pain, diarrhea and constipation, and heartburn
  2. Genitourinary manifestations, including dysuria, urinary frequency, urgency, and pelvic pain
  3. Cardiovascular symptoms, including dyspnea, chest pain, and dysrhythmias
  4. Visual disturbances, including blurred vision and dry eyes
  5. Neurologic symptoms, including forgetfulness and concentration problems

INTERPROFESSIONAL COLLABORATIVE CARE
- Management includes:
  1. Antidepressant drugs approved for fibromyalgia nerve pain (e.g., duloxetine [Cymbalta], nilnacipran (Savella); amitriptyline [Elavil, Apo-Amitriptyline], trazodone [Desyrel], or nortriptyline [Pamelor])
  2. Antiseizure drugs used to manage chronic neuropathic pain like gabapentin (Neurontin) or pregabalin (Lyrica)
  3. Physical therapy and regular exercise, which includes stretching, strengthening, and low-impact aerobic exercise
  4. Complementary and alternative therapies, such as tai chi, acupuncture, hypnosis, and stress management, may help some patients with symptom relief.

FLAIL CHEST

OVERVIEW
- Flail chest is the inward movement of the thorax during inspiration, with outward movement during expiration, usually involving only one side of the chest.
- It results from two neighboring ribs broken in two or more places, leaving a segment of the chest wall loose.
- Flail chest often occurs with blunt trauma from high-speed vehicular crashes. Another cause is bilateral separations of the ribs from their cartilage connections without an actual rib fracture during cardiopulmonary resuscitation (CPR).
- Gas exchange, the ability to cough, and the ability to clear secretions are impaired.

INTERPROFESSIONAL COLLABORATIVE CARE
Assessment: Noticing
- Assess the patient for and document:
  1. Paradoxical chest movement ("sucking inward" of the loose chest area during inspiration and a "puffing out" of the same area during expiration)
  2. Pain
  3. Dyspnea
  4. Cyanosis
  5. Tachycardia
  6. Hypotension

Interventions: Responding
  1. Humidified oxygen
  2. Pain management
  3. Promotion of lung expansion through deep breathing and positioning
  4. Secretion clearance by coughing and tracheal aspiration
  5. Psychosocial support
  6. Intubation with mechanical ventilation and positive end-expiratory pressure (PEEP)
  7. Surgical stabilization (only in extreme cases of flail chest)
- Monitor the patient's:
  1. Vital signs, oxygen saturation, and arterial blood gases
  2. Fluid and electrolyte balance
  3. Central venous pressure

FLUID OVERLOAD

OVERVIEW
- Fluid overload, also called *overhydration,* is an excess of body fluid.
- It is a clinical sign of a problem in which fluid intake or retention is greater than the body's fluid needs.
- The most common type of fluid overload is hypervolemia because the problems result from excessive fluid in the extracellular fluid (ECF) space.
  1. Most problems caused by fluid overload are related to fluid volume excess in the vascular space or to dilution of specific electrolytes and blood components.
  2. Causes of fluid overload are related to excessive intake or inadequate excretion of fluid and include:
     a. Excessive fluid replacement
     b. Kidney failure (late phase)
     c. Heart failure
     d. Long-term corticosteroid therapy
     e. Syndrome of inappropriate antidiuretic hormone (SIADH)

  f. Psychiatric disorders with polydipsia
  g. Water intoxication

INTERPROFESSIONAL COLLABORATIVE CARE
Assessment: Noticing
 1. Assess the patient for and document:
  a. Skin and mucous membrane changes
  b. Pitting edema occurs in dependent areas and joints and skin around bony prominences (ankles, elbows, metacarpals, metatarsals).
  c. Skin is pale and cool to touch; skin and puncture sites from needle sticks may "weep" as fluid tries to escape through the skin.
 2. Cardiovascular changes
  a. Bounding pulse quality
  b. Elevated blood pressure
  c. Decreased pulse pressure
  d. Elevated central venous pressure and distended neck veins
  e. Weight gain
 3. Respiratory changes
  a. Tachypnea (increased respiratory rate)
  b. Shallow respirations
  c. Dyspnea (shortness of breath) that increases with exertion or in the supine position
  d. Moist crackles present on auscultation
  e. Decreased peripheral oxygenation (SpO_2)
 4. Neuromuscular changes
  a. Altered level of consciousness
  b. Headache
  c. Visual disturbances
  d. Skeletal muscle weakness
  e. Paresthesias
 5. GI changes
  a. Increased motility
  b. Enlarged liver
 6. Laboratory tests
  a. Normal serum electrolytes (or slightly low sodium)
  b. Decreased hemoglobin and hematocrit from dilution
  c. Low serum protein levels may contribute to fluid overload or be the result of fluid overload.
Interventions: Responding
RESTORE NORMAL FLUID BALANCE
 1. Assess particularly for symptoms of pulmonary edema and heart failure that may indicate a need for increased surveillance or additional interventions.

2. Collaborate with health care team members to set daily intake (restriction) and output goals and inform the physician when goals are at risk for not being met.

! NURSING SAFETY PRIORITY: Critical Rescue

Assess the patient with fluid overload at least every 2 hours to recognize pulmonary edema, which can occur very quickly and can lead to death. If indications of worsening fluid overload are present (bounding pulse, increasing neck vein distention, presence of crackles in lungs, increasing peripheral edema, reduced urine output), respond by notify the health care provider.

1. Provide drug therapy
   a. High-ceiling (loop) diuretics, such as furosemide (Lasix, Furoside)
   b. If there is concern that too much sodium and other electrolytes would be lost using loop diuretics or if the patient has SIADH, conivaptan (Vaprisol) or tolvaptan (Samsca) may be prescribed.
2. Monitor patient for response to restricted fluid or sodium intake and drug therapy, especially weight loss and increased urine output.
3. Observe for manifestations of electrolyte imbalance.
   a. Changes in electrocardiographic patterns
   b. Changes in sodium and potassium values
4. Collaborate with the dietitian to meet fluid and sodium restriction goals.

PREVENT INJURY
- Reduce the risk for pressure ulcers in patients with edema by using a pressure-reducing or pressure-relieving overlay on the mattress and over bony prominences (e.g., heel protectors, padding at elastic bands for holding oxygen delivery devices in place).
- Assess skin pressure areas, especially the coccyx, elbows, hips, and heels, daily for signs of redness or open areas and document findings.
- Assist the patient to change positions at least every 2 hours.

FOOD POISONING

OVERVIEW
- Food poisoning is caused by ingestion of infectious organisms in food. Unlike gastroenteritis, food poisoning is not directly communicable from person to person and incubation periods are shorter.

- Prevention occurs with good handwashing and properly handling and processing food. Food poisoning is caused by over 250 pathogens.
- Examples of food poisoning are:
  1. Staphylococcal food poisoning
     a. *Staphylococcus* grows in meats and dairy products and can be transmitted by human carriers.
     b. Symptoms of staphylococcal infection include abrupt onset of vomiting, diarrhea, and abdominal cramping, usually 2 to 4 hours after the ingestion of contaminated food.
     c. The diagnosis is made when stool culture yields 100,000 enterotoxin-producing staphylococci.
     d. Treatment includes oral or IV fluids if the fluid volume is grossly depleted.
  2. *Escherichia coli* infection
     a. Some strains cause disease by making a substance called *Shiga toxin*. The bacteria that make these substances are called *Shiga toxin-producing E. coli,* or STEC for short. Enterohemorrhagic strains of *E. coli* (EHEC) and STEC can cause serious complications, such as hemorrhagic colitis and hemolytic-uremic syndrome.
     b. Symptoms include vomiting, diarrhea, abdominal cramping, and fever.
     c. Treatment includes IV fluids.
  3. Botulism
     a. Botulism is a severe, life-threatening food poisoning associated with a high mortality rate; it is most commonly acquired from improperly processed canned foods.
     b. The incubation period is 18 to 36 hours, and the illness may be mild or severe.
     c. *Clostridium botulinum* enters the bloodstream from the intestines and causes symptoms of diplopia, dysphagia, dysphonia, respiratory muscle paralysis, nausea, vomiting, and diarrhea or constipation.
     d. The diagnosis is made by the history and stool culture revealing *C. botulinum;* the serum may be positive for toxins.
     e. Treatment of botulism includes trivalent botulism antitoxin (types A, B, and E), stomach lavage, IV fluids, and tracheostomy with mechanical ventilation if respiratory paralysis occurs.

! NURSING SAFETY PRIORITY: Action Alert

To prevent botulism, teach patients the importance of discarding cans of food that are punctured or swollen or with defective seals. Remind them to check for expiration dates and to not use any canned food that has expired. Containers for home-canned foods must be sterilized by boiling for 20 minutes to destroy *C. botulinum* spores before canning.

4. Salmonellosis
   a. *Salmonellosis* is a bacterial infection; its incubation is 8 to 48 hours after ingestion of contaminated food or drink.
   b. Symptoms last 3 to 5 days and include fever, nausea, vomiting, cramping abdominal pain, and severe diarrhea, which may be bloody.
   c. Diagnosis is made by stool culture.
   d. Treatment is based on symptoms; antibiotics are used if the patient becomes bacteremic.
   e. *Salmonellosis* can be transmitted by the *five Fs: F*lies, *F*ingers, *F*ood, *F*eces, and *F*omites; strict handwashing is essential to avoid transmission.

 FRACTURE: MOBILITY CONCEPT EXEMPLAR   **F**

OVERVIEW

- A fracture is a break or disruption in the continuity of a bone and often results in impaired MOBILITY and pain.
- Fractures are identified by the extent of the break.
  1. *Complete fracture:* The break is across the entire width of the bone in such a way that the bone is divided into two distinct sections.
  2. *Incomplete fracture:* The fracture does not divide the bone into two portions because the break is through only part of the bone.
- Fractures are also described by the extent of associated soft-tissue damage.
  1. A *simple fracture* does not extend through the skin and therefore has no visible wound.
  2. An *open (compound) fracture* has a disrupted skin surface that causes an external wound.
- Fractures are also described by their cause.
  1. *Pathologic (spontaneous) fractures* occur after minimal trauma to a bone that has been weakened by disease.
  2. *Fatigue (stress) fractures* result from excessive strain and stress on the bone.
  3. *Compression fractures* are produced by a loading force applied to the long axis of cancellous bone.
- Bone healing occurs in five stages.
  1. Stage 1 occurs within 24 to 72 hours after the injury, with hematoma formation at the site of the fracture.

2. Stage 2 occurs in 3 days to 2 weeks, when granulation tissue begins to invade the hematoma, stimulating the formation of fibrocartilage.
3. Stage 3 of bone healing usually occurs within 2 to 6 weeks as a result of vascular and cellular proliferation. The fracture site is surrounded by new vascular tissue known as a *callus* that begins the nonbony union.
4. Stage 4 usually takes 3 to 8 weeks as the callus is gradually resorbed and transformed into bone.
5. Stage 5 consists of bone consolidation and remodeling. This stage can continue for up to 1 year.

- Bone healing requires adequate nutrition, especially calcium, phosphorus, vitamin D, and protein.

Considerations for Older Adults Patient-Centered Care

Bone healing is often affected by the aging process. Bone formation and strength rely on adequate nutrition. Calcium, phosphorus, vitamin D, and protein are necessary for the production of new bone. For women, the loss of estrogen after menopause decreases the body's ability to form new bone tissue. Chronic diseases can also affect the rate at which bone heals. For instance, peripheral vascular diseases, such as arteriosclerosis, reduce arterial circulation to bone. Thus the bone receives less oxygen and fewer nutrients, both of which are needed for repair.

- Acute complications of fractures include:
  1. *Acute compartment syndrome* (ACS) is a serious condition in which increased pressure within one or more tissue compartments causes massive compromise of circulation to the area. The most common sites for the problem in patients experiencing musculoskeletal trauma are the compartments in the lower leg and forearm. Edema fluid forms and is trapped within the compartment pressing on nerves (causing pain) and blood vessels, preventing adequate tissue perfusion and oxygenation. Without treatment, ACS can lead to infection, loss of motor function, contracture formation, and release of myoglobin, leading to renal failure. Treatment is by surgical fasciotomy.

❗ NURSING SAFETY PRIORITY: Critical Rescue

Acute kidney injury from muscle breakdown (rhabdomyolysis) is a potentially fatal complication of compartment syndrome. It occurs when large or multiple compartments are involved. Injured muscle tissues release myoglobin (muscle protein) into the circulation, where it can clog the renal tubules. Report oliguria and discolored urine; both are signs of rhabdomyolysis and acute kidney injury.

2. *Crush syndrome* (CS) results from an external crush injury that compresses one or more compartments in the leg, arm, or pelvis. It is a potentially life-threatening, systemic complication that results from hemorrhage and edema after a severe fracture injury. Management involves early recognition and IV fluids.

3. *Hypovolemic and hemorrhagic shock*: Bone is very vascular. Therefore bleeding is a risk with bone injury. In addition, trauma can cut nearby arteries and cause hemorrhage, resulting in rapidly developing hypovolemic shock.

4. *Fat embolism syndrome* (FES) is a serious complication in which fat globules are released from the yellow bone marrow into the bloodstream within 12 to 48 hours after an injury. These emboli clog small blood vessels that supply vital organs, most commonly the lungs, and impair organ perfusion. FES usually results from long bone fractures and pelvic bone or fracture repair, but it is occasionally seen in patients who have a total joint replacement. Manifestations include decreased level of consciousness, anxiety, respiratory distress, tachycardia, tachypnea, fever, hemoptysis, and petechiae, a macular, measles-like rash that may appear over the neck, upper arms, or chest and abdomen.

5. *Venous thromboembolism* (VTE) includes deep vein thrombosis (DVT) and pulmonary embolism (PE). It is the most common complication of lower extremity surgery or trauma and the most common fatal complication of musculoskeletal surgery.

6. Infection is possible with fractures because the trauma disrupts the body's defense system. Wound infections may range from superficial skin infections to deep wound abscesses. Osteomyelitis (bone infection) is more common with open fractures when skin integrity is lost and after surgical repair of a fracture.

• Chronic complications of fractures

1. *Ischemic necrosis,* sometimes referred to as *aseptic* or *avascular necrosis* (AVN) or *osteonecrosis,* can occur when the blood supply to the bone is disrupted.

2. *Delayed union* is a fracture that has not healed within 6 months of injury. Some fractures never achieve union; that is, they never completely heal (nonunion). Others heal incorrectly (malunion).

3. *Complex regional pain syndrome (CRPS),* formerly called reflex sympathetic dystrophy (RSD), is a poorly understood

dysfunction of the central and peripheral nervous systems that leads to severe, chronic pain. Genetic factors may play a role in the development of this devastating complication. CRPS most often results from fractures or other traumatic musculoskeletal injury and commonly occurs in the feet and hands.

INTERPROFESSIONAL COLLABORATIVE CARE

Assessment: Noticing
- Obtain patient history, including:
  1. Cause of the fracture
  2. Events leading to the fracture and immediate postinjury care
  3. Drug history, including substance and alcohol abuse
  4. Medical history
  5. Occupation and recreational activities
  6. Nutritional history
- Assess the patient for and document:
  1. Life-threatening complications of the respiratory, cardiovascular, and neurologic systems (priority assessment)
  2. Fracture site:
     a. Change in bone alignment
     b. Neurovascular status (pulse, warmth, movement, and sensation) distal to fracture

---

! NURSING SAFETY PRIORITY: Action Alert

Swelling at the fracture site is rapid and can result in marked neurovascular compromise due to decreased arterial perfusion. Assess skin color and temperature, sensation, mobility, pain, and pulses distal to the fracture site and document. Compare and document differences in extremity circulation, movement, and sensation.

---

  3. Soft-tissue damage: color, width, length, depth, drainage, and appearance of surrounding skin
  4. Amount of overt bleeding
  5. Muscle spasm
- Diagnostic tests for fractures may include:
  1. X-rays
  2. Computed tomography (CT) scanning
  3. Magnetic resonance imaging (MRI)

Analysis: Interpreting
- The priority collaborative problems for patients with fractures include:
  1. Acute pain due to broken bone(s), soft-tissue damage, muscle spasm, and edema

2. Decreased mobility due to pain, muscle spasm, and soft-tissue damage
3. Potential for neurovascular compromise related to impaired tissue perfusion
4. Potential for infection related to a wound caused by an open fracture

Planning and Implementation: Responding

MANAGE ACUTE PAIN

❗ NURSING SAFETY PRIORITY: Critical Rescue

For any patient who experiences trauma in the community, first call 911 and assess for airway, breathing, and circulation (ABCs, or primary survey). Then, provide lifesaving care if needed before being concerned about the fracture.

- After a head-to-toe assessment (secondary survey) and patient stabilization by the prehospital team, pain is managed with IV opioids such as fentanyl, hydromorphone (Dilaudid), or morphine sulfate. Cardiac monitoring for patients older than 50 years is established before drug administration.
- To prevent further tissue damage, reduce pain, and increase circulation, the prehospital or emergency team immobilizes the fracture by splinting.
  1. An air splint or any object or device that extends to the joints above and below the fracture to immobilize it can be used as a **splint**. Sterile gauze is placed loosely over open areas to prevent further contamination of the wound.
  2. In the emergency department (ED), primary health care provider (PHCP) office, or urgent care center, fracture management begins with reduction and immobilization of the fracture while attending to continued pain assessment and management.

NONSURGICAL MANAGEMENT

- Fracture management begins with immobilization of the fracture site and reduction (realignment of the bone ends for proper healing). Generally, rib fractures do not require immobilization with binding or bracing.
  1. *Closed reduction* is the manipulation of the bone ends for realignment while applying a manual pull, or traction, on the bone.
  2. *Splints and orthopedic boots/shoes* may be used to immobilize certain areas of the body, such as the scapula or clavicle or foot and ankle.
  3. *Casts* are rigid devices that immobilize the affected body part while allowing other body parts to move. A cast allows early

mobility, correction of deformity, prevention of deformity, and reduction of pain.

  a. The most common cast material is fiberglass.

  b. Special considerations for casts include:

    (1) Arm cast

      i. When a patient is in bed, elevate the arm above the heart to reduce swelling; the hand should be higher than the elbow.

      ii. When the patient is out of bed, support the arm with a sling placed around the neck so that the weight is distributed over a large area of the shoulders and trunk, not just the neck.

    (2) A leg cast may require the patient to use an ambulatory aid.

      i. A boot may be removed for hygiene but should be in place for all weight bearing.

      ii. Elevate the affected leg on pillows when the patient is in bed or in a chair to reduce swelling.

4. Splint or brace

  a. A brace is more typical treatment for neck or vertebral fracture.

  b. A splint may be used to immobilize the wrist during part of the day to keep the extremity in a neutral position.

- Cast care involves:

1. Ensuring that the cast is not too tight by inserting a finger between the cast and the skin

2. Notifying the health care provider when the cast is too tight so that it can be cut with a cast cutter to relieve pressure or allow tissue swelling; the cast may be bivalve (cut lengthwise into two equal pieces) if bone healing is almost complete. Either half of the cast can be removed for inspection or for provision of care. The two halves are then held in place by an elastic bandage wrap.

3. Inspecting the cast daily for drainage, alignment, and fit:

  a. Describing and documenting any drainage on the cast in the medical record

  b. Notifying the health care provider immediately about any sudden increases in the amount of drainage or change in the integrity of the cast

4. Assessing for and reporting complications from injury, casting, or immobility:

  a. Infection

  b. Circulation impairment

  c. Peripheral nerve damage

  d. Skin breakdown

  e. Pneumonia or atelectasis

  f. Thromboembolism

- *Traction* is the application of a pulling force to a part of the body to provide reduction, alignment, and rest. It is also used to decrease muscle spasm and prevent or correct deformity and tissue damage.
  1. Types of traction
     a. *Skin traction* involves the use of a Velcro boot (Buck's traction), belt, or halter securely placed around a body part to decrease painful muscle spasms. Weight is limited to 5 to 10 pounds (2.3 to 4.5 kg) to prevent injury to the skin.
     b. *Skeletal traction* uses pins, wires, tongs, or screws that are surgically inserted directly into bone to allow the use of longer traction time and heavier weights, usually 15 to 30 pounds (6.8 to 13.6 kg). It aids in bone realignment.
  2. Care for the patient in traction includes:
     a. Inspecting the skin at least every 8 hours for signs of irritation or inflammation
     b. Removing (when possible) the belt or boot that is used for skin traction every 8 hours to inspect under the device

! NURSING SAFETY PRIORITY: Action Alert

When patients are in traction, weights usually are not removed without a prescription. They should not be lifted manually or allowed to rest on the floor. Weights should be freely hanging at all times. Teach this important point to UAP on the unit, to other personnel such as those in the radiology department, and to visitors.

     c. Inspecting the points of entry of pins and wires or pin sites for signs of inflammation or infection at least every 8 hours
     d. Following agency policy for pin site care
     e. Checking traction equipment to ensure its proper functioning and inspecting all ropes, knots, and pulleys at least every 8 to 12 hours for loosening, fraying, and positioning
     f. Checking the weight for consistency with the health care provider's prescription
     g. Reporting patient complaints of severe pain from muscle spasm to the health care provider when body realignment fails to reduce the discomfort
     h. Assessing neurovascular status of the affected body part at least every 4 hours and more often if indicated

DRUG THERAPY

- For patients with chronic, severe pain, opioid and nonopioid drugs are alternated or given together to manage pain both centrally in the brain and peripherally at the site of injury.

1. For severe or multiple fractures, patient-controlled analgesia (PCA) with morphine, fentanyl, or hydromorphone (Dilaudid) is used.
2. *Meperidine (Demerol) **should never be used** because it has toxic metabolites that can cause seizures and other complications. Most hospitals no longer use this drug.*
3. Oxycodone and oxycodone with acetaminophen (Percocet) or hydrocodone with acetaminophen (Norco, Vicodin, Lortab) are common oral opioid drugs that are very effective for most patients with fracture pain.
4. NSAIDs are given to decrease associated tissue inflammation; however, they can slow bone healing.

PHYSICAL THERAPY
- Collaborate with the physical therapist (PT) to assist with pain control and edema reduction by using:
  1. Ice/heat packs
  2. Electrical muscle stimulation
  3. Special treatment such as dexamethasone iontophoresis
     a. **Iontophoresis** is a method for absorbing dexamethasone, a synthetic steroid, through the skin near the painful area to decrease inflammation and edema. A small device delivers a minute amount of electricity via electrodes placed on the skin.

MANAGEMENT OF CHRONIC REGIONAL PAIN SYNDROME
- The first priority for managing CRPS is pain relief.
- Nurses play an important role in interprofessional collaborative care, which includes drug therapy and a variety of nonpharmacologic modalities.

SURGICAL MANAGEMENT
- *Open reduction with internal fixation* (ORIF) permits early mobilization. Open reduction allows direct visualization of the fracture site, and internal fixation uses metal pins, screws, rods, plates, or prostheses to immobilize the fracture during healing. An incision is made to gain access to the broken bone and allow implanting one or more devices into bone tissue.
- *External fixation* involves fracture reduction and the percutaneous implantation of pins into the bone. The pins are then held in place by an external metal frame to prevent bone movement but allow patient mobility. A disadvantage of external fixation is the increased risk for pin site infection and osteomyelitis.
- Provide preoperative care and explain if a device or cast will be used after surgery to maintain alignment.
- Provide postoperative care and:
  1. Monitor neurovascular status at least every hour for the first 24 hours after surgery and then as often as agency policy, surgeon preference, and patient condition indicate

2. Communicate neurovascular compromise or other complications urgently to the provider

3. Promote self-management and mobility in collaboration with the physical therapist

- Additional procedures may be needed when surgical repairs are not successful and the bone does not heal (nonunion).

   1. *Electrical bone stimulation* may be noninvasive or invasive. It involves using electrical current stimulators near or into a fracture site. This procedure, when used for about 6 months, has resulted in bone healing for some patients.

   2. *Bone grafting* is the use of bone chips from the patient, a cadaver donor, or a living donor and packing or wiring the chips between the bone ends to facilitate union.

   3. *Low-intensity pulsed ultrasound (Exogen therapy)* involves the application of ultrasound treatments for about 20 minutes each day to the fracture site.

PROMOTE MOBILITY

Many patients with musculoskeletal trauma, including fractures, are referred by their primary health care provider for rehabilitation therapy with a PT (usually for lower extremity injuries) and/or occupational therapist (OT) (usually for upper extremity injuries). The timing for this referral depends on the nature, severity, and treatment modality of the fracture(s) or other musculoskeletal trauma.

- The use of crutches or a walker increases MOBILITY and assists in ambulation.
- The patient may progress to using a walker or cane after crutches.
- *Crutches* are the most commonly used ambulatory aid for many types of lower extremity musculoskeletal trauma (e.g., fractures, sprains, amputations).
- A *walker* is most often used by the older patient who needs additional support for balance.
- A *cane* is sometimes used if the patient needs only minimal support for an affected leg.

PREVENTING AND MONITORING FOR NEUROVASCULAR COMPROMISE

- Perform neurovascular (NV) assessments (also known as "circ checks" or CMS assessments) frequently before and after fracture treatment.
- Patients who have extremity casts, splints with elastic bandage wraps, and ORIF or external fixation are especially at risk for NV compromise.
- If PERFUSION to the distal extremity is impaired, the patient reports impaired COMFORT, impaired MOBILITY, and decreased SENSORY PERCEPTION. If these symptoms are allowed to progress, patients are at risk for ACS.

> **❗ NURSING SAFETY PRIORITY: Critical Rescue**
>
> Monitor for and document early signs of ACS. Assess for the "six Ps" including pain, pressure, paralysis, paresthesia, pallor, and pulselessness (rare or late stage). Pain is increased even with passive motion and may seem out of proportion to the degree of injury. Analgesics that had controlled pain become less effective or noneffective. Numbness and tingling or paresthesias are often one of the first signs of the problem. The affected extremity then becomes pale and cool as a result of decreased arterial perfusion to the affected area. Capillary refill is an important assessment of perfusion but may not be reliable in an older adult because of arterial insufficiency. Losses of movement and function and decreased pulses or pulselessness are late signs of ACS! Fortunately, ACS is not common, but it creates an emergency situation when it does occur.

- If ACS is suspected, notify the primary health care provider immediately, and if possible, implement interventions to relieve the pressure.
- If ACS is verified, the surgeon may perform a fasciotomy, or opening in the fascia, by making an incision through the skin and subcutaneous tissues into the fascia of the affected compartment.

PREVENTING INFECTION
- With open fractures, use aseptic technique for dressing changes.
- *Immediately notify the primary health care provider if you observe inflammation and purulent drainage.*
- For most patients with an open fracture, the primary health care provider prescribes one or more broad-spectrum antibiotics prophylactically and performs surgical débridement of any wounds as soon as possible after the injury. First-generation cephalosporins, clindamycin (Cleocin), and gentamycin are commonly used. In addition to systemic antibiotics, local antibiotic therapy through wound irrigation is commonly prescribed, especially during débridement.

Care Coordination and Transition Management
- Collaborate with the case manager or the discharge planner in the hospital to plan care for the patient with a fracture who is being discharged.

Teamwork and Collaboration: Informatics

Be sure to communicate current status and the plan of care to the health care agency receiving the patient. Ensure all drugs are current and accurate in the record.

- Assess the patient's ability to safely use a wheelchair or ambulatory aid.
- Arrange for a home health care nurse to check that the home is safe and that the patient and family are able to follow the interdisciplinary plan of care.
- Provide verbal and written instructions on the care of bandages, splints, casts, or external fixators.
- Emphasize the importance of follow-up visits with the health care provider and other therapists.
- Teach the patient and family about:
  1. Care of the extremity after removal of the cast
     a. Remove scaly, dead skin carefully by soaking; do not scrub.
     b. Move the extremity carefully. Expect discomfort, weakness, and decreased range of motion (ROM).
     c. Support the extremity with pillows or an orthotic device until strength and movement return.
     d. Exercise as instructed by the physical therapist.
  2. Wound assessment and dressing
  3. Recognition of complications and when and where to seek professional health care if complications occur

FRACTURES OF SPECIFIC SITES

- *Nose:* Bone or cartilage displacement typically associated with traumatic injury. Management is usually a closed reduction within 6 hours of injury.

! NURSING SAFETY PRIORITY: Critical Rescue

CSF drainage from nares or ear canals may indicate a skull fracture. When CSF is present in drainage, a yellow halo will surround spots of blood on filter paper. Immediately report positive findings to the health care provider.

- *Clavicular, self-healing:* A splint or bandage is used for immobilization.
- *Scapular:* A commercial immobilizer is used until the fracture heals, usually in 2 to 4 weeks.
- *Proximal humerus:* When impacted, the injury is usually treated with a sling for immobilization; when displaced, the fracture often requires ORIF with pins or prosthesis.
- *Humeral shaft:* Correction is achieved by closed reduction and application of a hanging-arm cast or splint.
- *Elbow (olecranon):* Correction by closed reduction and application of a cast. ORIF is performed for displaced fractures, and a splint is worn during the healing phase.

- *Forearm:* The ulna without accompanying injury is corrected with closed reduction and casting. If it is displaced, ORIF with intramedullary rods or plates and screws is required.
- *Wrist and hand:* Injury is most commonly to the carpal scaphoid bone, which is corrected by closed reduction and casting for 6 to 12 weeks. If the bone does not heal, ORIF with bone grafting is performed.
- *Distal radius (wrist; Colles' fracture):* Fracture of the distal radius is managed by closed reduction followed by splinting or a cast although complex fractures may require ORIF.
- *Metacarpals and phalanges (fingers):* Metacarpal fractures are immobilized for 3 to 4 weeks. Phalangeal fractures are immobilized in finger splints for 10 to 14 days.
- *Hip (intracapsular):* This fracture involves the upper third of the femur within the joint capsule. Injury is managed with surgical repair.
- *Hip (extracapsular):* This fracture involves the upper third of the femur outside of the joint capsule. Injury is managed by surgical repair, depending on the exact location of the fracture; ORIF may include an intramedullary rod, pins, prostheses (for femoral head or neck fractures), or a compression screw. Buck's traction may be applied before surgery to reduce muscle spasm.

Considerations for Older Adults

- Older adults are at risk for hip fracture because of physiologic aging changes, reduced vision, disease processes, drug therapy, and environmental hazards.
- These fractures occur most often in older adults with osteoporosis.
- Other disease processes, such as foot disorders and changes in cardiac function, increase the risk for hip fracture.
- Drugs such as diuretics, cardiac drugs, antidepressants, sedatives, opioids, and alcohol are factors that increase the risks for falling in older adults. Use of three or more drugs at the same time drastically increases the risk for falls.
- The older adult is more likely to have complications from the fracture and its management.

! NURSING SAFETY PRIORITY: Action Alert

Patients who have a hemiarthroplasty are at risk for hip dislocation or subluxation. Be sure to prevent hip adduction and rotation to keep the operative leg in proper alignment. Regular pillows or abduction devices can be used for patients who are confused or restless. If straps are used to hold the device in place, make sure that they are not too tight and check the skin for signs of pressure. Perform neurovascular assessments to ensure that the device is not interfering with arterial circulation or peripheral nerve conduction.

- *Lower two-thirds of the femur:* This is usually managed surgically by ORIF with nails, rods, or a compression screw. When extensive bone fragmentation or severe tissue trauma is found, external fixation may be employed.
- *Patellar (knee cap) fracture:* This is usually repaired by closed reduction and casting or internal fixation with screws.
- *Tibia and fibula:* These are corrected with closed reduction with casting for 8 to 10 weeks; internal fixation with nails or a plate and screws, followed by a long leg cast for 4 to 6 weeks; or external fixation for 6 to 10 weeks followed by application of a cast.
- *Ankle:* Closed, open, and combined closed and open techniques may be used, depending on the severity and extent of the fracture. An arthrodesis (fusion) is a surgical procedure used when the bone does not heal.
- *Foot or phalanges:* These are managed with closed or open reduction. Crutches are used for ambulation.
- *Ribs and sternum:* These fractures have the potential to puncture the lungs, heart, or arteries by bone fragments or ends. There is risk for deep chest injury such as pulmonary contusion, pneumothorax, and hemothorax (conditions listed separately in this text). Fractures of the lower ribs may damage underlying organs, such as the liver, spleen, or kidneys. These fractures tend to reunite spontaneously without splinting or surgical intervention.
- *Pelvis:* Pelvic fractures are the second most common cause of death from trauma. The major concern related to pelvic injury is venous oozing or arterial bleeding. Loss of blood volume leads to hypovolemic shock. When a non–weight-bearing part of the pelvis is fractured, management can be as minimal as bedrest on a firm mattress or bed board. A weight-bearing pelvis fracture requires external fixation with multiple pins, ORIF, or both. Progression to weight bearing depends on the stability of the fracture after fixation.
- *Compression fractures of the vertebrae (spine):* These fractures are associated with severe pain, deformity (kyphosis), and possible neurologic compromise. Nonsurgical management includes

bedrest, analgesics, nerve blocks, and physical therapy to maintain muscle strength. Compression fractures that remain painful and impair mobility may be surgically treated with vertebroplasty or kyphoplasty, in which bone cement is injected through the skin (percutaneously) directly into the fracture site to provide stability and immediate pain relief.

FROSTBITE

OVERVIEW
- Frostbite is a significant cold-related injury that occurs as a result of inadequate insulation against cold weather.
- Contributors to frostbite include wearing wet clothing, fatigue, dehydration, poor nutrition, smoking, alcohol consumption, and impaired peripheral circulation.

INTERPROFESSIONAL COLLABORATIVE CARE
Assessment: Noticing
- Severity of frostbite is related to the degree of tissue freezing and the resultant damage it produces.
  1. *Frostnip* is a superficial cold injury with initial pain, numbness, and pallor of the affected area. It is easily remedied with application of warmth and does not induce tissue damage.
  2. *First-degree frostbite* is the least severe type of frostbite, with hyperemia of the involved area and edema formation.
  3. *Second-degree frostbite* has large, fluid-filled blisters that develop with partial-thickness skin necrosis.
  4. *Third-degree frostbite* is a full-thickness injury that appears as small blisters containing dark fluid and an affected body part that is cool, numb, blue, or red and does not blanch.
  5. *Fourth-degree frostbite* is severe, with no blisters or edema; the part is numb, cold, and bloodless. Full-thickness necrosis extends into the muscle and bone.

Interventions: Responding
- Recognize frostbite by observing for a white, waxy appearance of exposed skin, especially on the nose, cheeks, and ears.
- Seek shelter from the wind and cold.
- Use body heat to warm up superficial frostbite-affected areas by placing warm hands over the affected areas on the face or placing cold hands under the arms in the axillary region.

Hospital Care
- Rapidly rewarm in a water bath at a temperature range of 104° to 108°F (40° to 42°C) or by using hot towels.
- Provide analgesic agents, especially IV opiates, and IV rehydration.

❗ NURSING SAFETY PRIORITY: Action Alert

Dry heat should never be applied, nor should the frostbitten areas be rubbed or massaged as part of the warming process. These actions produce further tissue injury.

- Handle the injured areas gently, and elevate them above heart level if possible to decrease tissue edema.
- Use splints to immobilize extremities during the healing process.
- Assess the patient at least hourly for the development of compartment syndrome.
- Immunize the patient for tetanus prophylaxis.
- Apply only loose, nonadherent, sterile dressings to the damaged areas.
- Avoid compression of the injured tissues.
- Topical and systemic antibiotics may be prescribed.
- Management of severe, deep frostbite requires the same types of surgical intervention as deep or severe burns.

G

GASTRITIS

OVERVIEW

- Gastritis is inflammation of the gastric mucosa.
- Gastritis can be erosive (causing ulcers) or nonerosive.
- Prostaglandins provide a protective mucosal barrier. If there is a break in the barrier, mucosal injury occurs, allowing hydrochloric acid to diffuse into the mucosa and injure small vessels, resulting in edema, bleeding, and erosion of the gastric lining.
- Gastritis can be classified as acute or chronic.
  1. *Acute gastritis,* the inflammation of gastric mucosa or submucosa, may result from food poisoning; the onset of infection (*Helicobacter pylori*, *Escherichia coli*); after exposure to local irritants such as alcohol, aspirin, nonsteroidal anti-inflammatory drugs (NSAIDs), or bacterial endotoxins; after ingestion of corrosive substances; or from the lack of stimulation of normal gastric secretions.
     a. Gastritis related to food poisoning often occurs within 5 hours of eating contaminated food.
     b. Complete regeneration and healing usually occurs within a few days without any residual damage.
  2. *Chronic gastritis* is an inflammatory process that persists until the mucosal lining becomes thin and atrophies, the parietal

(acid-secreting) cells decrease function, and the source of intrinsic factor needed for vitamin B12 absorption is lost.

a. Chronic gastritis is associated with an increased risk for stomach cancer, gastric ulcer formation, and upper GI bleeding.

b. Three subtypes of chronic gastritis are:
   (1) Type A is associated with the inflammation of the glands and the fundus and body of the stomach. It is associated with autoantibodies to parietal cells and intrinsic factor.
   (2) Type B usually affects the glands of the antrum but may involve the entire stomach. Type B is the most common form of chronic gastritis caused by *H. pylori* infection.
   (3) Chronic atrophic gastritis affects all layer of the stomach and includes intestinal metaplasia (abnormal tissue development).

INTERPROFESSIONAL COLLABORATIVE CARE
Assessment: Noticing
- Assess and document signs and symptoms:
  1. Epigastric discomfort, pain, or cramping
  2. Anorexia, dyspepsia, nausea, and vomiting
  3. Hematemesis, melena
- Presence of risk factors or conditions associated with gastric inflammation:
  1. Gastric infection, particularly *H. pylori*
  2. Chronic or excessive use of corticosteroids or NSAIDs
  3. Anorexia or malnutrition
  4. Autoimmune disease
  5. Occupational exposure to benzene, lead, or nickel
  6. Chronic local irritants like alcohol, radiation therapy, and smoking
  7. Chronic comorbidities including kidney disease (uremia) or systemic inflammatory disease like Crohn's disease

Interventions: Noticing
- Gastritis is a very common health problem in the United States. A balanced diet, regular exercise, and stress-reduction techniques can help prevent it.
- Acute gastritis is treated symptomatically and supportively.
- Eliminating the causative factors, such as *H. pylori* infection if present, is the primary treatment approach.
- H_2-receptor antagonists, such as famotidine (Pepcid) and nizatidine (Axid), are typically used to block gastric secretions.

- Proton pump inhibitors (PPIs), such as omeprazole (Prilosec), are used to reduce gastric acid secretion.
- Antacids are used as buffering agents.
- A common drug regimen for *H. pylori* infection is PPI-triple therapy, which includes a PPI, such as lansoprazole (Prevacid), plus two antibiotics, such as metronidazole (Flagyl) and tetracycline (Ala-Tet, Panmycin, Nu-Tetra), or clarithromycin (Biaxin, Biaxin XL) and amoxicillin (Amoxil, Amoxi) for 10 to 14 days.
- Instruct the patient to avoid using drugs associated with gastric irritation, including corticosteroids and NSAIDs, or provide gastroprotective agents when irritants are used therapeutically.
- If the patient experienced bleeding with symptomatic blood loss, blood transfusion may be needed. Fluid replacement is indicated for less severe blood loss or symptoms of hypovolemia from low oral intake.
- Diet and lifestyle therapy to avoid tobacco, alcohol, and foods that contribute to gastric irritation, such as those with caffeine, high levels of acid (e.g., tomatoes, citrus fruits), "hot" spices, and large volumes during a meal.
- Teach techniques to reduce stress and discomfort, such as progressive relaxation, cutaneous stimulation, guided imagery, and distraction.

GASTROENTERITIS

OVERVIEW

- Gastroenteritis is an increase in the frequency and water content of stools and vomiting as a result of inflammation of the mucous membranes of the stomach and intestines, primarily affecting the small bowel.
- The inflammation of gastroenteritis is caused by a viral or bacterial infection.
- Norovirus is the leading cause of foodborne disease causing gastroenteritis.
- Common microbes causing bacterial gastroenteritis are *Campylobacter, E. coli,* and *Shigellosis.*

INTERPROFESSIONAL COLLABORATIVE CARE
Assessment: Noticing

- Patient history can provide information about potential cause.
  1. Recent travel outside the United States or a recent meal at a restaurant associated with an outbreak of gastroenteritis
  2. Nausea and vomiting
  3. The time of onset of bloody, mucus-filled, watery, or foul-smelling stool or diarrhea with accompanying abdominal cramping or pain

4. Fever with associated malaise, myalgia, or headache
5. Dehydration exhibited by poor skin turgor, dry mucous membranes, orthostatic blood pressure changes, hypotension, changes in mentation, and oliguria
6. Positive result of a stool culture

Interventions: Noticing

- Provide fluid replacement therapy.
    1. Administer oral rehydration therapy with water. A recommended replacement is 6 teaspoons of sugar and 2 teaspoons of salt in a liter of water.
    2. Administer IV fluids and electrolytes for severe dehydration.
    3. Check vital signs and orthostatic blood pressure as clinically indicated.
    4. Record intake and output and daily weight.
- Depending on the type of gastroenteritis, notify the local health department.
- Provide drug therapy as ordered.
    1. Antibacterials are given for bacterial causes of gastroenteritis caused by an organism susceptible to therapy. Viral gastroenteritis, characterized by a shorter duration of illness (less than 72 hours), is treated symptomatically.
    2. Avoid drugs that slow or reduce gastric motility; evacuation of the infecting organism contributes to cure.
    3. Diarrhea that continues for 10 days is probably not caused by gastroenteritis, and an investigation for other causes is done.
- Promote skin protection from stool. Teach the patient to:
    1. Avoid toilet paper and harsh soaps and to gently clean the area with warm water and absorbent material, followed by thorough, gentle drying.
    2. Apply cream, oil, or gel to a damp, warm washcloth or flushable wipe for removing excrement adhering to excoriated skin.
- Teach the patient to avoid transmission of the infecting microbe.
    1. Wash hands after each bowel movement for at least 30 seconds.
    2. Do not share eating utensils, glasses, and dishes.
    3. Do not prepare or handle food that will be consumed by others; the public health department can advise about return to employment if it includes food handling.
    4. Maintain clean bathroom facilities to avoid exposure to stool.
    5. Inform the health care provider if symptoms persist beyond 3 days.
    6. Follow written instructions for antibiotics, if ordered, including the dose, schedule of administration, and side effects.

GASTROESOPHAGEAL REFLUX DISEASE: NUTRITION CONCEPT EXEMPLAR

OVERVIEW

- The most common upper gastrointestinal (GI) disorder in the United States, gastroesophageal reflux disease (GERD), occurs most often in middle-aged and older adults but can affect people of any age.
- Gastroesophageal reflux (GER) occurs as a result of backward flow (reflux) of stomach contents into the esophagus. GERD is the chronic and more serious condition that arises from persistent GER. GERD can interfere with NUTRITION.
- Reflux exposes the esophageal mucosa to the irritating effects of acidic gastric contents, resulting in inflammation.
- Chronic inflammation from acid, frequent and recurrent reflux episodes, and a longer duration of GERD can result in pain, coughing, hoarseness, wheezing at night, bronchitis, and dysphagia.
- *Dyspepsia* (also called *heartburn* or *pyrosis*), the primary symptom of GERD, is described as a substernal or retrosternal burning sensation that tends to move up and down the chest in a wavelike fashion; severe heartburn may radiate to the neck or jaw or may be felt in the back. It can resemble angina, the pain associated with *acute coronary syndrome* (ACS).

INTERPROFESSIONAL COLLABORATIVE CARE

Assessment: Noticing

- Record patient information related to eating and positioning.
  1. Location, quality, onset, and duration of dyspepsia or esophageal pain
     a. Dyspepsia (known also as indigestion) and regurgitation are the main symptoms of GERD, although symptoms may vary in severity. See Chart 2-9 for key features of GERD.
  2. Chest or upper abdominal pain aggravated by bending over, straining, or lying in a recumbent position
- Ask whether he or she has been newly diagnosed with bronchitis or asthma or has experienced dysphagia, chronic cough, morning hoarseness, or pneumonia. These symptoms suggest severe reflux reaching the pharynx or mouth or pulmonary aspiration.
- Access results of upper endoscopy, 48-hour esophageal pH monitoring, or esophageal manometry (motility testing).
- Evaluate whether obesity or body habitus (large belly) contributes to positional reflux.

G

| **Chart 2-9** | **Key Features Gastroesophageal Reflux Disease** |

- Dyspepsia (indigestion)
- Regurgitation (may lead to aspiration or bronchitis)
- Coughing, hoarseness, or wheezing at night
- Water brash (hypersalivation)
- Dysphagia
- Odynophagia (painful swallowing)
- Epigastric pain
- Generalized abdominal pain
- Belching
- Flatulence
- Nausea
- Pyrosis (heartburn)
- Globus (feeling of something in back of throat)
- Pharyngitis
- Dental caries (severe cases)

Analysis: Interpreting
- The priority collaborative problems for the patient with GERD include:
  1. Potential for compromised NUTRITION status due to dietary selection
  2. Acute pain due to reflux of gastric contents

Planning and Implementation: Responding

BALANCING NUTRITION
- Interventions are designed to optimize NUTRITION status, decrease symptoms experienced with GERD, and prevent complications. Nursing care priorities focus on teaching the patient about proper dietary selections that provide optimum nutrients and that do not contribute to reflux.
- Balance nutrition in collaboration with the patient and dietitian.
  1. Explore the patient's meal plan and food preferences.
  2. Plan diet modifications to reduce GERD symptoms by limiting or eliminating food that decreases the pressure of the lower esophageal sphincter (LES) and irritates inflamed tissue, including:
     a. Avoid chocolate, peppermint, fatty (especially fried) foods, and carbonated beverages
     b. Eat small meals that are not spicy or acidic
     c. Avoid eating for 3 hours (or more) before bedtime
     d. Limit or eliminate alcohol and tobacco

IMPROVE COMFORT
- Encourage lifestyle changes.
  1. If the patient is obese, examine approaches to weight reduction with the patient.
  2. Promote smoking cessation and reduced alcohol intake.
  3. Instruct the patient to elevate the head of the bed by 6 inches to prevent nighttime reflux.
  4. Remain upright after meals for 1 to 2 hours.
  5. Encourage the patient to avoid wearing tight-fitting clothing and working in a bent-over or stooped position.
- Drug therapy
  1. PPIs are the main treatment for GERD and provide effective, long-acting inhibition of gastric acid secretion.

Considerations for Older Adults

Patient-Centered Care

Research has found that long-term use of PPIs may increase the risk for hip fracture, especially in older adults. PPIs can interfere with calcium absorption and protein digestion and therefore reduce available calcium to bone tissue. Decreased calcium makes bones more brittle and likely to fracture, especially as adults age.

G

  2. H_2 histamine receptor blockers are sometimes used instead of PPIs to reduce gastric acid production, provide symptom improvement, and support healing of the inflamed esophageal tissue.
  3. Antacids are used to neutralize gastric acids.

ENDOSCOPIC THERAPIES
- The Stretta procedure, a nonsurgical method, can replace surgery for GERD when other measures are not effective.
- Patients who are very obese or have severe symptoms may not be candidates for this procedure.
- In the Stretta procedure, the physician applies radiofrequency (RF) energy through the endoscope using needles placed near the gastroesophageal junction. The RF energy decreases vagus nerve activity, thus reducing discomfort for the patient.

SURGICAL MANAGEMENT
- Laparoscopic Nissen fundoplication is a minimally invasive surgery that is the standard surgical approach for treatment of severe GERD.

Care Coordination and Transition Management
- Remind the patient to make appropriate dietary selections that enhance nutrition and decrease symptoms associated with GERD.

- For patients with nonsurgical GERD, teach about signs and symptoms of more serious complications such as esophageal stricture and Barrett's esophagus.

GENDER REASSIGNMENT

OVERVIEW

- Discomfort with one's natal sex is gender dysphoria.
- The term "transgender" is often used as an umbrella description for all people whose gender identity and presentation do not conform to social expectations. More commonly, transgender describes patients who self-identify as the opposite gender or a gender that does not match their natal sex.
- Another common term is transsexual, which generally describes a person who has modified his or her natal body to match the appropriate gender identity, either through cosmetic, hormonal, or surgical means.
- Transgender individuals (also referred to as trans-people) encounter frequent discrimination and face numerous stressful situations related to their identity. Sources of stress such as job discrimination and harassment have an impact on patients' physical and psychological health.

INTERPROFESSIONAL COLLABORATIVE CARE

Assessment: Noticing

1. How he or she prefers to be addressed during the nursing history and physical assessment
2. How care may affect sexual identity or treatment for transgender transition; it may be that the nurse will have to discuss this topic with a provider expert before delivering care to maintain trust and provide sensitive, individualized interventions
3. Level and sources of stress that may affect health care or can be reduced with health promotion interventions

Interventions: Noticing

- Interventions for transgender individuals who experience gender dysphoria include one or more of these options:
  1. Changes in gender expression that may involve living part-time or full-time in another gender role
  2. Psychotherapy to explore gender identity and expression, improving body image, or strengthening coping mechanisms
  3. Hormone therapy to feminize or masculinize the body
     a. Transgender patients often take hormone therapy for many years.
     b. Teach them that ongoing follow-up with a qualified health care professional is needed to maintain health and detect any complications, such as diabetes or cardiovascular problems, as early as possible.

4. Surgery to change primary and/or secondary sex characteristics such as the breasts/chest, facial features, internal and/or external genitalia

☤ Gender Health Considerations

- Unique needs regarding sexual health and prevention and treatment of sexually related infections of lesbian, gay, bisexual, and transgender (LGBT) patients should be identified and addressed by the nurse.
- Because of discrimination, health care inequities, and health care provider lack of understanding, the overall health status of individuals in these populations may be poor. LGBT individuals may have difficulty finding health care that identifies and addresses their particular risks and concerns.
- Taking a health history that provides opportunity for the patient to identify his or her sexual orientation, sexual identity, and sexual activity is essential to care. Especially among transgender individuals, opportunities for physical examination are avoided or missed by both the patient and care provider because of fears of being misunderstood or inadequately prepared to give or receive appropriate care.

SURGICAL MANAGEMENT
- **Gender** or **sex reassignment surgery (SRS)** also known as gender-affirming surgery or gender-confirming surgery.
- Genital surgeries "below the waist" are the most invasive procedures. The criteria for genital surgery depend on the type of surgery being requested.
  1. Most surgeons (usually urologists or plastic surgeons) require 12 months of hormone therapy plus one or two referrals from qualified psychotherapists for male-to-female (MtF) patients.
  2. Feminizing surgeries are performed for MtF patients to create a functional and/or aesthetic (cosmetic) female anatomy, including:
     a. Breast/chest surgeries, such as breast augmentation (mammoplasty to increase breast tissue)
     b. Genital surgeries, such as partial penectomy (removal of the penis), orchiectomy (removal of the testes), vaginoplasty, and labiaplasty-vulvoplasty (creation of a vagina and labia/vulva), clitoroplasty (creation of a clitoris)
     c. Other surgeries, such as facial feminizing surgery (to achieve feminine facial contour), liposuction (fatty tissue removal),

G

often from the waist or abdominal area, vocal feminizing surgery, and other body-contouring procedures

3. The same requirements of hormonal therapy and psychiatric evaluation are needed for female-to-male (FtM) patients.
4. Masculinizing surgeries are performed for FtM patients to create a functional and/or aesthetic male anatomy, including:
   a. Breast/chest surgeries, usually a bilateral mastectomy (removal of both breasts) and chest reconstruction
   b. Genital surgeries, such as a hysterectomy and bilateral BSO, vaginectomy (removal of the vagina), phalloplasty (creation of an average-size male penis) with ureteroplasty (creation of a urethra) or metoidioplasty (creation of a small penis using hormone-enhanced clitoral tissue), and scrotoplasty (creation of a scrotum) with insertion of testicular prostheses
   c. Other surgeries, such as liposuction, pectoral muscle implants, and other body-contouring procedures
5. Pre- and postoperative care includes:
   a. Using culturally sensitive and accurate language when communicating with transgender patients; use pronouns that match the patient's physical appearance and dress unless the patient requests a specific term
   b. Provide preoperative care for a patient having a vaginoplasty, including teaching about bowel preparation, food and fluid intake, hair removal methods, and the need for informed consent

- Monitor for potentially life-threatening complications of gender reassignment surgery, such as fistula development, bleeding, and wound infection.

 ## GLAUCOMA: SENSORY PERCEPTION EXEMPLAR

OVERVIEW

- Glaucoma is a group of ocular diseases resulting in increased intraocular pressure (IOP) that can result in loss of visual SENSORY PERCEPTION.
- The normal IOP is 10 to 21 mm Hg, maintained when there is a balance between production and outflow of aqueous humor.
- If the IOP becomes too high, pressure on blood vessels, results in poorly oxygenated photoreceptors; combined with compression on nerve fibers IOP can lead to ischemic injury and permanent blindness.
- In most types of glaucoma, vision is lost gradually and painlessly from the periphery to the central area.

- Types of glaucoma:
  1. *Primary:* The structures involved in circulation and reabsorption of the aqueous humor undergo direct pathologic changes from aging, heredity, and central retinal vessel occlusion.
     a. *Primary open-angle glaucoma* (POAG) has reduced outflow of aqueous humor through the chamber angle. Because the fluid cannot leave the eye at the same rate it is produced, IOP gradually increases.
     b. *Primary angle-closure glaucoma* (PACG, also called *acute glaucoma*) has a sudden onset and is an emergency.
  2. *Secondary:* Glaucoma results from other problems within the eye, such as uveitis, iritis, trauma, and ocular surgeries.
  3. *Associated:* Glaucoma results from systemic disease, such as diabetes mellitus and hypertension.

INTERPROFESSIONAL COLLABORATIVE CARE
Assessment: Noticing
- Assess for manifestations of early glaucoma
  1. Increased ocular pressure measured by tonometry
  2. Reduced accommodation
- Assess for late manifestations of glaucoma
  1. Peripheral visual field losses
  2. Decreased visual acuity not correctable with glasses
  3. Appearance of halos around lights
- Opthalmoscopic examination shows cupping and atrophy of the optic disc.

Analysis: Interpreting
- The priority collaborative problems for patients with glaucoma include:
  1. Decreased visual acuity due to glaucoma
  2. Need for health teaching due to treatment regimen for glaucoma

Planning and Implementation: Responding
SUPPORT VISUAL ACUITY VIA HEALTH TEACHING
- Teach the patient that loss of visual SENSORY PERCEPTION from glaucoma can be prevented by early detection, lifelong treatment, and close monitoring.
- Use of ophthalmic drugs that reduce ocular pressure can delay or prevent damage.
- Drug therapy for glaucoma focuses on reducing IOP with eye drops; drug therapy does not improve lost vision.
  1. Prostaglandin agonists dilate blood vessels to drain aqueous fluid and include bimatoprost (Lumigan), latanoprost (Xalatan), and travoprost (Travatan).
  2. Adrenergic agonists block production of aqueous humor and include apraclonidine (Iopidine), brimonidine (Alphagan), and dipivefrin (Propine).

3. Beta-adrenergic blockers block production of aqueous fluid and include betaxolol (Betoptic), carteolol (Cartrol, Ocupress), levobunolol (Betagan), and timolol (Betimol, Timoptic, Timoptic GFS for extended release).

4. Cholinergic agonists increase the outflow of fluid and slow aqueous fluid production; products include carbachol (Carboptic, Isopto Carbachol, Miostat), echothiophate (Phospholine Iodide), and pilocarpine (Adsorbocarpine, Akarpine, Isopto Carpine, Ocu-Carpine, Ocusert, Piloptic, Pilopine, Pilostat).

5. Carbonic anhydrase inhibitors directly and strongly reduce aqueous fluid production and include brinzolamide (Azopt) and dorzolamide (Trusopt).

6. There are also combination agents that use drugs from more than one of the above categories such as brimonidine tartrate and timolol maleate (Combigan).

- Teach the patient:
  1. The importance of instilling the drops on time and not skipping doses
  2. To wait 5 to 15 minutes between drug instillations when more than one drug is prescribed to prevent one drug from "washing out" or diluting another drug
  3. The technique of punctal occlusion (placing pressure on the corner of the eye near the nose) immediately after eye drop instillation to prevent systemic absorption of the drug
  4. About the need for good handwashing, keeping the eye drop container tip clean, and avoiding touching the tip to any part of the eye

❗ NURSING SAFETY PRIORITY: Drug Alert

Most eyedrops used for glaucoma therapy can be absorbed systemically and cause systemic problems. It is critical to teach punctal occlusion to patients using eyedrops for glaucoma therapy.

- Surgery is used when drugs for the patient with open-angle glaucoma are not effective in controlling IOP. The two most common procedures are laser trabeculoplasty and trabeculectomy to improve the outflow of aqueous fluid.

Care Coordination and Transition Management

- Reinforce teaching about self-management, especially the techniques for eye drop instillation.
- For the patient who has had surgery, teach the signs and symptoms of choroidal detachment and hemorrhage. These can occur after coughing, sneezing, straining at stools, or Valsalva maneuver.

- Refer to community agencies and resources for assistance in adapting to vision impairment.

GLOMERULONEPHRITIS, ACUTE

OVERVIEW

- Acute glomerulonephritis is a group of diseases that injure and inflame the glomerulus, the part of the kidney that filters blood.
- It can be categorized as primary or secondary.
  1. Primary glomerular nephritis
     a. Many causes are infectious. One example is the syndrome that occurs with *streptococcus* infection. Microbes can be bacterial, viral, or fungal.
     b. Excessive inflammation can also cause primary acute glomerulonephritis.
     c. *Rapidly progressive glomerulonephritis,* a subtype of this condition, develops over several days and causes a rapid and significant loss of kidney function.
  2. Secondary glomerulonephritis is a part of a systemic disorder that includes kidney involvement.
     a. Examples of multi-system disease that are associated with this chronic condition are systemic lupus erythematosus, small vessel vasculitis, Wegener's granulomatosis, and other inflammatory conditions that alter immunity.
     b. Chronic infections from HIV and metastatic cancers can also cause this secondary condition.

INTERPROFESSIONAL COLLABORATIVE CARE

Assessment: Noticing

- Record patient information.
  1. History of recent infections, particularly skin and upper respiratory infections
  2. Recent travel or activities with exposure to viruses, bacteria, fungi, or parasites
  3. Diagnosis of systemic diseases, especially those associated with inflammation or autoimmunity
- Assessment findings include:
  1. Presence of symptoms indicating systemic volume overload: extra heart sound (i.e., S_3 gallop), neck vein engorgement, edema, and crackles in the lungs with tachypnea and dyspnea or orthopnea
  2. Changes in urine color (typically smoky, reddish brown, or tea-colored urine), clarity, or odor; and altered patterns of urination such as dysuria, urgency, and incontinence
  3. Decreased urine output
  4. Mild to moderate hypertension

5. Changes in weight
6. Fatigue, malaise, and activity intolerance
7. Abnormal urinalysis including leukocyte esterase, nitrogen, red blood cells (RBCs), white blood cells (WBCs), low creatinine, and presence of protein, casts, or cells
8. Increased blood urea nitrogen (BUN) and serum creatinine levels
9. Positive cultures from urine, blood, sputum, skin, or throat
10. Serologic testing for antistreptolysin O titers, C3 complement levels, immunoglobulin G, antinuclear bodies, and circulating immune complexes
11. Results of percutaneous needle biopsy of the kidney to provide a precise diagnosis

Interventions: Responding

- Manage infection by administering anti-infective agents.
- Balance intake and output; fluid intake may be restricted to the previous 24-hour urinary output plus 500 to 600 mL for insensible fluid loss.
- Hypertension, circulatory overload, and edema may be managed with diuretics or fluid and sodium restrictions.
- Avoid electrolyte imbalance and protein overload during kidney dysfunction with dietary adjustments in collaboration with the dietitian.
- Support education and blood pressure management for dialysis or plasmapheresis used to filter out antigen-antibody complexes and manage uremia or fluid and electrolyte imbalances.
- Provide health teaching, including:
  1. Reviewing prescribed drug instructions, including purpose, timing, frequency, duration, and side effects
  2. Ensuring that the patient and family understand dietary and fluid modifications. Offer assistance with coping with fluid restrictions, such as a mouth moisturizer or mouth swabs. In some situations ice chips or hard candy may be used to offer relief from a dry mouth.
  3. Advising the patient to measure weight and blood pressure daily and to notify the health care provider of any sudden changes
  4. Instructing the patient about peritoneal or vascular access care if short-term dialysis is required to control excess fluid volume or uremic symptoms

GLOMERULONEPHRITIS, CHRONIC

OVERVIEW

- Chronic glomerulonephritis, or *chronic nephritic syndrome,* is the diagnostic name given to changes in kidney tissue that develop over decades of infection, hypertension, inflammation, or poor kidney blood flow.

- Nephrons become damaged and are lost; proteinuria occurs; kidney tissue atrophies and the ability to filter blood is reduced.
- The process eventually results in chronic kidney disease (CKD) and uremia, requiring dialysis or transplantation.

INTERPROFESSIONAL COLLABORATIVE CARE
Assessment: Noticing
- Record the patient's history about health problems, including systemic disease, kidney or urologic problems, and infectious diseases, especially streptococcal infections and recent exposure to infection.
- Assess for:
  1. Presence of symptoms indicating systemic volume overload: the cardiac extra sound of an S_3 gallop, neck vein engorgement, edema, and crackles in the lungs with tachypnea
  2. Uremic symptoms such as changes in concentration, slurred speech, ataxia, tremors, bruising, and rash or itching
  3. Changes in urine and elimination, including amount, frequency of voiding, and changes in urine color, clarity, and odor
  4. Changes in activity tolerance and comfort
  5. Abnormal urinalysis, especially proteinuria
  6. Abnormal BUN, serum creatinine, and estimated glomerular filtration rate (eGFR) electrolyte values
  7. Ultrasound or radiographic findings of kidney size (usually small)
  8. Vital signs (especially hypertension and irregular heart rhythm) and weight

Interventions: Responding
- Management of chronic glomerulonephritis is similar to management for CKD, including dialysis when kidneys fail to adequately filter the blood.
- Treatment consists of dietary modification, fluid intake sufficient to prevent reduced blood flow volume to the kidneys, and drug therapy to temporarily control the symptoms of uremia.

GONORRHEA

OVERVIEW
- Gonorrhea is a sexually transmitted bacterial infection caused by *Neisseria gonorrhoeae*.
- It is transmitted by direct sexual contact with mucosal surfaces (vaginal intercourse, orogenital contact, or anogenital contact).
- The first symptoms of gonorrhea may appear 3 to 10 days after sexual contact with an infected person.

- The disease can be present without symptoms and can be transmitted or progress without warning.
- In women, ascending spread of the organism can cause pelvic infection (pelvic inflammatory disease [PID]), endometritis (endometrial infection), salpingitis (fallopian tube infection), and pelvic peritonitis.

INTERPROFESSIONAL COLLABORATIVE CARE
Assessment: Noticing
- Obtain patient information about:
  1. Sexual history that includes sexual orientation and sites of intercourse
  2. Allergies to antibiotics
  3. Symptoms in men
     a. Dysuria
     b. Penile discharge (profuse, yellowish-green fluid or scant, clear fluid)
     c. Urethritis
     d. Pain or discomfort in the prostate, seminal vesicles, or epididymal regions
  4. Symptoms in women
     a. Vaginal discharge (yellow, green, profuse, odorous)
     b. Urinary frequency
     c. Dysuria and urethral discharge
  5. Anal manifestations (in men or women)
     a. Itching and irritation
     b. Rectal discharge or bleeding
     c. Diarrhea
     d. Painful defecation
- Assess for and document:
  1. Oral cavity manifestations
     a. Reddened throat
     b. Ulcerated lips
     c. Tender gingivae
     d. Blisters in the throat
  2. Tenderness of the lower abdomen
  3. Manifestations of disseminated *gonococci* infection (DGI)
     a. Fever
     b. Chills
     c. Skin lesions on hands and feet
     d. Joint pain, with or without swelling, heat, or redness
- Diagnostic testing may include:
  1. Nucleic acid amplification test (NAAT) using samples from vagina or male urethra
  2. Gram staining and cultures from a smear from penile discharge or from a vaginal swab

❗ NURSING SAFETY PRIORITY: Critical Rescue

All patients with gonorrhea should be tested for syphilis, chlamydia, hepatitis B and C, and HIV infection because they may have been exposed to multiple sexually transmitted diseases (STDs). Sexual partners who have been exposed in the past 30 days should be examined and specimens for culture should be obtained.

Interventions: Responding
- Drug therapy for uncomplicated gonorrhea is ceftriaxone plus azithromycin.
- Disseminated gonorrhea infection requires hospitalization and IV antibiotics, typically for 48 hours, followed by 7 days of oral antibiotics.
- Sexual partners also must be treated.
- A test of cure is not required but the patient should be advised to return for a follow-up examination if symptoms persist after treatment.
- This condition must be reported to the local health department by the health care provider.
- Teach the patient about:
  1. Transmission and treatment of gonorrhea
  2. Prevention of re infection
  3. Complications of chronic gonorrhea
     a. PID
     b. Ectopic pregnancy
     c. Infertility
     d. Chronic pelvic pain
  4. Avoiding sexual activity until the antibiotic therapy is completed
  5. Condom use if abstinence is not possible
  6. The need for all sexual contacts to be examined for STDs
- Encourage patients to express their feelings during assessments and teaching sessions.
- Provide privacy for teaching and maintain confidentiality of medical records.

GOUT

OVERVIEW
- Gout, or *gouty arthritis,* is a systemic disease in which urate crystals deposit in the joints and other body tissues, causing inflammation.
- There are two major types of gout.
  1. *Primary gout* results from one of several inborn errors of purine metabolism that allows the production of uric acid to

exceed the excretion capability of the kidneys. Urate is deposited in synovium and other tissues, resulting in inflammation. A number of patients have a family history of gout. It is most common in middle-aged and older men and postmenopausal women.

2. *Secondary gout* results from excessive uric acid crystals that are present in the blood (hyperuricemia) as a result of another disease, condition, or treatment. Causes include renal insufficiency, diuretic therapy, "crash" diets, certain chemotherapeutic agents, and diseases such as multiple myeloma and certain carcinomas. Treatment for secondary gout focuses on management of the underlying disorder.

- There are three clinical stages of primary gout:
  1. *Asymptomatic hyperuricemic stage,* in which there are no symptoms but the serum uric acid level is elevated.
  2. *Acute stage,* in which the patient experiences excruciating pain and inflammation in one or more small joints, usually the metatarsophalangeal joint of the great toe, called *podagra.*
  3. *Chronic tophaceous stage,* which occurs after repeated episodes of acute gout have caused deposits of urate crystals under the skin and within the major organs, particularly in the kidney system; this stage can begin between 3 and 40 years after the initial gout symptoms occur.

INTERPROFESSIONAL COLLABORATIVE CARE
Assessment: Noticing
- For acute gout, assess for and document joint inflammation and pain.
- For chronic gout, assess for and document history of disease duration and:
  1. Presence of tophi (skin deposits of urate crystals) on the outer ear and near the joints of the digits of both hands and feet
  2. Infected skin areas
  3. Manifestations of kidney (stones) or kidney dysfunction
     a. Severe pain
     b. Changes in urine output
- Diagnostic assessment may include:
  1. Serum uric acid level
  2. Urinary uric acid levels
  3. Kidney function tests (in chronic gout)
  4. Synovial fluid aspiration (arthrocentesis)
Interventions: Responding
- Drug therapy during acute attacks is a combination of colchicine (Colcrys) and an NSAID, such as indomethacin (Indocin, Novomethacin ♣) or ibuprofen (Motrin, Amersol ♣) for acute gout.

IV colchicine works within 12 hours. The patient takes oral medications until the inflammation subsides, usually for 4 to 7 days.
- Drug therapy for chronic gout is allopurinol (Zyloprim) or febuxostat (Uloric) to promote uric acid secretion and its production.
- Other drugs to manage chronic gout are probenecid (Benemid, Benuryl ✦), a uricosuric, and pegloticase (Krystexxa), an enzyme that converts uric acid to a chemical that can be excreted.

❗ NURSING SAFETY PRIORITY: Action Alert

Aspirin should be avoided because it inactivates the effects of the drug therapy.

- Nutritional therapy is a low-purine diet and teaching patient to avoid foods that precipitate attacks like organ or red meats and shellfish or oily fish with bones (sardines).
- Teach the patient to drink plenty of fluids, especially water.

✳️ GUILLAIN-BARRÉ SYNDROME: IMMUNITY CONCEPT EXEMPLAR

OVERVIEW
- Guillain-Barré syndrome (GBS) is an *acute inflammatory* disorder that affects axons and/or myelin of the peripheral nervous system resulting from altered IMMUNITY.
- Antibodies attack the myelin sheath that surrounds the axons of the peripheral neurons resulting in slowed or absent impulses leading to impaired mobility and sensory perception.
- Three stages make up the acute course:
  1. *Acute or initial period* begins with the onset of the first definitive symptoms and ends when no further deterioration is noted (usually 1 to 4 weeks).
  2. *Plateau period* is a time of little change and lasts several days to 2 weeks.
  3. *Recovery phase* is thought to coincide with re-myelination and axonal regeneration and occurs gradually over 4 to 48 months. Patients with chronic GBS do not recover and have permanent neurologic defects.
- GBS is often associated with bacterial infection, especially infection with *Campylobacter jejuni*. Influenza, Epstein-Barr, Zika, and cytomegalovirus (CMG) viral infections have also been associated with GBS.
- There are also reports of some vaccines increasing the risk for GBS slightly, but epidemiologic evidence is weak.

INTERPROFESSIONAL COLLABORATIVE CARE

Assessment: Noticing

- Obtain a health history, recording GBS symptoms in chronologic order.
- Assess for:
  1. Comfort, numbness, and paresthesias
  2. Muscle weakness or paralysis and loss of reflexes in arms and legs
  3. Low BP or poor BP control, bradycardia, and other signs of autonomic nervous system derangements
  4. Blurred or double vision
  5. Cranial nerve involvement that impairs swallowing or airway clearance
  6. Respiratory compromise or failure:
     a. Decreased peripheral oxygenation (Spo_2)
     b. Dyspnea, tachypnea, or paradoxical breathing
     c. Decreased breath sounds from reduced tidal volume or vital capacity
     d. Increased oral secretions, inability to swallow, or compromised airway patency
  7. Bowel and bladder incontinence
  8. Altered coping manifested by anxiety, fear, anger, or depression
  9. Protein in cerebrospinal fluid without leukocytosis
  10. Electrophysiologic studies (EPSs) demonstrating demyelinating neuropathy

Analysis: Interpreting

- The priority collaborative problems for patients with GBS typically include:
  1. Potential for respiratory and/or cardiovascular distress or failure due to thoracic muscle weakness and hypotension
  2. Decreased mobility due to skeletal muscle weakness

Planning and Implementation: Responding

PREVENT RESPIRATORY AND/OR CARDIOVASCULAR DISTRESS OR FAILURE

- Frequent assessment of the respiratory system (airway, breathing, effort, and lung sounds)
  1. Positioning
  2. Suction; note sputum appearance
  3. Supplemental oxygenation to maintain Spo_2 greater than 92%
  4. Frequent monitoring of VS with peripheral oxygenation
  5. Implementing aspiration precautions
  6. Observe for dyspnea, air hunger, adventitious breath sounds, cyanosis, and confusion
  7. Administer humidified air or oxygen, as appropriate
  8. Administer bronchodilator treatments, as appropriate

• Treat immunity alterations with plasma exchange or immuno-globulin. There is no benefit to using both therapies.

1. *Plasmapheresis* (*apheresis*) removes the circulating antibodies thought to be responsible for the disease. Nursing interventions for the patient undergoing plasmapheresis include:

   a. Providing information and reassurance
   b. Monitoring for complications of plasmapheresis: hypovolemia, hypokalemia, hypocalcemia, temporary circumoral and distal extremity paresthesia, muscle twitching, nausea, and vomiting
   c. Monitoring intake and output and weighing the patient after the procedure to detect dehydration or overhydration as a result of treatment
   d. Administering shunt care to maintain patency and prevent infections

❗ NURSING SAFETY PRIORITY: Critical Rescue

If a shunt is used, use these interventions to avoid infection and harm from clotting or bleeding.

• Check shunt patency by palpating a thrill or auscultating a bruit every 2 to 4 hours.
• Avoid taking blood pressure and venipuncture for intravenous catheter placement or collection of blood specimen from the extremity used for shunt.
• Keep double bulldog clamps at the bedside to prevent high-volume blood loss if shunt is dislodged.
• Observe the puncture site for bleeding or ecchymosis (bruising).
• Maintain sterile, occlusive dressing at the insertion site.

2. Intravenous immunoglobulin therapy (IVIG) is equally effective as plasmapheresis but is safer and immediately available. Infuse slowly initially to detect major adverse effects early.

   a. Minor adverse effects from IVIG are chills, mild fever, myalgia, and headache.
   b. Major complications from IVIG are anaphylaxis, aseptic meningitis, retinal necrosis, and acute kidney injury and failure.

IMPROVE MOBILITY AND PREVENT COMPLICATIONS OF IMMOBILITY

1. Collaborate with the patient, family, physical and occupational therapists (PT/OT), speech-language pathologist (SLP), and dietitian to develop interventions that prevent complications of immobility and to address temporary deficits in self-care.

2. Monitor the patient's response to activity, provide rest between activities, and reduce the frequency or duration of activity if intolerant.
3. Collaborate with the dietitian to optimize nutritional intake and assist with meals as needed.
4. Monitor intake and output for balance, and assess the patient for urinary retention every shift.
5. Monitor for complications of immobility: atelectasis, pneumonia, pressure ulcers, and venothromboembolism.
6. Manage pain to improve mobility.

Care Coordination and Transition Management

1. Provide a detailed plan of care at the time of discharge for patients to be transferred to a long-term care or rehabilitation facility (rehabilitation may be lengthy).
2. Assess the patient's and family's knowledge and understanding of the disease and provide information and emotional support for this devastating condition with an uncertain outcome in terms of function.
3. Refer the patient to local agencies or national neurologic organizations such as the Guillain-Barré Foundation for assistance in the home setting and educational materials.

H

HEADACHE, MIGRAINE
OVERVIEW

- A migraine headache is a syndrome of recurrent episodic head pain that can last 4 to 72 hours, characterized by throbbing, intense unilateral pain on one side of the head and can be accompanied by nausea and sensitivity to light, sound, or head movement.
- The cause of migraine headaches is likely a combination of neuronal hyper-excitability and vascular, genetic, hormonal, and environmental factors that result in cerebral vasodilation followed by a sterile brain tissue inflammation.
- Three categories of migraine headache are migraine with aura (classic migraine), migraine without aura, and atypical migraine.
  1. An *aura* is a sensation such as visual changes that signals the onset of a headache or seizure. In a migraine, the aura occurs immediately before the migraine episode.
  2. *Atypical migraines* are less common and include menstrual and cluster migraines.

INTERPROFESSIONAL COLLABORATIVE CARE

- The priority of care is pain management
  1. Prevention includes interventions and education to reduce migraine episodes.

a. Drugs may be used when migraine occurs more than twice per week, interferes with activities of daily living (ADLs), or is not relieved with acute treatment.

b. Migraine-preventive drugs include nonsteroidal anti-inflammatory drugs (NSAIDs), beta-adrenergic blockers, calcium channel blockers, onabotulinum toxin A (Botox), and antiepileptics.

2. Abortive therapy is aimed at alleviating pain during the aura phase or soon after a headache starts. Examples of migraine abortive drugs are:

a. Acetaminophen and NSAIDs; the addition of caffeine to these drugs in some over-the-counter (OTC) agents results in vasoconstriction to enhance symptom relief

b. Antiemetics or prokinetics to relieve nausea and vomiting

c. Triptan or ergotamine preparations are used with severe pain and can be taken orally sublingually, inhaled, or as a suppository (e.g., Cafergot, Migergot, Ergomar SL, Medihaler ergotamine)

! NURSING SAFETY PRIORITY: Drug Alert

Teach patients taking triptan drugs to take them as soon as migraine symptoms develop. Instruct patients to report angina (chest pain) or chest discomfort to their health care providers immediately to prevent cardiac damage from myocardial ischemia. Remind them to use contraception (birth control) while taking the drugs because the drugs may not be safe for women who are pregnant. Teach them to expect common side effects that include flushing, tingling, and a hot sensation. These annoying sensations tend to subside after the patient's body gets used to the drug. Triptan drugs should not be taken with selective serotonin reuptake inhibitor (SSRI) antidepressants or St. John's wort, an herb used commonly for depression.

3. Trigger avoidance and management can reduce the frequency or severity of migraines by identifying and stopping exposure to dietary and environmental factors that contribute to migraines such as:

a. Tyramine-containing products, such as pickled products, caffeine, beer, and wine

b. Preservatives and artificial sweeteners

c. Instruct the patient to keep a diary to link exposures to migraine symptoms

4. Complementary and integrative health therapies associated with symptom relief include acupressure and acupuncture,

yoga, meditation, massage, exercise, yoga, and biofeedback. Vitamin B$_2$ (riboflavin) and magnesium supplement to maintain normal serum values have a role in migraine prevention.

HEARING LOSS: SENSORY PERCEPTION CONCEPT EXEMPLAR

OVERVIEW
- Hearing loss, an auditory SENSORY PERCEPTION impairment or loss, is a common handicap worldwide and categorized as follows:
  1. *Conductive hearing loss* is a result of obstruction of sound wave transmission such as a foreign body in the external canal, a retracted or bulging tympanic membrane, or fused bony ossicles.
  2. *Sensorineural hearing loss* is a result of a defect in the cochlea, the eighth cranial nerve, or the brain. Also, exposure to loud noise or music damages the cochlear hair and this type of hearing loss. *Presbycusis* is a sensorineural hearing loss that occurs as a result of aging.
  3. *Mixed conductive-sensorineural hearing loss* has components of both conductive and sensorineural loss.
- About one-third of people between the ages of 65 and 75 years have a hearing loss. As many as one-half of people older than 85 years have some degree of hearing loss.
- The type and cause of hearing loss determine the degree to which loss can be corrected and the amount of hearing that can return.

INTERPROFESSIONAL COLLABORATIVE CARE
Assessment: Noticing
- Obtain patient information about:
  1. Any differences in his or her ears or hearing and whether the changes occurred suddenly or gradually, including:
     a. Feeling of ear fullness or congestion
     b. Dizziness or vertigo
     c. Tinnitus
     d. Difficulty hearing sounds or understanding conversations, especially in a noisy room
  2. Age
  3. Occupational or leisure exposure to loud or continuous noises
  4. Current or previous use of ototoxic drugs
  5. History of external ear or middle ear infection and whether eardrum perforation occurred with the infection
  6. History of ear trauma
  7. Whether any family members are hearing impaired
  8. Recent upper respiratory infection and allergies affecting the nose and sinuses

- Assess for and document:
  1. External ear features (pinna) including size and position
  2. Abnormal otoscopic and Rinne or Weber (tuning fork) test findings by the provider
  3. Psychosocial issues
     a. Social isolation
     b. Depression, fear, and despair
- Diagnostic studies include audiometry to determine the type and extent of hearing loss and imaging to determine possible causes.

Analysis: Interpreting

- The priority collaborative problems for the patient with any degree of hearing impairment include:
  1. Decreased hearing ability due to obstruction, infection, damage to the middle ear, or damage to the auditory nerve
  2. Decreased functional ability (communication) due to difficulty hearing

Planning and Implementation: Responding

INCREASE HEARING

  1. Promote early detection to help correct reversible problems causing the hearing loss.
  2. Administer drug therapy to correct an underlying pathologic change or to reduce side effects of problems occurring with hearing loss, including antibiotic therapy for infection.
  3. Administer antivertiginous drugs to decrease dizziness when this symptom accompanies hearing loss.
  4. Apply hearing-assistive devices:
     a. Telephone amplifiers
     b. Therapy dogs
     c. Portable audio amplifiers
     d. Collaborate with the audiologist to promote safe, effective use of a hearing aid
        (1) Remind the patient that background noise will be amplified along with voices and that a new hearing aid requires a period of adjustment.
        (2) Teach him or her to care for the hearing aid by:
            i. Cleaning the ear mold with mild soap and water while avoiding excessive wetting
            ii. Cleaning debris from the hole in the middle of the part that goes into the ear with a toothpick or a pipe cleaner
            iii. Turning off the hearing aid and removing the battery when not in use
            iv. Keeping extra batteries on hand and replacing the battery often
            v. Avoiding dropping the hearing aid or exposing it to temperature extremes

H

      vi. Adjusting the volume to the lowest setting that allows hearing to prevent feedback squeaking

      vii. Avoiding use of hair and face products that may damage the receiver

MAXIMIZE COMMUNICATION

1. Use best practices for communicating with a hearing-impaired patient, including:
   a. Positioning yourself directly in front of the patient
   b. Making sure that the room is well lighted
   c. Getting the patient's attention before you begin to speak
   d. Moving closer to the better hearing ear
   e. Speaking clearly and slowly
   f. Keeping hands and other objects away from your mouth when talking to the patient
   g. Attempting to have conversations in a quiet room with minimal distractions
   h. Having the patient repeat your statements rather than just indicating assent
   i. Rephrasing sentences and repeating information to aid in understanding
   j. Using appropriate hand motions
   k. Writing messages on paper if the patient is able to read

2. Have the patient use hearing-assistive devices described earlier.

3. Manage anxiety and promote social interaction by:
   a. Enhancing communication, as described earlier
   b. Working with the patient to identify his or her most satisfying activities and social interactions and determine the amount of effort necessary to continue them
   c. Suggesting the use of closed captioning for television programming

SURGICAL MANAGEMENT

- The type of operative procedure selected depends on the cause of the hearing loss.

   1. *Tympanoplasty* reconstructs the middle ear. The procedures vary from simple reconstruction of the eardrum (myringoplasty or type I tympanoplasty) to replacement of the ossicles within the middle ear (type II tympanoplasty).

   2. *Stapedectomy* is the removal of the head and neck of the stapes and, less often, the footplate. After removal of the bone, a small hole is drilled or made with a laser in the footplate, and a prosthesis in the shape of a piston is connected between the incus and the footplate.

   3. A totally implanted device is placed to treat bilateral moderate to severe sensorineural hearing loss.

- Provide routine preoperative care, including:
  1. Assuring the patient that hearing loss immediately after surgery is normal because of canal packing
  2. Reinforcing the information provided by the surgeon
- Provide routine postoperative care, including:
  1. Adhering to routine postoperative care, as described in Part One
  2. Keeping the dressing clean and dry, using sterile technique for changes
  3. Keeping the patient flat, with the head turned to the side and the operative ear facing up for at least 12 hours after surgery
  4. Using communication techniques for the hearing impaired
  5. Giving prescribed antibiotics to prevent infection
  6. Giving prescribed analgesics
  7. Giving prescribed antivertiginous drugs
  8. Assessing for and reporting complications (stapedectomy, implanted devices)
     a. Asymmetric appearance or drooping of features on the affected side of the face
     b. Changes in facial perception of touch and in taste, as reported by patient
  9. Assisting the patient with ambulating
  10. Reminding the patient to move his or her head slowly when changing position to avoid vertigo
  11. Teaching the patient about care and activity restrictions
      a. Not using small objects, such as cotton-tipped applicators, matches, toothpicks, or hairpins, to clean the external ear canal
      b. Washing the external ear and canal daily in the shower or while washing the hair
      c. Blowing the nose gently
      d. Not occluding one nostril while blowing the nose
      e. Sneezing with the mouth open
      f. Wearing sound protection around loud or continuous noises
      g. Avoiding activities with high risk for head or ear trauma, such as wrestling, boxing, motorcycle riding, and skateboarding; wearing head and ear protection when engaging in these activities
      h. Keeping the volume on head receivers at the lowest setting that allows hearing
      i. Frequently cleaning objects that come into contact with the ear (e.g., headphones, telephone receivers)
      j. Avoiding environmental conditions with rapid changes in air pressure

H

Care Coordination and Transition Management
- Teach patients who have persistent vertigo and their families to determine the best ways to maintain adequate self-care abilities, maintain a safe environment, decide about assistance needs, and provide needed care.
- Give patients written instructions about how to take drugs and when to return for follow-up care.
- Teach patients how to instill eardrops and irrigate the ears, and obtain a return demonstration.
- Support patients by listening to their concerns and recognizing the emotional response to hearing loss.
- Provide information about public and private agencies that offer hearing evaluations, education, information, and counseling for patients with hearing disorders.

 HEART FAILURE: PERFUSION CONCEPT EXEMPLAR

OVERVIEW
- Heart failure (HF), also called *pump failure,* is the chronic inability of the heart to work effectively to support systemic PERFUSION.
- Basic cardiac physiologic mechanisms such as ejection fraction, stroke volume, cardiac output, and contractility are altered in HF.
- It is a common chronic health problem, with acute exacerbations, often requiring frequent hospitalizations.
- The major types of HF are:
  1. *Left-sided HF,* characterized by decreased perfusion from low cardiac output and pulmonary congestion is further subdivided into systolic HF and diastolic HF:
     a. *Systolic HF* with reduced ejection fraction (HFrEF) results when the heart is unable to contract forcefully enough during systole to eject adequate amounts of blood into the circulation.
        (1) The ejection fraction drops from a normal of 50% to 70% to below 40%.
        (2) Vascular volume and pressure increase in the pulmonary system causing lung edema or "congestion."
     b. *Diastolic HF* with preserved ejection (HFpEF) occurs when the left ventricle is unable to relax adequately during diastole preventing the ventricle from filling with sufficient blood to ensure an adequate cardiac output.
        (1) Although the ejection fraction is more than 40%, the ventricle becomes less compliant over time.
        (2) Diastolic failure represents 20% to 40% of all HF and is associated with older age and women with chronic hypertension.

2. *Right-sided HF* occurs when the right ventricle is unable to empty completely. Right HF in the absence of left HF is most often the result of pulmonary problems. Increased volume and pressure develop in the systemic veins resulting in peripheral edema.

3. *High-output failure* can occur when cardiac output remains normal or above normal and is caused by increased metabolic needs or hyperkinetic conditions such as septicemia, anemia, and hyperthyroidism.

• When cardiac output is insufficient to meet the demands of the body, compensatory mechanisms operate to improve cardiac output. Although these mechanisms may initially increase cardiac output, they eventually have a damaging effect on pump function. Compensatory mechanisms contribute to increased myocardial oxygen consumption, leading to worsening signs and symptoms of HF. Compensatory mechanisms include:

1. Sympathetic nervous system stimulation: increased heart rate, increased force of contraction, and arterial vasoconstriction that increases afterload.

2. Renin-angiotensin-aldosterone system (RAAS) activation: when perfusion to the kidney decreases during HF, these hormones are released to increase water and sodium reabsorption; angiotensin also increases arterial constriction or afterload.

3. Synthesis and release of B-type natriuretic peptide (BNP) from the overstretched atrium. BNP acts on kidneys to promote diuresis and vasodilation, decreasing preload.

4. Vascular endothelial cells secrete endothelin, a potent vasoconstrictor, increasing peripheral resistance and hypertension, increasing afterload and worsening HF.

5. Myocardial hypertrophy in response to inflammatory and growth factors released by poorly perfused myocardium and other tissues initially sustains cardiac output but, overtime, the myofibrils may not receive sufficient oxygen and nutrients, contributing to fibrosis and myofibril dysfunction; capillary or collateral vessel development may not be sufficient for adequate blood supply to the enlarged muscle.

Considerations for Older Adults

Patient-Centered Care

Heart failure is a common problem among older adults. The use of certain drugs can contribute to the development or exacerbation of the problem in this population. For example, long-term use of NSAIDs for arthritis and other chronic pain can cause fluid and sodium retention. NSAIDs may cause peripheral vasoconstriction and increase the toxicity of diuretics and angiotensin-converting enzyme inhibitors (ACEIs). Thiazolidinediones (TZDs) (e.g., pioglitazone [Actos]) used for diabetics also cause fluid and sodium retention. Rosiglitazone (Avandia), another TZD drug, has recently been found to cause acute myocardial infarction (AMI) in patients with type 2 diabetes. These drugs should be used with caution and restrictions in the older adult population.

- The American College of Cardiology (ACC) and American Heart Association (AHA) have developed evidence-based guidelines for staging and managing HF as a chronic, progressive disease. The New York Heart Association (NYHA) functional classification system is used to describe symptoms a patient may exhibit. These categorical approaches to HF help clinicians select and intensify treatment and prognosticate complications or terminal HF.

INTERPROFESSIONAL COLLABORATIVE CARE
Assessment: Noticing
- Assessment findings include:
  1. History of hypertension, acute coronary syndrome, heart valve disease, or other myocardial disease such as myocarditis; myocardial infarction is a common cause of HF.
  2. Dyspnea, orthopnea, breathlessness, exertional dyspnea, paroxysmal nocturnal dyspnea
  3. Decreased oxygen saturation (Spo_2) or Pao_2
  4. Increased respiratory rate and work of breathing including use of accessory muscles
  5. Crackles or wheezes on lung auscultation
  6. Cough with or without frothy sputum
  7. Dysrhythmias, especially tachycardia
  8. Weight gain, with more than 1 pound per day or 3 pounds per week indicating potential fluid retention (e.g., edema) and a need for consultation with a physician or advanced practice nurse
  9. Peripheral edema: an adult can gain 4 to 7 L of fluid (10 to 15 pounds or 4 to 7 kg) before pitting edema occurs; the abdomen can hold volumes of more than 10 L.

❗ NURSING SAFETY PRIORITY: Action Alert

Edema is an extremely unreliable sign of HF. Be sure that accurate daily weights are taken at the same time every morning to document fluid retention. Weight is the most reliable indicator of fluid gain and loss! Use weight gain and loss as well as intake and output to establish goals of care.

10. Decreased mentation, restlessness, or anxiety
11. Increased heart size and vascular or interstitial fluid on chest radiograph
12. S_3 or S_4 heart sounds
13. Cardiomegaly by palpation, electrocardiograph (ECG), chest radiograph, or echocardiography
14. Increased serum BNP
15. Increased abdominal girth
16. Jugular venous distention
17. Enlarged liver and spleen, especially with right-sided HF
18. Reduced kidney function including oliguria and increased blood urea nitrogen (BUN) and serum creatinine
19. Anxiety and depression or other markers of psychological distress
20. Electrolyte imbalance or presence of anemia (reduced hemoglobin means reduced oxygen carrying capacity and further compromise of tissue perfusion)

Considerations for Older Adults

Patient-Centered Care

Thyroxin (T_4) and thyroid-stimulating hormone (TSH) levels should be assessed in patients who are older than 65 years, have atrial fibrillation, or have evidence of thyroid disease. HF may be caused or aggravated by hypothyroidism or hyperthyroidism.

H

Analysis: Interpreting
- The priority collaborative problems for most patients with HF include:
  1. Decreased gas exchange due to ventilation/perfusion imbalance
  2. Potential for decreased PERFUSION due to inadequate cardiac output
  3. Fatigue due to hypoxemia
  4. Potential for pulmonary edema due to left-sided HF

Planning and Implementation: Responding
INCREASING GAS EXCHANGE
- The purpose of collaborative care is to help promote gas exchange.
- Interventions include:
  1. Monitoring for decreased gas exchange by assessing respiratory rate, rhythm, and character with breath sounds and cognitive status every 1 to 4 hours
  2. Providing supplemental oxygen to maintain Spo$_2$ at 90% or greater

3. Placing the patient experiencing respiratory difficulty in a high Fowler's position with pillows under each arm to maximize chest expansion and improve oxygenation
4. Encouraging the patient to deep breathe and re-position himself or herself every 2 hours while awake and in bed

---

! NURSING SAFETY PRIORITY: Action Alert

Provide the necessary amount of supplemental oxygen within a range prescribed by the primary health care provider to maintain oxygen saturation at 90% or greater. If the patient has dyspnea, place in a high Fowler's position with pillows under each arm to maximize chest expansion and improve gas exchange. Re-positioning and performing coughing and deep-breathing exercises every 2 hours helps to improve gas exchange and prevents atelectasis. Interprofessional collaboration with the respiratory therapist is important to plan the most effective methods for assisting with ventilation.

INCREASING PERFUSION
- Collaborative care begins with nonsurgical interventions, but the patient may need surgery if these are not successful in meeting optimal outcomes.
  Nonsurgical Management
- Administer drug therapy to improve perfusion by enhancing cardiac output. Monitor for therapeutic and adverse effects.
  1. Drugs that reduce afterload (relax arterioles) are:
     a. Angiotensin-converting enzyme inhibitors (ACEIs) or angiotensin receptor blockers (ARBs) reduce arterial constriction. These drugs also suppress the RAAS, which decreases fluid and sodium retention (causing diuresis and preload reduction). Monitor blood pressure (BP) to achieve the therapeutic goal. Monitor serum potassium level for hyperkalemia, serum creatinine level for kidney dysfunction, and the patient for development of a cough.
     b. A new combination medication, sacubitril/valsartan (Entresto), has demonstrated a reduction in death and hospitalization in patients with HF with a decreased ejection fraction. Entresto is a first-in-class medication as an angiotensin receptor neprilysin inhibitor (ARNI). It is used in place of an ACEI or ARB and should not be given in patients with a history of angioedema.

! NURSING SAFETY PRIORITY: Drug Alert

ACEIs and ARBs are started slowly and cautiously. The first dose may be associated with a rapid drop in BP. Patients at risk for hypotension usually have an initial systolic BP less than 100 mm Hg, are older than 75 years, have a serum sodium level less than 135 mEq/L, or are volume depleted. Monitor BP every hour for several hours after the initial dose and each time the dose is increased. Immediately report to the health care provider and document a systolic blood pressure of less than 90 mm Hg (or designated protocol level). If this problem occurs, place the patient flat and elevate legs to increase cerebral perfusion and promote venous return.

   c. Diuretics are the first-line drug of choice in older adults with HF and fluid overload. These drugs enhance the renal excretion of sodium and water by reducing circulating blood volume, decreasing preload, and reducing systemic and pulmonary congestion. The type and dosage of diuretic prescribed depend on the severity of HF and renal function. Loop diuretics such as furosemide (Lasix), torsemide (Demadex), and bumetanide (Burinex) are most effective for treating fluid volume overload.

     (1) Human B-type natriuretic peptides such as nesiritide (Natecor) are used to diurese patients during acute exacerbation of HF. These drugs cause renal excretion of sodium (water follows) as well as vasodilation. These drugs reduce preload and afterload.

     (2) Spironolactone (Aldactone) is a potassium-sparing diuretic added during later stages of HF because it provides additional RAAS blockade (blocks aldosterone) and boosts diuresis.

   d. Venous vasodilators (e.g., nitrates) can be used to return venous vasculature to a more normal capacity as well as decrease the volume of blood returning to the heart.

   e. Digoxin improves contractility and can be used to improve symptoms in later stages.

   f. Other positive inotropes used during acute exacerbation of HF include milrinone (Primacor), dobutamine (Dobutrex), and levosimenden (Simdax).

   g. Beta-adrenergic blockers (commonly referred to as beta blockers) improve the condition of some patients in HF. *Beta blockers must be started slowly for HF.* Patients in acute HF should not be started on these drugs. Carvedilol (Coreg),

H

metoprolol succinate (Toprol XL, Betaloc), and bisoprolol (Zebeta) are approved for treatment of chronic HF.

h. Ivabradine (Corlanor) is used for the treatment of stabilized, chronic HF. It slows the heart rate by inhibiting a specific channel in the sinus node.

i. Oxygen therapy can be used to maintain or increase Spo_2 above 92%.

2. For patients with *diastolic* HF, drug therapy has not been as effective. Calcium channel blockers, ACEIs, and beta blockers have been used with various degrees of success.

- Use diet therapy to reduce sodium and fluid overload and promote ideal body weight.

    1. Collaborate with the dietitian and patient to select foods that meet a heart-healthy, sodium-restricted diet to avoid fluid retention. Increase the patient's intake of potassium-rich foods if using a loop or thiazide diuretic.

- Fluid restriction and monitoring

    1. Limit the patients in AHA class 3 or 4 to 2 L/day of fluids, including intravenous (IV) fluids; other HF patients may be restricted to 2.5 to 3 L/day. Weigh the patient every morning before breakfast using the same scale; weight is the most reliable indicator of fluid gain or loss (1 kg of weight gain or loss equals 1 lb of fluid retained or lost).

    2. Monitor and record intake and output and report or intervene when intake exceeds output by more than 500 mL.

    3. Monitor for and prevent potassium deficiency from diuretic therapy. If the patient's potassium level is below 4 mEq/L, a potassium supplement may be prescribed.

    4. Recognize that patients with kidney problems may develop hyperkalemia, especially with the use of potassium supplements, ACEIs, or potassium-sparing diuretics. Kidney problems are indicated by a creatinine level higher than 1.8 mg/dL.

- Monitor patient responses to other options to treat HF.

    1. Continuous positive airway pressure (CPAP) improves sleep apnea (oxygen desaturation) and supports cardiac output and ejection fraction.

    2. Cardiac resynchronization therapy (CRT) uses a permanent pacemaker alone or in combination with an implantable cardioverter-defibrillator to provide biventricular pacing.

    3. *CardioMems implantable monitoring system* can be inserted into the pulmonary artery and allows the patient to take a daily reading of the pulmonary artery pressure. This data is transmitted to the provider's office and allows for management and adjustment of medications.

4. Investigative stem cell and gene therapy replaces damaged myocytes or genes by a series of injections into the left ventricle.

DECREASING FATIGUE
- The most common symptom reported by patients with HF is fatigue. The purpose of collaborative care is to regulate energy, prevent fatigue, and optimize function.
  1. Provide periods of uninterrupted physical rest.
  2. Assess the patient's response to increased activity. Check for changes in BP, pulse, and SpO_2 before and after an episode of new or increased activity.
  3. Consult cardiac rehabilitation services for both inpatient care and for transition to home care.
  4. Consider emotional exhaustion or anxiety as sources of physical fatigue and intervene with social support or referral to a mental health specialist.
  5. Depression is a common comorbidity in patients with chronic HF and is associated with noncompliance. Screen patients with HF for depression and refer them to a mental health care provider to assist with self-management, including management of fatigue, which is a disabling symptom of depression.

PREVENTING OR MANAGING PULMONARY EDEMA
- Monitor for symptoms of fluid overload.
- New onset pulmonary edema and acute HF exacerbation may be the result of acute coronary syndrome; monitor troponin levels and ECG for myocardial ischemia.
- New onset dysrhythmias, especially atrial fibrillation and abnormal ventricular beats, can further decrease cardiac output and exacerbate HF; monitor heart rate and rhythm with new onset fatigue or oxygen desaturation.

H

! NURSING SAFETY PRIORITY: Critical Rescue

Assess for and report early symptoms such as crackles in the lung bases, dyspnea at rest, disorientation, and confusion, especially in older patients. Document the precise location of the crackles because the level of the fluid progresses from the bases to higher levels in the lungs as the condition worsens. The patient in acute pulmonary edema is typically extremely anxious, tachycardic, and struggling for air. As pulmonary edema becomes more severe, he or she may have a moist cough productive of frothy, blood-tinged sputum; and his or her skin may be cold, clammy, or cyanotic.

SURGICAL MANAGEMENT
- Heart transplantation is the ultimate choice for end-stage HF.
- Ventricular assist devices can improve cardiac output in patients who are not candidates for heart transplant or are awaiting transplantation.
- Surgical therapies to reshape the left ventricle in patients with HF include:
  1. Partial left ventriculectomy
  2. Endoventricular circular patch
  3. Acorn cardiac support device
  4. Myosplint
- Care for the HF patient who is receiving a surgical intervention or ventricular assist device to improve HF is similar to patients receiving coronary revascularization or other open heart surgery. Specific monitoring and interventions include:
  1. Assessing the patient with HF for acute pulmonary edema. Clinical manifestations include decreased oxygen saturation (Spo$_2$); dyspnea; extreme anxiety; tachycardia; moist cough productive of frothy sputum; cold, clammy, cyanotic skin; crackles in lung bases; disorientation; and confusion.
  2. Administering rapid-acting diuretics as prescribed
  3. Providing oxygen and maintaining the patient in a high Fowler's position
  4. Administering morphine sulfate intravenously to manage pain while dilating peripheral veins (preload), decrease anxiety, and reduce the work of breathing
  5. Administering other drugs such as bronchodilators and vasodilators
  6. Monitoring vital signs closely, including pulse oximetry
  7. Monitoring intake and output; weighing daily

Care Coordination and Transition Management
- Collaborate with the case manager or social worker to assess the patient's needs for health care resources (e.g., home care nurse) and social support (family and friends to help with care if needed), and facilitate appropriate placement.
- Encourage the patient to stay as active as possible and develop a regular exercise program; investigate the possibility of a rehabilitation program referral.
- Instruct the patient to watch for and report to the primary health care provider:
  1. Chest pain or pronounced dyspnea while exercising or a decrease in exercise tolerance that persists for 2 or 3 days
  2. Weight gain of more than 3 pounds in 1 week or 1 to 2 pounds overnight
  3. Excessive fatigue unrelieved by sleep

4. Cold symptoms (cough) lasting more than 3 to 5 days
5. Frequent urination at night
6. Development of dyspnea or angina at rest, or worsening angina
7. Increased swelling in the feet, ankles, and hands

- Provide oral and written instructions concerning drugs.
- Teach the patient and caregiver how to take and record the pulse rate and BP to help monitor response to drug and exercise regimens.
- Instruct the patient to weigh himself or herself each day in the morning.
- Review the signs and symptoms of dehydration and hyper- and hypokalemia for patients taking diuretics and provide information on foods high in potassium.
- Recommend that the patient restrict dietary sodium, provide written instructions on low-salt diets, and identify food flavorings to use as a substitute for salt, such as lemon, garlic, and herbs.
- Discuss the importance of advance directives with the patient or family. If resuscitation is desired, the family should know how to activate the Emergency Medical System and how to provide CPR until an ambulance arrives. If CPR is not desired, the patient and family should be given resources on what to do and how to respond in the event of declining patient condition.

HEMOPHILIA

OVERVIEW

- Hemophilia is an inherited clotting disorder that leads to excessive bleeding.
- Two different clotting factor deficiencies result in hemophilia.
  1. *Hemophilia A (classic hemophilia)* is a deficiency of factor VIII (factor 8)and accounts for 80% of cases of hemophilia.
  2. *Hemophilia B (Christmas disease)* is a deficiency of factor IX (factor 9) and accounts for 20% of cases of hemophilia.

⚕ Genetic/Genomic Considerations

- Hemophilia is an X-linked recessive trait. Women who are carriers (able to pass on the gene without actually having the disorder) have a 50% chance of passing the hemophilia gene to their daughters (who then are carriers) and to their sons (who then have hemophilia). Affected men will pass the gene onto daughters, all of whom will be carriers, but not to their sons.
- About 30% of hemophilia arises from a new gene mutation and has no family history.

INTERPROFESSIONAL COLLABORATIVE CARE

* Assess for and document:
  1. Excessive bleeding from minor cuts, bruises, or abrasions
  2. Joint and muscle hemorrhages that lead to disabling long-term problems
  3. A tendency to bruise easily or experience prolonged nosebleeds
  4. Prolonged and potentially fatal hemorrhage after surgery
  5. Prolonged partial thromboplastin time (PTT), a normal bleeding time, and a normal prothrombin time (PT)
* Management of hemophilia generally occurs at a comprehensive care center and includes hemostasis during bleeding episodes, use of factor replacement products and medications, and rehabilitation for patients with joint injury from bleeding.
  1. The bleeding problems of hemophilia A are managed by prophylactic, scheduled, or intermittent infusions of synthetic factor VIII.
* Hemophilia B is managed with infusions of recombinant factor IX.

HEMATOPOIETIC STEM CELL TRANSPLANTATION

OVERVIEW

* Hematopoietic stem cell transplantation (HSCT), sometimes called *bone marrow transplantation (BMT),* is standard treatment for the patient with leukemia who has a closely matched donor and who is in temporary remission after induction therapy.
* HSCT is used also for lymphoma, multiple myeloma, aplastic anemia, sickle cell disease, and many solid tumors.
* HSCT started with the use of allogeneic bone marrow transplantation (transplantation of bone marrow from a sibling or matched unrelated donor) and has advanced to the use of human leukocyte antigen (HLA)-matched stem cells from the umbilical cords of unrelated donors. Transplants are classified by the source of stem cells.
* Transplantation has five phases: stem cell obtainment, conditioning regimen, transplantation, engraftment, and post-transplantation recovery.
  1. Obtaining stem cells: Stem cells are taken either from the patient directly (*autologous stem cells*), an HLA-identical twin (*syngeneic stem cells*), or from an HLA-matched person (*allogeneic stem cells*).

⊕ Cultural and Spiritual Considerations

Patient-Centered Care

About 70% of people on the bone marrow donor lists are white. The chance of finding an HLA-matched unrelated donor is estimated at 30% to 40% for white people, but for African

Americans the chance is less than 20% because there are fewer African Americans among registered donors. Although blood types are common in all racial groups, tissue types can be very different among racial and ethnic groups. Nationally, efforts are made to publicize the need for donors from all cultural backgrounds. Help in this effort by providing accurate information and dispelling myths.

    a. *Bone marrow harvesting* occurs after a suitable donor is identified by tissue typing in the operating room, where 500 to 1000 mL of marrow is removed through multiple aspirations from the iliac crests. The donor's marrow regrows within a few weeks.

    b. *Peripheral blood stem cell (PBSC) harvesting* requires three phases: mobilization, collection by apheresis, and reinfusion. During the mobilization phase, chemotherapy or hematopoietic growth factors are given to the patient for an autologous collection.

    c. *Cord blood harvesting* involves obtaining stem cells from umbilical cord blood of newborns.

2. The conditioning regimen "wipes out" the patient's own bone marrow, thus preparing him or her for optimal graft take and rids the person of cancer cells (*myeloablation*) with high doses of chemotherapy and, occasionally, radiation therapy over 5 to 10 days.

    a. Adverse effects from high dose chemotherapy are common.

    b. Severe immunosuppression from the regimen leaves the patient vulnerable to infection.

3. The transplantation of thawed marrow, PBSCs, or umbilical cord blood cells are infused through the patient's central catheter like an ordinary blood transfusion.

4. Engraftment or the successful "take" of the transplanted cells in the patient's bone marrow occurs after the transfused PBSCs and marrow cells circulate briefly in the peripheral blood. The stems cells find their way to the marrow-forming sites of the patient's bones and establish residency there.

    a. Monitoring of engraftment involves checking the patient's blood for "*chimerism*," which is the presence of blood cells that show a different genetic profile or marker from those of the patient. Mixed chimerism is the presence of both the patient's cells and those from the donor. Regressive chimerism with increasing percentages of the patient's cells indicates graft failure.

    b. When engraftment is successful, only the donor's cells are present.

5. Post-transplant recovery is difficult.
   a. Infection and poor clotting with bleeding are severe problems because the patient remains without bone marrow cells to provide white blood cells (WBCs) and platelets until the transfused cells grow and engraft.
   b. Other complications of HSCT include failure to engraft, development of graft-versus-host disease (GVHD), and veno-occlusive disease (VOD).
      (1) *Failure to engraft* occurs when the donated stem cells fail to grow in the bone marrow and function properly.
      (2) *GVHD* occurs mostly in allogeneic transplants but also can occur in autologous transplants.
         i. The immunocompetent cells of the donated marrow recognize the patient's (recipient) cells, tissues, and organs as foreign and start an immunologic attack against them. The graft is actually trying to attack the host tissues and cells.
         ii. Although all host tissues can be attacked and harmed, the tissues usually damaged are the skin, eyes, intestinal tract, liver, female genitalia, lungs, immune system, and musculoskeletal system.
         iii. Management of GVHD involves limiting the activity of donor T cells by using drugs to suppress immunity such as cyclosporine, tacrolimus, methotrexate, corticosteroids, mycophenolate mofetil (Cellcept, MMF), and antithymocyte globulin (ATG).
      (3) *VOD* is the blockage of liver blood vessels by clotting and inflammation (phlebitis) and occurs in about one-fifth of patients with HSCT, usually within 30 days of the HSCT.
         i. Patients who received high-dose chemotherapy, especially with alkylating agents, are at risk for life-threatening liver complications.
         ii. Symptoms include jaundice, pain in the right upper quadrant, ascites, weight gain, and liver enlargement.

HEMORRHOIDS

OVERVIEW

- Hemorrhoids are unnaturally swollen or distended veins in the anorectal region that are common and not significant unless they cause pain or bleeding.
- Internal hemorrhoids cannot be seen on inspection of the perianal area and lie above the anal sphincter.

- External hemorrhoids can be seen on inspection and lie below the anal sphincter.
- Prolapsed hemorrhoids can become thrombosed or inflamed, or they can bleed.
- Common causes are increased abdominal pressure associated with pregnancy, constipation with straining, obesity, HF, prolonged sitting or standing, strenuous exercise, and weight lifting.

INTERPROFESSIONAL COLLABORATIVE CARE

Assessment: Noticing
- Assessment findings include:
  1. Bleeding, which is characteristically bright red and found on toilet tissue or outside the stool
  2. Pain associated with thrombosis
  3. Itching
  4. Mucous discharge
- Diagnosis is made by inspection, digital examination, and proctoscopy, if needed.

Interventions: Responding
NONSURGICAL MANAGEMENT
- Conservative management focuses on reducing symptoms and includes:
  1. Application of cold packs to the anorectal area
  2. Topical anesthetics such as lidocaine (Xylocaine) or corticosteroid cream to be used for short term relief of pain and itching
  3. Treatment to avoid/manage constipation: fluids, high-fiber diet, fiber supplements, stool softeners, and bowel stimulants
  4. Teaching the patient to cleanse the anal area with moistened cleaning tissues and to gently dab the area rather than wipe

SURGICAL MANAGEMENT
- Ultrasound, laser removal, or other outpatient procedures may be indicated for prolapsed or thrombosed hemorrhoids. Monitor for bleeding and pain postoperatively. Warm compresses or sitz bath can promote comfort during recovery.

H

! NURSING SAFETY PRIORITY: Action Alert

Tell the patient who has had surgical intervention for hemorrhoids that the first postoperative bowel movement may be very painful. Be sure that someone is with or near the patient when this happens. Some patients become light-headed and diaphoretic and may have syncope related to a vasovagal response.

HEMOTHORAX

OVERVIEW

- Hemothorax is blood loss into the chest cavity and is a common result of blunt chest trauma or penetrating injuries. It can be combined with a pneumothorax.
  1. A simple hemothorax is a blood loss of less than 1000 mL.
  2. A massive hemothorax is a blood loss of more than 1000 mL.
- Bleeding can occur with rib and sternal fractures causing lung contusions and lacerations in addition to the hemothorax.
- Physical assessment findings depend on the size of the hemothorax and include:
  1. Respiratory distress
  2. Reduced breath sounds
  3. Blood in the pleural space (seen on a chest x-ray and confirmed by diagnostic thoracentesis)

INTERPROFESSIONAL COLLABORATIVE CARE

- Interventions aimed at removing the blood include front and back chest tube insertion.
- A hemothorax may require an open thoracotomy to repair torn vessels and to evacuate the chest cavity.
- Nursing interventions include:
  1. Monitoring vital signs and reporting when signs of hypoperfusion or hypotension occur
  2. Carefully monitoring chest tube drainage for blood loss >150 to 200 mL/hour for 3 to 4 hours
  3. Measuring intake and output and replacing output with IV fluids or blood products
  4. Assessing the patient's response to the chest tubes and managing pain
- Blood collected through closed chest drainage systems can be infused back into the patient after processing if needed.

 HEPATITIS: IMMUNITY CONCEPT EXEMPLAR

OVERVIEW

- Hepatitis is the widespread inflammation of liver cells, most commonly from altered IMMUNITY caused by viral infection.
- Liver inflammation persisting longer than 6 months is considered *chronic hepatitis.*
- Toxins can result in enlargement of the liver and congestion with inflammatory cells; typical toxins are chemicals, drugs, and some herbs.
- Hepatitis may occur as a secondary infection during the course of other viral infections, such as cytomegalovirus, Epstein-Barr virus, herpes simplex virus, and varicella-zoster virus.

- Fulminant hepatitis is a failure of the liver cells to regenerate, with progression of the necrotic process that is often fatal.
- Viral hepatitis is most commonly caused by one of five common viruses. Many patients have multiple infections, especially the combination of HBV with hepatitis C virus, hepatitis D, or human immunodeficiency virus (HIV) infection.
  1. Hepatitis A virus (HAV)
     a. HAV is a ribonucleic acid (RNA) virus of the enterovirus family. It is a hardy virus and survives on human hands. HAV is spread by the fecal-oral route, consuming contaminated food, or by person-to-person contact (e.g., oral-anal sexual activity). Unsanitary water, shellfish caught in contaminated water, and food contaminated by food handlers infected with HAV are all potential sources of infection.
     b. It is characterized by a mild course and often goes unrecognized. HAV is the most common type of viral hepatitis.
     c. The incubation period is usually 15 to 50 days.
  2. Hepatitis B virus (HBV)
     a. HBV is a double-shelled particle containing deoxyribonucleic acid (DNA) composed of a core antigen (HBcAg), a surface antigen (HBsAg), and another antigen found within the core (HBeAg) that circulates in the blood.
     b. HBV is transmitted through broken skin or mucous membranes by infected blood and body fluids.
     c. HBV is spread by:
        (1) Unprotected sexual intercourse with an infected partner
        (2) Sharing needles, syringes, or other drug-injection equipment
        (3) Sharing razors or toothbrushes with an infected individual
        (4) Accidental needle sticks or injuries from sharp instruments primarily in health care workers (low incidence)
        (5) Blood transfusions (that have not been screened for the virus, before 1992)
        (6) Hemodialysis
        (7) Direct contact with the blood or open sores of an infected individual
        (8) Birth (spread from an infected mother to baby during birth)
     d. The clinical course is varied, with an insidious onset and mild symptoms (such as anorexia, nausea, vomiting, fever, fatigue, and dark urine with light stool).
     e. The incubation period is generally between 25 and 180 days and blood tests confirm the disease.

H

3. Hepatitis C virus (HCV)
   a. The causative virus is an enveloped, single-strand RNA virus that is transmitted blood to blood.
   b. HCV is spread by contaminated items such as illicit IV drug needles, blood and blood products and transplanted organs received before 1992, needle stick injury with HCV-contaminated blood, tattoos, and sharing of intranasal cocaine paraphernalia.
   c. It is not transmitted by casual contact or intimate household contacts. However, those infected should not share razors, toothbrushes, or pierced earrings because there may be microscopic blood on these items.
   d. The average incubation period is 7 weeks, and it can lead to cirrhosis.
4. Hepatitis D virus (delta hepatitis or HDV)
   a. HDV is an RNA virus that needs the helper function of HBV for viral replication. HDV co-infects with HBV.
   b. Incubation period is 14 to 56 days.
   c. HDV is transmitted primarily by parenteral routes.
5. Hepatitis E virus (HEV)
   a. HEV is caused by fecal contamination of food or water.
   b. The incubation period is 15 to 64 days.

INTERPROFESSIONAL COLLABORATIVE CARE
- Prevention of hepatitis includes administration of hepatitis A and B through vaccination.
- Care of the patient with hepatitis includes preventing immunity-related complications.

Assessment: Noticing
- Record patient information:
   1. Known exposure to persons with hepatitis infection or a contaminated water source
      a. Crowded living conditions increase transmission occurrence
      b. Health care work increases exposure to hepatitis
      c. Travel to another country
      d. Unprotected sexual activity (with someone with a hepatic infection)
   2. Blood transfusions or organ transplantation
   3. History of hemodialysis
   4. Injectable drug use
   5. Recent ear or body piercing or tattooing
   6. Recent ingestion of shellfish
   7. HIV infection
   8. History of alcohol abuse or illicit intravenous or intranasal drug use

- Assessment findings for viral hepatitis include:
  1. Abdominal pain
  2. Changes in skin or sclera (icterus)
  3. Fever, arthralgia (joint pain) or myalgia (muscle pain), and lethargy or malaise
  4. Diarrhea or constipation, clay-colored stools
  5. Dark or amber-colored urine
  6. Nausea and vomiting
  7. Pruritus (itching)
  8. Liver tenderness in the right upper quadrant
  9. Elevated serum liver enzymes
  10. Elevated total bilirubin (serum and urine)
  11. Serologic markers for hepatitis A, B, C, or D
- The signs and symptoms of toxic and drug-induced hepatitis depend on the causative agent.
- Patients may be angry about being sick and being fatigued; may feel guilty about having exposed others to the disease; may be embarrassed by the isolation and hygiene precautions that are necessary; and may be worried about the loss of wages, cost of hospitalization, and general financial issues.
- Family members may be afraid of contracting the disease and therefore distance themselves from the patient. Counsel about the value of hepatitis vaccination.
- Liver biopsy may be used to confirm the diagnosis of hepatitis and to establish the stage and grade of liver damage.

Analysis: Interpretation

- The priority collaborative problems for patients with hepatitis include:
  1. Weight loss due to complications associated with the inflammation of the liver
  2. Fatigue due to decreased metabolic energy production
  3. Potential for infection related to state of immunocompromised

Planning and Implementation: Responding

- The patient with viral hepatitis can be mildly or acutely ill depending on the severity of the inflammation. Most patients are not hospitalized, although older adults and those with dehydration may be admitted for a short-term stay. The plan of care for all patients with viral hepatitis is based on measures to rest the liver, promote CELLULAR REGULATION and regeneration, strengthen IMMUNITY, and prevent complications, if possible.

PROMOTE NUTRITION

- The patient with hepatitis may decline food due to general malaise, anorexia, abdominal discomfort, or nausea.
  1. Determine food preferences that are high in calories and carbohydrates.
  2. Provide small, frequent meals and high-calorie snacks as needed.

- Address fatigue.
  1. Maintain physical rest alternating with periods of activity to promote liver cell regeneration by reducing the liver's metabolic needs.
  2. Individualize the patient's plan of care and change it to reflect the severity of symptoms, fatigue, and the results of liver function tests and enzyme determinations.
  3. Drugs of any kind are used sparingly for patients with hepatitis to allow the liver to rest. An antiemetic to relieve nausea may be prescribed. However, due to the life-threatening nature of chronic hepatitis B and hepatitis C, a number of drugs are given, including antiviral and immunomodulating drugs.

REDUCE THE POTENTIAL FOR INFECTION
  1. Teach the patient and caregivers about proper handwashing.
  2. Restrict visitors who have active infection or have recently been exposed to such.
  3. Monitor for development of a fever and report increasing temperature or changes in white blood cell count to the primary health care provider.

Care Coordination and Transition Management
- Liver transplantation may be performed for patients with end-stage liver disease from chronic hepatitis.
- Provide health teaching.
  1. Give patients information about modes of viral transmission.
  2. Maintain adequate sanitation and personal hygiene such as washing hands before eating and after using the toilet and avoid sharing of bed linens, towels, eating utensils, or drinking glasses.
  3. If traveling in underdeveloped or nonindustrialized countries, drink only bottled water. Avoid food washed or prepared with tap water, such as raw vegetables, fruits, and soups. Avoid ice.
  4. Do not share needles for injection, body piercing, or tattooing.
  5. Do not share razors, nail clippers, toothbrushes, or Waterpiks or other hygiene items that may have blood of body fluids that convey infective microbes.
  6. Use a condom (male or female) during sexual intercourse, or abstain from this activity.
  7. Cover cuts or sores with occlusive bandages.
  8. If ever infected with hepatitis, never donate blood, organs, or other body tissue.

HERNIA

OVERVIEW
- A hernia is a weakness in the abdominal muscle wall through which a segment of bowel or other abdominal structure protrudes.

- Congenital or acquired muscle weakness and increased intra-abdominal pressure contribute to hernia formation.
- Hernias are labeled by anatomic location, combined with the severity of protrusion.
  1. An *indirect inguinal hernia* is a sac formed from the peritoneum that contains a portion of the intestine or omentum; in men, indirect hernias can become large and descend into the scrotum.
  2. A *direct inguinal hernia* passes through a weak point in the abdominal wall.
  3. A *femoral hernia* occurs through the femoral ring as a plug of fat in the femoral canal that enlarges and pulls the peritoneum and the bladder into the sac.
  4. An *umbilical hernia* is congenital (infancy) or acquired as a result of increased intra-abdominal pressure, most often in obese persons.
  5. An *incisional (ventral) hernia* occurs at the site of a previous surgical incision as a result of inadequate healing, postoperative wound infection, inadequate nutrition, or obesity.
- Hernias can also be classified by intervention.
  1. A *reducible hernia* allows the contents of the hernia sac to be reduced or placed back into the abdominal cavity.
  2. An *irreducible,* or *incarcerated, hernia* cannot be reduced or placed back into the abdominal cavity. It requires immediate surgical evaluation.
  3. A *strangulated hernia* results when the blood supply to the herniated segment of the bowel is cut off by pressure from the hernia ring, causing ischemia and obstruction of the bowel loop; this can lead to bowel necrosis and perforation, which are surgical emergencies.

INTERPROFESSIONAL COLLABORATIVE CARE
Assessment: Noticing
- Assess for a hernia when the patient is lying down and again when the patient is standing. If a hernia is reducible, it may disappear when the patient is lying flat.
- Listen for bowel sounds (absence may indicate gastrointestinal [GI] obstruction).

Interventions: Noticing
- A truss (a pad with firm support) may be used for patients who are poor surgical risks.
- Herniorrhaphy, the surgical treatment of choice, involves replacing the contents of the hernia sac into the abdominal cavity and closing the opening.
- Hernioplasty reinforces the weakened muscular wall with a mesh patch.

- Provide preoperative and postoperative care and instruct the patient to:
  1. Avoid coughing, but encourage deep breathing
  2. For inguinal hernia repair, wear a scrotal support and elevate the scrotum with a soft pillow when in bed
  3. Avoid bladder and bowel distention by:
     a. Using techniques to stimulate voiding, such as assisting a man to stand
     b. Avoiding constipation and teaching the patient to avoid straining with stool during healing
- Teach the patient:
  1. How to care for the incision if surgery corrects the muscle defect
  2. To limit activity, including avoiding lifting and straining, for several weeks after surgery
  3. To report to the health care provider symptoms such as fever and chills, wound drainage, redness or separation of the incision, and increasing incisional pain

HERNIA, HIATAL
OVERVIEW
- Hiatal hernias, also called *diaphragmatic hernias,* involve the protrusion of the stomach through the esophageal hiatus (opening) of the diaphragm into the chest.
- There are two major types of hiatal hernias.
  1. *Sliding hernia* occurs when the esophagogastric junction and a portion of the fundus of the stomach slide upward through the esophageal hiatus into the thorax, with the hernia moving freely and sliding into and out of the thorax with changes in position or increases in intra-abdominal pressure.
  2. *Paraesophageal,* or *rolling, hernia,* occurs when the gastroesophageal junction stays below the diaphragm but the fundus and portions of the greater curvature of the stomach roll through the esophageal hiatus and into the thorax beside the esophagus; risk for volvulus, obstruction, and strangulation are high.

INTERPROFESSIONAL COLLABORATIVE CARE
Assessment: Noticing
- Assessment findings include:
  1. Symptoms of gastroesophageal reflux disease (GERD), dysphagia, heartburn, chest or esophageal pain, belching
  2. A feeling of fullness, breathlessness, or suffocation after eating
  3. Increased symptoms when in a supine position
  4. Confirmation via a barium swallow study with fluoroscopy is the most specific diagnostic test.

Interventions: Responding

NONSURGICAL MANAGEMENT

- Drug therapy includes the use of a proton pump inhibitor to control esophageal reflux and its symptoms.
- Diet therapy include avoiding fatty foods, caffeine, carbonation, chocolate, alcohol, spicy foods, and acidic foods such as orange juice.
- Encourage the patient to eat small-volume meals and consume liquids between meals to avoid abdominal distention.
- Lifestyle therapy includes attaining or sustaining ideal body weight because obesity increases intra-abdominal pressure.
- Elevate the head of the bed 6 or more inches.
- Instruct the patient to remain upright for several hours after eating, and to avoid straining or excessively vigorous exercise and wearing tight or constrictive clothing.

SURGICAL MANAGEMENT

- Elective surgery is indicated when the risk of complications such as aspiration are high or damage from chronic reflux is severe.
- Surgical approaches for sliding hernias involve reinforcement of the lower esophageal sphincter (LES) to prevent reflux through fundoplication, or the wrapping of a portion of the stomach fundus around the distal esophagus to anchor it and reinforce the LES.
- Provide preoperative and postoperative care and:
  1. Provide safe and effective care for the patient with a chest tube if a transthoracic approach was used.
  2. Assess for complications of surgery, such as temporary dysphagia, gas bloat syndrome, atelectasis or pneumonia, and obstruction of the NG tube.
  3. Prevent aspiration and respiratory complications with positioning, early ambulation, and use of incentive spirometry and deep breathing while providing adequate pain relief.
  4. Elevate the head of the bed at least 30 degrees.
  5. Teach the patient to support the incisional area during coughing and deep breathing.
  6. Ensure correct placement and patency of the NG tube.
  7. Reinforce dietary restrictions and nutritional goals.

Care Coordination and Transition Management

- Advise the patient:
  1. To avoid lifting and restrict stair climbing for 3 to 6 weeks after surgical repair
  2. To inspect the surgical wound daily and report the incidence of swelling, redness, tenderness, or discharge to the physician
  3. About the importance of reporting fever or other signs of infection to the surgeon

H

4. To avoid people with respiratory infection because prolonged coughing can cause the incision to break open (dehisce)
5. To stop smoking; inform about strategies for smoking cessation
6. About diet modifications, including weight goals, eating small portions, avoiding irritating foods and liquids, and reporting recurrence of reflux symptoms to the physician
7. To avoid straining and prevent constipation; stool softeners or bulk laxatives may be needed

HERPES, GENITAL

OVERVIEW

- Genital herpes (GH) is an acute, recurring, incurable viral disease.
- The two types of herpes simplex virus (HSV) are diagnosed and treated with the same interventions. The two types are:
    1. Type 1 (HSV-1) causes most nongenital lesions such as cold sores and about one-third of GH infections.
    2. Type 2 (HSV-2) causes most of the genital lesions.

> **! NURSING SAFETY PRIORITY: Action Alert**
>
> Either type of virus can produce oral or genital lesions through oral-genital contact with an infected person.

- The incubation period is 2 to 20 days, with the average period being 1 week; many people do not have symptoms during this time.
- Recurrences are not caused by re-infection but by reactivation of dormant virus. Recurrent episodes are usually less severe and of shorter duration than the primary infection. However, there is viral shedding and the patient is infectious with each outbreak of vesicles.
- Long-term complications of GH include the risk of neonatal transmission and an increased risk for acquiring HIV infection.

INTERPROFESSIONAL COLLABORATIVE CARE

Assessment: Noticing

- Obtain patient information about:
    1. The sensation of itching or tingling felt in the skin 1 to 2 days before the outbreak
    2. Presence of painful urination or urinary retention
    3. Factors that can trigger virus re-activation such as stress, fever, sunburn, poor nutrition, menses, and sexual activity
- Assess for and document:
    1. The presence of *vesicles* (blisters) or painful erosions in a typical cluster on the penis, scrotum, vulva, vagina, cervix, or perianal region
    2. Swelling of inguinal lymph nodes or other symptoms of infection such as headache, malaise or fever

- Diagnostic tests for GH include:
  1. Viral culture or polymerase chain reaction (PCR) assay of the lesions from blister fluid
  2. Serology testing to identify the HSV type, including type-specific rapid assays

Interventions: Responding

- GH is treated with oral antiviral medications such as acyclovir (Zovirax, Avirax), famciclovir (Famvir), or valacyclovir (Valtrex).

❗ NURSING SAFETY PRIORITY: Drug Alert

The drugs do not cure the infection; they decrease the severity of symptoms, promote healing, and decrease the frequency of recurrent outbreaks.

- Emphasize the risk for neonatal infection to all patients, both male and female.
- Teach patients to avoid transmission by:
  1. Adhering to suppressive therapy
  2. Abstaining from sexual activity while lesions are present
  3. Using condoms during all sexual exposures

❗ NURSING SAFETY PRIORITY: Action Alert

Remind patients to abstain from sexual activity while lesions are present. Urge condom use during sex because of the risk for HSV transmission. Viral shedding can occur even when lesions are not present. Teach the patient about how and when to use condoms.

---

  4. Keeping the skin in the genital region clean and dry
  5. Washing hands thoroughly after contact with lesions and laundering towels that have had direct contact with lesions
  6. Wearing gloves when applying ointments
- Help patients and their partners cope with the diagnosis by assessing the patient's and partner's emotional responses to the diagnosis of GH.

✳ HIV AND AIDS: IMMUNITY CONCEPT EXEMPLAR

OVERVIEW

- Human immunodeficiency virus (HIV) infection and disease can progress to acquired immune deficiency syndrome (AIDS). This common chronic disorder of impaired immunity is a serious worldwide epidemic (World Health Organization [WHO], 2015).

The time from the beginning of HIV infection to development of AIDS ranges from months to years. The range depends on how HIV was acquired, which additional health problems the patient has, personal factors, and interventions.

- A diagnosis of AIDS requires that the adult be HIV positive and have either a CD4+ T-cell count of less than 200 cells/mm³ or less than 14% (even if the total CD4+ count is above 200 cells/mm³) or one of 27 opportunistic infections or conditions.
    1. The HIV virus must first enter the host's bloodstream and then "hijack" certain cells, especially the *CD4+* T-cell, also known as the *CD4+* cell, *helper/inducer T-cell*, or *T4-cell*.
    2. When HIV enters a CD4+ T-cell, it can then create more virus particles. These new viral particles are able to infect more cells, repeating the cycle as long as there are new host cells to infect.
- Everyone who has AIDS has an HIV infection; however, not everyone who has an HIV infection has AIDS.

⊕ Cultural and Spiritual Considerations

Patient-Centered Care

Most new HIV infections reported in the United States and Canada occur in racial and ethnic minority groups, particularly among blacks/African Americans and Hispanics (CDC, 2015b). More culturally sensitive efforts targeted to these groups for prevention and treatment are needed.

Veterans' Health Considerations

The Veteran's Health Administration (VHA), a major health care provider in the United States, has found that a significant number of veterans have undiagnosed HIV disease. As a result, in 2009, the VHA eliminated the need for written consent for including HIV screening as part of routine testing. Despite the directive, only about 9% of veterans treated annually at VHA facilities have ever been tested (Gant-Clark et al., 2015). When asked, most veterans believed that they were HIV negative because they thought the test had already been done as part of routine testing and that the VHA would have notified them of positive results. This false sense of security has major implications because of the high prevalence of risky behaviors such as substance abuse and unsafe sexual practices among the VHA patient population. When interacting with veterans and discussing the issue of being aware of their HIV status as part of disease prevention, be sure to inform them that HIV screening is available to them through the VHA.

INTERPROFESSIONAL COLLABORATIVE CARE

Assessment: Noticing

The adult who has HIV disease is monitored on a regular basis for changes in immunity or health status that indicate disease progression and the need for intervention. The frequency of monitoring varies from every 2 to 6 months based on disease progression and responses to treatment. Continuing assessment is crucial to ensure that the drugs continue to work optimally because the patient may have medication issues or problems related to disease in many organ systems. Assess for subtle changes so any problems can be found early and treated.

- Determine risk for HIV/AIDS by asking focused questions about sexual history and drug-injecting activities.
- Ask the patient about when the HIV infection was diagnosed and what symptoms led to that diagnosis.
- Determine the extent of AIDS by defining illness and presence of opportunistic infections and malignancies, including when it started, the severity of symptoms, associated problems, and any interventions to date. All body systems are affected in AIDS.
- *AIDS dementia complex (ADC)* (also called *HIV-associated dementia complex*) is a result of infection of cells within the central nervous system by HIV, causing cognitive, motor, and behavioral impairments that range from barely noticeable to severe dementia.
- *AIDS wasting syndrome* is characterized by diarrhea, malabsorption, anorexia, and oral and esophageal lesions that contribute to persistent weight loss and an emaciated appearance.
- See Chart 2-10 for key features of AIDS.

Laboratory Assessment

- Lymphocyte counts: Patients with AIDS are often leukopenic, with a WBC count of less than 3500 cells/mm^3, and lymphopenic (<1500 lymphocytes/mm^3).
- CD4+ T-cell and CD8+ T-cell counts: in patients with AIDS, the ratio of CD4+ to CD8+ T-cells is low (less than 2:1), and this low ratio is associated with more disease symptoms.
- Antibody-antigen tests: A positive HIV antibody test means that the patient has been infected with the HIV virus, not that he or she has HIV disease or AIDS. Antibodies cannot be detected until 21 or more days after HIV exposure.
- Viral load testing directly measures the actual amount of HIV viral RNA particles present in 1 mL of blood. An uninfected adult has no viral load for HIV. A positive viral load test can measure as few as 40 HIV particles/mL. High viral loads can be greater than 80,000 HIV particles/mL. The higher the viral load, the greater the risk for transmission.

Chart 2-10 Key Features of AIDS

Immunologic Signs and Symptoms
Low white blood cell counts:
- CD4+/CD8+ ratio <2
- CD4+ count <200/mm^3
- Hypergammaglobulinemia
- Opportunistic infections
- Lymphadenopathy
- Fatigue

Integumentary Signs and Symptoms
- Dry skin
- Poor wound healing
- Skin lesions
- Night sweats

Respiratory Signs and Symptoms
- Cough
- Shortness of breath

Gastrointestinal Signs and Symptoms
- Diarrhea
- Weight loss
- Nausea and vomiting

Central Nervous System Signs and Symptoms
- Confusion
- Dementia
- Headache
- Fever
- Visual changes
- Memory loss
- Personality changes
- Pain
- Seizures

Opportunistic Infections
Protozoal infections:
- Toxoplasmosis
- Cryptosporidiosis
- Isosporiasis
- Microsporidiosis
- Strongyloidiasis
- Giardiasis

Fungal infections:
- Candidiasis
- *Pneumocystis jiroveci* pneumonia
- Cryptococcosis
- Histoplasmosis
- Coccidioidomycosis

Bacterial infections:
- *Mycobacterium avium* complex infection
- Tuberculosis
- Nocardiosis

Viral infections:
- Cytomegalovirus
- Herpes simplex virus
- Varicella-zoster virus

Malignancies
- Kaposi's sarcoma
- Non-Hodgkin's lymphoma
- Hodgkin's lymphoma
- Invasive cervical carcinoma

Analysis: Interpreting

- The priority interprofessional collaborative problems for patients with AIDS are:
  1. Potential for infection as a result of reduced immunity
  2. Inadequate gas exchange due to anemia, respiratory infection
  3. Pain due to neuropathy, myelopathy, cancer, or infection
  4. Inadequate nutrition due to increased metabolic need, nausea, vomiting, diarrhea, difficulty chewing or swallowing, or anorexia
  5. Diarrhea due to infection, food intolerance, or drugs
  6. Potential for reduced tissue integrity due to KS, infection, reduced nutrition, incontinence, immobility, hyperthermia, or cancer
  7. Cognitive decline due to ADC, central nervous system infection, or cancer
  8. Potential for psychosocial distress due to living with a life-threatening chronic disease that affects all aspects of life

Planning and Implementation: Responding

PREVENT INFECTION

- Teach patients to avoid exposure to infectious disease and what to do if symptoms of an infection or malignancy appear.
- Instruct about modes of transmission and preventive behaviors (e.g., guidelines for safer sex; not sharing toothbrushes, razors, and other potentially blood-contaminated articles).
- Combination antiretroviral therapy (cART) is the treatment for HIV and AIDS:
  1. Nucleoside reverse transcriptase inhibitors (NRTIs)
  2. Non-nucleoside reverse transcriptase inhibitors (NNRTIs)
  3. Protease inhibitors (PIs)
  4. Integrase inhibitors
  5. Fusion inhibitors
  6. Entry inhibitors

H

! NURSING SAFETY PRIORITY: Drug Alert

Ensure that cART drugs are not missed, delayed, or administered in lower-than-prescribed doses in the inpatient setting. Teach patients the importance of taking their drugs exactly as prescribed to maintain the effectiveness of cART drugs. Even a few missed doses per month can promote drug resistance (remember the 90% rule).

ENHANCE GAS EXCHANGE

- With HIV and AIDS, gas exchange can decrease related to anemia, respiratory infection (*P. jiroveci* pneumonia [PCP], cytomegalovirus [CMV] pneumonitis), pulmonary Kaposi's sarcoma (KS), or anemia.

1. Communicate with the primary health care provider when rate and depth of respirations are not within the normal range or new adventitious breath sounds occur.
2. Implement oxygen therapy when pulse oximetry is not within the normal range.
3. Administer antibiotics if respiratory complications are related to a pulmonary infection.

MANAGE PAIN

- Provide pain management for chronic pain related to neuropathy, myelopathy, cancer, or infection.
  1. Arthralgia and myalgia respond to NSAIDs.
  2. Chronic pain of peripheral neuropathy responds to:
     a. Tricyclic antidepressants, such as amitriptyline (Elavil)
     b. Anticonvulsant drugs, such as gabapentin (Neurontin) or carbamazepine (Tegretol)
  3. General pain at end of life can be managed with opioids
     a. Weaker opioids, such as oxycodone or codeine
     b. Stronger opioids, such as morphine, hydromorphone (Dilaudid), or transdermal fentanyl (Duragesic)
  4. Provide comfort measures:
     a. Pressure-relieving mattress pads
     b. Warm baths or other forms of hydrotherapy
     c. Massage
     d. Application of heat or cold to painful areas
     e. Use of lift sheets to avoid pulling or grasping the patient with joint pain
     f. Frequent position changes

ENHANCE NUTRITION

- Avoid protein and calorie deficiencies related to increased metabolic need, nausea, vomiting, diarrhea, difficulty chewing or swallowing, or anorexia. Because there are many factors for poor nutrition in AIDS, diagnostic procedures are needed to determine the cause. Once the cause is determined, appropriate therapy is initiated. For example, in candidal esophagitis, nutrition is affected by swallowing difficulties.
  1. Collaborate with the dietitian to optimize food intake or nutritional supplementation.
     a. Assess food preferences and any dietary cultural or religious practices.
     b. Monitor weight, intake and output, and calorie count to detect weight gain/loss.
     c. Teach the patient about a high-calorie, high-protein, nutritionally sound diet.

    d. Encourage the patient to avoid dietary fat.

    e. Administer prescribed supplemental vitamins, fluid, or supplements.

    f. Provide prescribed tube feedings or total parenteral nutrition.

MINIMIZE DIARRHEA

- For most patients with AIDS and diarrhea, symptom management is all that is available. Antidiarrheals such as diphenoxylate hydrochloride (Diarsed ✿, Lomotil) or loperamide (Imodium), given on a regular schedule, provide some relief. Consult with the dietitian and teach about appropriate foods.

RESTORE SKIN INTEGRITY

- Maintain skin integrity and promote healing of impaired skin related to KS of the skin, mucous membranes, and internal organs; infection; altered nutritional state; incontinence; immobility; hyperthermia; or cancer.
- KS is the most common skin lesion. Lesions may be localized or widespread; monitor for progression and keep weeping lesions clean and dressed.
    1. Lesions are managed with local radiation, intralesional or systemic chemotherapy, or cryotherapy. Lesions also respond well to antiretroviral therapy.
    2. Make-up, long-sleeved shirts, and hats may help maintain a normal appearance.

ENHANCE COGNITION

- Maintain a safe environment when confusion (acute and chronic) related to ADC, central nervous system infection, or cancer occurs.
    1. Assess baseline neurologic and mental status.
    2. Evaluate the patient for subtle changes in memory, ability to concentrate, affect, and behavior.
    3. Re-orient the confused patient to person, time, and place.
    4. Remind the patient of your identity and explain what is to be done at any given time.
    5. Give information and directions in short, uncomplicated sentences.
    6. Involve the patient in planning the daily schedule.
    7. Ask relatives or significant others to bring in familiar items from home.
    8. Make the environment safe and comfortable.
    9. Administer prescribed psychotropic drugs, antidepressants, or anxiolytics.
    10. Assess the patient with neurologic manifestations for increased intracranial pressure (ICP).

ADDRESS PSYCHOSOCIAL DISTRESS

- Patients diagnosed with HIV disease have many issues that can lead to psychosocial distress in the forms of depression, anxiety,

H

fear, isolation, and loss. The disease is chronic, debilitating, and fatal.

1. Provide a climate of acceptance for patients with AIDS by promoting a trusting relationship; maintain respectful communication.
2. Help patients express feelings and identify positive attributes.
3. Allow for privacy, but not avoiding or isolating the patient.
4. Encourage self-care, independence, control, and decision making by helping him or her set short-term, attainable goals and offering praise when goals are achieved.
5. Maintain social contact and assist with identifying support systems, including those already in place and those that need to be arranged.

Care Coordination and Transition Management

- The management of HIV/AIDS as a chronic disease occurs in many settings, most often at home.
- Hospitalizations occur during periods of severe infection or other acute exacerbations of symptoms.
- As the illness becomes more severe, the patient may need referral to a long-term care facility, home care agency, or hospice.
- In collaboration with the social worker, dietitian, and others, work with patients to plan what will be needed and how they will manage at home with self-care and ADLs.
- Teach the patient, family, and significant others about:
  1. Modes of HIV transmission and preventive behaviors
  2. Guidelines for safer sex; urge all patients who are HIV positive to use condoms and other precautions during sexual intimacy, even if the partner is also HIV positive
  3. Not sharing toothbrushes, razors, and other potentially blood-contaminated articles
  4. Signs of infection and when to seek medical help
  5. Teach patients with protein-calorie malnutrition what foods to include in the diet to promote better NUTRITION.
  6. Protection against infection transmission by:
     a. Avoiding crowds and other large gatherings of people where someone may be ill
     b. Not sharing personal toilet articles, such as toothbrushes or razors with others
     c. Washing hands thoroughly with an antimicrobial soap before eating or drinking, after touching a pet, after shaking hands with anyone, returning home from any outing, and after using the toilet
     d. Washing dishes between uses with hot sudsy water or using a dishwasher
     e. Not drinking water, milk, juice, or other cold liquids that have been standing for longer than an hour

    f. Not reusing cups and glasses without washing

    g. Not changing pet litter boxes; if unavoidable, using gloves and washing hands immediately

    h. Avoiding turtles and reptiles as pets

7. Support psychosocial integrity.

    a. Urge all patients who are HIV positive to inform their sexual partners of their HIV status.

    b. Respect the patient's right to inform or not to inform family members about his or her HIV status.

    c. Ensure the confidentiality of the patient's HIV status.

    d. Use a nonjudgmental approach when discussing sexual practices, sexual behaviors, and recreational drug use.

    e. Encourage the patient to express his or her feelings about a change in health status or the diagnosis of an "incurable" disease.

    f. Allow patients who have a change in physical appearance to express feelings of loss and mourn this change.

HYDROCELE

OVERVIEW

- A hydrocele usually is a painless cystic mass filled with a straw-colored fluid that forms around the testis.
- It is caused by impaired lymphatic drainage of the scrotum, leading to swelling of the tissue surrounding the testes.

INTERPROFESSIONAL COLLABORATIVE CARE

- Unless the swelling becomes large and uncomfortable or begins to impair blood flow to the testis, no treatment is necessary.
- When a hydrocele is large, uncomfortable, or cosmetically unacceptable, intervention is done by one of the following two methods:
  1. Drainage through a needle and syringe
  2. Surgical removal
- Provide postoperative care, including:
  1. Explaining the importance of wearing a scrotal support (jock strap) for the first 24 to 48 hours after surgery to keep the dressing in place and to prevent edema
  2. Assessing for pain and wound complications (infection or bleeding)
  3. Instructing the patient to schedule a follow-up visit with the surgeon
  4. Instructing the patient to stay off his feet for several days and to limit physical activity for a week
  5. Reassuring the patient that this swelling is normal and eventually subsides

HYDRONEPHROSIS, HYDROURETER, AND URETHRAL STRICTURE

OVERVIEW

- Several disorders obstruct the outflow of urine.
- In hydronephrosis, the kidney becomes enlarged as urine accumulates in the renal pelvis and the calyces. Obstruction within the pelvis or ureteropelvic junction results in renal pelvic distention, and extensive damage to the vasculature and renal tubules can result.
- Hydroureter is the obstruction of the ureter and obstruction of urine outflow to the bladder.
- A urethral stricture is the most distal point of obstruction, with bladder distention occurring before hydroureter and hydronephrosis.
- Urinary tract obstruction causes structural damage to the urinary tract with potential for subsequent infection and kidney failure.
- Causes of hydronephrosis and hydroureter include tumors, stones, trauma, congenital structural defects, and retroperitoneal fibrosis.
- Urethral stricture occurs from chronic inflammation.

INTERPROFESSIONAL COLLABORATIVE CARE

- Management includes:
  1. Recording history of kidney or urologic disorders, including pelvic radiation or surgery
  2. Documenting pattern of urination, including amount and frequency, and communicating decreases in urine flow
  3. Describing urine, including color, clarity, and odor
  4. Reporting new symptoms, including flank or abdominal pain, chills, fever, and malaise
  5. Re-establishing urine flow with irrigation of drainage device
  6. Managing flank, abdominal, or ureteral pain
  7. Monitoring urinalysis for protein, bacteria, or WBCs
  8. Anticipating an enlarged ureter or kidney on ultrasound, x-ray, or computed tomography (CT) scan
  9. Preparing the patient and managing recovery if a urologic procedure to restore urine flow, such as a stent placement, or a nephrostomy drain to divert urine flow is performed

HYPERALDOSTERONISM

OVERVIEW

- Hyperaldosteronism is increased secretion of aldosterone (mineralocorticoid excess) by the adrenal glands.
- Primary hyperaldosteronism (Conn's syndrome) results from excessive secretion of aldosterone from one or both adrenal glands and is most often caused by a benign adrenal tumor (adrenal adenoma).

- Secondary hyperaldosteronism is caused by high levels of angiotensin II that are stimulated by high plasma renin levels. Kidney hypoxemia, diabetic nephropathy, and excessive use of some diuretics can result in secondary hyperaldosteronism.
- Regardless of the cause, hyperaldosteronism is manifested by hypernatremia, hypokalemia, metabolic alkalosis, hypervolemia, and hypertension.

INTERPROFESSIONAL COLLABORATIVE CARE
Assessment: Noticing
- Obtain patient information about:
  1. Headache
  2. Fatigue
  3. Muscle weakness or paresthesia from electrolyte imbalance
- Assess for and document:
  1. Hypertension
  2. Elevated serum levels of sodium
  3. Low serum levels of potassium
- Diagnostic assessment includes:
  1. Serum electrolyte levels
  2. Serum renin levels
  3. Serum aldosterone levels (high)
  4. Imaging with CT scans or magnetic resonance imaging (MRI)

Interventions: Responding
- Adrenalectomy of one or both adrenal glands is the most common treatment for early-stage hyperaldosteronism.
  1. Provide preoperative care and:
     a. Correct the serum fluid and electrolyte imbalances by administering prescribed potassium supplements, potassium-sparing diuretics, or aldosterone antagonists.
     b. Manage preoperative hypertension.
  2. Provide postoperative care and:
     a. Teach the patient about corticosteroid (also called glucocorticoid) replacement (replacement is lifelong if both adrenal glands are removed).
     b. Instruct the patient to wear a medical alert bracelet while he or she is taking corticosteroids.
- For patients who do not have surgery and must remain on spironolactone therapy to control hypokalemia and hypertension, teach them about:
  1. Avoiding potassium supplements and foods rich in potassium
  2. Reporting symptoms of fluid and electrolyte imbalance
     a. Mouth dryness, thirst
     b. Changes in quantity or concentration of urine output

H

   c. Lethargy, drowsiness or neuromuscular changes, including weakness

3. Side effects of spironolactone therapy
   a. Gynecomastia
   b. Diarrhea
   c. Drowsiness
   d. Headache
   e. Rash, urticaria (hives)
   f. Confusion
   g. Erectile dysfunction
   h. Hirsutism
   i. Amenorrhea

HYPERCALCEMIA

OVERVIEW

- Hypercalcemia is a total serum calcium level above 10.5 mg/dL or 2.62 mmol/L.
- Because the normal range for serum calcium is so narrow, even small increases have severe effects.
- The effects of hypercalcemia occur first in excitable tissues.
- Common causes of hypercalcemia include:
  1. Actual calcium excesses
     a. Excessive oral intake of calcium
     b. Excessive oral intake of vitamin D
     c. Kidney failure
     d. Use of thiazide diuretics
  2. Relative calcium excesses
     a. Hyperparathyroidism
     b. Malignancy
     c. Hyperthyroidism
     d. Immobility
     e. Use of corticosteroids
     f. Dehydration

INTERPROFESSIONAL COLLABORATIVE CARE

Assessment: Noticing

- Assess for and document:
  1. Cardiovascular changes, which are the most serious and life threatening
     a. Irregular or increased heart rate and BP (early)
     b. Slow heart rate (late or severe)
     c. Cyanosis and pallor from impaired blood flow and hyper-coagulation
        (1) Assess hand and foot temperature, color, and capillary refill

2. Neuromuscular changes, which include:
   a. Severe muscle weakness
   b. Decreased deep tendon reflexes without paresthesia
   c. Altered level of consciousness (confusion, lethargy, coma)
3. Intestinal changes, which include:
   a. Constipation, anorexia, nausea, vomiting, and abdominal pain
   b. Hypoactive or absent bowel sounds
   c. Increased abdominal size

Interventions: Responding

- Restore calcium balance and prevent additional increases in calcium by:
  1. Discontinuing IV solutions containing calcium (lactated Ringer's solution)
  2. Discontinuing oral drugs containing calcium or vitamin D (e.g., calcium-based antacids, OTC vitamin supplements)
  3. Discontinuing thiazide diuretics that increase kidney calcium resorption
  4. Administering drug therapy to reduce circulating calcium and monitor effects with serum calcium levels:
     a. IV normal saline (0.9% sodium chloride) to dilute serum levels and promote elimination
     b. Diuretics that enhance calcium excretion, such as furosemide (Lasix, Furoside ✦)
     c. Calcium chelators (calcium binders) like plicamycin (Mithracin) or penicillamine (Cuprimine, Pendramine ✦)
     d. Drugs that inhibit calcium resorption from bone
        (1) Calcitonin (Calcimar)
        (2) Bisphosphonates
  5. Anticipate hemodialysis or blood ultrafiltration for rapid calcium reduction when levels are life threatening
  6. Consider cardiac monitoring to evaluate changes in the T waves, QT interval, and heart rate and rhythm
  7. Encouraging weight-bearing exercise to slow bone resorption in chronic conditions of hypercalcemia

HYPERCORTISOLISM (CUSHING'S DISEASE; ADRENAL GLAND HYPERFUNCTION): FLUID AND ELECTROLYTE EXEMPLAR

OVERVIEW

- Cushing's disease is the excess secretion of cortisol from the adrenal cortex leading to impaired FLUID AND ELECTROLYTE BALANCE and associated with a problem in the:
  1. Anterior pituitary gland (excess adrenocorticotropic hormone [ACTH])

2. Hypothalamus (excess corticotrophin hormone [CRH])
3. Adrenal cortex (commonly from a benign adrenal adenoma)
- Glucocorticoid therapy also can lead to hypercortisolism.
- *Adrenal hyperfunction* can also result in hyperaldosteronism, excessive androgen production, and *pheochromocytoma* or excess catecholamines.
- Excess cortisol affects metabolism and all body systems to some degree:
  1. Immune dysfunction with reduced lymphocytes and lymph tissue and inactive forms of WBCs
  2. Altered fat metabolism leading to truncal obesity, "buffalo hump," and "moon face"
  3. Hyperglycemia from insulin resistance
  4. Osteoporosis from excessive bone resorption
  5. Increased androgen production leading to acne, hirsutism, clitoral hypertrophy, and oligomenorrhea
  6. Thrombocytopenia (reduced platelets) and bleeding
  7. Skeletal muscle wasting leading to thin extremities and decreased activity
  8. Changes in skin (thinning) and impaired wound healing
- The most common cause of Cushing's disease is a pituitary adenoma.

INTERPROFESSIONAL COLLABORATIVE CARE
Assessment: Noticing
- Obtain patient information about:
  1. History of all health problems and drug therapies
  2. Age, gender, and usual weight
  3. Changes in weight, diet, or eating behaviors
  4. Change in activity or sleep patterns, fatigue, and muscle weakness
  5. Bone pain or a history of fractures
  6. Infections, particularly increased frequency or severity
  7. Easy bruising
  8. Cessation of menses
  9. GI ulcers
- Assess for and document:
  1. General appearance
     a. Buffalo hump on shoulder, central fat, moon face
     b. Thin arms and legs, generalized muscle wasting and weakness
  2. Skin changes
     a. Bruises
     b. Thin, translucent skin
     c. Wounds that have not healed

    d. Reddish purple striae ("stretch marks") on the abdomen, thighs, and upper arms
    e. Acne
    f. Fine coating of hair over the face and body
  3. Cardiac changes
    a. Tachycardia
    b. Hypertension
    c. Edema and evidence of hypervolemia
  4. Musculoskeletal changes
    a. Decreased muscle mass, especially in arms and legs
    b. Osteoporosis is common
  5. Glucose metabolism
    a. Fasting blood glucose levels are high
  6. Immune changes
    a. Infection risk is increased
  7. Emotional lability, mood swings, irritability, confusion, depression
- Diagnostic assessment includes:
  1. Blood, salivary, and urine cortisol levels
  2. Dexamethasone suppression testing
  3. Serum electrolyte values (increased sodium, decreased calcium, decreased potassium)
  4. X-rays, CT scans, or MRI to identify tumors of the adrenal or pituitary glands, lung, GI tract, or pancreas

Analysis: Interpreting
- The priority problems for patients with Cushing's disease or Cushing's syndrome are:
  1. Fluid overload due to hormone-induced water and sodium retention
  2. Potential for injury due to skin thinning, poor wound healing, and bone density loss
  3. Potential for infection due to hormone-induced reduced immunity
  4. Potential for acute adrenal insufficiency

Planning and Implementation: Responding
RESTORE FLUID VOLUME BALANCE
- Prevent fluid overload leading to pulmonary edema and HF:
  1. Monitor for indicators of increased fluid overload (bounding pulse, increasing neck vein distention, lung crackles, increasing peripheral edema, reduced urine output) at least every 2 hours.
  2. Administer drug therapy that interfere with ACTH production or adrenal hormone synthesis (Metyrapone [Metopirone], aminoglutethimide [Elipten, Cytadren], and ketoconazole) or manages hypercortisolism resulting from a pituitary adenoma (pasireotide [Signifor]).

3. Nutrition therapy for the patient with hypercortisolism may involve restrictions of both fluid and sodium intake to control fluid volume.
4. Monitor intake and output and weight to assess therapy effectiveness. Fluid retention may not be visible. Rapid weight gain is the best indicator of fluid retention and overload. Each 1 lb (about 500g) of weight gained (after the first half pound) equates to 500 mL of retained water.

PREVENT INJURY

- Injury is related to skin breakdown, bone fractures, and GI bleeding.
- Prevent skin injury by:
  1. Assessing the patient's skin for reddened areas, excoriation, breakdown, and edema
  2. Using pressure-relieving intervention during bed rest, including re-positioning or assisting with turns every 2 hours
  3. Teaching the patient activities to avoid trauma
     a. Use a soft toothbrush.
     b. Use an electric shaver.
     c. Keep the skin clean and dry it thoroughly after washing.
     d. Use a moisturizing lotion.
     e. Use tape sparingly and take care when removing it.
- Prevent pathologic fractures by:
  1. Using a lift sheet to move the patient instead of grasping him or her
  2. Reminding the patient to call for help when ambulating
  3. Reviewing the use of ambulatory aids (walkers or canes), if needed
  4. Keeping rooms free of extraneous objects that may cause a fall
  5. Teaching UAP to use a gait belt when ambulating the patient
  6. Teaching the patient about safety issues and dietary support for bone health
- Prevent GI bleeding by:
  1. Implementing prescribed drug therapy
     a. Antacids
        (1) H_2 histamine receptor blockers like ranitidine (Zantac, Apo-Ranitidine ✦), famotidine (Pepcid), or nizatidine (Axid)
        (2) Proton pump inhibitors like omeprazole (Losec ✦, Prilosec) or esomeprazole (Nexium)
     b. Encourage the patient to reduce or eliminate habits that contribute to gastric irritation, such as:
        (1) Consuming alcohol or caffeine
        (2) Smoking
        (3) Using NSAIDs

PREVENT INFECTION
- Continually assess the patient for the presence of infection.
    1. Monitor the daily CBC with differential WBC count and absolute neutrophil count (ANC) to detect and report abnormal values.
    2. Inspect the mouth during every shift for mucosal integrity.
    3. Assess the lungs every 8 hours for crackles, wheezes, or reduced breath sounds.
    4. Assess all urine for odor and cloudiness.
    5. Ask the patient about any urgency, burning, or pain present on urination.
    6. Take vital signs at least every 4 hours to assess for fever.
- Urge the patient to cough and deep breathe or to perform sustained maximal inhalations every 1 to 2 hours while awake.
- Teach the patient about radiation therapy for hypercortisolism caused by pituitary adenomas and:
    1. Observe for any changes in the patient's neurologic status, such as headache, elevated BP or pulse, disorientation, or changes in pupil size or reaction.
    2. Assess for skin dryness, redness, flushing, or alopecia at the radiation site.

PREVENT ACUTE ADRENAL INSUFFICIENCY
- The patient most at risk for acute adrenal insufficiency is the one who has Cushing's syndrome as a result of glucocorticoid drug therapy.
- If the drug is stopped, even for a day or two, the atrophied adrenal glands cannot produce the glucocorticoids and the patient develops acute adrenal insufficiency, a life-threatening condition.

> **! NURSING SAFETY PRIORITY: Drug Alert**
>
> Teach patients who are taking a corticosteroid for longer than a week to not stop the drug suddenly. Gradual drug tapering should be done under the care of the primary health care provider.

SURGICAL MANAGEMENT
- When adrenal hyperfunction results from increased pituitary secretion of ACTH, removal of a pituitary adenoma may be done.
- When hypercortisolism is caused by adrenal tumors, a partial or complete adrenalectomy (removal of the adrenal gland) may be performed by open abdominal procedures or laparoscopic procedures.
- Provide preoperative care and:
    1. Implement prescribed drug and diet therapy to correct electrolyte imbalances.

2. Monitor blood potassium, sodium, and chloride levels for abnormal values.

3. Monitor ECG for dysrhythmias related to electrolyte imbalance.

4. Monitor blood glucose levels and manage hyperglycemia.

5. Prevent infection with hand washing and aseptic technique.

6. Implement fall prevention measures with changes in mental status.

7. Teach the patient about the care needs after surgery and the need for long-term drug therapy.

- Provide postoperative care and:

1. Assess the patient every 15 minutes for shock (e.g., hypotension, a rapid and weak pulse, decreasing urine output) during the first 6 hours.

2. Monitor vital signs and other hemodynamic variables to detect hypervolemia/hypovolemia.
   a. Central venous pressure
   b. Intake and output
   c. Daily weights
   d. Serum electrolyte levels

Care Coordination and Transition Management

- Teach the patient who must take corticosteroid replacement drugs after surgery to:

1. Take the drug in divided doses, with the first dose in the morning and the second dose between 4:00 and 6:00 PM and to take the drug with food.

2. Weigh daily, record it, and compare with previous weights.
   a. Call the health care provider if more than 3 pounds are gained in a week or more than 1 to 2 pounds is gained within 24 hours.

3. Increase the dosage as directed for increased physical stress or severe emotional stress, including surgery, dental work, influenza, fever, pregnancy, and family problems.

4. *Never skip a dose of the drug.* If the patient has persistent vomiting or severe diarrhea and cannot take the drug by mouth for 24 to 36 hours, he or she must call the physician. If the patient cannot reach the physician, he or she must go to the nearest emergency department because an injection may be needed in place of the usual oral drug.

5. Always wear his or her medical alert bracelet or necklace.

6. Make regular visits for health care follow-up.

7. Urge attention to hand washing and personal hygiene to reduce exposure to transmissible disease.

8. Avoid crowds or others with infections.

9. Encourage the patient and all people living in the same home to maintain recommended vaccine schedule, including annual influenza vaccinations.

- The patient with hypercortisolism usually has muscle weakness and fatigue for some weeks after surgery and remains at risk for falls and other injury.
- Immediately after returning home, the patient may need a support person to stay and provide more attention than could be given by a visiting nurse or home care aide.

HYPERKALEMIA
OVERVIEW

- Hyperkalemia is a serum potassium level greater than 5 mEq/L (5 mmol/L).
- The normal range for serum potassium values is narrow, so even slight increases above normal values can affect excitable tissues, especially the heart.
- The consequences of hyperkalemia can be life threatening, and the imbalance usually is not seen in people with normally functioning kidneys.
- Causes include:
  1. Intake of potassium-containing foods or drugs
     a. Salt substitutes
     b. Potassium chloride
     c. Potassium-sparing diuretics
  2. Rapid infusion of potassium-containing IV solution
  3. Transfusions of whole blood or packed cells
  4. Adrenal insufficiency (Addison's disease, adrenalectomy)
  5. Tissue damage (crushing injuries, burns)
  6. Acidosis
  7. Hyperuricemia
  8. Chronic or acute kidney disease
- The problems that occur with hyperkalemia are related to how rapidly ECF potassium levels increase. Sudden rises in serum potassium cause severe problems at potassium levels between 6 and 7 mEq/L. When serum potassium rises slowly, problems may not occur until potassium levels reach 8 mEq/L or higher.

INTERPROFESSIONAL COLLABORATIVE CARE
Assessment: Noticing

- Obtain patient information about:
  1. Age
  2. Chronic illnesses (particularly kidney disease and diabetes mellitus)
  3. Recent medical or surgical treatment

4. Urine output, including the frequency and amount of voiding
5. Drug use, particularly potassium-sparing diuretics and ACE inhibitors (ACEIs)
6. Nutrition history to determine the intake of potassium-rich foods or the use of salt substitutes that contain potassium
7. Palpitations, skipped heartbeats, and other cardiac irregularities
8. Muscle twitching and weakness in the leg muscles
9. Unusual tingling or numbness in the hands, feet, or face
10. Recent changes in bowel habits, especially diarrhea
- Assess for and document:
  1. Cardiovascular changes
     a. Bradycardia
     b. Hypotension
     c. ECG changes
        (1) Tall, peaked T waves
        (2) Prolonged PR intervals
        (3) Flat or absent P waves
        (4) Wide QRS complexes
  2. Neuromuscular changes, early
     a. Skeletal muscle twitches
     b. Tingling and burning sensations followed by numbness in the hands and feet and around the mouth
  3. Neuromuscular changes, late
     a. Muscle weakness
     b. Flaccid paralysis first in hands and feet, then moving higher
  4. Intestinal changes
     a. Increased motility
     b. Hyperactive bowel sounds
     c. Frequent watery bowel movements
  5. Laboratory data: serum potassium level greater than 5 mEq/L

Interventions: Responding
- Interventions for hyperkalemia are aimed at rapidly reducing the serum potassium level, preventing recurrences, and ensuring patient safety during the electrolyte imbalance.
- Drug therapy
  1. IV therapy
     a. Discontinuing potassium-containing infusions
     b. Keeping the IV catheter open
     c. Administering IV preparation of 100 mL of 10% to 20% glucose with 10 to 20 units of regular insulin
  2. Withholding oral potassium supplements
  3. Potassium-excreting diuretics, such as furosemide
  4. Sodium polystyrene sulfonate (Kayexalate) exchange resins
- Hemodialysis or ultrafiltration

- Nursing care priorities include:
  1. Cardiac monitoring for early recognition of dysrhythmias and other manifestations of hyperkalemia on cardiac function

---

! NURSING SAFETY PRIORITY: Critical Rescue

Notify the health care provider or Rapid Response Team if the patient's heart rate falls below 60 beats/min or if the T waves become spiked.

---

  2. Collaborating with the dietitian to reduce dietary potassium intake by reading product packages and avoiding foods high in potassium including many salt substitute products, preserved meats, dried fruit, and large volumes of dark green vegetables or beans

HYPERLIPIDEMIA
OVERVIEW

- Hyperlipidemia is a condition of elevated serum lipid levels, including total cholesterol, low density lipoproteins (LDL), and triglycerides.
- High density lipoproteins (HDL) reduce hyperlipidemia; these cholesterol particles act as scavengers moving LDL out of the blood and into the liver for metabolism.
- Hyperlipidemia contributes to the formation of atherosclerotic plaque.
- Patients with metabolic syndrome and diabetes experience increased total cholesterol, LDL, and triglycerides, contributing to early atherosclerosis and cardiovascular events like heart attack or stroke.

INTERPROFESSIONAL COLLABORATIVE CARE

- Hyperlipidemia is treated with lifestyle interventions (e.g., diet, exercise) and drugs, typically statins (e.g., atorvastatin [Lipitor], fluvastatin [Mevacor], lovastatin [Pravachol], and simvastatin [Zocor]).

HYPERMAGNESEMIA
OVERVIEW

- *Hypermagnesemia* is a serum magnesium level above 2.6 mEq/L or 1.07 mmol/L.
- Magnesium is a membrane stabilizer, therefore, symptoms of hypermagnesemia occur as a result of reduced membrane excitability when serum magnesium levels exceed 4 mEq/L (1.6 mmol/L).

INTERPROFESSIONAL COLLABORATIVE CARE
Assessment: Noticing
- Assess:
  1. Cardiac changes of bradycardia, peripheral vasodilation, and hypotension
     a. ECG changes show a prolonged PR interval with a widened QRS complex.
     b. Patients with severe hypermagnesemia are in grave danger of cardiac arrest.
  2. CNS change of drowsiness, lethargy, or coma
  3. Neuromuscular changes of reduced or absent deep tendon reflexes and weak or absent voluntary skeletal muscle contractions

Interventions: Responding
- Restore magnesium balance by
  1. Stopping magnesium oral and parental supplementation
  2. Administering magnesium-free IV fluids and diuretic drugs to excrete this mineral
  3. When cardiac problems are severe, giving calcium may reverse the cardiac effects of hypermagnesemia

HYPERNATREMIA

OVERVIEW
- Hypernatremia is a serum sodium level greater than 145 mEq/L and is often accompanied by changes in fluid volume; sodium levels influence water balance because "where sodium goes, water follows."
- It makes excitable tissues more easily excited, a condition known as irritability, and leads to cellular dehydration.
- Common causes include:
  1. Actual sodium excesses
     a. Hyperaldosteronism
     b. Kidney failure
     c. Corticosteroids
     d. Cushing's syndrome or disease
     e. Excessive oral sodium ingestion
     f. Excessive administration of sodium-containing IV fluids
  2. Relative sodium excesses
     a. Restricted oral intake; "nothing by mouth" status; inability to perform ADL or self-manage oral intake
     b. Increased rate of metabolism (fever, surgery, burns, injury/trauma, infection, and sepsis)
     c. Hyperventilation
     d. Excessive diaphoresis (heat stroke, heat exhaustion)
     e. Watery diarrhea (food poisoning, gastrointestinal infection)
     f. Dehydration

INTERPROFESSIONAL COLLABORATIVE CARE

Assessment: Noticing

- Assess for and document:
  1. Nervous system changes
     a. Altered cognition such as decreased attention span and recall of recent events
     b. Agitation or confusion
     c. Lethargy, drowsiness, stupor, or coma (when accompanied by fluid overload)
  2. Musculoskeletal changes
     a. Muscle twitching and irregular muscle contractions (mild hypernatremia)
     b. Muscle weakness and reduced hand grip strength
  3. Cardiovascular changes that differ with fluid status
     a. High sodium with hypovolemia leads to increased pulse rate, hypotension, and reduced quality of peripheral pulses.
     b. High sodium with euvolemia or hypervolemia leads to normal or bounding pulses, neck vein distention, and elevated diastolic BP.
  4. Respiratory changes occur with hypervolemia.
     a. Pulmonary edema: lung crackles, dyspnea, tachypnea
     b. Decreased peripheral SpO_2

Interventions: Responding

- Increase fluid intake when hypernatremia is caused by fluid loss.
- Restrict fluid intake when hypervolemic hypernatremia occurs.
- Drug therapy includes diuretics that promote sodium loss, such as furosemide (Lasix, Furoside ✤) or bumetanide (Bumex).
- Measure fluid intake and output and ensure that the goals of therapy are communicated to health care team members.
- Dietary sodium restriction may be needed to prevent sodium excess.
- Priorities for nursing care of the patient with hypernatremia include monitoring the patient's response to therapy and preventing hyponatremia and dehydration.
  1. Prevent fluid overload, leading to pulmonary edema and HF.
     a. Monitor for indicators of increased fluid overload at least every 2 hours.

❗ NURSING SAFETY PRIORITY: Critical Rescue

Pulmonary edema can occur very quickly and can lead to death. Notify the health care provider about decrease in peripheral oxygen saturation or increased work of breathing (rate and depth of respirations) or ineffective breathing (hypoventilation) that can occur with fluid overload.

   2. Prevent skin and tissue injury from edema or reduced mobility.
   3. Monitor for patient response to diuretic drug therapy.
      a. Weigh the patient daily.
      b. Document intake and output.
      c. Establish intake and output goals with health care provider.
   4. Observe for manifestations of sodium imbalance.
      a. Changes in nerve, muscles, or cardiac excitability
      b. Changes in serum and urine sodium levels
   5. Promote nutrition therapy by teaching patients and families about:
      a. Sodium restriction
      b. Fluid restriction

HYPERPARATHYROIDISM

OVERVIEW

- Hyperparathyroidism results from increased levels of parathyroid hormone (PTH) that act directly on the kidney, causing increased kidney resorption of calcium and increased phosphate excretion. These processes cause hypercalcemia (excessive calcium) and hypophosphatemia (inadequate phosphate).
- Primary hyperparathyroidism results when one or more parathyroid glands do not respond to the normal feedback mechanisms for serum calcium levels. The most common cause is a benign tumor in the parathyroid gland.
- Secondary hyperparathyroidism is a response to the hypocalcemia associated with chronic kidney disease (CKD) or vitamin D deficiency, which leads to hyperplasia of the parathyroid glands.
- In bone, excessive PTH levels increase bone *resorption* (bone loss of calcium) by decreasing *osteoblastic* (bone production) activity and increasing *osteoclastic* (bone destruction) activity. This process releases calcium and phosphorus into the blood and reduces bone density.

INTERPROFESSIONAL COLLABORATIVE CARE

Assessment: Noticing

- Obtain patient information about:
   1. Bone fractures; joint, bone, and muscle pain
   2. GI problems of anorexia, nausea, vomiting, epigastric pain, constipation, and weight loss
   3. History of radiation treatment to the head or neck
   4. History of kidney stones
- Assess for and document:
   1. Waxy pallor of the skin
   2. Bone deformities in the extremities and back
   3. GI manifestations of anorexia, nausea, vomiting, epigastric pain or constipation

4. Fatigue and lethargy
5. Confusion, coma (severe hyperparathyroidism)
6. Diagnostic studies that include results for:
   a. Serum electrolyte levels, especially calcium and phosphorus
   b. Serum PTH and urine cyclic adenosine monophosphate (cAMP) levels
   c. X-rays with calcium deposits in joints or blood vessels, renal stones, or bone loss or abnormal lesions
   d. CT with or without arteriography
   e. Loss of bone density in a DEXA scan

Interventions: Responding

NONSURGICAL MANAGEMENT

- Intravenous fluids followed by a loop diuretic (furosemide [Lasix]) are used most often for reducing symptomatic serum calcium levels in patients.
- When symptoms are severe or related to parathyroid cancer, drug therapy includes:
  1. Cinacalcet (Sensipar) to decrease serum calcium
  2. Oral phosphates to interfere with dietary calcium absorption
- Interventions to manage symptoms and complications from hyperparathyroidism include:
  1. Evaluating cardiac rate, rhythm, and waveforms with continuous ECG monitoring
  2. Measuring intake and output 2 to 4 hours during hydration therapy
  3. Closely monitoring serum calcium levels for return to safe range
  4. Assessing for tingling and numbness in the hands, feet, and around the mouth to detect hypocalcemia early
  5. Preventing injury by implementing fall precautions to avoid fracture and injury to hypo-dense bones

QSEN SAFETY, EVIDENCE-BASED PRACTICE

Ensure patients are evaluated for fall risk on admission, with any change in health status, and when cognition or balance decreases. Use a standard, reliable, and valid risk assessment tool.

SURGICAL MANAGEMENT

- Surgical management of hyperparathyroidism is parathyroidectomy.
  1. All four parathyroid glands are examined for enlargement.
  2. If a tumor is present on one side but the other side is normal, the surgeon removes the glands containing tumor and leaves the remaining glands on the opposite side intact.
  3. If all four glands are diseased, they are all removed.

- Provide preoperative care and:
  1. Promote near-normal calcium levels before surgery occurs.
  2. Teach about neck support by having the patient place both hands behind his or her neck to assist in elevating the head.
- Provide postoperative care and:
  1. Closely observe the patient for respiratory distress that may occur from calcium derangements, compression of the trachea by hemorrhage, or swelling of neck tissues.
  2. Ensure that emergency equipment, including suction and oxygen is at the bedside.

! NURSING SAFETY PRIORITY: Critical Rescue

If severe swelling occurs and the airway begins to be obstructed, notify the Rapid Response Team and prepare for an emergent tracheostomy. Most institutions have an emergent tracheostomy tray; equipment may also be available on the Code Cart.

---

  3. Check serum calcium levels immediately after surgery and every 4 hours thereafter until calcium levels stabilize.
  4. Monitor for manifestations of hypocalcemia.
     a. Tingling and twitching in the extremities and face indicating onset of tetany
     b. Positive Trousseau's or Chvostek's sign (tetany; see *Hypocalcemia*)
  5. Assess for damage to the recurrent laryngeal nerve with changes in voice patterns and hoarseness.
- If all four parathyroid glands are removed, the patient will need lifelong treatment with calcium and vitamin D because the resulting *hypoparathyroidism* is permanent.

HYPERPITUITARISM

OVERVIEW

- Hyperpituitarism is hormone oversecretion that occurs with pituitary tumors or hyperplasia.
- Tumors occur most often in the anterior pituitary cells that produce growth hormone, prolactin (PRL), and ACTH.
  1. Overproduction of growth hormone results in acromegaly, manifested by increased skeletal thickness, hypertrophy of the skin, and enlargement of all visceral organs.
  2. Excessive PRL inhibits secretion of sex hormones in men and women and results in galactorrhea, amenorrhea, and infertility.

3. Excess ACTH over stimulates the adrenal cortex, resulting in excessive production of corticosteroids, mineralocorticoids, and androgens, which leads to the development of Cushing's disease.

⚝ Genetic/Genomic Considerations

One cause of hyperpituitarism is multiple endocrine neoplasia, type 1 (MEN1), in which there is inactivation of the suppressor gene *MEN1* (Online Mendelian Inheritance in Man [OMIM], 2016). MEN1 has an autosomal dominant inheritance pattern and may result in a benign tumor of the pituitary, parathyroid glands, or pancreas. In the pituitary, this problem causes excessive production of growth hormone and acromegaly. Ask a patient with acromegaly whether either parent also has this problem or has had a tumor of the pancreas or parathyroid glands.

INTERPROFESSIONAL COLLABORATIVE CARE
Assessment: Noticing
- Obtain patient information about changes in appearance and target organ function:
  1. Family history of endocrine problems
  2. Change in appearance: lip or nose size, gain or change in hat, glove, ring, or shoe size
  3. Fatigue and lethargy
  4. Arthralgias (joint pain)
  5. Headaches and changes in vision
  6. Menstrual changes (e.g., amenorrhea, irregular menses, difficulty in becoming pregnant)
  7. Changes in sexual functioning (e.g., decreased libido, painful intercourse, impotence)
  8. Loss of or change in secondary sexual characteristics
  9. Weight gain or loss (unplanned)
- Assess for and document:
  1. Changes in the facial features (e.g., increases in lip and nose sizes; prominent brow ridge; increases in head, hand, and foot sizes); moon face
  2. Extremity muscle wasting
  3. Acne
  4. Hirsutism
  5. Striae
  6. Hypertension
  7. Areas of uneven pigmentation or hyperpigmentation
  8. Dysrhythmias, including tachycardia or bradycardia

- Diagnostic testing may include:
  1. Blood test for hormone levels (any or all may be elevated)
  2. MRI of the head
  3. Hormone suppression tests

Interventions: Responding

NONSURGICAL INTERVENTIONS

- Drug therapy may be used alone or in combination with surgery and/or radiation.
  1. Dopamine agonists bromocriptine (Parlodel) and cabergoline (Dostinex) stimulate dopamine receptors in the brain and inhibit the release of growth hormone and PRL.
  2. Other agents used for acromegaly are the somatostatin analogs, especially octreotide (Sandostatin) and lanreotide (Somatuline), and a growth hormone receptor blocker, pegvisomant (Somavert).
- Gamma knife or stereotactic radiation therapy may be used to manage some conditions.

SURGICAL MANAGEMENT

- Surgical removal of the pituitary gland and tumor (hypophysectomy) is the most common treatment for hyperpituitarism.
- A minimally invasive trans-nasal or a trans-sphenoidal hypophysectomy is the most commonly used surgical approach. With a trans-sphenoidal approach, the surgeon makes an incision just above the upper lip and reaches the pituitary gland through the sphenoid sinus.
- A craniotomy may be needed if the tumor cannot be reached by a trans-sphenoidal approach.
- Provide preoperative care and:
  1. Explain that hypophysectomy decreases hormone levels, relieves headaches, and may reverse changes in sexual functioning.
  2. Remind the patient that body changes, organ enlargement, and visual changes are not usually reversible.
  3. Explain that because nasal packing is present for 2 to 3 days after surgery, it will be necessary to breathe through the mouth, and a "mustache dressing" ("drip pad") will be placed under the nose.
  4. Instruct the patient not to brush teeth, cough, sneeze, blow the nose, or bend forward after surgery.
- Provide postoperative care and:
  1. Monitor neurologic responses hourly for the first 24 hours and then every 4 hours and document any changes in vision, mental status, altered level of consciousness, or decreased strength of the extremities.

2. Observe for complications such as transient diabetes insipidus, cerebrospinal fluid (CSF) leakage, infection, and increased ICP.
   a. Excess urine output may indicate onset of diabetes insipidus.
   b. Any postnasal drip may indicate leakage of CSF.
   c. Assess nasal drainage for quantity, quality, and odor; send a sample to the laboratory for testing because the presence of glucose may confirm CSF drainage.
3. Keep the head of the bed elevated.
4. Instruct the patient to avoid transient elevated ICP from coughing, straining, or placing head below heart (bending at waist).
5. Perform frequent oral rinses and apply lip moisturizer.
6. Assess for manifestations of meningitis:
   a. Headache
   b. Fever
   c. Nuchal (neck) rigidity
7. Teach the patient self-administration of the prescribed hormones.

✴ HYPERTENSION: PERFUSION CONCEPT EXEMPLAR

OVERVIEW

- Hypertension is high BP and ultimately causes problems with cell, tissue, and organ PERFUSION.
- Hypertension is a BP above 140/90 mm Hg. In adults aged 60 years or older, hypertension is above 150/90 mm Hg. Patients with diabetes and heart disease should have a BP below 130/90 mm Hg to avoid perfusion complications.
- Hypertension reduces perfusion to heart, brain, kidney, eyes (retinal; vision), and tissues in the periphery.
- Classifications of hypertension:
  1. Essential (primary) hypertension is the most common type and is not caused by an existing health problem. However, a number of risk factors can increase a person's likelihood of becoming hypertensive, including: family history of hypertension, age older than 60 years, hyperlipidemia, stress, and smoking.
  2. Secondary hypertension results from specific diseases such as kidney disease, primary aldosteronism, Cushing's disease, brain tumors, and some drugs, such as estrogen-containing oral contraceptives, glucocorticoids, mineralocorticoids, and sympathomimetics.
  3. Malignant hypertension is a severe type of elevated BP that rapidly progresses. Symptoms include: morning headaches, blurred vision, and dyspnea and/or symptoms of uremia (accumulation in the blood of substances ordinarily eliminated in the urine). Systolic BP is greater than 200 mm Hg. Diastolic BP

H

is greater than 150 mm Hg or greater than 130 mm Hg when there are pre-existing complications. Unless intervention occurs promptly, kidney failure, left ventricular heart failure, or stroke may occur.

🌐 Cultural Considerations

The prevalence of hypertension in African Americans in the United States is among the highest in the world and is constantly increasing. When compared with Euro-Americans, they develop high blood pressure earlier in life, making them much more likely to die from strokes, heart disease, and kidney disease (Mozaffarian et al., 2016). The exact reasons for these differences are not known. Raising awareness of hypertension through education within African-American communities, including the importance of receiving treatment and controlling blood pressure, has been somewhat successful (Mozaffarian et al., 2016). Because of the prevalence in the African-American population, the JNC-8 Guideline differentiates first-line therapy based on race (Davis, 2015).

🌐 Gender Health Considerations: Patient-Centered Care

A higher percentage of men than women have hypertension until 45 years of age. From ages 45 to 64, the percentages of men and women with hypertension are similar. After age 64, women have a higher percentage of the disease (Mozaffarian et al., 2016). The causes for these differences are not known.

INTERPROFESSIONAL COLLABORATIVE CARE
Assessment: Noticing
- Record patient information
  1. BP in both arms while sitting
  2. Age
  3. Race or ethnic origin
  4. Family history of hypertension
  5. Dietary intake pattern, including alcohol
  6. Smoking
  7. Exercise habits
  8. Past and present history of cardiovascular, kidney disease, and diabetes
  9. Drug use (prescribed, OTC, and illicit)
  10. Peripheral pulse rate, rhythm, and force
  11. Psychosocial stressors

- Assess for hypertensive symptoms
  1. When a diagnosis of hypertension is made, most people have no symptoms
  2. Headache, dizziness, facial flushing, or fainting
  3. Edema
  4. Nosebleeds
  5. Vision changes or retinal changes on funduscopic examination
  6. Signs of kidney injury, such as elevated BUN or creatinine levels or low urine output
  7. Physical findings related to vascular damage, including atherosclerosis, acute coronary syndrome, peripheral arterial disease, stroke, chronic kidney disease, blindness, and HF
     a. Abdominal, carotid, or femoral bruits
     b. Dysrhythmias, tachycardia, sweating, and pallor
     c. Decreased or absent peripheral pulses
     d. Cardiomegaly or left ventricular hypertrophy
  8. Diagnostic assessment
     a. No laboratory tests are diagnostic of essential hypertension, several laboratory tests can assess possible causes of secondary hypertension.
     b. Kidney disease can be diagnosed by the presence of protein, red blood cells, pus cells, and casts in the urine; elevated levels of BUN and serum creatinine; and estimated or calculated glomerular filtration rate.
     c. Urinary test results are positive for the presence of catecholamines in patients with a pheochromocytoma (tumor of the adrenal medulla).
     d. An elevation in levels of serum corticoids and 17-ketosteroids in the urine is diagnostic of Cushing's disease.
     e. An ECG can determine atrial and ventricular hypertrophy, which is one of the first ECG signs of heart disease resulting from hypertension.

Analysis: Interpreting
- The priority collaborative problems for most patients with hypertension are:
  1. Need for health teaching due to the plan of care for hypertension management
  2. Potential for decreased adherence due to side effects of drug therapy and necessary changes in lifestyle

Planning and Implementation: Responding
HEALTH TEACHING
- Assist with planning and implementing lifestyle changes, including the regular evaluation of BP outside of office visits.
- In collaboration with the health care team, teach the patient to:
  1. Restrict sodium intake in the diet per the ACC/AHA guidelines.

2. Reduce weight, if overweight or obese.
3. Use alcohol sparingly (no more than one drink a day for women and two drinks a day for men).
4. Exercise 3 to 4 days a week for 40 minutes each day per ACC/AHA guidelines.
5. Use relaxation techniques to decrease stress.
6. Stop smoking and tobacco use.

- Drug therapy is individualized for each patient, with consideration given to culture, age, other existing illness, severity of BP elevation, and cost of drugs and follow-up.
  1. The most common drugs to control hypertension are:
     a. Diuretics
     b. Calcium channel blockers (CCBs)
     c. Angiotensin-converting enzyme inhibitors (ACEIs)
     d. Angiotensin II receptor blockers (ARBs)
  2. Diuretics are the first type of drugs for managing hypertension. Three basic types of diuretics are used to decrease blood volume and lower blood pressure:
     a. Thiazide diuretics, such as hydrochlorothiazide (Microzide, Urozide), inhibit sodium, chloride, and water reabsorption in the distal tubules while promoting potassium, bicarbonate, and magnesium excretion. Thiazide diuretics are considered the drug of choice for uncomplicated hypertension due to their low cost and high effectiveness.
     b. Loop (high-ceiling) diuretics, such as furosemide (Lasix, Apo-Furosemide) and torsemide (Demadex), inhibit sodium, chloride, and water reabsorption in the ascending loop of Henle and promote potassium excretion.
     c. Potassium-sparing diuretics, such as spironolactone (Aldactone), triamterene (Dyrenium), and amiloride (Midamor), act on the distal renal tubule to inhibit reabsorption of sodium ions in exchange for potassium, thereby retaining potassium in the body. When used, they are typically in combination with another diuretic or antihypertensive drug to conserve potassium.

Considerations for Older Adults

Loop diuretics are not used commonly for older adults as initial antihypertensive therapy because they can cause dehydration and orthostatic hypotension. These complications increase the patient's risk for falls. Teach families to monitor for and report patient dizziness, falls, or confusion to the health care provider as soon as possible and discontinue the medication.

3. CCBs, such as verapamil hydrochloride (Calan, Nu-Verap SR) and amlodipine (Norvasc), lower blood pressure by interfering with the transmembrane flux of calcium ions. This results in vasodilation, which decreases blood pressure.
   a. Some CCBs should not be administered with grapefruit juice.
   b. CCBs are most effective in older adults and African Americans.
4. ACEIs, known as the "-pril" drugs, are also used as single or combination agents in the treatment of hypertension. These drugs block the action of the ACE as it attempts to convert angiotensin I to angiotensin II, one of the most powerful vaso-constrictors in the body. This action also decreases sodium and water retention and lowers peripheral vascular resistance, both of which lower blood pressure.
   a. ACEIs include captopril (Capoten), lisinopril (Prinivil, Zestril), and enalapril (Vasotec).
   b. The most common side effect of this group of drugs is a nagging, dry cough.

❗ NURSING SAFETY PRIORITY: Drug Alert

Instruct the patient receiving an ACEI for the first time to get out of bed slowly to avoid the severe hypotensive effect that can occur with initial use. Orthostatic hypotension may occur with subsequent doses, but it is usually less severe. If dizziness continues or there is a significant decrease in the systolic blood pressure (more than a change of 20 mm Hg), notify the primary health care provider or teach the patient to notify the primary health care provider. The older patient is at the greatest risk for postural hypotension because of the cardiovascular changes associated with aging.

---

5. ARBs selectively block the binding of angiotensin II to recep-tor sites in the vascular smooth muscle and adrenal tissues by competing directly with angiotensin II but not inhibiting ACE. Examples of drugs in this group are candesartan (Atacand), valsartan (Diovan), losartan (Cozaar), and azilsar-tan (Edarbi).
   a. ARBs can be used alone or in combination with other anti-hypertensive drugs.
   b. These drugs provide an option for patients who report a nagging cough associated with ACEIs.

6. Beta-adrenergic blockers can also be used in the treatment of hypertension. Beta blockers are often the drug of choice for hypertensive patients with ischemic heart disease (IHD) because the heart is the most common target of end-organ damage with hypertension.

PROMOTE ADHERENCE TO THE PLAN OF CARE
- Patients who require medications to control essential hypertension usually need to take them for the rest of their lives.
- Patients who do not adhere to antihypertensive treatment are at high risk for target organ damage and hypertensive crisis.

Care Coordination and Transition Management
- Provide educational information for hypertension control, especially:
  1. Salt/sodium restriction
  2. Weight maintenance or reduction
  3. Self-awareness for healthy food selections such as the DASH or Mediterranean diets
  4. Stress reduction or coping strategies
  5. Alcohol restriction
  6. Exercise program
  7. Taking prescribed antihypertensive drugs even in the absence of symptoms
  8. Regular ongoing follow-up with health care provider
- Give oral and written information on drug therapy, including:
  1. Rationale for use, dose, and time of administration
  2. Side effects and vigilance for drug interactions
  3. The value of BP control to avoid serious adverse health consequences like stroke
- Instruct the patient and family members in the technique of BP monitoring at home and record values to share with scheduled provider interactions.
- Refer the patient to home care agency if necessary.

HYPERTHYROIDISM

OVERVIEW
- Hyperthyroidism is excessive thyroid hormone secretion from the thyroid gland.
- The manifestations of hyperthyroidism are called *thyrotoxicosis.*
- Thyroid hormones cause hypermetabolism and increased sympathetic nervous system activity.
- The most common cause is Graves' disease, an autoimmune disorder in which antibodies are made and bind to the thyroid stimulating hormone (TSH) receptor sites on thyroid tissue. The bound thyroid-stimulating immunoglobulins (TSIs) increase the number of glandular cells, resulting in overproduction of thyroid hormones.

⚕ Genetic/Genomic Considerations

Susceptibility to Graves' disease is associated with several gene mutations (*GRD1*, *GRD2*, *GRDX1*, *GRDX2*). The pattern of inheritance is autosomal recessive with sex limitation to females. Graves' disease is associated with other autoimmune disorders, such as diabetes mellitus, vitiligo, and rheumatoid arthritis, and often occurs in both members of identical twins. Ask the patient with Graves' disease whether any other family members also have the problem.

- Other causes of thyrotoxicosis from hyperthyroidism include benign or malignant tumors and excessive use of thyroid replacement drugs.
- *Thyroid storm,* or *thyroid crisis,* is a life-threatening condition of an extreme hyperthyroidism that occurs when the condition is uncontrolled or triggered by stressors such as trauma, infection, diabetic ketoacidosis, and pregnancy. Key manifestations include fever, tachycardia, and systolic hypertension.

INTERPROFESSIONAL COLLABORATIVE CARE
Assessment: Noticing
- Obtain patient information about:
  1. Heat intolerance—a hallmark of hyperthyroidism
  2. Age, gender, usual weight, and any unplanned weight loss
  3. Increased appetite
  4. Increased number of daily bowel movements
  5. Palpitations or chest pain
  6. Dyspnea (with or without exertion)
  7. Changes in vision, especially exophthalmos (specific to Graves' disease)
  8. Fatigue, weakness
  9. Insomnia (common)
  10. Irritability, depression
  11. Amenorrhea or a decreased menstrual flow (common)
  12. Changes in libido
  13. Previous thyroid and neck surgery or radiation therapy to the neck
  14. Past and current drugs, especially the use of thyroid hormone replacement or antithyroid drugs
- Assess for and document:
  1. Exophthalmos (Graves' disease)
  2. Photophobia, double vision, blurring
  3. Eyelid retraction or eyeball lag (the upper eyelid pulls back faster than the eyeball when the patient gazes upward)

H

    4. Presence or absence of a goiter (enlarged thyroid gland)
    5. Hypertension
    6. Dysrhythmias and tachycardia
    7. Fine, soft, silky hair
    8. Warm, moist skin
    9. Tremor
   10. Psychosocial issues or changes, including:
       a. Wide mood swings
       b. Irritability
       c. Decreased attention span
       d. Mild-to-severe hyperactivity
- Diagnostic assessment may include:
    1. Blood tests for:
       a. Triiodothyronine (T_3)
       b. Thyroxin (T_4)
       c. TSH
       d. Thyrotropin receptor antibodies (TSH-rAbs) (Graves' disease)
    2. Thyroid scan (radionuclide)
    3. Ultrasonography of the thyroid gland
    4. ECG with tachycardia, atrial fibrillation, T-wave changes

Interventions: Responding

- Interventions are described for Graves' disease because it is the most common form of hyperthyroidism. The goals of management are to restore cellular regulation by decreasing the effect of thyroid hormone on cardiac function during the acute phase and, both acutely and for long-term, reduce thyroid hormone secretion.

NONSURGICAL MANAGEMENT

- Monitoring, including:
    1. Measure apical pulse and BP at least every 4 hours and reporting status changes in a timely manner.
    2. Instruct the patient to report palpitations, dyspnea, chest pain, or dizziness immediately.
    3. Check temperature at least every 4 hours and report fever in a timely manner.
    4. Immediately report hyperthermia and hypertension to the provider because these signs precede thyroid storm.

> **! NURSING SAFETY PRIORITY: Critical Rescue**
>
> Immediately report a temperature increase of even 1°F (0.3°C) because it may indicate impending thyroid crisis.

    5. Promote comfort by keep the environment cool and linens dry.
    6. Administer drug therapy:

a. Antithyroid drugs
   (1) Methimazole (Tapazole)
   (2) Propylthiouracil (PTU)

> **! NURSING SAFETY PRIORITY: Drug Alert**
>
> Methimazole can cause birth defects and should not be used during pregnancy, especially during the first trimester. Instruct women to notify their health care provider if pregnancy occurs.

b. Supportive drug therapy with propranolol (Inderal, Detensol ✦) to relieve diaphoresis, anxiety, tachycardia, and palpitations
c. Radioactive iodine (RAI) therapy typically administered in an outpatient setting as an oral drug
   (1) Do not use in pregnant women because RAI crosses the placenta and can damage the fetal thyroid gland.
   (2) May take 4 to 8 weeks for results
   (3) May cause some patients to experience hypothyroidism as a result of the treatment
   (4) Some radioactivity is present in the patient's body fluids and stool for a few weeks after therapy; radiation precautions are needed to prevent exposure to family members and other people.
- Thyroid storm or thyroid crisis requires emergency management; even with optimal management, it can result in death.
  1. A life-threatening, uncontrolled hyperthyroidism can result in rapid onset of symptoms and life-threatening complications.
  2. Stressors such as trauma, infection, diabetic ketoacidosis, and pregnancy can cause thyroid storm. Thyroid crisis can also occur after thyroid surgery if thyroid hormone reduction drug therapy was not used.
  3. *Key symptoms include fever, tachycardia, and systolic hypertension.* The patient may have abdominal pain, nausea, vomiting, and diarrhea. Often he or she is very anxious and has tremors.
  4. Emergency measures to prevent death from thyroid storm vary with the intensity and type of changes. Interventions focus on maintaining airway patency, providing adequate ventilation, reducing fever, and stabilizing the hemodynamic status.

SURGICAL MANAGEMENT
- Surgery to remove all (total thyroidectomy) or part of the thyroid gland (subtotal thyroidectomy) is used to manage Graves' disease, when a goiter compresses the trachea or esophagus, or when hyperthyroidism does not respond to therapy.
- A thyroidectomy is typically performed under general anesthesia using a minimally invasive approach.

H

- After a total thyroidectomy, patients must take lifelong thyroid hormone replacement.
- Provide preoperative care and:
  1. Administer antithyroid drugs and iodine preparations to decrease the secretion of thyroid hormones and reduce thyroid size and vascularity.
  2. Ensure that hypertension, dysrhythmias, and tachycardia are controlled before surgery.
  3. Teach the patient to support the neck when coughing or moving by placing both hands behind the neck when moving.
- Providing postoperative care and monitoring for complications:
  1. Use pillows to support the head and neck to avoid neck extension.
  2. Place the patient, while he or she is awake, in a semi-Fowler's position.
  3. Prevent complications from airway obstruction or respiratory distress by:
     a. Listening for laryngeal stridor (harsh, high-pitched respiratory sounds)
     b. Ensuring that oxygen and suctioning equipment are nearby and in working order
     c. Assessing for laryngeal damage resulting in hoarseness or a weak voice

---

! NURSING SAFETY PRIORITY: Critical Rescue

If symptoms of airway obstruction such as stridor, dyspnea, or decreased oxygenation occur, notify the Rapid Response Team.

---

  4. Monitor for hemorrhage.
     a. Inspect the neck dressing and behind the patient's neck for blood at least every 2 hours for the first 24 hours.
     b. Assess drainage for amount, color, and character.
  5. Avoid injury from concurrent parathyroid removal or injury resulting in hypocalcemia and tetany.
     a. Ask the patient hourly about any tingling around the mouth or of the toes and fingers.
     b. Assess for muscle twitching.
     c. Ensure calcium gluconate or calcium chloride is available.

Care Coordination and Transition Management
- Teach the patient and family about:
  1. The manifestations of hyperthyroidism and instruct them to report an increase or recurrence of symptoms
  2. The manifestations of hypothyroidism and the need for thyroid hormone replacement

3. The need for regular follow-up because hypothyroidism can occur several years after RAI therapy
4. Prescribed drugs, including side effects
5. Inspecting the incision area and reporting redness, tenderness, drainage, or swelling to the surgeon
6. Possible continued mood changes, reassuring the patient and family that these effects will decrease with continued treatment

HYPOCALCEMIA

OVERVIEW

- Hypocalcemia is a total serum calcium (Ca^{2+}) level less than 9 mg/dL or 2.25 mmol/L.
- Because the normal blood level of calcium is so low, any change in calcium levels has major effects on function.
- Common causes of hypocalcemia include:
  1. Decreased vitamin D intake
  2. Complication of chemotherapy
  3. Hypoparathyroidism
  4. Certain types of leukemia or blood disorders
  5. Chronic renal failure
  6. Alcoholism
  7. Certain drugs such as diuretics and estrogen replacement therapy
  8. Excessive laxative use
  9. Consuming excess phosphate
- Low serum calcium levels increase sodium movement across excitable membranes, allowing depolarization to occur more easily and at inappropriate times.
- The more rapidly hypocalcemia occurs and the more severe it is, the more likely life-threatening manifestations will occur.

Gender Health Considerations

Postmenopausal women are at risk for chronic calcium loss. This problem is related to reduced weight-bearing activities and a decrease in estrogen levels. As they age, many women decrease weight-bearing activities such as running and walking, which allows osteoporosis to occur at a more rapid rate. Also, the estrogen secretion that protects against osteoporosis diminishes.

INTERPROFESSIONAL COLLABORATIVE CARE

Assessment: Noticing

- Assess for and document dietary intake of calcium or calcium supplement.

- Evaluate low serum calcium levels and related symptoms of:
  1. Neuromuscular changes (most common)
     a. Paresthesias with sensations of tingling and numbness
     b. Muscle twitches, painful cramps, and spasms
     c. Anxiety, irritability
     d. Positive Trousseau's sign: Place a BP cuff around the upper arm, inflate the cuff to greater than the patient's systolic pressure, and keep the cuff inflated for 1 to 4 minutes. Under these hypoxic conditions, a positive Trousseau's sign occurs when the hand and fingers go into spasm in palmar flexion.
     e. Positive Chvostek's sign: Tap the face just below and in front of the ear (over the facial nerve) to trigger facial twitching of one side of the mouth, nose, and cheek.
  2. Cardiovascular changes
     a. Bradycardia or tachycardia
     b. Weak, thready pulse
     c. Hypotension (severe hypocalcemia)
     d. ECG changes (prolonged ST interval, prolonged QT interval)
  3. GI changes
     a. Hyperactive bowel sounds
     b. Abdominal cramping
     c. Diarrhea
  4. Skeletal changes (thin, brittle, and fragile bones)
     a. Overall loss of height
     b. Unexplained bone pain

Interventions: Responding
- Restore calcium balance
  1. Administer drug therapy with:
     a. Direct calcium replacement (oral and IV)
     b. Drugs that enhance the absorption of calcium, such as vitamin D
  2. Collaborate with the dietitian to provide and teach about a high-calcium diet
- Promote safety during severe hypocalcemia by:
  1. Managing the environment to reduce stimulation, such as keeping the room quiet or adjusting lighting
  2. Instituting seizure precautions including placing emergency equipment (e.g., oxygen, suction) at the bedside
  3. Instituting fall precautions and gentle handling when fragile bones occur with prolonged hypocalcemia.

HYPOKALEMIA

OVERVIEW
- Hypokalemia is a serum potassium level less than 3.5 mEq/L (3.5 mmol/L).

- With hypokalemia, the cell membranes of all excitable tissues, such as nerve and muscle, are less responsive to normal stimuli.
- Rapid reduction of serum potassium levels results in dramatic changes in function, whereas gradual reductions may not show changes in function until the level is very low.
- Older adults are more vulnerable to hypokalemia because of risk factors of chronic conditions and drug therapy that contribute to this electrolyte imbalance.
- Common causes include:
    1. Actual potassium deficits
        a. Inappropriate or excessive use of drugs
            (1) Diuretics
            (2) Digitalis-like agents
            (3) Corticosteroids
        b. Increased secretion of cortisol or aldosterone
        c. Diarrhea
        d. Vomiting
        e. Wound drainage (especially gastrointestinal)
        f. Prolonged nasogastric suction
        g. Heat-induced excessive diaphoresis
        h. Kidney disease impairing reabsorption of potassium
        i. Nothing by mouth status
    2. Relative potassium deficits
        a. Alkalosis
        b. Hyperinsulinism
        c. Hyperalimentation
        d. Total parenteral nutrition
        e. Water intoxication

INTERPROFESSIONAL COLLABORATIVE CARE
Assessment: Noticing
- Obtain patient information about:
    1. Drugs, especially diuretics, corticosteroids, digoxin, and potassium supplements
    2. Presence of acute or chronic disease, especially cardiac or kidney conditions
    3. Diet history
- Assess for and document:
    1. Respiratory changes:

! NURSING SAFETY PRIORITY: Critical Rescue

Assess the respiratory status of a patient who has hypokalemia at least every 3 hours because respiratory insufficiency is a major cause of death for these patients.

  a. Breath sounds
  b. Respiratory effort including rate and depth of respiration
  c. Oxygen saturation
  d. Color of nail beds and mucous membranes
2. Musculoskeletal changes that indicate weakness
  a. Weak hand grasps
  b. Lethargy, inability to complete ADLs
  c. Flaccid paralysis
3. Cardiovascular changes
  a. Rapid, thready pulse that is difficult to palpate
  b. Dysrhythmias and ECG changes
    (1) ST-segment depression
    (2) Flat or inverted T waves
    (3) Increased U waves

! NURSING SAFETY PRIORITY: Critical Rescue

Dysrhythmias can lead to death, particularly in older adults. Report new onset dysrhythmias and all ECG changes consistent with hypokalemia to the physician or Rapid Response Team.

  c. Orthostatic hypotension
4. Neurologic changes
  a. Altered mental status
  b. Irritability and anxiety
  c. Lethargy, acute confusion, coma
5. GI changes of reduced peristalsis leading to:
  a. Hypoactive or absent bowel sounds
  b. Abdominal distension
  c. Nausea, vomiting
  d. Constipation

Interventions: Responding
RESTORE POTASSIUM BALANCE
1. Administer oral and IV potassium replacement therapy or drugs to reduce urinary loss of potassium.
  a. In the presence of persistent hypokalemia despite replacement therapy, evaluate and consider replacing magnesium.

! NURSING SAFETY PRIORITY: Drug Alert

The maximum recommended infusion rate is 5 to 10 mEq/hr; this rate is not to exceed 20 mEq/hr. In accordance with National Patient Safety Goals (NPSGs), potassium is not given by IV push to avoid causing cardiac arrest.

   b. Oral potassium preparations have a strong, unpleasant taste that is difficult to mask; give the drug during or after a meal or dilute it with nearly any patient-preferred liquid.

   c. Potassium-sparing diuretics like spironolactone (Aldactone, Novo-Spiroton ✦) may be used to slow potassium loss.

2. Monitor patient response to potassium replacement therapy, including cardiac and neurologic derangements from too rapid or delayed replacement therapy.

3. Collaborate with the dietitian for nutrition therapy to increase dietary potassium intake.

4. Institute fall precautions as a safety measure.

5. Perform respiratory monitoring at least hourly for severe hypokalemia.

   a. Respiratory effort, including rate and depth (checking for increasing rate and decreasing depth)

   b. Oxygen saturation by pulse oximetry

HYPOMAGNESEMIA

OVERVIEW

- Hypomagnesemia is a serum magnesium (Mg^2) level below 1.8 mEq/L or 0.74 mmol/L.
- It is most often caused by decreased absorption of dietary magnesium or increased kidney magnesium excretion from thiazide diuretics.

INTERPROFESSIONAL COLLABORATIVE CARE

Assessment: Noticing

- Assess serum magnesium levels and symptoms of low magnesium.
  1. Cardiovascular changes, including hypertension, atherosclerosis, hypertrophic left ventricle, and a variety of dysrhythmias
  2. Neuromuscular changes, including hyperactive deep tendon reflexes, numbness and tingling, and painful muscle contractions
     a. Low magnesium often occurs with low calcium.
     b. Positive Chvostek's and Trousseau's signs may be present when hypocalcemia co-occurs.
  3. Intestinal changes, including paralytic ileus from decreased intestinal smooth muscle contraction, anorexia, nausea, constipation, and abdominal distention are common.

Interventions: Responding

RESTORE MAGNESIUM BALANCE

1. Magnesium is replaced with oral or IV magnesium sulfate ($MgSO_4$)

H

    a. Assess deep tendon reflexes at least hourly in the patient receiving IV magnesium to monitor effectiveness and prevent hypermagnesemia.

    b. If hypocalcemia is also present, drug therapy to increase serum calcium levels is prescribed.

2. Stop drugs that promote magnesium loss at least until balance is restored.

HYPONATREMIA

OVERVIEW

* Hyponatremia is a serum sodium (Na^+) level less than 136 mEq/L (136 mmol/L), and it often occurs with fluid volume imbalances; sodium levels influence water balance because "where sodium goes, water follows."
* The problems caused by hyponatremia involve reduced excitable membrane depolarization and cellular swelling.
* The cells especially affected are those involved in cerebral, neuromuscular, intestinal smooth muscle, and cardiovascular functions.
* Common causes of hyponatremia include:
  1. Actual sodium deficits
     a. Excessive diaphoresis
     b. Diuretics (high-ceiling diuretics)
     c. Wound drainage (especially gastrointestinal)
     d. Decreased secretion of aldosterone
     e. Hyperlipidemia
     f. Kidney disease (scarred distal convoluted tubule)
     g. Nothing by mouth
     h. Low-salt diet
     i. Cerebral salt-wasting syndrome
     j. Hyperglycemia
  2. Relative sodium deficits (dilution)
     a. Excessive ingestion of hypotonic fluids
     b. Psychogenic polydipsia
     c. Freshwater submersion accident
     d. Kidney failure (nephrotic syndrome)
     e. Irrigation with hypotonic fluids
     f. Syndrome of inappropriate antidiuretic hormone secretion
     g. HF

INTERPROFESSIONAL COLLABORATIVE CARE

Assessment: Noticing

* Assess for and document:
  1. Cerebral changes
     a. Acute confusion

     b. Reduced level of cognition
     c. Seizure activity
  2. Neuromuscular changes
     a. General muscle weakness, especially in arms and legs
     b. Diminished deep tendon reflexes

> **! NURSING SAFETY PRIORITY: Critical Rescue**
>
> If the patient has muscle weakness, immediately check respiratory effectiveness such as SpO_2 and consciousness or cognition. Ventilation depends on adequate strength of respiratory muscles.

  3. GI changes
     a. Increased motility
     b. Diarrhea
     c. Abdominal cramping
     d. Hyperactive bowel sounds
  4. Cardiovascular changes
     a. Hyponatremia with hypovolemia
       (1) Rapid, weak, thready pulse
       (2) Reduced peripheral pulses
       (3) Hypotension
     b. Hyponatremia with hypervolemia
       (1) Full, bounding pulse
       (2) Normal or high BP
       (3) Edema

Interventions: Responding
RESTORE SODIUM BALANCE
  1. Drug therapy
     a. Discontinue or reduce drugs that increase sodium loss, such as loop diuretics and thiazide diuretics.
     b. If hyponatremia with a fluid deficit, anticipate administering IV saline infusion to restore both sodium and fluid volume; severe hyponatremia may be treated with small-volume infusions of hypertonic (2% to 3%) saline.
     c. If hyponatremia with fluid excess, anticipate using osmotic diuretics that promote the excretion of water rather than sodium, such as mannitol (Osmitrol) or conivaptan (Vaprisol).
     d. If hyponatremia caused by inappropriate secretion of antidiuretic hormone (ADH), anticipate therapy that includes agents that antagonize ADH, such as lithium and demeclocycline (Declomycin).
  2. Monitor the amount and quality of oral and IV intake and urine output.

3. Evaluate serum and urine lab results for electrolyte panel and osmolality.
4. Weigh daily.
5. Observe for manifestations and complications of electrolyte imbalance in neurologic, muscular, GI, and cardiovascular health, including ECG patterns.
6. Collaborate with the dietitian to increase sodium intake and, if prescribed, restrict fluid intake.
7. Provide skin protection interventions if the patient with hyponatremia has decreased consciousness, muscle weakness leading to reducing mobility, or edema.
8. Teach patients and families about fluid and electrolyte balance and symptoms of hyponatremia.

HYPOPARATHYROIDISM

OVERVIEW
- Hypoparathyroidism is a rare endocrine disorder in which parathyroid function is decreased, resulting in a deficiency of circulating PTH levels.
- The main result is hypocalcemia.
- There are two forms:
  1. *Iatrogenic hypoparathyroidism,* the most common form, is caused by the removal of all parathyroid tissue during surgical removal of the thyroid or parathyroid glands.
  2. *Idiopathic hypoparathyroidism* is rare and probably caused by an autoimmune problem.
- Severe hypomagnesemia from malabsorption syndromes, CKD, and malnutrition may cause hypoparathyroidism.

INTERPROFESSIONAL COLLABORATIVE CARE
Assessment: Noticing
- Obtain patient information about:
  1. Any head or neck surgery, injury, or radiation therapy
  2. Presence of mild tingling and numbness around the mouth or in the hands and feet
  3. Presence of muscle cramps and spasms of the hands and feet
- Assess for and document hypocalcemia signs or symptoms:
  1. Symptoms of tetany from hypocalcemia, including numbness or tingling (mild) or cramping and spasms (moderate or severe)
     a. Positive Chvostek's or Trousseau's sign (see *Hypocalcemia*)
  2. Irritability, psychosis, or seizures
  3. Bands or pits encircling the crowns of the teeth indicating a loss of tooth calcium and enamel

- Diagnostic tests for hypoparathyroidism include:
  1. Serum electrolyte tests, vitamin D and PTH levels
  2. CT scan of the brain (may show calcium deposits) and neck
  3. Urine cAMP levels

Interventions: Responding

- Management focuses on correcting hypocalcemia, vitamin D deficiency, and hypomagnesemia.
  1. For severe hypocalcemia, IV calcium is given as a 10% solution of calcium chloride or calcium gluconate over 10 to 15 minutes.
  2. Long-term calcium therapy includes oral calcium of 0.5 to 2 g daily in divided doses.
  3. For vitamin D deficiency, oral calcitriol (Rocaltrol), 0.5 to 2 mg daily emergently followed by oral ergocalciferal daily.
  4. Acute hypomagnesemia is corrected with 50% magnesium sulfate in 2 mL doses up to 4 g daily.
- Promote self-management.
  1. Inform the patient and family about the drug regimen and need for ongoing monitoring and adjustments.
  2. Collaborate with the dietitian to identify and include foods high in calcium but low in phosphorus (milk, yogurt, and processed cheeses are avoided because of their high phosphorus content).
  3. Advise the patient to wear a medical alert bracelet.
  4. Teach the patient about for manifestations of hypocalcemia, especially numbness or tingling around the mouth and a positive Chvostek's sign or Trousseau's sign.

HYPOPITUITARISM

OVERVIEW

- Hypopituitarism is a deficiency of one or more anterior pituitary hormones, resulting in metabolic problems and sexual dysfunctions that vary depending on the under-secreted hormones.
- Decreased production of all anterior pituitary hormones is a rare condition known as panhypopituitarism.
- Usually, there is a decrease in the secretion of one hormone (selective hypopituitarism) and a lesser decrease in the other hormones.
- Deficiencies of ACTH and TSH are the most life threatening because they result in a corresponding decrease in the secretion of vital hormones from the adrenal and thyroid glands.
- Other deficiencies include gonadotropins (luteinizing hormone [LH] and follicle stimulating hormone [FSH]), growth hormone
- Causes of hypopituitarism include pituitary tumors, severe malnutrition or rapid loss of body fat, shock or severe hypotension, head trauma, brain tumors or infection, radiation or surgery of the head and brain, and AIDS.

1. Idiopathic hypopituitarism has an unknown cause.
2. Postpartum hemorrhage is the most common cause of pituitary infarction, which results in decreased hormone secretion. This clinical problem is known as Sheehan's syndrome.

INTERPROFESSIONAL COLLABORATIVE CARE
Assessment: Noticing
- Assess for and document changes in physical appearance and target organ dysfunction:
  1. Loss of secondary sexual characteristics (men)
     a. Facial and body hair loss
     b. Impotence
     c. Decreased libido
  2. Loss of secondary sexual characteristics (women)
     a. Absence of menstrual periods
     b. Painful intercourse (dyspareunia)
     c. Infertility
     d. Decreased libido
     e. Breast atrophy
     f. Decreased amount or absence of axillary and pubic hair
  3. Neurologic changes
     a. Loss of visual acuity, especially peripheral vision
     b. Temporal headaches
     c. Diplopia (double vision)
     d. Ocular muscle paralysis, limiting eye movement
- Diagnostic assessment may include:
  1. Blood levels of pituitary hormones
  2. Hormone stimulation testing
  3. MRI of the head
  4. Angiography (brain)
Interventions: Responding
- Management of the patient with hypopituitarism focuses on replacement of deficient hormones.
- Instruct the patient about the hormone replacement method and regimen.
  1. Men with gonadotropin deficiency receive sex steroid replacement therapy with androgens (testosterone) parenterally or with transdermal testosterone patches.
     a. High doses are used until virilization (presence of male secondary sex characteristics) occurs, and then maintenance doses are used.
     b. Side effects may include gynecomastia (development of breast tissue in men), acne, baldness, and prostate enlargement.
     c. Fertility is difficult to achieve and requires additional therapy.

2. Women who have gonadotropin deficiency receive hormone replacement with a combination of estrogen and progesterone.
   a. Combined estrogen and progestin are used, usually orally or by transdermal patch.
   b. Complications include hypertension and deep vein thrombosis.
   c. Additional therapy is needed for fertility.
3. Adult patients with growth hormone deficiency may be treated with injections of growth hormones.
4. ACTH and TSH are not replaced; instead thyroid hormone and cortisol are given.

✳ HYPOTHYROIDISM: CELLULAR REGULATION CONCEPT EXEMPLAR

OVERVIEW

- Hypothyroidism is the underproduction of thyroid hormones by the thyroid gland, resulting in altered CELLULAR REGULATION from decreased whole-body metabolism.
- Most cases of hypothyroidism in the United States occur as a result of thyroid surgery and radioactive iodine (RAI) treatment of hyperthyroidism.
- Worldwide, hypothyroidism is common in areas where the soil and water have little natural iodide, a mineral essential to normal thyroid function.
- Other causes of hypothyroidism include autoimmune thyroid destruction; infection of thyroid tissue; congenital absence or hypoplasia of thyroid tissues; neck surgery, irradiation, or trauma; and a wide variety of drugs.
- Women are affected much more often than men.
- Myxedema coma is a rare, serious complication of untreated or poorly treated hypothyroidism.
  1. Myxedema is characterized by changes in the patient's appearance from the formation of non-pitting edema, especially around the eyes, hands, feet, and between shoulder blades.
  2. This type of edema is mucinous; it is filled with proteins and sugars rather than water alone.
  3. Myxedema coma, sometimes called "hypothyroid crisis," is a rare, serious complication with a mortality rate of 60%.
     a. The decreased metabolism causes the heart muscle to become flabby and the chamber size to increase similar to HF.
     b. Decreased cardiac output and decreased perfusion to the brain and other vital organs, which makes the already slowed cellular metabolism worse, resulting in multiple tissue and organ failure.

H

INTERPROFESSIONAL COLLABORATIVE CARE

Assessment: Noticing

- Obtain patient information about:
    1. Energy levels including activity levels and amount of time sleeping now compared with the previous time period of assessment
    2. Generalized weakness, anorexia, muscle aches, and paresthesias
    3. Constipation
    4. Cold intolerance (use of more blankets at night or sweaters and extra clothing, even in warm weather)
    5. Change in libido
    6. Heavy, prolonged menses or amenorrhea
    7. Impotence and infertility
    8. Current or previous use of drugs known to interfere with thyroid function, such as lithium, amiodarone, aminoglutethimide, sodium or potassium perchlorate, thiocyanates, or cobalt
    9. Medical history, including prior treatment for hyperthyroidism and the specific treatment
    10. Recent weight gain
- Assess for and document:
    1. Physical signs and symptoms
        a. Coarse features
        b. Non-pitting edema around the eyes, in hands, feet and between shoulder blades.
        c. Blank expression
        d. Thick tongue and vocal hoarseness (from myxedematous deposits)
        e. Slow muscle movement
        f. Slurred or unclear speech with slow response to questions
        g. Bradycardia
        h. Hypotension
        i. Slow respiratory rate
        j. Low core body temperature (less than 97°F or 36.1°C)
        k. Presence or absence of a goiter
    2. Psychosocial assessment and issues may include:
        a. Depression
        b. Lethargy, apathy, drowsiness
        c. Reduced attention span and memory
    3. Diagnostic blood and imaging results including:
        a. Triiodothyronine (T_3)
        b. Thyroxin (T_4)
        c. TSH levels

Analysis: Interpreting
- The priority problems for patients who have hypothyroidism are:
  1. Decreased GAS EXCHANGE and oxygenation as a result of decreased energy, obesity, muscle weakness, and fatigue
  2. Hypotension and reduced perfusion as a result of decreased heart rate from decreased myocardial metabolism
  3. Reduced cognition as a result of reduced brain metabolism and formation of edema
  4. Potential for the complication of myxedema coma

Planning and Implementation: Responding
IMPROVE GAS EXCHANGE
- Observe and record the rate and depth of respirations.
- Measure oxygen saturation by pulse oximetry.
- Apply oxygen if the patient has hypoxemia.
- Auscultate the lungs for a decrease in breath sounds or presence of crackles.
- If hypothyroidism is severe, the patient may require ventilatory support.
- Severe respiratory distress occurs with myxedema coma.

PREVENT HYPOTENSION
- The patient may have decreased blood pressure, bradycardia, and dysrhythmias.
- Nursing priorities are monitoring for condition changes and preventing complications.
- Drug therapy to restore cellular regulation is the mainstay of management for hypothyroidism.
- The patient requires lifelong thyroid hormone replacement; the most commonly used drug is levothyroxine (Synthroid, Levothroid, Levoxyl, Unithroid, generic).
  1. Therapy is started with a low dose that is gradually increased over a period of weeks.
  2. The patient with more severe symptoms of hypothyroidism is started on the lowest dose of thyroid hormone replacement because starting at too high a dose or increasing the dose too rapidly can cause severe hypertension, HF, and myocardial infarction.
     a. Teach patients and the families of patients who are beginning thyroid replacement hormone therapy to take the drug exactly as prescribed and not to change the dose or schedule without consulting the health care provider.
     b. Assess the patient for chest pain and dyspnea during initiation of therapy.
  3. Dosage is determined by blood levels of TSH and the patient's physical responses.

4. Monitor for and teach the patient and family about the manifestations of hyperthyroidism/excess treatment, including:
   a. Tachycardia
   b. Intolerance to heat
   c. Difficulty sleeping
   d. Diarrhea
   e. Excessive weight loss
   f. Fine tremors of the hands

SUPPORT COGNITION

- Observe for and record the presence and severity of lethargy, drowsiness, memory deficit, poor attention span, and difficulty communicating.
- These problems should decrease with thyroid hormone treatment, and mental awareness usually returns to the patient's normal level within 2 weeks.
- Orient the patient to person, place, and time, and explain all procedures slowly and carefully.

PREVENT MYXEDEMA COMA

1. *Myxedema coma* is a severe and life-threatening form of hypothyroidism in which the patient's overall metabolism slows to the point that cardiac and respiratory arrest can occur.
2. Factors leading to myxedema coma include acute illness, surgery, chemotherapy, discontinuing thyroid replacement therapy, and the use of sedatives or opioids.
3. Signs and symptoms include:
   a. Respiratory failure
   b. Coma
   c. Hypotension
   d. Hyponatremia
   e. Hypothermia
   f. Hypoglycemia
4. Emergency care of the patient with myxedema coma includes:
   a. Maintaining a patent airway and instituting aspiration precautions
   b. Supporting bradycardia and hypotension with IV fluids
   c. Giving levothyroxine IV as prescribed
   d. Giving glucose IV as prescribed
   e. Giving corticosteroids as prescribed
   f. Monitoring vital signs hourly and reporting significant or symptomatic changes
   g. Managing hypothermia with warm blankets or a warming device
   h. Monitoring for changes in mental status and reporting decreased consciousness in a timely manner

Care Coordination and Transition Management

- Hypothyroidism is usually a chronic condition and the patient may live in any type of environment. Ensure that whoever is responsible for overseeing the patient's daily care is aware of the condition and understands its treatment.
- The patient who has a decreased attention span may need help from family, friends, or a home care aide with the drug regimen.
- Develop a plan for drug therapy so that doses are neither missed nor duplicated.
- Teach the patient and family about hormone replacement therapy and its side effects.
    1. Emphasize the need for lifelong drugs.
    2. Review the manifestations of both hyperthyroidism and hypothyroidism.
    3. Teach the patient to wear a medical alert bracelet and to sustain health provider contact, follow-up blood tests, and the need for periodic re-evaluation during changes in health and with aging.
    4. Instruct the patient to carefully evaluate OTC drugs and fiber preparations because thyroid hormone preparations interact with many other drugs.
- Teach the family to orient the patient often and to explain everything clearly, simply, and as often as needed when activity tolerance and cognitive changes have not resolved from initial manifestations of hypothyroidism.
- Teach the patient to monitor himself or herself for therapy effectiveness by assessing the need for sleep and the frequency of bowel elimination.
    1. When the patient requires more sleep and is constipated, the dose of replacement hormone may need to be increased.
    2. When the patient has difficulty getting to sleep and has more bowel movements than normal for him or her, the dose may need to be decreased.

I

✸ INFECTION: IMMUNITY CONCEPT EXEMPLAR

OVERVIEW

- A pathogen is any microorganism (also called an agent) capable of producing disease.
- Infections can be communicable (transmitted from person to person [e.g., influenza]) or not communicable (e.g., peritonitis).
- Transmission of infection requires three factors:
    1. Reservoir (or source) of infectious agents

2. Susceptible host with a portal of entry
3. Mode of transmission
- The patient's immune status plays a large role in determining risk for infection.
- Immunity is resistance to infection; it is usually associated with the presence of antibodies or cells that act on specific microorganisms (Chart 2-11).
- Pathogens can enter the body through many routes of transmission, such as the respiratory tract where microbes in droplets can be sprayed into the air when infected persons sneeze, talk, or cough. These droplets are then inhaled by a susceptible host where the pathogens can localize in the lungs or distribute throughout the body via the lymphatic system or the blood stream. Pathogens can also enter the body via the gastrointestinal (GI) tract, genitourinary tract, breaks in the skin, and the bloodstream.
- For infection to be transmitted from an infected source to a susceptible host, a transport mechanism is required:
1. Contact transmission (indirect and direct)
2. Droplet transmission
3. Airborne transmission

Chart 2-11	**Factors that May Increase Risk for Infection in the Older Patient**

Factor	Aging-Associated Changes or Conditions
• Immune system	• Decreased antibody production, lymphocytes, and fever response
• Integumentary system	• Thinning skin, decreased subcutaneous tissue, decreased vascularity, slower wound healing
• Respiratory system	• Decreased cough and gag reflexes
• Gastrointestinal system	• Decreased gastric acid and intestinal motility
• Chronic illness	• Diabetes mellitus, chronic obstructive pulmonary disease, neurologic impairments
• Functional/cognitive impairments	• Immobility, incontinence, dementia
• Invasive devices	• Urinary catheters, feeding tubes, IV devices, tracheostomy tubes
• Institutionalization	• Increased person-to-person contact and transmission

- Prevention of infection and detecting signs and symptoms of infection as early as possible are integral elements of care.
- Infection acquired in the inpatient health care setting (not present or incubating at admission) is termed a health care–associated infection (HAI). HAIs can be endogenous (from a patient's flora) or exogenous (from outside the patient, often from the hands of health care workers, tubes, or implants).
- Health care workers' hands are the primary way in which infection is transmitted from patient to patient or staff to patient. Hand hygiene refers to both hand washing and alcohol-based hand rubs (ABHRs) ("hand sanitizers").
- Standard Precautions are based on the belief that all body excretions, secretions, and moist membranes and tissues, excluding perspiration, are potentially infectious (Chart 2-12).
    1. As barriers to potential or actual infections, personal protective equipment (PPE) is used. PPE refers to gloves, isolation gowns, face protection (masks, goggles, face shields), and powered air-purifying respirators (PAPRs) or N95 respirators.

! NURSING SAFETY PRIORITY: Action Alert

Remember that gloves are an essential part of infection control and should always be worn as part of Standard Precautions. Either hand washing or use of ABHRs should be done before donning and after removing gloves. The combination of hand hygiene and wearing gloves is the most effective strategy for preventing infection transmission!

MULTIDRUG-RESISTANT ORGANISM INFECTIONS AND COLONIZATIONS

Antibiotics have been available for many years. These drugs were commonly prescribed for conditions that did not need them or were given at higher doses and for longer periods of time than were necessary. As a result, a number of microorganisms have become resistant to certain antibiotics; that is, drugs that were once useful no longer control these infectious agents (multidrug-resistant organisms [MDROs]). Common MDROs are:

- Methicillin-resistant *Staphylococcus Aureus* (MRSA)
    1. MRSA is spread by direct contact and invades hospitalized patients through indwelling urinary catheters, vascular access devices, open wounds, and endotracheal tubes.
    2. It is susceptible to only a few antibiotics, such as IV vancomycin (Lyphocin, Vancocin) and oral linezolid (Zyvox). A newer IV antibiotic, ceftaroline fosamil (Teflaro), is the first cephalosporin approved to treat MRSA.

Chart 2-12 Transmission-Based Infection Control Precautions

Precautions (in addition to Standard Precautions)
Airborne Precautions
1. Private room required with monitored negative airflow (with appropriate number of air exchanges and air discharge to outside or through HEPA filter); keep door(s) closed
2. Special respiratory protection:
   • Wear PAPR for known or suspected TB
   • Susceptible persons not to enter room of patient with known or suspected measles or varicella unless immune caregivers are not available
   • Susceptible persons who must enter room must wear PAPR or N95 HEPA filter*
3. Transport: patient to leave room only for essential clinical reasons, wearing surgical mask

Droplet Precautions
1. Private room preferred: if not available, may cohort with patient with same active infection with same microorganisms if no other infection present; maintain distance of at least 3 feet from other patients if private room not available
2. Mask: required when working within 3 feet of patient
3. Transport: as previously discussed

Contact Precautions
1. Private room preferred: if not available, may cohort with patient with same active infection with same microorganisms if no other infection present
2. Wear gloves when entering room
3. Wash hands with antimicrobial soap before leaving patient's room
4. Wear gown to prevent contact with patient or contaminated items, or if patient has uncontrolled body fluids; remove gown before leaving room
5. Transport: patient to leave room only for essential clinical reasons; during transport, use needed precautions to prevent disease transmission
6. Dedicated equipment for this patient only (or disinfect after use before taking from room)

HEPA, High-efficiency particulate air; *PAPR,* powered air-purifying respirator; *TB,* tuberculosis; *VRE,* vancomycin-resistant *Enterococcus.*
*Before use: training and fit testing required for personnel.

- Vancomycin-resistant *Enterococcus* (VRE)
  1. *Enterococci* are bacteria that live in the intestinal tract and are important for digestion. When they move to another area of the body, such as during surgery, they can cause an infection, which is usually treatable with vancomycin.
  2. In recent years, many of these infections have become resistant to the drug, and VRE results. Risk factors for this infection include prolonged hospital stays, severe illness, abdominal surgery, enteral nutrition, and immunosuppression. Place patients with VRE infections on Contact Precautions to prevent contamination from body fluids.
- Carbapenem-resistant *Enterobacteriaceae* (CRE)
  1. CRE is a family of pathogens that are difficult to treat because they have a high level of resistance to carbapenem antibiotics caused by enzymes that break down the antibiotics.
  2. Patients who are high risk for CRE include those in ICUs or nursing homes and patients who are immunosuppressed, including older adults.

INTERPROFESSIONAL COLLABORATIVE CARE
Assessment: Noticing
- Assess and document patient history including:
  1. Risks for altered immune status such as age, history of tobacco or alcohol use, current illness or disease, poor nutritional status, or current therapies such as chemotherapy or radiation.
  2. Ask the patient if they have recently been in a hospital or nursing home and if they have had any recent invasive testing (such as a colonoscopy).
  3. Travel history
  4. Sexual history
  5. Type and location of symptoms

PHYSICAL ASSESSMENT
- Common signs and symptoms are associated with specific sites of infection.
- Fever (generally above 101°F [38.3°C], chills, and malaise are primary indicators of systematic infection.
- Lymphadenopathy (enlarged lymph nodes), pharyngitis, and GI disturbance (usually diarrhea or vomiting) are often associated with infection.

LABORATORY ASSESSMENT
- The definitive diagnosis of an infectious disease requires identification of a microorganism in the tissues of an infected patient.

- The best procedure for identifying a microorganism is culture, or isolation of the pathogen by cultivation in tissue cultures or artificial media.
- A white blood cell (WBC) count is often done for the patient with a suspected infection.

Analysis: Interpreting

- The priority collaborative problem for patients with an infection is fever related to the immune response triggered by the pathogen. In addition, the patient has a potential for developing severe sepsis, systemic inflammatory response syndrome (SIRS), and septic shock.

Planning and Implementation: Responding

MANAGING FEVER

- The primary concern is to eliminate the underlying cause of the fever and destroy the causative microorganism.

   Drug Therapy
- Antimicrobials (called anti-infective agents) are the cornerstone of drug therapy.

❗ NURSING SAFETY PRIORITY: Drug Alert

Before administering an antimicrobial drug, check to see that the patient is not allergic to it. Be sure to take an accurate allergy history before drug therapy begins to prevent possible life-threatening reactions, such as anaphylaxis.

- Antipyretic drugs (such as acetaminophen [Tylenol, Ace-Tabs]) are often given to reduce fever. These drugs often mask fever, which makes it difficult to monitor the course of the disease. As a result, antipyretics are not always prescribed.

   Other Interventions
- External cooling using hypothermia blankets or ice packs can be effective for reducing a high fever. Assess for shivering because this can be an indication that the patient is being cooled too quickly.
- Monitor fluid balance because fluid volume loss is increased in a patient with a fever.

Care Coordination and Transition Management

- Patients with infections may be cared for in the home (group or individual), hospital, nursing home, or ambulatory care setting, depending on the type and severity of the infection.
   1. Explaining the disease and making certain that the patient understands what is causing the illness are the primary purposes of health teaching.
   2. For the patient who is discharged to the home setting to complete a course of antimicrobial therapy, the importance of

adherence to the planned drug regimen needs to be stressed. Explain the importance of both the timing of doses and the completion of the planned number of days of therapy.
3. Many patients are discharged with an infusion device to continue drug therapy at home or in other inpatient facilities.

INFLUENZA, SEASONAL AND PANDEMIC
OVERVIEW
- Seasonal influenza, or "flu," is a highly contagious, acute viral respiratory infection that can occur at any age.
- Pandemic influenza is the term used to describe viral infections that are highly contagious, typically mutate for animal or birds infections such that humans have no immunity, and have the potential to spread globally with concerning morbidity and mortality.
  1. Examples of pandemic influenza occurrences include the 1918 "Spanish" flu and the 2009 "swine" or H1N1 flu.
  2. A new strain of bird ("avian") flu, H5Ni, is being monitored for potential pandemic implications.
- Influenza infection can lead to complications of pneumonia or death, especially in older adults and debilitated or immunocompromised patients.

INTERPROFESSIONAL COLLABORATIVE CARE
Assessment: Noticing
- The prioritized care reduces risk of infection through vaccination, hand washing, and community and personal quarantine to avoid droplet spread of the virus. Adults are contagious from 24 hours before symptoms occur and up to 5 days after they begin.
- The rapid influenza diagnostic test can be used to confirm influenza diagnosis, but it has a high false-negative rate and diagnosis is usually based on symptoms combined with community awareness of other cases.
- Symptoms typically have a sudden onset:
  1. Severe headache
  2. Fever, chills, fatigue, weakness, muscle aches
  3. Sore throat, cough, watery nasal discharge
  4. Influenza Type B can lead to nausea, vomiting, and diarrhea
  5. Rapid progression to shortness of breath and pneumonia
Interventions: Responding
- Vaccination for everyone older than 3 months of age
  1. Seasonal vaccination, usually in late fall, contains antigens for the three or four expected strains.
  2. Influenza vaccination is administered as an IM injection (Fluvirin, Fluzone).

- For infected patients, provide supportive care and strategies to reduce transmission.
  1. Promote social distance or quarantine/isolation to decrease the spread of the virus.
  2. Provide fluids and rest to promote recovery.
  3. Consider administration of antiviral agents given within 12 to 24 hours of symptom onset to reduce the severity or duration of influenza; these agents include oseltamivir (Tamiflu), peramivir (Rapivab), and zanamivir (Relenza) for those not vaccinated or to shorten the duration of the disease.
  4. Anticipate hospitalization for frail or immunocompromised patients, infants, and older adults, who require respiratory support or close monitoring to prevent complications.

IRRITABLE BOWEL SYNDROME
OVERVIEW
- Irritable bowel syndrome (IBS) is a functional GI disorder that causes chronic or recurrent diarrhea, constipation, and/or abdominal pain and bloating.
- Increased or decreased bowel transit times result in changes in the normal *bowel elimination* pattern to one of these classifications: diarrhea (IBS-D), constipation (IBS-C), or alternating diarrhea and constipation (IBS-M).
- The etiology is unclear and a combination of environmental, immunologic, genetic, hormonal, and stress factors have a role in the development and course of IBS.

INTERPROFESSIONAL COLLABORATIVE CARE
Assessment: Noticing
- Assess for and document:
  1. Fatigue, malaise
  2. Abdominal pain, cramps, particularly pain in the left lower quadrant
  3. Changes in the bowel pattern (diarrhea, constipation, or an alternating pattern of both) or consistency of stools and the passage of mucus
  4. Food intolerance
  5. Serum albumin, CBC, erythrocyte sedimentation rate, and *Helicobacter pylori* testing to detect infection and nutritional deficits
  6. Occult blood or melena
  7. The Rome III staging used by the provider to address the symptoms and frequency of symptoms

Interventions: Responding
- Diet therapy includes:
  1. Suggesting a symptom diary to help identify triggers and bowel habits

    2. Helping the patient identify and eliminate foods associated with exacerbations

    3. Consulting with the dietitian to promote intake of fiber and fluid

       a. Teaching the patient to ingest 30 to 40 g of fiber daily

       b. Teaching the patient to drink 8 to 10 glasses of liquid per day

- Drug therapy includes:

    1. Bulk-forming laxatives, such as psyllium hydrophilic (Metamucil), may be taken at mealtimes with a glass of water to prevent dry, hard, or liquid stools.

    2. Lubiprostone (Amitiza) or linaclotide (Linzess) can be used to increase intestinal fluid and promote bowel elimination in IBS-C.

    3. Antidiarrheal agents such as loperamide (Imodium) may be used to decrease cramping and frequency of stools.

    4. Alosetron (Lotronex), a serotonin-selective (5-HT_3) drug, may be used with caution for women with diarrhea-predominant IBS-D; it has many drug-drug interactions.

    5. Patients with IBS who have bloating and abdominal distention without constipation may be prescribed rifaximin (Xifaxan), an antibiotic with little systemic absorption.

    6. For IBS in which pain is the predominant symptom, tricyclic antidepressants, such as amitriptyline (Elavil), have also been used successfully.

    7. Complementary and alternative therapy includes:

       a. Probiotics to reduce bacteria and alleviate GI symptoms of IBS

       b. Peppermint oil capsules to reduce GI symptoms

       c. Stress management such as meditation, imagery, and/or yoga to decrease GI symptoms

K

  KIDNEY DISEASE, CHRONIC: ELIMINATION CONCEPT EXEMPLAR

K

OVERVIEW

- Chronic kidney disease (CKD) is a progressive, irreversible disorder when kidney function does not recover (Taal et al., 2015). It is defined as abnormalities in kidney structure or function that alter health and are present for longer than 3 months (KDIGO, 2013).

- CKD is classified in five stages based on the glomerular filtration rate (GFR) category:

    1. *Stage 1:* At risk for CKD. Normal kidney function with a GFR greater than 90 mL/min. Kidney function is normal, but the

patient has sufficient risk factors to require screening and ongoing monitoring of kidney function.

2. *Stage 2:* Mild CKD. GFR is reduced to 60 to 89 mL/min. The focus of care is to reduce risk factors for kidney disease.

3. *Stage 3:* Moderate CKD. GFR 30 to 59 mL/min. The focus of care is to slow progression of the disease through diet and increase vigilance to avoid hypoperfusion, toxins, and other risk factors.

4. *Stage 4:* Severe CKD. GFR 15 to 29 mL/min. The intensity of the care is increased to manage complications (anemia, hypertension) and prepare for eventual renal replacement therapy.

5. *Stage 5:* End-stage kidney disease (ESKD); renal replacement therapy (dialysis) is started. Alternatively, kidney transplantation is performed.

- The risk for progression of CKD, ESKD, and mortality is increased when urine albumin increases.
- Albumin in the urine is a marker of kidney damage whereas GFR reflects kidney function.
- Three albuminuria stages also are considered in evaluating CKD. These stages are defined by the albumin-to-creatinine ratio in urine.
  1. The first stage (A1) is a none to mildly increased albumin, up to 29 mg/g creatinine (<3 mg/mmol) and is sometimes called *microalbuminuria.*
  2. The second (A2) stage has values of 30 to 300 mg/g creatinine (3 to 30mg/mmol).
  3. The stage of greatest kidney damage (A3) has values > 300mg/g creatinine (>30 mg/mmol).
- The combined values help identify adults at risk for progression of CKD and its complications, and to guide interventions.
- CKD with greatly reduced GFR causes many problems, including abnormal urine production, severe disruption of FLUID AND ELECTROLYTE BALANCE, and metabolic abnormalities.
  1. Kidney changes
     a. Because healthy nephrons become larger and work harder, urine production and water ELIMINATION are sufficient to maintain essential homeostasis until about three fourths of kidney function is lost.
     b. As the disease progresses, the ability to produce diluted urine is reduced, resulting in urine with a fixed osmolarity (*isosthenuria*).
  2. Metabolic changes
     a. Creatinine comes from proteins in skeletal muscle. The rate of creatinine excretion depends on muscle mass, physical activity, and diet. Creatinine is partially excreted by the

kidney tubules, and a decrease in kidney function leads to a buildup of serum creatinine.

b. Early in CKD, the patient is at risk for *hyponatremia* (sodium depletion) because there are fewer healthy nephrons to reabsorb sodium and sodium is lost in the urine.

c. In the later stages of CKD, kidney excretion of sodium is reduced as urine production decreases. Then sodium retention and high serum sodium levels (*hypernatremia*) occur.

d. Hyperkalemia results from an increase in potassium load, including ingestion of potassium in drugs, failure to restrict potassium in the diet, blood transfusions, and excess bleeding.

e. Other metabolic changes in CKD include changes in pH (metabolic acidosis), calcium (hypocalcemia) and phosphorus (hyperphosphatemia) imbalances, and vitamin D insufficiency.

   (1) Renal osteodystrophy is skeletal demineralization manifested by bone pain, pseudo fractures, sclerosis of the spine, skull demineralization, osteomalacia, reabsorption of bone, and loss of tooth lamina.

   (2) Hypophosphatemia results in parathyroid dysfunction and accelerates bone loss.

3. Cardiac changes

   a. *Hypertension* is common in most patients with CKD. It may be either the cause or the result of CKD. Hyperlipidemia, heart failure, uremic cardiomyopathy, and pericarditis may also occur.

4. Hematologic and immunity changes

   a. Anemia is common in patients in the later stages of CKD and worsens CKD symptoms.

   (1) The causes of anemia include a decreased erythropoietin level with reduced red blood cell (RBC) production, decreased RBC survival time from uremia, and iron and folic acid deficiencies. The patient may have increased bleeding or bruising as a result of impaired platelet function.

5. Gastrointestinal changes

   a. Uremic stomatitis, anorexia, peptic ulcer disease, nausea, and vomiting

   b. Altered mouth and GI tract flora (microbiome) affect mucous membrane integrity and immunity

K

INTERPROFESSIONAL COLLABORATIVE CARE

• Because patients with CKD are at risk for so many adverse outcomes (not just ESKD), the interprofessional care team includes many specialists and health care providers (e.g., nephrologists, nephrology nurses, pharmacists, registered dietitians, mental health therapists, physical therapists, case managers, social workers, clergy or pastoral care workers).

Assessment: Noticing

- Obtain patient information about:
    1. Age (because a reduction in the number and function of nephrons occurs with age)
    2. Height and weight, including recent weight gain or loss
    3. Current and past medical conditions
    4. Drugs, prescription and OTC
    5. Family history of kidney disease
    6. Dietary and nutritional habits, including food preferences
    7. History of GI problems, such as nausea, vomiting, anorexia, diarrhea, or constipation
    8. Recent injuries and abnormal bruising or bleeding
    9. Activity intolerance, weakness, and fatigue
    10. Detailed urinary elimination history
- Assess for and document:
    1. Neurologic symptoms
        a. Changes in mentation or new lethargy
        b. Changes in sensation or weakness in extremities indicating uremic neuropathy
    2. Cardiovascular symptoms of CKD result from fluid overload, hypertension, or cardiac disease
        a. Extra heart sounds (particularly S_3)
        b. Peripheral edema
    3. Respiratory symptoms of CKD vary.
        a. Breath that smells like urine (uremic fetor or halitosis)
        b. Kussmaul pattern or deep sighing or yawning to release carbon dioxide, compensating for metabolic acidosis
        c. Tachypnea or shortness of breath
        d. Lung sounds congruent with pulmonary edema (crackles) or pleural effusion (rub)
    4. Hematologic symptoms
        a. Anemia with fatigue, pallor, and shortness of breath with exertion
        b. Abnormal bleeding (skin, GI, vaginal); bruising, petechiae
    5. GI symptoms
        a. Mouth ulceration
        b. Abdominal pain or cramping
        c. Nausea or vomiting
    6. Urinary symptoms
        a. Change in urinary amount, frequency, and appearance of urine
        b. Proteinuria or hematuria

7. Skin symptoms
   a. Yellow coloration from pigment deposition; darkening of skin for some African Americans
   b. Severe itching (pruritus)
   c. Uremic frost, a layer of uremic crystals from evaporated sweat on the face, eyebrows, axilla, and groin (rare)
   d. Bruises or purple patches and rashes
8. Immunologic considerations
   a. Increased susceptibility to infections
9. Psychosocial considerations because CKD affects family relations, social activity, work patterns, body image, and sexual activity
   a. Anxiety and depression are common responses to CKD.
   b. Self-management is essential to attain optimal health outcomes.

- Diagnostic testing may include:
   1. Serum creatinine, BUN, sodium, potassium, calcium, phosphorus, bicarbonate, hemoglobin, and hematocrit
   2. Urinalysis
   3. A 24-hour urinalysis for creatinine to calculate GFR
   4. Ultrasound, computed tomography (CT) scan, or x-ray to detect small and fibrotic kidneys

Analysis: Interpreting

- The priority problems for patients with CKD include:
   1. Fluid overload due to the inability of diseased kidneys to maintain body fluid balance
   2. Potential for pulmonary edema due to fluid overload
   3. Decreased cardiac function due to reduced stroke volume, dysrhythmias, fluid overload, and increased peripheral vascular resistance
   4. Weight loss due to inability to ingest, digest, or absorb food and nutrients as a result of physiologic factors
   5. Potential for infection due to skin breakdown, immunity-related kidney dysfunction, or malnutrition
   6. Potential for injury due to effects of kidney disease on bone density, blood clotting, and drug elimination
   7. Fatigue due to kidney disease, anemia, and reduced energy production
   8. Anxiety due to change in health status, economic status, relationship status, role function, and threat of death
   9. Potential for depression due to chronic illness

Planning and Implementation: Responding

- The overall goal of care is to slow the rate of disease progression and preserve elimination for as long as possible.

K

MANAGE FLUID VOLUME
- Achieve and maintain acceptable fluid balance with drug therapy, nutrition therapy, fluid restriction, and dialysis.
  1. Prevent fluid overload with diuretics and, if needed, fluid restriction.
  2. Monitor weight daily.
  3. Monitor serum electrolytes.
  4. Measure and record intake and output and report concerning imbalances to provider.

PREVENT PULMONARY EDEMA
  1. Assess for early signs of pulmonary edema, such as restlessness, dyspnea, decreased peripheral oxygenation (Spo_2), and crackles.
  2. If the patient is dyspneic, placing the patient in a high Fowler's position and giving oxygen to maximize lung expansion and improve gas exchange
  3. Assess cardiovascular system for fluid overload: S_3 heart sounds, peripheral edema, jugular venous distention, tachycardia, hypotension, or hypertension.
  4. Provide drug therapy.
     a. Diuretics for stages 1 through 4 CKD; monitor for ototoxicity with loop diuretics
     b. Morphine to reduce myocardial oxygen demands; monitor for respiratory depression
     c. Vasodilators such as nitroglycerin

INCREASE CARDIAC OUTPUT
- Cardiac output alterations are related to hypovolemia or hypervolemia, dysrhythmias, cardiomyopathy, pericarditis and greater peripheral vascular resistance influenced by CKD.
  1. Determine and assist in attaining BP goals typically around 130/80 mm Hg
     a. Administer calcium channel blockers, ACE inhibitors, alpha- and beta-adrenergic blockers, and vasodilators.
  2. Teach the family to measure the patient's BP and weight daily and to bring these records when visiting the physician, nurse, or nutritionist.
  3. Monitor the patient for decreased cardiac output, heart failure, congestive heart failure, and dysrhythmias.
     a. Notify provider with increasing peripheral edema or decreasing peripheral pulses.
     b. Teach the patient and family about the relationships between diet, drug therapy, and cardiovascular health.
  4. Consider decreased cognitive status an emergency and notify the Rapid Response Team or provider.

ENHANCE NUTRITION
- The nutritional need and diet restrictions for the patient with CKD vary according to the degree of remaining kidney function and the type of renal replacement therapy used.
  1. Common changes include control of protein intake; fluid intake limitation; restriction of potassium, sodium, and phosphorus intake; taking vitamin and mineral supplements; and eating enough calories to meet metabolic demand.
  2. Consult with the nutritionist to provide nutritional teaching and planning and to assist the patient in adapting the diet to food preferences, ethnic background, and budget.

PREVENT INFECTION
- Infection is related to skin breakdown, immunomodulation from uremia, exposure to blood borne pathogens during hemodialysis treatment, and malnutrition.
- Monitor for signs of infection, including:
  1. Temperature (fever, but hypothermia can occur especially with altered perfusion)
  2. Lymph node enlargement
  3. Positive culture or serum markers (e.g., markers for hepatitis)
  4. Tenderness, redness, or drainage at dialysis access site or other areas of impaired skin integrity
  5. Abnormal WBC count and differential

PREVENT INJURY
- Potential for injury is related to effects of kidney disease on bone density, blood clotting, and drug elimination.
  1. Implement falls precaution.
  2. Use skin pressure reduction strategies to reduce risk for pressure ulcer formation.
  3. Interprofessional collaboration with the pharmacist to adjust drug doses to avoid toxicity from reduced renal clearance
  4. Administer drugs to control hyperphosphatemia to prevent renal osteodystrophy.
  5. Avoid drugs that interfere with clotting such as aspirin.
  6. Monitor the patient closely for drug-related complications.
  7. Teach the patient to avoid certain drugs that can increase kidney damage, such as nonsteroidal anti-inflammatory drugs (NSAIDs), antibiotics, antihypertensives, and diuretics, in the presence of hypovolemia.
  8. Instruct the patient to avoid compounds containing magnesium.
  9. Administer opioid analgesics cautiously because the effects may last longer, and uremic patients are sensitive to the respiratory depressant effects.

K

MINIMIZE FATIGUE
- Fatigue is related to kidney disease, anemia, and reduced energy production.
  1. Establish patient preferences to conserve energy and preserve the ability to perform self-care, retain interest in surroundings, and sustain mental concentration.
  2. Provide vitamin and mineral supplementation.
  3. Administer erythropoietin to maintain hemoglobin 7 to 9 g/dL3; administer iron supplements to maintain safe levels of hemoglobin and hematocrit (hematocrit goal is usually 27% to 28%).
  4. Monitor dietary intake (improved appetite challenges patients in their attempts to maintain protein and potassium) and fluid restriction.

REDUCE ANXIETY
- Anxiety is related to threat to or change in health status, economic status, relationships, role function, systems, or self-concept; situational crisis; threat of death; lack of knowledge about diagnostic tests, disease process, treatment; loss of control; or disrupted family life.
  1. Observe the patient's behavior for signs of anxiety.
  2. Evaluate the patient's support system.
  3. Explain all procedures, tests, and treatments.
  4. Provide instruction on kidney function and kidney failure.
  5. Encourage the patient to discuss current problems, fears, or concerns and to ask questions.
  6. Facilitate discussion with family members concerning the patient's prognosis and potential impacts on the patient's lifestyle.

RECOGNIZE AND MANAGE DEPRESSION
  1. Use a valid and reliable depression screening tool to evaluate the need for additional assessment or intervention for depression.
  2. Provide opportunity for the patient to express feelings about the disease, prognosis, and challenges with self-management.
  3. Promote sleep, especially minimizing sleep interruptions during hospitalization.

RENAL REPLACEMENT THERAPY
- Renal replacement therapy is needed when the symptoms of kidney disease present complications that are potentially life-threatening or that pose continuing discomfort to the patient.
- *Hemodialysis* removes excess fluid and waste products and restores chemical and electrolyte balance. It is based on the principle of diffusion, in which the patient's blood is circulated through a semipermeable membrane that acts as an artificial kidney.
  1. Dialysis settings include the acute care facility, free-standing centers, and the home.
  2. Total dialysis time is usually 12 hours per week, which usually is divided into three 4-hour treatments.

3. A vascular access route is needed to perform hemodialysis.
   a. Long-term vascular access for hemodialysis is accomplished by arteriovenous (AV) fistula or graft.
   b. Temporary vascular access for hemodialysis is accomplished by a specially designed catheter inserted into the subclavian, internal jugular, or femoral vein.
   c. Complications of vascular access include:
      (1) Thrombosis or stenosis
      (2) Infection
      (3) Ischemia
      (4) Loss of patency
- Nurses are specially trained to perform hemodialysis.
- Post-dialysis care includes:
  1. Closely monitoring for side effects: hypoglycemia, hypotension, headache, nausea, malaise, vomiting, dizziness, and muscle cramps
  2. Obtaining the patient's weight and vital signs
  3. Avoiding invasive procedures for 4 to 6 hours because of anticoagulation used during dialysis
  4. Monitoring for signs of bleeding
  5. Monitoring laboratory results
- Complications of hemodialysis include:
  1. Dialysis disequilibrium caused by rapid shifts of electrolytes
  2. Infection, particularly hepatitis

Considerations for Older Adults

- Stage 5 CKD or CKD requiring dialysis occurs most often in people older than 65 years of age.
- Patients older than 65 years receiving dialysis have a greater risk than younger patients for dialysis-induced hypotension. Older adults require more frequent monitoring of vital signs and level of consciousness during and after dialysis.

- *Peritoneal dialysis* (PD), an alternative and slower dialysis method, is accomplished by the surgical insertion of a silicone rubber catheter (Tenckhoff catheter) into the abdominal cavity to instill dialysis solution into the abdominal cavity.
- Candidates for PD include:
  1. Patients who are unable to tolerate anticoagulation
  2. Patients who lack vascular access
  3. Patients without peritoneal adhesions and without extensive abdominal surgery
- The PD process occurs by means of a transfer of fluid and solutes from the bloodstream through the peritoneum.

K

- The types of PD include intermittent, continuous ambulatory (CAPD), automated, and others; the type is selected based on patient ability and lifestyle.
- Complications of PD include:
  1. Pain
  2. Poor dialysate flow
  3. Leakage of the dialysate
  4. Exit site and tunnel infection and peritonitis
- Nursing interventions include:
  1. Implementing and monitoring PD therapy and instilling, dwelling, and draining the solution, as ordered
  2. Maintaining PD flow data and monitoring for negative or positive fluid balances
  3. Obtaining baseline and daily weights
  4. Monitoring laboratory results to measure the effectiveness of the treatment
  5. Maintaining accurate intake and output records
  6. Taking vital signs every 15 to 30 minutes during initiation of PD
  7. Performing an ongoing assessment for signs of respiratory distress or pain
- Kidney transplantation is appropriate for selected patients with ESKD.
  1. Discussion about kidney transplant can occur at any time during CKD; it need not wait until Stage 5 or dialysis is started.

Care Coordination and Transition Management
- Case managers can plan, coordinate, and evaluate care.
  1. The physical and occupational therapist collaborates with the patient and family to evaluate the home environment and to obtain needed equipment before discharge.
  2. Refer the patient to home health nursing as needed.

! NURSING SAFETY PRIORITY: Action Alert

Teach patients with mild CKD that carefully managing fluid volume, blood pressure, electrolytes, and other kidney-damaging diseases by following prescribed drug and nutrition therapies can prevent damage and slow the progression to ESKD.

- Provide in-depth health teaching about diet and pathophysiology of kidney disease and drug therapy:
  1. Provide information and emotional support to assist the patient with decisions about treatment course, personal lifestyle, support systems, and coping.
  2. Teach the patient about the hemodialysis treatment.

3. Teach the patient about care of the vascular access.
4. Provide patients with home-based renal replacement therapy with extensive teaching and assist the patient to obtain the needed equipment and supplies. Emphasize the importance of strict sterile technique and of reporting manifestations of infection at any dialysis access site.
5. Assist the patient and family to identify coping strategies to adjust to the diagnosis and treatment regimen.
6. Instruct patients and family members in all aspects of diet therapy, drug therapy, and complications. Assist patients to schedule drugs so that drugs will not be unintentionally eliminated by dialysis.
7. Teach patients and family members to report complications, such as fluid overload, bleeding, and infection.
8. Stress that although uremic symptoms are reduced as a result of dialysis procedures, the patient will not return completely to his or her previous state of well-being.
9. Instruct the family to monitor the patient for any behaviors that may contribute to nonadherence to the treatment plan and to report such to the health care provider.
10. Refer the patient to a home health nurse and to local and state support groups and agencies such as the National Kidney Foundation.

KIDNEY DISEASE, POLYCYSTIC

OVERVIEW

- Polycystic kidney disease (PKD) is a genetic kidney disorder in which fluid-filled cysts develop in nephrons.
- Growing cysts damage the nephron (i.e., glomerular and tubular membranes), reducing kidney function and causing hypertension.
  1. The cysts do not filter blood; kidney failure will occur over time.
  2. The fluid-filled cysts are at increased risk for infection, rupture, and bleeding; they contribute to kidney stone formation.
  3. Each cystic kidney may enlarge to two to three times its normal size, causing discomfort and abdominal organ displacement.
- Cysts may occur in other tissues, such as the liver or blood vessels.

INTERPROFESSIONAL COLLABORATIVE CARE

Assessment: Noticing

- Obtain patient information about:
  1. Family history and genetic testing because PKD can be autosomal dominant (most common form of PKD with several

different subtypes) or autosomal recessive (more severe, with death typically occurring in early childhood)
  2. Current health status
  3. Changes in urine or pattern of urination
  4. Hypertension
- Assess for and document:
  1. Pain (flank or abdominal)
  2. Distended abdomen
  3. Enlarged, tender kidney on palpation
  4. Changes in urine, including hematuria, clarity, odor
  5. Changes in pattern of urination, including nocturia
  6. Dysuria
  7. Vital signs, noting hypertension and fever as needing intervention
  8. Edema
  9. Uremic symptoms: nausea, vomiting, pruritus, and fatigue
  10. Emotional responses such as anger, resentment, futility, sadness, or anxiety related to chronicity or inheritable condition
- Diagnostic studies may include:
  1. Urinalysis with findings of proteinuria and hematuria
  2. Urine culture and sensitivity if infection is suspected
  3. Serum creatinine and BUN to assess kidney function
  4. Renal sonography, CT scan, or MRI to assess the presence and size of cysts

Interventions: Responding
- Manage pain.
  1. Provide drug therapy.
     a. Administer analgesics for comfort; use NSAIDs cautiously.
     b. Administer antibiotics such as trimethoprim/sulfamethoxazole (Bactrim, Septra) or ciprofloxacin (Cipro) if a cyst infection is causing discomfort.
  2. Provide other interventions.
     a. Apply dry heat to the abdomen or flank.
     b. Teach relaxation or distraction techniques to self-manage pain and discomfort.
- Provide hypertension and fluid management.
  1. Administer antihypertensive agents, including ACE inhibitors, vasodilators, beta-blockers, and calcium channel blockers, as ordered.
  2. Administer diuretics, as ordered, to eliminate fluid overload.
  3. Monitor daily weight to detect fluid-related weight gain.
- Implement diet therapy with dietitian consultation to slow progression of kidney injury with fluid, sodium, and protein restrictions.
- Prevent constipation associated with fluid restriction and intestinal tract displacement from cysts with fiber intake and regular activity.

- Provide counseling, support, and teaching about health mainte-nance to promote self-management.

KIDNEY INJURY, ACUTE
OVERVIEW
- Acute kidney injury (AKI) is a rapid decrease in kidney function resulting in failure to maintain fluid, electrolyte, and acid-base balance, along with impaired urinary elimination with accumula-tion of metabolic wastes.
- AKI can result from conditions that reduce perfusion to the kid-neys (prerenal); damage kidney tissue (glomeruli, interstitial tis-sue, or tubules [intrarenal or intrinsic]); or obstruct urine outflow (postrenal); and combinations of these mechanisms of injury.
- AKI is associated with acute and severe illnesses and with in-creased mortality in acute and critical illnesses.
- AKI is defined by the extent of changes in serum creatinine and urine output because GFR is not accurate during acute and critical illness.
- The most current definition is from the Kidney Disease, Improving Global Outcomes group (KDIGO): an increase in serum creatinine by 0.3 mg/dL (26.2 mcmol/L) or more within 48 hours, or an increase in serum creatinine to 1.5 times or more from baseline, which is known or presumed to have occurred in the previous 7 days, or a urine volume of less than 0.5 mL/kilogram/hours for 6 hours.

INTERPROFESSIONAL COLLABORATIVE CARE
Assessment: Noticing
- Obtain patient information about:
  1. Exposure to nephrotoxins, such as antibiotics, ACE inhibitors, and NSAIDs
  2. History of diseases that contribute to impaired kidney function such as diabetes mellitus, systemic lupus erythematosus, and hypertension
  3. History of acute infections, including influenza, colds, gastro-enteritis, and sore throat or pharyngitis that contribute to glomerulonephritis
  4. Recent dehydration or intravascular volume depletion (from surgery or trauma) or the need for transfusion
  5. History of urinary obstructive disease, such as prostatic hyper-trophy or kidney stones
- Assess for and document:
  1. Mean arterial pressure < 65 mm Hg or symptoms of hypovo-lemia such as hypotension, tachycardia, decreased mentation, and low urine output

K

> **❗ NURSING SAFETY PRIORITY: Critical Rescue**
>
> In any acute care setting, preventing volume depletion and provid-
> ing intervention early when volume depletion occurs is a nursing
> priority. Reduced perfusion from volume depletion is a common
> cause of AKI. Recognize the manifestations of volume depletion
> (low urine output, decreased systolic blood pressure, decreased
> pulse pressure, orthostatic hypotension, thirst, rising blood osmo-
> lality). Intervene early with oral fluids, or if the patient is unable to
> take or tolerate oral fluid, request an increase in IV fluid rate from
> the provider to prevent permanent kidney damage.

2. Urine output less than 0.5 ml/kg for 2 or more hours or urine output less than 0.3 mL/kg/h for 6 or more hours
3. Abnormal or sharply increasing values for BUN and serum creatinine and electrolytes
4. Reduced, estimated, or measured creatinine clearance (GFR)
5. Protein in urine or signs of a urinary tract or kidney infection (dysuria, urgency, frequency, foul urine odor, flank pain)
6. Symptoms of fluid overload, including pulmonary edema (dyspnea, crackles, reduced Spo_2) and peripheral edema
7. Symptoms of electrolyte derangements, including nausea and vomiting, anorexia, impaired cognition, acute abnormalities in neuromuscular function, and ECG changes

- Diagnostic studies may include:
  1. Serum CBC (WBC for infection) and basic metabolic panel
  2. Urinalysis
  3. Urine and serum electrolytes, creatinine, and BUN
  4. Abdominal or pelvic ultrasound to assess the size of the kidneys and CT without contrast dye to identify obstruction
  5. Renal biopsy if immunologic disease is suspected

Considerations for Older Adults

Patient-Centered Care

Prevention of AKI in older adults first involves recognition of
their increased vulnerability to kidney injury. There is a 20%
greater rate of AKI among older adults in ICU compared with
younger adults. Structural and functional changes in the aging
kidney contribute to the risk for AKI. As kidneys age, there are
fewer nephrons, more sclerotic glomeruli, and renal artery arteriosclerosis leading to reducing renal blood flow and a decline
in GFR. Age-related changes in tubular function decrease the
ability to regulate sodium and potassium balance and to con-
centrate urine, increasing the risk for blood volume depletion.

- The use of multiple drugs is associated with drug-induced AKI, particularly in acute and critical care settings. Assess risk and take actions to reduce exposure to nephrotoxic agents, maintain euvolemia, avoid hypotension, evaluate drug-drug interactions for potential adverse kidney effects, and stop unnecessary drugs to maintain kidney function in older adults.

Interventions: Responding

- Avoid hypotension and maintain fluid balance (*euvolemia*) to prevent AKI and manage elimination.
- Monitor fluid and electrolyte status to detect imbalance and abnormal values. The patient may move from an oliguric phase (fluids and electrolytes are retained) to a diuretic phase, in which hypovolemia and electrolyte loss are the main problems during the course of AKI.
- Fluid challenges and diuretics are commonly used to promote fluid balance and kidney perfusion; avoid hypervolemia that can lead to lung or intestinal damage.
- With the interprofessional team, review drugs and drug-drug interactions to reduce nephrotoxicity.
- Communicate with the radiologist to avoid large doses or nephrotoxic contrast (dye) during imaging and ensure adequate hydration to clear contrast before and after imaging.
- Hypercatabolism during illness, surgery, or trauma results in the breakdown of muscle for protein, which leads to increased azotemia. Patients require increased calories.
- Indications for hemodialysis or PD in patients with AKI are symptomatic uremia (pericarditis or encephalopathy), persistent hyperkalemia or other electrolyte abnormalities, uncompensated metabolic acidosis, fluid overload, and uncontrolled inflammation (see *Kidney Disease, Chronic* for a discussion of dialysis).
- Continuous hemofiltration, an alternative to dialysis, may be used in the intensive care unit (ICU).

Care Coordination and Transition Management

- The needs of the patient depend on the status of the disease on discharge (see *Care Coordination and Transition Management* under *Kidney Disease, Chronic*).
- Follow-up care may include medical visits, laboratory tests, consultation with a nutritionist, temporary dialysis, home nursing care, and social work assistance.
- Be sure the primary care provider is aware of occurrence of AKI because it increases risk for CKD and may necessitate more frequent monitoring of kidney function or health status in the immediate post-hospitalization care.

L

LABYRINTHITIS
OVERVIEW
- Labyrinthitis is an infection of the labyrinth of the inner ear.
- Other causes include cholesteatoma (benign squamous cell overgrowth), complications of middle ear or inner ear surgery, and aftermath of a viral upper respiratory infection or mononucleosis.
- Manifestations include hearing loss, tinnitus, nystagmus on the affected side, and vertigo with nausea and vomiting.

INTERPROFESSIONAL COLLABORATIVE CARE
- Management includes supportive care with rest in a darkened room, antiemetics, and antivertiginous drugs.

LACERATIONS, EYE
OVERVIEW
- Lacerations are wounds caused by sharp objects and projectiles.
- The most commonly injured areas involved in eye lacerations are the eyelids and the cornea.

INTERPROFESSIONAL COLLABORATIVE CARE
1. Eyelid lacerations:
   a. Bleed heavily and look more severe than they are
   b. Are managed by closing the eye and applying a small icepack, checking visual acuity, and cleaning and suturing the eyelid
   c. Should be managed by an ophthalmologist if they involve the eyelid margin, affect the lacrimal system, involve a large area, or have jagged edges
2. Corneal lacerations:
   a. Are an emergency because eye contents may prolapse through the laceration
   b. Are manifested by severe eye pain, photophobia, tearing, decreased visual acuity, and inability to open the eyelid

> **! NURSING SAFETY PRIORITY: Action Alert**
>
> If an object is seen protruding from the eye, do not remove it. The object should be removed only by the ophthalmologist because it may be holding eye structures in place.

   c. Are managed with surgical repair and antibiotic therapy
   d. May require a corneal transplant if scarring alters vision
   e. May need *enucleation* (surgical eye removal) if the eye contents have prolapsed through the laceration or if the injury is severe

✳ LEIOMYOMAS (UTERINE FIBROIDS): SEXUALITY CONCEPT EXEMPLAR

OVERVIEW

- Uterine leiomyomas, also called *fibroids* or *myomas,* are benign, slow-growing solid tumors of the uterine myometrium (muscle layer) that can affect SEXUALITY.
- These tumors are classified according to their position in the layers of the uterus and anatomic position. The most common types are:
  1. *Intramural tumors,* contained in the uterine wall in the myometrium
  2. *Submucosal tumors* that protrude into the cavity of the uterus
  3. *Subserosal tumors* that protrude through the outer uterine surface and may extend into the broad ligament

INTERPROFESSIONAL COLLABORATIVE CARE

Assessment: Noticing

- Assessment findings include:
  1. No symptoms
  2. Abnormal uterine bleeding
  3. Reports of a feeling of pelvic pressure
  4. Constipation
  5. Urinary frequency or retention
  6. Increased abdominal size
  7. Dyspareunia (painful intercourse)
  8. Infertility
  9. Abdominal pain occurring with torsion of the fibroid around a connecting stalk or pedicle
  10. Uterine enlargement on abdominal, vaginal, or rectal examination

Analysis: Interpreting

- The priority collaborative problem for patients with uterine leiomyoma is:
  1. Potential for prolonged or heavy bleeding due to abnormal uterine growth.

Planning and Implementation: Responding

- Assess the significance of the diagnosis and surgery for the woman and her partner related to SEXUALITY. If treatment involves loss of the uterus, she may feel a great loss if she wishes to become pregnant. Many women relate their uterus to self-image and femininity or believe that their sexual function is related to their uterus.

MANAGE BLEEDING

Nonsurgical Management

- The patient who has no symptoms or who desires childbearing should be observed and examined for changes in the size of the leiomyoma every 4 to 6 months.

L

- Many fibroids spontaneously shrink after menopause and require no treatment.
- Mild leiomyoma symptoms can be managed with nonsteroidal anti-inflammatory drugs (NSAIDs), hormonal contraceptives, or a levonorgestrel intrauterine device (IUD).
- Artificial menopause and fibroid shrinkage can be induced with agonists to gonadotropin-releasing hormone (GnRH).
- Magnetic resonance imaging (MRI)–focused ultrasound pulsed into the uterus can destroy the fibroid.
- Uterine artery embolization or uterine fibroid embolization (UFE) involves the injection of embolic particles into the blood supply of the tumors, occluding the blood supply to the tumor and thereby causing its shrinkage and resorption.

Surgical Management

- Surgical management depends on whether future childbearing is desired, the age of the woman, the size of the fibroid, and the degree of symptoms.
- A *myomectomy* (removal of the leiomyomas with preservation of the uterus) is performed to preserve childbearing capabilities and relieve the symptoms.
- A *transcervical endometrial resection* (TCER) involves destroying the endometrium with a diathermy rectoscope or with radioablation. This procedure manages submucosal fibroids and menorrhagia.

! NURSING SAFETY PRIORITY: Critical Rescue

Monitor for rare but potential complications of hysteroscopic surgery, which include:

- Fluid overload (fluid used to distend the uterine cavity can be absorbed)
- Embolism
- Hemorrhage
- Perforation of the uterus, bowel, or bladder, and ureter injury
- Persistent increased menstrual bleeding
- Incomplete suppression of menstruation

Monitor for any indications of these problems, and report signs and symptoms such as severe pain and heavy bleeding to the surgeon immediately. Scarring may cause a small risk for complications in future pregnancies.

- *Hysterectomy,* surgical removal of the uterine body, is the usual surgical management in the older woman who has multiple leiomyomas and unacceptable symptoms. One of three approaches may be used: vaginal, abdominal, or laparoscopic.

1. *Total abdominal hysterectomy* (TAH) includes the removal of the uterus, ovaries, and fallopian tubes.
2. A *radical hysterectomy* involves removal of the uterus, lymph nodes, upper one-third of the vagina, and the surrounding tissues.

- Provide preoperative nursing care and:
  1. Listen to the patient's concerns about her sexuality
  2. Identify the patient's support system
- Provide postoperative care and:
  1. Assess and document vital signs with vaginal bleeding (more than one saturated perineal pad in 4 hours is concerning and needs to be reported to the health care provider; anticipate fluid or blood replacement therapy)
  2. Pay specific attention to:
     a. Abdominal bleeding at the incision site(s) (a small amount is normal)
     b. Urine output from urinary catheter for 24 hours or less (for open surgery) with a goal of greater than 0.5 mL/kg/hour urine output

Care Coordination and Transition Management

- Women identified as being at high risk for psychological problems may need long-term follow-up care or referral.
  1. They may need to be counseled about signs of depression. Intermittent sadness is normal, but continued feelings of low self-esteem or loss of interest or pleasure in usual activities and sex is not expected and should be evaluated.
  2. Provide written materials, and focus on the positive aspects of the woman's life to help decrease adverse psychological reactions.
- Provide teaching about wound care and follow-up.

 LEUKEMIA: IMMUNITY CONCEPT EXEMPLAR

OVERVIEW

- Leukemia is cancer with uncontrolled production of immature white blood cells (WBCs) in the bone marrow altering IMMUNITY. The bone marrow is overcrowded with immature, nonfunctional cells ("blast" cells) and production of normal blood cells is greatly decreased.
- Leukemia may be *acute*, with a sudden onset, or *chronic*, with a slow onset and symptoms that persist for years.
- Leukemias are classified as one of two major cell types and classification of cell types and subtypes guides treatment:
  1. *Lymphocytic (lymphoblastic) leukemias* have cells from lymphoid pathways.

2. *Myelocytic (myelogenous) leukemias* have abnormal cells originating in myeloid pathways.

- The basic problem causing leukemia involves damage to genes controlling cell growth. This damage then changes cells from a normal to a malignant (cancer) state. Analysis of the bone marrow of a patient with acute leukemia shows abnormal chromosomes about 50% of the time.
- Possible risk factors for the development of leukemia include ionizing radiation, viral infection, exposure to chemicals and drugs, disorders such as myelodysplastic syndrome or Fanconi's anemia, genetic factors, immunologic factors, environmental factors, older age, and the interaction of these factors.
- Leukemic cells can invade all tissues and organs and lead to infection or hemorrhage when untreated.

INTERPROFESSIONAL COLLABORATIVE CARE
Assessment: Noticing

- Obtain patient information about:
  1. Age
  2. Exposure to agents or ionizing radiation that increase the risk for leukemia
  3. Recent history of frequent or severe infections (e.g., influenza, pneumonia, bronchitis) or unexplained fevers
  4. A tendency to bruise or bleed easily or for a long period, including hematuria and gastrointestinal (GI) bleeding; platelet function is often decreased with leukemic disorders
  5. Weakness and fatigue or related symptoms of headaches, behavior changes, increased somnolence, decreased attention span, lethargy, muscle weakness, loss of appetite, or weight loss
- Assess for and document:
  1. Signs of infection, particularly in the respiratory, skin, and urinary systems
     a. Increased respiratory rate, dyspnea, cough or abnormal breath sounds
     b. Skin ulcer formation
     c. Urgent, frequent, bloody, or painful urination
  2. Skin changes from bleeding or reduced perfusion
     a. Pallor and coolness to the touch
     b. Pale conjunctiva and palmar creases
     c. Bruising or petechiae
     d. Mouth sores that do not heal
  3. GI changes from bleeding or decreased perfusion
     a. Nausea and anorexia
     b. Weight loss

    c. Rectal fissures
    d. Bloody stools
    e. Reduced bowel sounds, constipation
    f. Enlarged liver or spleen
    g. Abdominal distension or tenderness
4. Central nervous system (CNS) changes from bleeding or reduced perfusion
    a. Cranial nerve dysfunction
    b. Papilledema
    c. Seizures or coma
5. Miscellaneous changes
    a. Bone and joint tenderness
    b. Lymph node enlargement
    c. Fatigue or activity intolerance from anemia
6. Psychosocial issues and concerns, especially anxiety and fear about the diagnosis, treatment, and outcome
7. Abnormal complete blood count (CBC), including:
    a. Decreased hemoglobin and hematocrit levels
    b. Low platelet count and abnormal coagulation values (INF, aPTT)
    c. WBC count (low, normal, or elevated) and differential
- Diagnosis of leukemia is based on findings from a bone marrow biopsy. The leukemia type is diagnosed by cell surface antigens and chromosomal or gene markers.

Analysis: Interpreting
- The priority collaborative problems for patients with acute myelogenous leukemia (AML), the most common type of acute leukemia seen in adults, include:
  1. Potential for infection due to decreased immunity and chemotherapy
  2. Potential for injury due to poor clotting from thrombocytopenia
  3. Fatigue due to decreased gas exchange and increased energy demands

PREVENT INFECTION
- Prevent infection due to decreased immunity and chemotherapy. Infection is a major cause of death in the patient with leukemia because the WBCs are immature and cannot function or WBCs are depleted from chemotherapy, leading to sepsis.
  1. Prevent auto- and cross-contamination with best practices in infection control.
  2. Teach and support self-management to avoid situations of increased risk for infection transmission.
  3. Communicate early and urgently to the provider if the patient has signs of infection, particularly if neutropenia is present.

L

4. Administer drug therapy to treat leukemia. Drug therapy occurs in three phases:
   a. Induction to achieve a rapid, complete remission. Combination chemotherapeutic drugs are used, generally over 7 days of hospitalization
      (1) These drugs can result in severe neutropenia and risk for infection.
      (2) They are also associated with adverse effects of alopecia, nausea, vomiting, diarrhea, stomatitis, and kidney, liver, and cardiac toxicity.
   b. Consolidation with drugs that may be the same as induction but reduced doses or different drugs with the intent to cure
   c. Maintenance therapy may be prescribed for months or years to maintain remission.

! NURSING SAFETY PRIORITY: Critical Rescue

A temperature elevation of even 1°F (or 0.5°C) above baseline is significant for a patient with leukopenia and indicates infection until it has been proven otherwise. Monitor patients with reduced IMMUNITY closely to recognize indications of infection. When any temperature elevation is present in a patient with leukemia, respond by reporting it to the health care provider immediately, and implement standard infection protocols.

5. *Hematopoietic stem cell transplantation or bone marrow transplant* may be considered, depending on the disease subtype and the patient's response to induction therapy.
   a. This therapy requires a conditioning regimen (radiation, chemotherapy) to ensure absence of cancer and reduce the patient's immune response to transplanted cells resulting in *pancytopenia* (few circulating blood cells).
   b. Engraftment is the successful "take" of the transplanted cells in bone marrow, taking about 14 days.
   c. Complications include failure to engraft, graft versus host disease, bleeding, hemorrhagic shock, and death.

MINIMIZE INJURY
- Minimize risk for injury due to thrombocytopenia and chemotherapy.
   1. Poor clotting from decreased platelets and coagulation factors can lead to excessive bleeding.
   2. Monitor laboratory values daily especially CBC, to assess bleeding risk.

3. Implement institutional bleeding precautions for patients to communicate risk.

DECREASE FATIGUE

- Conserve energy related to fatigue, decreased gas exchange, and increased energy demands.
  1. Nutrition therapy can help meet caloric intake goals; consult the dietitian.
  2. Use institutional policy to transfuse red blood cells (RBCs) and other blood products.
  3. Administer drug therapy with colony-stimulating growth factors to reduce the duration of anemia and neutropenia.
  4. Actively manage the periods of rest and activity to meet patient-centered goals of care.

Care Coordination and Transition Management

- Teach the patient and family about:
  1. Measures to prevent infection
  2. The importance of continuing therapy and medical follow-up
  3. The symptoms of infection and when to seek provider advice
  4. The precautions to avoid injury, and detect and manage problematic bleeding when clotting is impaired
  5. Care of the central catheter if in place at discharge
- Make referrals to resources for psychological and financial support and for role and self-esteem adjustment.
- Assess the patient's need for a home care nurse, aide, or equipment.

LIVER, FATTY

OVERVIEW

- Fatty liver is caused by the accumulation of fats in and around hepatic cells.
- Causes include chronic alcohol abuse, diabetes, obesity, and elevated lipid profile.
- The patient usually has no symptoms; the typical finding is elevated serum liver enzymes.
- Assess for signs of cirrhosis (see *Cirrhosis*).
- MRI, ultrasound, or liver biopsy confirms the diagnosis.

INTERPROFESSIONAL COLLABORATIVE CARE

L

- Interventions are aimed at removing the underlying cause of the infiltration and include administration of lipid-lowering drugs and dietary restriction of fats.
- Monitoring liver function tests regularly evaluates treatment effectiveness or progression of disease.

LYME DISEASE
OVERVIEW
- Lyme disease is a reportable systemic infection transmitted by deer ticks infected with a spirochete, *Borrelia burgdorferi*.
- The disease can be prevented by avoiding heavily wooded areas or areas with thick underbrush; by wearing long-sleeved tops, long pants, and socks; and by using an insect repellent on skin and clothing when in an area where infected ticks are likely to be found.

INTERPROFESSIONAL COLLABORATIVE CARE
- Symptoms appear in three stages:
  1. Stage I symptoms appear in 3 to 30 days after the tick bite and resemble the flu with a distinctive rash
     a. Fever, chills, headache, swollen lymph nodes, joint and muscle ache
     b. Spreading, oval or circular rash (erythema migrans)
  2. Stage II symptoms appear 2 to 12 weeks after the tick bite
     a. Cardiac symptoms of carditis: dysrhythmia, dizziness, palpitations, and dyspnea
     b. Neurologic symptoms of meningitis, cranial nerve paralysis, or peripheral neuritis
  3. Stage III, chronic persistent Lyme disease, occurs weeks to years after the tick bite
     a. Arthralgia and arthritis (may be the only symptom of Lyme disease)
     b. Memory and cognitive problems
     c. Fatigue
     d. Enlarged lymph nodes (lymphadenopathy)
- Management of acute or chronic infection consists of antibiotic therapy with the type or duration of antibiotic varying with the stage of Lyme disease.
- Management of joint inflammation is similar to that for rheumatoid arthritis.
- Vaccination against Lyme disease is available and should be encouraged for adults living in high-risk areas.

LYMPHOMA, HODGKIN'S AND NON-HODGKIN'S
OVERVIEW
- Lymphomas (also called *malignant lymphomas*) are cancers of the lymphoid tissues with abnormal overgrowth of lymphocytes. Lymphomas are cancers of committed lymphocytes rather than stem cell precursors (as in leukemia). The two major adult forms of lymphoma are Hodgkin's lymphoma (HL) and non-Hodgkin's lymphoma (NHL).
- HL usually starts in a single lymph node or a single chain of nodes and contains a specific cancer cell type, the Reed-Sternberg cell. HL often spreads predictably from one group of lymph nodes to the next.

- NHL includes all lymphoid cancers that do not have the Reed-Sternberg cell. There are more than 60 subtypes of NHL divided into either indolent or aggressive lymphoma.
- HL affects any age group, but it is most common among teens and young adults and among adults in their 50s and 60s. NHL is more common in men and older adults.
- The most common manifestation of any lymphoma is *lymphadenopathy,* or large but painless lymph node or nodes.
- Other manifestations may include fever, drenching night sweats, and unexplained weight loss.
- Lymph node biopsy provides the basis for an exact diagnosis classified by subtype and staged to determine the extent of the disease and individualize therapy.
- Computerized tomography (CT), MRI, and positron emission tomography (PET) scan are useful to also determine the extent of disease and patient response to therapy.

INTERPROFESSIONAL COLLABORATIVE CARE
- HL is one of the most treatable types of cancer. Generally for stage I and stage II disease, the treatment is external irradiation of involved lymph node regions. With more extensive disease, irradiation and combination chemotherapy are used to achieve remission.
- Treatment options for patients with NHL vary based the subtype of the tumor, international prognostic index (IPI) score, stage of the disease, performance status, and overall tumor burden. Options include combinations of chemotherapy drugs, targeted therapies, localized radiation therapy, radiolabeled antibodies, hematopoietic stem cell transplantation, and investigational agents.
- Nursing management of the patient undergoing chemotherapy treatment for HL or NHL focuses on the side effects of therapy, especially:
  1. Decreasing risk for infection, anemia, and bleeding from drug- or radiation-induced pancytopenia
  2. Reducing GI distress from treatment, including drug therapy to reduce nausea, vomiting, constipation, or diarrhea
  3. Detecting early organ dysfunction, including cardiac, liver, and kidney damage resulting from treatment and to adjust treatment as ordered
- Nursing management of the patient undergoing radiation therapy for HL or NHL focuses on decreasing the adverse effects of therapy, especially:
  1. Skin problems at the site of radiation
  2. Fatigue and taste changes
  3. Permanent sterility after receiving radiation to the abdomino-pelvic region or extensive chemotherapy; some cancer centers offer sperm and egg storage for reproductive options
  4. Specific interventions listed under *Cancer.*

M

MACULAR DEGENERATION

OVERVIEW

- Macular degeneration is the deterioration of the macula (the area of central vision) resulting in impaired visual SENSORY PERCEPTION.
- Age-related macular degeneration (AMD) has two types.
  1. Dry AMD is caused by gradual blockage of retinal capillaries, which allows retinal cells in the macula to become ischemic and necrotic. Central vision declines first, but eventually the person loses all central vision.
  2. Wet AMD is caused by the growth of new blood vessels in the macula, which have thin walls and leak blood and fluid.
- Exudative macular degeneration is also wet, but it can occur at any age. The condition may occur only in one eye or in both eyes. Patients have a sudden decrease in vision after a serous detachment of pigment epithelium in the macula.
- The loss of central vision reduces the ability to read, write, recognize safety hazards, and drive.

INTERPROFESSIONAL COLLABORATIVE CARE

- Management of dry AMD aims to slow the progression of vision loss and maximize remaining visual sensory perception. There is no cure.
  1. Dietary intake of antioxidants, vitamin B12, lutein, and zeaxanthin can slow disease progression.
  2. Suggest alternative strategies (e.g., large-print books, public transportation) and referrals to community organizations that provide a wide range of adaptive equipment.
- See *Visual Impairment (Reduced Vision)* for more discussion of patients' care needs.
- Management of wet macular degeneration focuses on slowing the process and identifying further changes in visual perception.
  1. Laser therapy to seal the leaking blood vessels in or near the macula can limit the extent of the damage.
  2. Vascular endothelial growth factor inhibitors (VEGFIs) injected monthly into the vitreous can also slow disease progression.

MALABSORPTION SYNDROME

OVERVIEW

- Malabsorption syndrome is associated with a variety of disorders and intestinal surgical procedures.

- Physiologic mechanisms limit absorption of nutrients as a result of one or more abnormalities:
  1. Bile salt deficiencies
  2. Enzyme deficiencies
  3. Presence of bacteria
  4. Disrupted mucosal lining of the small intestine
  5. Altered lymphatic or vascular circulation
  6. Decreased gastric or intestinal surface area

INTERPROFESSIONAL COLLABORATIVE CARE

- Signs and symptoms include chronic diarrhea, steatorrhea, weight loss, fatigue, bloating and flatus, easy bruising, anemia, bone pain, and edema.
- Interventions focus on avoiding dietary substances that aggravate malabsorption, supplementing nutrients, and surgical or nonsurgical management of the primary causative disease.

MALNUTRITION: NUTRITION CONCEPT EXEMPLAR

OVERVIEW

- Malnutrition, also called *undernutrition,* results from inadequate NUTRITION, increased nutrient loss, and increased nutrient requirements; it is a multinutrient problem.
- Inadequate nutrient intake can be linked to:
  1. Poverty
  2. Lack of education
  3. Substance abuse
  4. Decreased appetite or a decline in functional ability to eat
  5. Infectious diseases such as tuberculosis (TB) or HIV
  6. Diseases that produce diarrhea and infections leading to anorexia
  7. Chemotherapy
  8. Vomiting causes decreased intestinal absorption with increased nutrient loss
- Eating disorders can lead to malnutrition
  1. Anorexia nervosa (self-induced starvation) and bulimia nervosa (binge eating followed by purging behavior such as self-induced vomiting) also lead to malnutrition
- *Protein-energy malnutrition* (PEM), also known as *protein-calorie malnutrition,* may present in three forms.
  1. *Marasmus* is a calorie malnutrition in which body fat and protein are wasted. Serum proteins are often preserved.
  2. *Kwashiorkor* is a lack of protein quantity and quality in the presence of adequate calories. Body weight is normal, and serum levels of proteins are low.

M

3. *Marasmic-kwashiorkor* is a combined protein and energy malnutrition.

Considerations for Older Adults

Patient-Centered Care

Older adults in the community or in any health care setting are most at risk for poor nutrition, especially PEM. Risk factors include physiologic changes of aging, environmental factors, and health problems.

INTERPROFESSIONAL COLLABORATIVE CARE

Assessment: Noticing

- Assess for signs and symptoms of malnutrition, including:
  1. Leanness and cachexia
  2. Decreased activity tolerance and lethargy
  3. Intolerance to cold
  4. Edema
  5. Dry, flaking skin; dermatitis; or other skin impairment
  6. Poor wound healing
  7. Infections, particularly postoperative
- Collaborate with the dietician to assess:
  1. Usual daily food intake
  2. Eating behaviors
  3. Change in appetite
  4. Recent weight changes
- A weight loss of 5% or more in 30 days, a weight loss of 10% in 6 months, or a weight that is below ideal may indicate malnutrition.

! NURSING SAFETY PRIORITY: Action Alert

When assessing for malnutrition, assess for difficulty or pain in chewing or swallowing. Unrecognized dysphagia is a common problem among nursing home residents and can cause malnutrition, dehydration, and aspiration pneumonia. Ask the patient whether any foods are avoided and why. Ask unlicensed assistive personnel (UAP) to report any choking while the patient eats. Record the occurrence of nausea, vomiting, heartburn, or any other symptoms of discomfort while eating.

- Interpret laboratory data carefully with regard to the total patient. Laboratory data can supply objective data that can support subjective data and identify deficiencies.

Analysis: Interpreting

- The priority collaborative problem for the patient with malnutrition is:
  1. Weight loss due to inability to digest food or absorb nutrients.

Planning and Implementation: Responding

IMPROVE NUTRITION

  1. Collaborate with the dietitian to set caloric and protein intake goals.
  2. Adapt meal choices and times to reflect patient preferences.
  3. Provide nutrition supplements.
  4. Administer vitamins and minerals as prescribed to avoid nutrient deficits.
  5. Maintain a daily calorie count, and weigh the patient daily. Evaluate whether nutrients consumed are sufficient to meet basal and stress-related energy needs.
  6. Evaluate nutritional indices at least weekly: skin intactness, weight, serum albumin, electrolytes, renal function, hemoglobin and hematocrit, and white blood cell (WBC) count.

! NURSING SAFETY PRIORITY: Action Alert

Malnourished ill patients often need to be encouraged to eat. Instruct UAP who are feeding patients to keep food at the appropriate temperature and to provide mouth care before feeding. Assess for other needs, such as pain management, and provide interventions to make the patient comfortable. Pain can prevent patients from enjoying their meals. Remove bedpans, urinals, and emesis basins from sight. Provide a quiet environment conducive to eating. Soft music may calm those with advanced dementia or delirium. Appropriate time should be taken so that the patient does not feel rushed through a meal.

- Ensure best practices with enteral feeding
  1. Total enteral nutrition (TEN) or tube feedings can be administered through one of the available gastrointestinal (GI) tubes.
     a. A nasoenteric tube is any feeding tube inserted nasally and advanced into the GI tract. These tubes are used for short term enteral feedings (less than 4 weeks).

M

    b. Enterostomal feeding tubes are used for long-term enteral feeding, directly accessing the GI tract using various surgical, endoscopic, and laparoscopic techniques.

    c. Tube feedings are administered by bolus feeding, continuous feeding, and cyclic feeding.

2. Complications of TEN include:

    a. Obstructed tube

    b. Tube misplacement or dislodgement

    c. Abdominal distension

    d. Nausea or vomiting

    e. Diarrhea

    f. Refeeding syndrome

!   **NURSING SAFETY PRIORITY: Action Alert**

If enteral tubes are misplaced or become dislodged, the patient is likely to aspirate. Aspiration pneumonia is a life-threatening complication associated with TEN, especially for older adults. Observe for increasing temperature and pulse, as well as for other signs of dehydration such as dry mucous membranes and decreased urinary output. Auscultate lungs every 4 to 8 hours to check for diminishing breath sounds, especially in lower lobes. Patients may become short of breath and report chest discomfort. A chest x-ray confirms this diagnosis and treatment with antibiotics is started.

Chart 2-13   **Best Practice for Patient Safety & Quality Care**
Maintaining a Patent Feeding Tube

- Flush the tube with 20 to 30 mL of water (or the amount prescribed by the health care provider or dietitian):
  - At least every 4 hours during a continuous tube feeding
  - Before and after each intermittent tube feeding
  - Before and after drug administration (use warm water)
  - After checking residual volume
- If the tube becomes clogged, use 30 mL of water for flushing, applying gentle pressure with a 50-mL piston syringe.
- Avoid the use of carbonated beverage, except for existing clogs *when water is not effective*. Do not use cranberry juice.
- Whenever possible, use liquid medications instead of crushed tablets unless liquid forms cause diarrhea;

make sure that the drug is compatible with the feeding solution.
- Do not mix drugs with the feeding product before giving. Crush tablets as finely as possible and dissolve in warm water. *(Check to see which tablets are safe to crush. For example, do not crush slow-acting [SA] or slow-release [SR] drugs.)*
- Consider use of automatic flush feeding pump such as Flexiflo or Kangaroo.

Care Coordination and Transition Management
- Malnutrition is often diagnosed when the patient is admitted to the acute care hospital or shortly after hospitalization if complications such as poor wound healing or sepsis occur.
- The malnourished patient will need resources at home for aggressive nutrition support.
- It is important to educate the patient and family about the following:
  1. Reinforce the importance of adhering to the prescribed diet
  2. Review any drugs the patient may be taking.
  3. If taking an iron preparation, teach the importance of taking the drug immediately before or during meals.
  4. Caution the patient that iron can cause constipation.
  5. For the patient already susceptible to constipation, emphasize the importance of measures for prevention, including adequate fiber intake, adequate fluids, and exercise; teach the family or other caregiver how to continue these therapies.

MASTOIDITIS

OVERVIEW
- Mastoiditis is a progression of an infection of the middle ear (otitis media) to include temporal bone.
- Manifestations include swelling behind the ear and pain with minimal movement of the tragus, the pinna, or the head. Cellulitis develops on the skin or external scalp over the mastoid process, and the ear is pushed sideways and down.
- Otoscopic examination shows a red, dull, thick, immobile eardrum with or without perforation.
- Other manifestations include low-grade fever, malaise, ear drainage, loss of appetite, and enlarged lymph nodes.
- Hearing loss is common.

M

INTERPROFESSIONAL COLLABORATIVE CARE

- Management involves IV antibiotics and surgical removal of the infected tissue if the infection does not respond to antibiotic therapy. A simple or modified radical mastoidectomy with tympanoplasty is the most common treatment.
- Complications of surgery include damage to cranial nerves VI and VII, decreasing the patient's ability to look sideways (cranial nerve VI) and causing a drooping of the mouth on the affected side (cranial nerve VII). Other complications include vertigo, meningitis, brain abscess, chronic purulent otitis media, and wound infection.

MELANOMA

OVERVIEW

- Melanomas are pigmented cancers arising in the melanin-producing epidermal cells.
- Melanoma is highly metastatic, and a person's survival depends on early diagnosis and treatment.
- Risk factors include genetic predisposition, excessive exposure to ultraviolet (UV) light, and the presence of one or more precursor lesions that resemble unusual moles.
- It occurs most often among light-skinned races and people older than 60 years.

INTERPROFESSIONAL COLLABORATIVE CARE

Assessment: Noticing

- Obtain patient information about:
  1. Age and ethnicity/race
  2. Family history of skin cancer
  3. Any past surgery for removal of skin growths
  4. Recent changes in the size, color, or sensation of any mole, birthmark, wart, or scar
  5. Sun exposure
  6. Exposure to arsenic, coal tar, pitch, radioactive waste, or radium
- Assess for and document all lesions for:
  1. Location, size, and color
  2. Surface features (ABCDE)
     a. *A*symmetry of shape
     b. *B*order irregularity
     c. *C*olor variation within one lesion
     d. *D*iameter greater than 6 mm
     e. *E*xudate presence and quality
- Diagnosis is made based on biopsy findings.

Interventions: Responding

SURGICAL MANAGEMENT

- Surgical intervention is the management of choice for melanoma.

1. *Excision* is used for the biopsy of small lesions, and a sentinel node biopsy can determine whether tumor spread has started.
2. *Wide excision* for deeper melanoma often involves removing full-thickness skin in the area of the lesion. Subcutaneous tissues and lymph nodes may also be removed, and grafting may be needed for wound closure.

NONSURGICAL MANAGEMENT

- Drug therapy may involve systemic chemotherapy, biotherapy, or targeted therapy.
  1. Systemic chemotherapy with a combination of agents; the general management issues for care of patients undergoing chemotherapy are presented under *Cancer*
  2. Biotherapy with interferon
  3. Targeted therapy with experimental drugs such as a CTLA-4 receptor blocker
- Radiation therapy for melanoma may be helpful for patients with metastatic disease when used in combination with systemic corticosteroids. General management issues for care of patients undergoing radiation therapy are presented under *Cancer*.

MELANOMA, OCULAR

OVERVIEW

- Melanoma is the most common malignant eye tumor in adults and is associated with exposure to UV light. Because of its rich blood supply, a melanoma can spread easily into nearby tissue and the brain.
- Manifestations may not be readily apparent, and the tumor may be discovered during a routine examination.
- Manifestations vary with the exact location and may include blurred vision, reduced visual acuity, increased intraocular pressure (IOP), change in iris color, and visual field loss.
- Diagnostic tests usually include ultrasonography or magnetic resonance imaging (MRI) scan.
- Management depends on the tumor's size and growth rate and on the condition of the other eye:
  1. *Enucleation* (surgical removal of the entire eyeball) with insertion of a ball implant to provide a base for fitting the socket prosthesis (in about 1 month)
  2. *Radiation therapy* using an implanted radioactive disk to reduce the size and thickness of melanoma; but this is associated with complications of vitreous hemorrhage, retinopathy, glaucoma, necrosis of the sclera, and cataract formation

M

MÉNIÈRE'S DISEASE

OVERVIEW

- Ménière's disease has three features: tinnitus, one-sided sensori-neural hearing loss, and vertigo; these occur in attacks that can last for several days.
- It is caused by an excess of endolymphatic fluid that distorts the entire inner-ear canal system.

INTERPROFESSIONAL COLLABORATIVE CARE

Nonsurgical Management

- Teach patients about attack prevention strategies, including:
  1. Making slow head movements to prevent worsening of the vertigo
  2. Stopping smoking because nicotine constricts blood vessels
  3. Reduced sodium intake can decrease the endolymphatic fluid volume
- Administer drug therapy and monitor patient response to control the vertigo, including:
  1. Mild diuretics
  2. Antihistamines like diphenhydramine hydrochloride (Benadryl, Allerdryl)
  3. Antivertiginous drugs like meclizine (Antivert, Bonamine)
  4. Antiemetics to control nausea associated with vertigo
  5. Intratympanic therapy with gentamycin and corticosteroid to control infection or inflammation
- Use of pulse pressure treatments, such as the Meniett device, to apply low-pressure micropulses to the inner ear for 5 minutes three times daily

Surgical Management

- Surgical procedures such as a labyrinthectomy resects the vestibular nerve or removes the labyrinth.

MENINGITIS

OVERVIEW

- Meningitis is inflammation of the meninges that surround the brain and spinal cord.
- Viral meningitis is the most common type, followed by bacterial, fungal, and protozoa infections.
- Vaccinations can prevent *Neisseria meningitides* and *Haemophilus influenzae* meningeal infections.

❗ NURSING SAFETY PRIORITY: Action Alert

People ages 16 through 21 years have the highest rates of infection from life-threatening *N. meningitides* meningococcal infection. The Centers for Disease Control and Prevention (CDC) recommends an initial meningococcal vaccine between ages 11 and 12 years with a booster at age 16 years. Adults are advised to get an initial or booster vaccine if living in a shared residence (residence hall, military barracks, group home), traveling or residing in countries where the disease is common, or are immunocompromised due to a damaged or surgically removed spleen or a serum complement deficiency. If the patient's baseline vaccination status is unclear and the immediate risk for exposure to *N. meningitides* infection is high, the CDC recommends vaccination. It is safe to receive a booster as early as 8 weeks after the initial vaccine.

INTERPROFESSIONAL COLLABORATIVE CARE
Assessment: Noticing
- Obtain patient information about:
  1. Recent viral or respiratory diseases and exposure to communicable disease
  2. Head or spine surgery or trauma or ear, nose, or sinus infection
  3. Heart disease, diabetes mellitus, cancer, immunosuppressive therapy, and neurologic procedures that increase the risk for infection or invading organisms
- Assess for and document:
  1. Fever, nuchal rigidity (neck stiffness), headache, myalgia (muscle aches), and altered mental status
  2. Rash, especially on trunk or abdomen
  3. Photophobia or phonophobia (noise sensitivity)
  4. Kernig's and Brudzinski's signs, which are present in only a small percentage of patients with definite meningitis
  5. Seizure and focal neurologic deficits, especially with bacterial meningitis
  6. Complications of meningitis, including syndrome of inappropriate antidiuretic hormone (SIADH) or coagulopathy resulting in emboli that compromise peripheral circulation
- Diagnostic studies may include:
  1. Analysis of cerebrospinal fluid (CSF) for cell count, differential, protein, and culture; although antibiotic administration should *not* be delayed for this procedure, it is desirable to

M

complete the spinal fluid collection via lumbar puncture before the first dose of antibiotics
2. Complete blood count (CBC) with WBC differential and basic metabolic panel for kidney function and electrolytes
3. Computed tomography (CT) scan to detect increased intracranial pressure, abscess (encapsulated pus), or hydrocephalus

Interventions: Responding

- Assess and record the patient's neurologic status with vital signs and peripheral circulation at least every 4 hours. Level of consciousness is the most sensitive indicator of change in patient status.
- Assess and record with particular attention to cranial nerves III, IV, VI, VII, and VIII (pupillary response to light and ability to move eyes through four quadrants) to detect early concerning deterioration of the patient's condition.
- Administer drugs such as antimicrobials and analgesics as ordered.
- Maintain isolation precautions according to hospital policy.
- Implement institutional seizure precautions when indicated.
- Monitor for complications such as vascular compromise from emboli, shock, coagulation disorders, prolonged fever, and septic complications.
- Prevent occurrence with vaccinations, especially if traveling or living in shared residential spaces (e.g., group homes, dormitories, skilled nursing facilities).

METABOLIC SYNDROME

OVERVIEW

- Metabolic syndrome is the simultaneous presence of metabolic factors known to increase risk for developing type 2 diabetes and cardiovascular disease. Features of the syndrome include:
  1. Abdominal obesity: waist circumference of 40 inches (100 cm) or more for men and 35 inches (88 cm) or more for women
  2. Hyperglycemia: fasting blood glucose level of 100 mg/dL or more or on drug treatment for elevated glucose
  3. Abnormal A_{1C}: between 5.5% and 6.0%
  4. Hypertension: systolic blood pressure (BP) of 130 mm Hg or more or diastolic BP of 85 mg Hg or more or on drug treatment for hypertension
  5. Hyperlipidemia: triglyceride level of 150 mg/dL or more or on drug treatment for elevated triglycerides; high-density lipoprotein (HDL) cholesterol less than 40 mg/dL for men or less than 50 mg/dL for women
- Management consists of addressing each of the features (e.g., drug therapy for hypertension, hyperglycemia [diabetes], and hyperlipidemia) and teaching patients about the lifestyle changes that can improve health and reduce obesity.

MULTIDRUG-RESISTANT ORGANISMS (MDRO)

OVERVIEW

* Multidrug-resistant organisms (MDROs) are infectious agents that are no longer responsive to antibiotics.
* The most common MDROs are methicillin-resistant *Staphylococcus aureus* (MRSA), vancomycin-resistant *enterococcus* (VRE), carbapenem-resistant *enterococcus* (CRE), and *Neisseria gonorrhea.*
  1. MRSA is spread by direct contact and invades hospitalized patients through indwelling urinary catheters, vascular access devices, and endotracheal tubes. It is susceptible to only a few antibiotics, such as vancomycin (Lyphocin, Vancocin) and linezolid (Zyvox). A newer IV antibiotic, ceftaroline fosamil (Teflaro), is the first cephalosporin approved to treat MRSA.
  2. *Enterococci* are bacteria that live in the intestinal tract and are important for digestion. VRE can live on almost any surface for days or weeks and still be able to cause an infection. Contamination of toilet seats, door handles, and other objects is very likely for a lengthy period. The most common infections caused by VRE include wound infections, urinary tract infections (UTIs), and bloodstream infections.
  3. *Klebsiella* and *Escherichia coli* (*E. coli*) are types of *Enterobacteriaceae* that are located within the intestinal tract; these bacteria have become increasingly resistant to carbapenem antibiotics, which are most often given for abdominal infections.

INTERPROFESSIONAL COLLABORATIVE CARE

> **❗ NURSING SAFETY PRIORITY: Action Alert**
>
> To help prevent the transmission of an MDRO, change clothes before leaving work. Keep work clothes separate from personal clothes. Take a shower when you get home, if possible, to rid your body of any unwanted pathogens. Be careful not to contaminate equipment that is commonly used, such as your stethoscope.

* Experts suggest several strategies to decrease the incidence of this growing problem.
  1. Perform frequent hand hygiene, including using hand sanitizers.
  2. Use chlorohexidine (2% dilution) when bathing to prevent CRE or decrease colonization and other types of infections from MDROs.
  3. Stop administering multiple antimicrobials when a specific effective drug is identified from culture results.

M

4. Use best practices in infection control in hospital and other health care settings, including the use of personal protective equipment (staff and visitors) and cleaning surfaces and equipment.
5. Teach patients and primary health care providers to avoid the use of antibiotics to treat common viral illnesses such as colds.
6. Follow guidelines or best practices to ensure selection of the most effective antibiotic, the correct dose for the condition, and the duration of treatment.

✴ MULTIPLE SCLEROSIS: IMMUNITY CONCEPT EXEMPLAR

OVERVIEW

- Multiple sclerosis (MS) is a chronic disease caused by immune, genetic, and/or infectious factors that affect the myelin and nerve fibers of the brain and spinal cord.
- It is one of the leading causes of neurologic disability in young and middle-aged adults.
- MS is characterized by periods of remission and exacerbation (flare), which is commonly referred to as a relapsing-remitting course.
- Patients progress at different rates and over different lengths of time.
- As the severity and duration of the disease progress, the periods of exacerbation become more frequent.
- MS often mimics other neurologic diseases, which makes the diagnosis difficult and prolonged.
- The major types of MS are:
  1. Relapsing-remitting MS (RRMS), which is characterized as mild or moderate, depending on the degree of disability; symptoms develop and resolve in a few weeks to months, after which the patient may return to baseline.
  2. Primary progressive MS (PPMS), which is characterized by a steady and gradual neurologic deterioration without remission of symptoms; the patient has progressive disability with no acute attacks. Patients with this type of MS tend to be between 40 and 60 years old at onset of the disease.
  3. Secondary progressive MS (SPMS) begins with a relapsing-remitting course that later becomes steadily progressive. About half of all people with RRMS develop SPMS within 10 years. The current addition of disease-modifying drugs as part of disease management may decrease the development of SPMS.
  4. Progressive-relapsing MS (PRMS) is characterized by frequent relapses with partial recovery, but not a return to baseline. This type of MS is seen in only a small percentage of patients. Progressive, cumulative symptoms and deterioration occur over several years.

Gender Health Considerations

Patient-Centered Care

MS affects women two to three times more often than men, suggesting a possible hormonal role in disease development. Some studies show that the disease occurs up to four times more often in women than men (National Multiple Sclerosis Society, 2016).

INTERPROFESSIONAL COLLABORATIVE CARE

Assessment: Noticing

- Assess for and document:
  1. Progression of symptoms
  2. Factors that aggravate symptoms
     a. Stress
     b. Fatigue
     c. Overexertion
     d. Temperature extremes such as a hot shower or bath
  3. Motor function
     a. Fatigue
     b. Stiffness of legs
     c. Flexor spasms, clonus
     d. Increased deep tendon reflexes
     e. Positive Babinski's reflex
  4. Cerebellar function
     a. Ataxic gait
     b. Intention tremor (tremor when performing activity)
     c. Dysmetria (inability to direct or limit movement)
     d. Clumsy motor movements
  5. Cranial nerve function
     a. Hearing loss
     b. Facial weakness
     c. Swallowing difficulties (dysphagia)
     d. Tinnitus
     e. Vertigo
  6. Vision
     a. Decreased visual acuity
     b. Blurred vision
     c. Diplopia
     d. Scotoma (changes in peripheral vision)
     e. Nystagmus
  7. Sensation
     a. Hyperalgesia
     b. Paresthesia
     c. Facial pain

M

  d. Change in bowel and bladder function
  e. Impotence, difficulty sustaining an erection
  f. Decreased vaginal secretion
 8. Cognitive changes seen late in the course of the disease
  a. Memory loss
  b. Decreased ability to perform calculations
  c. Inattention
  d. Impaired judgment
 9. Psychosocial function
  a. Apathy, emotional lability, and depression
  b. Disturbed body image
- No single specific laboratory test is definitively diagnostic for MS. Collective results of a variety of tests are usually conclusive.
- Diagnostic testing may include:
 1. MRI to determine the presence of plaques in the central nervous system (CNS)
 2. Lumbar puncture for analysis of CSF

Analysis: Interpreting
- The priority collaborative problems for patients with MS include:
 1. Potential for infection/decreased IMMUNITY secondary to disease and drug therapy for disease management
 2. Decreased MOBILITY due to spasticity, tremors, and/or fatigue
 3. Decreased visual acuity and COGNITION due to dysfunctional central system nerves

Planning and Implementation: Responding
- The purpose of management is to modify effect of the disease on the immune system, prevent exacerbations, manage symptoms, improve function, and maintain quality of life.

MANAGING RISK FOR INFECTION AND DECREASED IMMUNITY
Drug therapy includes:
 1. Current therapies are designed to alter the immune system responses associated with MS
  a. Interferon-beta (Avonex, Betaseron, Rebif), immunomodulators that modify the course of the disease and have antiviral effects
  b. Glatiramer acetate (Copaxone), a synthetic protein that is similar to myelin-based protein
  c. Natalizumab (Tysabri), a monoclonal antibody that binds to WBCs to prevent further damage to the myelin
  d. Fingolimod (Gilenya), teriflunomide (Aubagio), or dimethyl fumarate (Tecfidera) to modulate the immune system
  e. Mitoxantrone (Novantrone), a chemotherapy drug, during worsening symptoms
  f. A combination of cyclophosphamide (Cytoxan) and methylprednisolone (Solu-Medrol) may be used for some patients

for immunosuppression during the onset and acute exacerbation of MS symptoms.

g. Ocrelizumab (Ocrevus) was recently approved for patients with PPMS and has shown positive effects on disease progression.

! NURSING SAFETY PRIORITY: Drug Alert

The interferons and glatiramer acetate (Copaxone) are subcutaneous injections that patients can self administer. Teach patients how to give and rotate the site of interferon-beta and glatiramer acetate injections because local injection site (skin) reactions are common. The first dose of these drugs is given under medical supervision to monitor for allergic response, including anaphylactic shock. Teach patients receiving these drugs to avoid crowds and people with infections. Remind them to report any sign or symptom associated with infection immediately to their primary health care provider.

IMPROVING MOBILITY
- The symptoms of MS that affect mobility include spasticity, tremor, and fatigue.
  1. Refer to rehabilitative services (physical and occupational therapy)
     a. Implementing an exercise program to strengthen and stretch muscles
     b. Using assistive devices, such as a cane, walker, or electric (Amigo) cart
  2. Adjunctive therapy to treat muscle spasticity and paresthesia
     a. For spasticity, the primary health care provider may prescribe baclofen (Lioresal), tizanidine (Zanaflex), diazepam (Valium, Apo-Diazepam), or clonazepam (Klonopin)
  3. Provide sufficient time to complete activities of daily living (ADLs); as a result of weakness and fatigue, the patient requires more time or assistance

MANAGING DECREASED VISUAL ACUITY AND COGNITION
- Alterations in visual acuity and cognition can occur at any time during the course of the disease process. Areas affected include attention, memory, problem solving, auditory reasoning, handling distractions, and visual perception.
  1. For diplopia: An eye patch that is alternated from eye to eye every few hours may relieve this condition.
  2. For peripheral vision deficits: Teach scanning techniques to help compensate for the visual deficit.

M

3. Complementary and integrative health therapies such as reflexology, massage, and yoga may be successful in decreasing symptoms of MS.
4. Marijuana has been used by some patients to relieve muscle spasm pain and is now legal for medical use in more than 20 US states and in Canada.

Care Coordination and Transition Management
- Self-management education includes:
  1. Avoiding factors that may exacerbate the symptoms including overexertion, extremes of temperatures (fever, hot baths, overheating, excessive chilling), humidity, and exposure to infection
  2. Providing drug information
  3. Encouraging the patient to follow the exercise program developed by the physical therapist (PT) and to remain independent in all activities for as long as possible
  4. Encouraging the patient to engage in regular social activities, obtain adequate rest, and manage stress
  5. Teaching the family strategies to cope with personality changes
  6. Reinforcing established bowel and bladder, skin care, and nutrition programs
  7. Identifying community organizations and support groups for education and to promote adaptive psychosocial coping

MYASTHENIA GRAVIS

OVERVIEW
- Myasthenia gravis (MG) is an acquired autoimmune disease characterized by muscle weakness. The thymus gland may be abnormal.
- MG is caused by an autoantibody attack on the acetylcholine receptors (AChRs) in the muscle end plate membranes. As a result, nerve impulses are reduced at the neuromuscular junction.
- There are two types of MG: ocular and generalized.
- MG manifestations can range from mild disturbances of the cranial and peripheral motor neurons to a rapidly developing, generalized weakness that may lead to death from respiratory failure.

INTERPROFESSIONAL COLLABORATIVE CARE
Assessment: Noticing
- Obtain patient information about:
  1. Muscular weakness that increases on exertion or as the day wears on and improves with rest (with a temporary increase in weakness sometimes noted after vaccination, menstruation, and exposure to extremes in environmental temperature)
  2. Family history of MG and thymus gland tumor

- Assess for and document:
  1. Symptoms related to involvement of the levator palpebrae or extraocular muscles
  2. Involvement of muscles for facial expression, chewing, and speech
  3. Proximal limb weakness that leads to difficulty climbing stairs, lifting heavy objects, or raising arms overhead
  4. Mild or severe neck weakness
  5. Difficulty sustaining a sitting or walking posture
  6. Respiratory distress
  7. Bowel and bladder incontinence
  8. Weakness of the pelvic and shoulder girdles (seen in Eaton-Lambert syndrome)
  9. Disturbed body image
  10. Feelings of loss, fear, helplessness, and grief
  11. Usual coping methods
- Diagnostic studies may include:
  1. Serum thyroid function tests because thyrotoxicosis can mimic MG
  2. Serum protein electrophoresis tests to evaluate the presence of autoantibodies
  3. Serum AChR antibodies
  4. Chest x-ray and CT scan to evaluate the thymus gland in the mediastinum
  5. Pharmacologic tests with the cholinesterase inhibitors edrophonium (Tensilon) and neostigmine (Prostigmin); anticipate a marked improvement of muscle tone that lasts 4 to 5 minutes
  6. Repetitive nerve stimulation of proximal nerves, the most common electrodiagnostic test performed to detect MG; alternatively, electromyography to test muscle contraction or single fiber contraction after electrical stimulation is used

Interventions: Responding

NONSURGICAL MANAGEMENT

- Maintain adequate respiratory functioning (ABCs [airway, breathing, circulation] of emergency care); intubation and mechanical ventilation may be needed during periods of acute exacerbation or drug-drug interactions.
- Administer drugs to reduce the symptoms of MG. Give these drugs for MG on time to avoid respiratory compromise and muscular weakness:
  1. Cholinesterase inhibitor drugs, also referred to as *anticholinesterase drugs* (typically pyridostigmine [Mestinon, Regonol]), prevent the breakdown of acetylcholine by enzymes in the neuromuscular junction, thereby increasing

M

the response of muscles to nerve impulses and improving strength.

a. The drug is given with a small amount of food to minimize GI side effects; meals are provided 45 minutes to 1 hour after taking the drug.

Emergency Care: Myasthenic Crisis

Myasthenic crisis is often caused by some type of infection. For other patients, increasing muscle weakness leads to an overdose of anticholinesterase drugs. As a result, the patient may experience a *mixed* crisis. The edrophonium test (Enlon, Tensilon), although not always conclusive, is an important procedure for differentiation. *Tensilon produces a temporary improvement in myasthenic crisis but worsening or no improvement of symptoms in cholinergic crisis.*

The priority for nursing management of the patient in myasthenic crisis is maintaining adequate respiratory function to promote GAS EXCHANGE. The acutely ill patient may need intensive nursing care for monitoring. He or she may require mechanical ventilation or other technologic support. Cholinesterase-inhibiting drugs are withheld because they increase respiratory secretions and are usually ineffective for the first few days after the crisis begins. Drug therapy is restarted gradually and at lower dosages.

Emergency Care: Cholinergic Crisis

In *cholinergic* crisis, do not give anticholinesterase drugs while the patient is maintained with mechanical ventilation. Atropine 1 mg IV may be given and repeated, if necessary. When atropine is prescribed, observe the patient carefully. Secretions can be thickened by the drug, which causes more difficulty with airway clearance and possibly the development of mucus plugs. Unless complications such as pneumonia or aspiration develop, the patient in crisis improves rapidly after the appropriate drugs have been given. Continue to provide assistance as necessary because he or she tires easily after minimal exertion.

2. Immunosuppresants including corticosteroids, methotrexate, a chemotherapeutic agent, or rituximab, a biologic agent effective against B-cells
3. Avoid drugs that contribute to muscle weakness
   a. Morphine or its derivatives, curare, quinine, quinidine, procainamide, hypnotics, or sedatives may increase weakness and should be avoided.

    b. Antibiotics such as neomycin, kanamycin, streptomycin, polymyxin B, and certain tetracyclines increase myasthenic symptoms by impairing transmitter release.

- Monitor the patient's responses to and vascular access for plasmapheresis. Plasmapheresis is a method by which autoantibodies are removed from the plasma.
- Promote mobility and in-bed positioning to maintain function.
- Assist with communication.
  1. Collaborate with the speech-language pathologist to develop communication strategies when needed.
  2. Instruct the patient to speak slowly and repeat information to verify that it is correct.
- Ensure adequate nutritional support.
  1. Provide small, frequent meals and high-calorie snacks. Record calorie counts.
  2. Measure intake and output, serum albumin levels, and daily weight.
  3. Assess for the onset of dysphagia. Implement aspiration precautions as needed.
  4. Promote or provide oral hygiene.
  5. Obtain a dietitian consultation to optimize nutrition.
- Maintain eye protection.
  1. Apply artificial tears to keep corneas moist and free from abrasion.
  2. Consider a lubricant gel and eye shield at bedtime.
  3. To help relieve diplopia, cover alternate eyes with a patch for 2 to 3 hours at a time.

SURGICAL MANAGEMENT
- Thymectomy may be performed early in the disease. Remission may not occur even with a thymectomy or may take up to 2 years to show effect.
- Provide routine preoperative care as outlined in Part One, including:
  1. Administering pyridostigmine (Mestinon), as ordered, to keep the patient stable throughout surgery
  2. If steroids have been used, administering before surgery but tapering postoperatively
  3. Giving antibiotics before and after surgery
- Provide routine postoperative care as outlined in Part One, including:
  1. Observing for signs of pneumothorax or hemothorax such as chest pain, sudden shortness of breath, diminished or absent breath sounds, and restlessness or a change in vital signs
  2. Focusing on respiratory health, including using spirometry, coughing, deep breathing, and frequent monitoring for respiratory distress
  3. Observing for signs and symptoms of wound infection
  4. Providing chest tube care if indicated

M

Care Coordination and Transition Management

- Promote self-management with education about the disease and expected outcomes, including the need to monitor for episodic exacerbations (worsening of symptoms). If rest does not relieve symptoms or respiratory distress occurs, contact the primary health care provider.
- Inform patients and family members about actors to avoid because they contribute to exacerbation, such as infection, stress, heat, and hard physical exercise.
- Teach the patient and family to monitor for these two types of crises:
  1. Myasthenic crisis: an exacerbation (flare-up or worsening) of the myasthenic symptoms caused by not enough anticholinesterase drugs
  2. Cholinergic crisis: an acute exacerbation of muscle weakness caused by too many anticholinesterase drugs
- Provide information concerning the drug regimen, and include the name, effects, side effects, and the importance of taking drugs on time and not missing doses.
- Refer the patient to community agencies and support groups such as the Myasthenia Gravis Foundation.

N

NEPHROTIC SYNDROME

OVERVIEW

- Nephrotic syndrome is a condition of increased glomerular permeability that allows larger molecules to pass through the membrane into the urine and be removed from the blood.
- It is commonly caused by changes in an immune or inflammatory process.
- The main features are severe proteinuria, hypoalbuminemia, hyperlipidemia, lipiduria, facial and periorbital edema, and derangements in blood pressure.

INTERPROFESSIONAL COLLABORATIVE CARE

- Treatment depends on what is causing the disorder (identified by renal biopsy) and may include:
  1. Angiotensin-converting enzyme inhibitors to preserve kidney function in early stages
  2. Cholesterol-lowering drugs and drugs to control hypercholesterolemia
  3. Anti-inflammatory and immunosuppressive agents such as a corticosteroid

4. Heparin to reduce clot formation and extension (clots form as part of the inflammatory response)
5. Diuretics
6. Diet changes, including fluid and sodium restriction

- Assess the patient's hydration status and monitor for dehydration. If the plasma volume is depleted, kidney problems worsen.
- Assess laboratory values for changes in kidney function, including serum blood urea nitrogen (BUN), creatinine, glomerular filtration rate, electrolytes, and urinalysis.

NEUROMA, ACOUSTIC
OVERVIEW

- An acoustic neuroma is a nonmalignant tumor of cranial nerve VIII (vestibulocochlear nerve, also known as the *auditory* or *acoustic* nerve). Damage to hearing, facial movements, and sensation can occur as the tumor grows.

INTERPROFESSIONAL COLLABORATIVE CARE

- Symptoms begin with tinnitus and progress to gradual sensorineural hearing loss in most patients. Constant, mild vertigo occurs later.
- Diagnosis is made by CT or MRI.
- Surgical removal is usually achieved by a craniotomy, and the remaining hearing is lost. See *Hearing Loss* for a review of care needs for the patient whose hearing is reduced.

O

 OBESITY: NUTRITION EXEMPLAR
OVERVIEW

- Obesity is not just one disease; it includes many conditions with varying causes. The terms *obesity* and *overweight* are often used interchangeably, but they refer to different health problems.
- Overweight: an increase in body weight for height compared with a reference standard, or up to 10% greater than ideal body weight (IBW) and a body mass index (BMI) of 25 to 29.
- Obesity: an excess amount of body fat when compared with lean body mass; an obese adult weighs at least 20% above the upper limit of the normal range for IBW and has a BMI of 30 or more.
  1. Normal body fat in men is 15% to 20% of body fat.
  2. Normal body fat in women is 18% to 32% of body fat.
- Morbid obesity: refers to a weight that has a severely negative effect on health; usually more than 100% above IBW and a BMI over 40.

- More than one-third of the US population is obese and around 10% of adults are morbidly obese. Obesity is the second leading cause of preventable deaths in the United States.
- Bariatrics is a branch of medicine that manages patients with obesity and its related diseases.
- Causes of obesity include high-fat and high-cholesterol diets, physical inactivity, drug treatment (corticosteroids, nonsteroidal anti-inflammatory drugs [NSAIDs]), dysregulation of hormones that affect appetite and fat metabolism, and familial or genetic factors.

Genetic/Genomic Considerations

Patient-Centered Care

Familial and genetic factors play an important role in obesity. When both parents are overweight, about 80% of their children will be overweight. If neither parent is overweight, fewer than 10% of the children will be overweight. In studies of non-identical twins, when one twin is obese, the second twin also is obese about 30% of the time. In studies of identical twins, when one twin is obese, the second twin also is obese about 80% of the time. These results indicate a strong genetic component to obesity along with lifestyle (environmental) influences.

Genetic composition may predispose some adults, but not others, to obesity. Leptin, the hormone encoded by the *ob* gene, appears to send a message to the brain that the body has stored enough fat. This message serves as a signal to stop eating. An abnormality of this gene has been found in some adults with obesity.

- Complications of obesity primarily affect the cardiovascular and respiratory systems. Excess weight can also cause degeneration of the musculoskeletal system, especially weight-bearing joints like hips and knees.

Chart 2-14 Common Complications of Obesity

- Type 2 diabetes mellitus
- Hypertension
- Hyperlipidemia (increased serum lipids)
- Coronary artery disease (CAD)
- Stroke
- Peripheral artery disease (PAD)
- Metabolic syndrome
- Obstructive sleep apnea

- Obesity hypoventilation syndrome
- Depression and other mental health/behavioral health problems
- Urinary incontinence
- Cholelithiasis (gallstones)
- Gout
- Chronic back pain
- Early osteoarthritis
- Decreased wound healing

O

INTERPROFESSIONAL COLLABORATIVE CARE
Assessment: Noticing
- Approach patients with obesity by using the acronym, RESPECT, created by The Ohio State University (Budd & Peterson, 2015):
  1. Create **R**apport in an **E**nvironment that is **S**afe.
  2. Ensure **P**rivacy.
  3. **E**ncourage realistic goals.
  4. Provide **C**ompassion.
  5. Utilize **T**act in conversation.
- In addition to a complete history regarding present and past health problems, collect this information about the patient in collaboration with the dietician:
  1. Usual food intake or 24-hour diet history recall
  2. Changes in eating behaviors or appetite
  3. Cultural and economic background
  4. Attitude toward food and current weight
  5. Drugs, including prescriptive, over-the-counter (OTC), and herbal or food additives
  6. Physical activity and functional ability
  7. Height and weight
  8. Waist-to-hip ratio or waist circumference; a ratio greater than 0.95 in men or greater than 0.8 in women or a waist greater than 40 inches indicates central obesity and high risk for cardiovascular conditions
  9. Determine arm and calf circumferences
  10. Comorbid or chronic conditions
  11. Family history of obesity
  12. Psychosocial assessment to determine emotional factors that might prevent successful therapy or that might be worsened by therapy; assess the patient's perception of current weight and weight reduction

Analysis: Interpreting
- The priority collaborative problem for the patient with obesity is:
  1. Weight gain due to excessive intake of calories.

Planning and Implementation: Responding
IMPROVING NUTRITION
  Nonsurgical Management
- Diet programs managed through close interaction among the patient, dietitian, nutritionist, and primary health care provider
- Exercise programs to include aerobic activity
- Drug therapy
- Anorectic drugs work to suppress appetite and reduce food intake.
    1. Lorcaserin (Belviq) acts on central serotonin receptors.
    2. Qsymia is a combination of phentermine and topiramate (an antiseizure drug).
    3. Orlistat (Xenical) works in the gastrointestinal tract to inhibit lipase and leads to partial hydrolysis of triglycerides. Because fats are only partially digested and absorbed, calorie intake is decreased.
- Sympathomimetic drugs suppress appetite and are used short-term with a structured weight management program.
    1. Phentermine hydrochloride (Adipex-P), diethylpropion hydrochloride (Tenuate, Tenuate Dospan), and phendimetrazine tartrate (Bontril PDM)

! NURSING SAFETY PRIORITY: Drug Alert

Patients with hypertension, heart disease, and hyperthyroidism should not take anorectic drugs because they may worsen their symptoms. These drugs are not prescribed for any patient taking psychoactive agents because they cause similar side effects. Teach patients who are candidates for sympathomimetic drugs about side effects, which include:
- Palpitations
- Diarrhea or constipation
- Restlessness
- Insomnia
- Dry mouth
- Blurred vision
- Change in sex drive or activity
- Anxiety

- Behavioral treatment to change habits around eating and weight management
  Surgical Management
- Surgery is indicated for the patient who is morbidly obese or who has a BMI greater than 35 with comorbidities that contribute to poor health.
    1. Bariatric surgical procedures include three types: gastric restrictive, malabsorption, or both. *Restrictive surgeries* decrease the volume capacity of the stomach to limit the amount of

food that can be eaten at one time. As the name implies, *mal-absorption procedures* interfere with the absorption of food and nutrients from the gastrointestinal (GI) tract.

    a. Most patients have laparoscopic adjustable gastric band (LAGB) surgery or the laparoscopic sleeve gastrectomy (LSG). Both procedures are classified as restrictive surgeries.

    b. The most common malabsorption surgery is the *Roux-en-Y gastric bypass*.

- Provide routine postoperative care after bariatric surgery and:

    1. Attend to airway management because a thick neck may lead to compromised airway.

    2. Monitor vital signs with peripheral oxygen saturation (SpO_2).

    3. Focus on patient and staff safety, using bariatric equipment to promote mobility and reduce skin complications.

    4. Monitor the patency of the nasogastric tube (NGT) and record the amount of drainage.

❗ NURSING SAFETY PRIORITY: Action Alert

Some patients who have bariatric surgery have an NGT put in place, especially after open surgical procedures. In gastroplasty procedures, the NGT drains both the proximal pouch and the distal stomach. Closely monitor the tube for patency. ***Never reposition the tube because its movement can disrupt the suture line!*** The NGT is removed on the second day if the patient is passing flatus.

---

    5. Monitor for symptoms of anastomotic leak if this process was part of the surgical approach. Symptoms of leak are increasing back, shoulder, or abdominal pain; restlessness; unexplained tachycardia; and oliguria (scant urine). Report any of these findings to the surgeon immediately. *Anastomotic leaks are the most common serious complication and cause of death after gastric bypass surgery.*

    6. Apply an abdominal binder to prevent wound dehiscence.

    7. Place the patient in a semi-Fowler's position for comfort.

    8. Use continuous positive airway pressure (CPAP) ventilation at night to improve ventilation and decrease risk for sleep apnea

    9. Implement best practices for maintaining skin integrity and observe skin folds for redness, excoriation, or breakdown.

    10. Observe for dumping syndrome, manifested by frequent, liquid stools after eating.

    11. Provide venothromboembolism prevention, including early mobility and sequential compression stockings and/or subcutaneous low molecular weight heparin.

12. Follow the institutional protocol about starting and advancing oral intake; avoid large volumes of liquid intake to avoid discomfort and stimulating hyperperistalsis.

Care Coordination and Transition Management

- Discuss community resources, such as Weight Watchers, Overeaters Anonymous, and Take Off Pounds Sensibly (TOPS).
- In collaboration with the nutritionist, provide health teaching regarding the diet and the importance of maintaining a healthy eating pattern.
- Encourage the patient to increase physical activity, decrease fat intake and reliance on drug use, establish a normal eating pattern in response to physiologic hunger, and address medical and psychological problems.
- Emphasize the necessity for follow-up after bariatric surgery to avoid complications and ensure safe weight loss.

Chart 2-15 Patient and Family Education: Preparing for Discharge

Teaching for the Patient After Bariatric Surgery

Nutrition: Diet progression, nutrient (including vitamin and mineral) supplements, hydration guidelines

Drug therapy: Analgesics and antiemetic drugs, if needed; drugs for other health problems

Wound care: Clean procedure for open or laparoscopic wounds; cover during shower or bath

Activity level: Restrictions, such as avoiding lifting; activity progression; return to driving and work

Signs and symptoms to report: Fever; excessive nausea or vomiting; epigastric, back, or shoulder pain; red, hot, and/or draining wound(s); pain, redness, or swelling in legs; chest pain; difficulty breathing

Follow-up care: Primary health care provider office or clinic visits, support groups and other community resources, counseling for patient and family

Continuing education: Nutrition and exercise classes; follow-up visits with dietitian

---

OBSTRUCTION, INTESTINAL: ELIMINATION EXEMPLAR

OVERVIEW

- Intestinal obstruction compromises ELIMINATION.
- Intestinal obstruction can be partial or complete and can occur in either the small or large intestine.

- Obstructions are classified as mechanical or nonmechanical.
  1. *Mechanical obstruction* occurs when the bowel is physically obstructed by problems outside the intestine (adhesions or hernias), in the bowel wall (strictures from radiation or inflammatory bowel disease like Crohn's disease), or in the lumen of the intestine (tumor, fecal impaction, fibrosis, intussusception, and volvulus).
  2. *Nonmechanical obstruction (paralytic or adynamic ileus)* occurs when peristalsis is decreased or absent, resulting in a slowing of the movement or a backup of intestinal content caused by physiologic, neurogenic, or chemical imbalances.
     a. Paralytic ileus is associated with opioids and other drugs, trauma, surgery, hypokalemia, peritonitis, and impaired perfusion (vascular insufficiency) to the bowel.
- Distention, edema, and increased capillary permeability occur with obstruction.
  1. Intestinal contents accumulate at and above the area of obstruction, leading to distension.
  2. With distension, peristalsis and intestinal secretions increase, leading to further distention and bowel edema.
  3. The changes in the bowel contribute to increased capillary permeability, and leakage of fluid and electrolytes into the interstitial space resulting in reduced circulatory blood volume (hypovolemia) and electrolyte imbalances.
  4. Edema in the bowel and surrounding issue can lead to increased intra-abdominal pressure and acute abdominal compartment syndrome, a complication that leads to bowel ischemia, injury, and necrosis.
  5. Vascular circulation to the bowel can become compromised with hypovolemia and with edema pressing on capillaries, leading to peritonitis and sepsis.
- It is a surgical emergency when there is obstruction with compromised blood flow.

INTERPROFESSIONAL COLLABORATIVE CARE
Assessment: Noticing
- Obtain patient information about:
  1. Medical history, including abdominal surgical procedures, radiation therapy, and bowel diseases such as Crohn's disease, ulcerative colitis, diverticular disease, gallstones, hernia repair, trauma, and peritonitis
  2. Diet history and drug use
  3. Bowel elimination patterns, including the presence of blood in the stool

4. Familial history of colorectal cancer
5. Nausea and vomiting, including the characteristics of emesis
- Assess for and document:
  1. The quality of abdominal pain, onset, and aggravating and alleviating factors associated with pain
  2. Vital signs, including symptoms of hypovolemia (tachycardia, hypotension, low urine output) or infections (fever)
  3. Abdominal distention (hallmark sign)
  4. Bowel sounds (borborygmi): high-pitched bowel sounds may be heard early in an obstructive process and absent bowel sounds in later stages
  5. Nausea, vomiting, and characteristics of emesis
     a. Obstruction above the ileum causes early and profuse vomiting of partially digested food and chyme, changing to watery contents containing bile and mucus.
     b. Obstruction in the large intestine produces vomitus with an orange-brown color and a foul odor caused by bacterial overgrowth, which may be fecal contamination.
  6. Presence or absence of stool or flatus and characteristics of stool
     a. No passage of stool (obstipation) or flatus, a characteristic of total small- and large-bowel mechanical obstruction
     b. Diarrhea may be present with a partial obstruction.
  7. Hiccups (singultus), which are common with all types of intestinal obstruction
- Diagnostic studies include:
  1. Computerized tomography (CT) scan
  2. A screening abdominal ultrasound may be used to evaluate the type of obstruction.

❗ NURSING SAFETY PRIORITY: Critical Rescue

The sudden change in abdominal pain from dull to sharp or local to generalized may indicate a perforation. Inform the physician immediately of this change in patient pain, along with current vital signs and oxygen status. A perforation is a surgical emergency.

Analysis: Interpreting
- The priority collaborative problems for patients with intestinal obstruction include:
  1. Potential for injury (e.g., peritonitis, acute injury, etc.) due to obstruction
  2. Acute pain due to obstruction

Planning and Implementation: Responding
- Interventions are aimed at uncovering the cause and relieving the obstruction to restore elimination.

DECREASING POTENTIAL FOR INJURY

Nonsurgical Management
- Decompress the GI tract by inserting or maintaining a gastric tube, which can be inserted nasally or orally.

❗ NURSING SAFETY PRIORITY: Action Alert

At least every 4 hours, assess the patient with an nasogastric tube (NGT) or orogastric tube (OGT) for proper placement of the tube, tube patency, and output (quality and quantity). Monitor the skin around the tube for irritation. Use a device that secures the tube to the nose or mouth to prevent accidental removal. Assess for peristalsis by auscultating for bowel sounds with the suction disconnected (suction masks peristaltic sounds).

1. Monitor and record quantity and character of nasogastric output every 4 hours.
2. Assess the skin for integrity at the site of tube insertion.
3. Mark the tube at the nares or lip to provide ongoing confirmation of placement.
4. Record the passage of flatus and the amount and character of bowel movements.
5. Inform the primary health care provider if outflow stops or becomes bloody.

- If paralytic or partial obstruction, drugs to enhance gastric mobility may be given.
- Obstruction caused by fecal impaction may resolve after disimpaction that can be manual or aided with enema administration.
- Intussusception (telescoping of bowel) and volvulus may resolve with hydrostatic pressure changes with manipulation under fluoroscopy.
- Administer fluid and electrolyte replacement.
    1. Administer intravenous (IV) fluid because of dehydration from NPO status, lack of normal reabsorption in the intestine, increased intestinal secretions, and NG suction.
    2. Monitor fluid status with vital signs, adequacy of urine output, and daily weight.

MANAGING PAIN
- Report uncontrolled or severe pain to the provider, including pain that significantly increases or changes from a colicky, intermittent type to constant discomfort.

- Administer stool softeners or stimulants with opioids unless the obstruction is complete.
- Provide a position of comfort, including the semi-Fowler's position, to relieve the pressure of abdominal distention and facilitate thoracic excursion and normal breathing patterns.
- Broad-spectrum antibiotics are given if surgery is anticipated.

SURGICAL MANAGEMENT
- Surgical management is required for complete mechanical obstruction and for many cases of incomplete mechanical obstruction.
- An exploratory laparotomy is performed to locate the obstruction and determine the nature of the problem.
- The specific surgical procedure performed depends on the cause and location of the obstruction. Examples of procedures include lysis of adhesions, colon resection with anastomosis for obstruction resulting from tumor or diverticulitis, and embolectomy or thrombectomy for intestinal infarction. A colon resection and colostomy may be necessary.

Care Coordination and Transition Management
- Patient and family education depend on the specific cause and treatment of the obstruction.
  1. Report signs that may indicate recurrent obstruction, including abdominal pain or distention, nausea, vomiting, or constipation (for nonmechanical obstruction after surgery or trauma).
  2. Develop a structured bowel regimen, such as a high-fiber diet or fiber supplements and daily exercise with sufficient oral intake of water for prevention of recurrences of fecal impaction.
- Information about incision care (if surgery was performed), drug therapy, and activity restriction is given to the patient and family.

OBSTRUCTION, UPPER AIRWAY

OVERVIEW
- Upper airway obstruction is an interruption in airflow through the nose, mouth, pharynx, or larynx. When gas exchange is impaired, airway obstruction can be life-threatening.
- Causes include:
  1. Tongue edema (surgery, trauma, angioedema as an allergic response to a drug)
  2. Tongue occlusion (e.g., loss of gag reflex, loss of muscle tone, unconsciousness, coma)
  3. Laryngeal edema
  4. Peritonsillar and pharyngeal abscess
  5. Head and neck cancer

6. Thick secretions
7. Stroke and cerebral edema
8. Smoke inhalation edema
9. Facial, tracheal, or laryngeal trauma
10. Foreign body aspiration
11. Burns of the head or neck area
12. Anaphylaxis

- Partial obstruction may have only subtle or general manifestations such as diaphoresis, tachycardia, and elevated blood pressure.
- To rule out a tumor, foreign body, or infection, diagnostic procedures, such as a chest x-ray, neck films, laryngoscopic examination, and CT scan, are performed.
- Observe for arterial blood gases (ABG) and symptoms related to low oxygenation or carbon dioxide retention, including restlessness, increasing anxiety, sternal retractions, a "seesawing" chest, abdominal movements, or a feeling of impending doom related to actual air hunger.
- Use pulse oximetry for ongoing monitoring of oxygen saturation to maintain values above 92%. Continually assess for stridor, cyanosis, and changes in level of consciousness.

> ! **NURSING SAFETY PRIORITY: Action Alert**
>
> Assess the oral care needs of the patient with risk factors for thickly crusted secretions daily. Ensure that whoever provides oral care understands the importance and the correct techniques for preventing secretion buildup and airway obstruction.

INTERPROFESSIONAL COLLABORATIVE CARE

- Management depends on the cause of the obstruction.
  1. Prevent airway obstruction from thick, hardened oral and nasopharyngeal secretions with regular oral hygiene and adequate hydration.
  2. For tongue occlusion or excessive secretions, slightly extend the patient's head and neck, insert a nasal or oral airway, then suction to remove secretions.
  3. For a foreign body, perform abdominal thrusts.
  4. For complete obstruction from edema, cancer, or abscesses, anticipate the need for direct visualization of the airway (laryngoscopy) by a provider or placement of an artificial airway, including:
     a. Cricoidectomy
     b. Endotracheal intubation
     c. Tracheotomy

OBSTRUCTIVE SLEEP APNEA

OVERVIEW

- Obstructive sleep apnea is a breathing disruption during sleep that lasts at least 10 seconds and occurs a minimum of five times in an hour.
- The most common cause of sleep apnea is upper airway obstruction by the soft palate or tongue. Factors that contribute to sleep apnea include obesity, a large uvula, a short neck, smoking, enlarged tonsils or adenoids, and oropharyngeal edema.
- The most accurate test for sleep apnea is an overnight sleep study in which the patient is directly observed while wearing a variety of monitoring equipment to evaluate the depth of sleep, type of sleep, respiratory effort, oxygen saturation, and muscle movement.

INTERPROFESSIONAL COLLABORATIVE CARE

- A common method to prevent airway collapse is the use of non-invasive positive-pressure ventilation (NPPV) to hold open the upper airways.
- A change in sleeping position, weight loss, or devices to prevent the tongue or neck anatomy from obstructing the airways may correct mild sleep apnea.

ORGAN TRANSPLANTATION

OVERVIEW

- Organs are transplanted to improve quantity or quality of life when an organ fails or to replace bone marrow associated with immunity dysregulation.
- Common organ transplants in the United States are kidney, pancreas, liver, heart, lung, and intestine. Sometimes double transplants of kidney/pancreas or heart/lung are performed.
- Vascularized composite allografts (VCAs) are now also possible, including face and hand transplantation.
- Transplant centers specialize in the surgical care and ongoing management of organ recipients.
- The patient for potential transplantation has extensive physiologic and psychological assessment and evaluation by primary health care providers and transplant coordinators.
- Generally, the patient has a chronic disabling condition that must be stabilized before transplant, but rapid progressive organ failure may result in organ transplantation.
- Donor organs are obtained primarily from deceased donors (trauma or other conditions) and living-related donors.

- Organs are distributed through a nationwide program—the United Network of Organ Sharing (UNOS). This system distributes donor organs based on regional considerations and patient acuity.
- Candidates with the highest level of acuity receive highest priority.
- Most organ recipients require life-long immune-modulation through drug therapy to avoid rejection of the transplanted organ.

ONCOLOGIC EMERGENCIES

OVERVIEW

- Acute complications of cancer or cancer therapy include sepsis and disseminated intravascular coagulopathy, syndrome of inappropriate antidiuretic hormone, spinal cord compression, hypercalcemia, superior vena cava syndrome, and tumor lysis syndrome.

INTERPROFESSIONAL COLLABORATIVE CARE

- Perform a total assessment each time the patient with cancer is seen to determine the level of cancer treatment side effects and whether an oncologic emergency exists.
  1. Sepsis
     a. *Sepsis*, or *septicemia*, is a condition in which organisms enter the bloodstream (bloodstream infection) and can result in septic shock, a life-threatening condition.
     b. Adults with cancer who have low white blood cell (WBC) counts and impaired immunity from cancer therapy are at risk for infection and sepsis. More information is found in *Shock, Sepsis*.
     c. Teach the patient and family about symptoms of infection and when to seek medical advice.
  2. Disseminated intravascular coagulopathy (DIC) is a problem with CLOTTING process. DIC is triggered by many severe illnesses, including cancer.
     a. Extensive, abnormal CLOTTING occurs throughout the small blood vessels of patients with DIC. This widespread clotting depletes circulating clotting factors and platelets. As this happens, extensive bleeding occurs.
     b. Use bleeding precautions for any patient with thrombocytopenia and impaired clotting.
     c. During the early phase of DIC, anticoagulants (especially heparin) are given to limit clotting and prevent the rapid consumption of circulating clotting factors. When DIC has progressed and hemorrhage is the primary problem, clotting factors are given.

> ## ❗ NURSING SAFETY ALERT: Patient-Centered Care
>
> DIC is a life-threatening problem with a high mortality rate even when proper therapies are instituted. Thus the best management of sepsis and DIC is prevention. Identify patients at greatest risk for sepsis and DIC. Practice strict adherence to aseptic technique during invasive procedures and during contact with nonintact skin and mucous membranes. Teach patients and families the early indicators of infection and when to seek assistance.

3. Syndrome of inappropriate antidiuretic syndrome (SIADH) occurs when tumors (typically lung, head, neck, and hematologic cancers) synthesize antidiuretic hormone (ADH, also called vasopressin) or when brain tumors stimulate ADH production in the pituitary.
   a. Hyponatremia often accompanies this condition.
   b. Restoration of fluid and electrolyte balance.
4. Spinal cord compression occurs either when a tumor directly enters the spinal cord or the spinal column, or when the vertebrae collapse from tumor degradation of the bone.
   a. Back pain, weakness, loss of sensation, urinary retention, and constipation are common presenting symptoms along with loss of or reduced deep tendon reflexes and reduced pinprick and vibratory sensations.
   b. Treatment is begun urgently to preserve function.
      (1) Treatment is often palliative with high-dose corticosteroids given first as an IV bolus to reduce swelling around the spinal cord and relieve symptoms followed by a tapered dose over time.
      (2) High-dose radiation may be used to reduce the size of the tumor in the area and relieve compression.
      (3) Surgery may be performed to remove the tumor and rearrange the bony tissue so less pressure is placed on the spinal cord, or to repair the spine if the spinal column is unstable.
5. Hypercalcemia occurs when tumors secrete parathyroid hormone, causing bone to release calcium, and from bone metastasis that stimulates bone breakdown.
   a. Vigorous IV hydration with normal saline at an infusion rate for 500 mL/hour (if cardiovascular function is normal) is used. Loop diuretics can promote calcium loss in urine.
   b. More information is found in *Hypercalcemia*.

6. Superior vena cava syndrome is cause when tumor growth compresses or clots obstruct blood flow in this large vessel that returns blood to the heart from the head, neck, and upper trunk.

   a. Early signs and symptoms include edema of the face, especially around the eyes (periorbital edema) and neck. Persistent engorgement results in erythema of the upper body, edema in the arms and hands, and dyspnea as the airway becomes obstructed.

   b. High dose radiation therapy can reduce tumor size and fibrinolytic therapy can dissolve thrombi. Following initial treatment, a metal stent placed in the vena cava can preserve perfusion.

7. Tumor lysis syndrome (TLS) occurs when large numbers of tumor cells are destroyed rapidly. The intracellular contents of damaged cancer cells, including potassium and purines (DNA components), are released into the bloodstream faster than the body can eliminate them.

   a. TLS is usually seen in patients with high-grade cancers that are growing quickly and in extensive cancers that are very responsive to treatment.

   b. Hydration prevents and manages TLS by diluting the serum potassium level and increasing the kidney flow rates. These actions prevent the precipitation of uric acid crystals, increase the excretion of potassium, and flush any kidney precipitates.

OSTEOARTHRITIS: MOBILITY CONCEPT EXEMPLAR

OVERVIEW

- Osteoarthritis (OA), sometimes called *osteoarthrosis* or *degenerative joint disease* (DJD), is the most common arthritis, with joint pain and loss of function leading to impaired MOBILITY.

- The disease includes progressive deterioration and loss of cartilage in one or more joints (articular or hyaline cartilage), especially the hips and knees, the vertebral column, and the hands.

  1. Enzymes, such as stromelysin, break down the articular matrix.

  2. As cartilage and the bone beneath the cartilage begin to erode, the joint space narrows and *osteophytes* (bone spurs) form.

  3. As the disease progresses, fissures, calcifications, and ulcerations develop and the cartilage thins.

  4. Cartilage disintegrates and pieces of bone and cartilage "float" in the diseased joint causing *crepitus,* a grating sound caused by the loosened bone and cartilage.

  5. Joints become painful and stiff and the body's normal repair process cannot overcome the rapid process of degeneration.

- Risk factors for OA include aging, genetics, obesity, joint trauma, metabolic and blood disorders, and smoking.

Considerations for Older Adults

As people age or experience joint injury, proteoglycans and water decrease in the joint. The production of synovial fluid, which provides joint lubrication and nutrition, also declines because of the decreased synthesis of hyaluronic acid and less body fluid in the older adult.

INTERPROFESSIONAL COLLABORATIVE CARE

Assessment: Noticing

- Obtain patient information about:
  1. Joint pain and function
     a. The nature and location of joint pain, stiffness, or swelling
     b. What relieves or increases pain or stiffness
     c. Any loss of mobility or difficulty in performing ADLs
  2. Age and gender
  3. Trauma or recurrent stress to joints from occupational and recreational activity or sports
  4. Weight history
  5. Smoking history
  6. Family history of arthritis
- Assess for and document:
  1. Chronic joint pain and stiffness
  2. Aggravating and relieving factors such as activity and rest
  3. Limitations in range of motion (ROM)
  4. Crepitus (a continuous grating sensation felt or heard as the joint goes through its ROM)
  5. Joint enlarged from bony hypertrophy
  6. Joint warmth or inflammation (indicates a secondary synovitis)
  7. Hand changes with Heberden's nodes (at the distal interphalangeal [DIP] joints) and Bouchard's nodes (at the proximal interphalangeal [PIP] joints)
  8. Joint effusions (excess joint fluid), especially in the knee
  9. Atrophy of skeletal muscle from disuse
  10. Compression of spinal nerve roots that produces radiating pain, stiffness, and muscle spasms in one or both extremities with vertebral involvement
  11. Reduced mobility and function
  12. Change in role and self-esteem
  13. Depression, anger, stress
- Imaging assessment may include x-rays or MRI.

Analysis: Interpreting
- The priority collaborative problems for patients with OA include:
  1. Chronic pain due to joint swelling and deterioration
  2. Potential for decreased mobility due to joint pain and muscle atrophy

Planning and Implementation: Responding
MANAGING CHRONIC PAIN

Nonsurgical Management
- Drug therapy
  1. Analgesic drugs
     a. Acetaminophen (Tylenol, Atasol) because OA is not primarily an inflammatory process
  2. Topical drug applications
     a. Lidocaine 5% patches
     b. Topical gel or cream (trolamine salicylate [Aspercreme] or diclofenac [Voltran])

> ### ❗ NURSING SAFETY PRIORITY: Drug Alert
>
> The standard ceiling dose of acetaminophen is 4000 mg each day. However, patients may be at risk for liver damage if they take more than 3000 mg daily, have alcoholism, or have liver disease. *Older adults are particularly at risk because of normal changes of aging, such as slowed excretion of drug metabolites.* Remind patients to read the labels of over-the-counter (OTC) or prescription drugs that could contain acetaminophen before taking them. Teach them that their liver enzyme levels may be monitored while taking this drug.

  3. NSAIDs as oral or topical agents
     a. Cyclooxygenase (COX)-2 inhibiting selective agents like celecoxib (Celebrex)
     b. Nonselective COX inhibiting agents like ibuprofen (Advil)

> ### ❗ NURSING SAFETY PRIORITY: Drug Alert
>
> All of the COX inhibiting drugs are thought to cause cardiovascular disease, such as myocardial infarction, and kidney problems. Older NSAIDs, such as ibuprofen, can cause severe GI side effects, bleeding, and acute kidney failure. Therefore they are prescribed at the lowest effective dose for a short period of time. Teach your patient about adverse effects from NSAIDs and the need to report them to his or her primary health care provider. Examples include having dark, tarry stools; shortness of breath; edema; frequent dyspepsia (indigestion); hematemesis (bloody vomitus); and changes in urinary output.

4. Joint injection (typically no more than three times per year)
   a. Cortisone
   b. Hyaluronic acid (HA): lubricating, synthetic joint fluid that replaces the body's natural HA, which is broken down by inflammation and aging.

- Nonpharmacologic measures
  1. Joint rest, using a joint immobilizer
  2. Balancing rest and activity to promote 8 to 10 hours of night-time sleep and avoid prolonged inactivity
  3. Position joint to avoid excessive flexion of involved joint and maintain normal extension.
     a. Teach the patient to position joints in their functional position to avoid flexion contracture formation.
     b. Supportive shoes or foot insoles can relieve pressure on painful metatarsal joints.
  4. Heat or cold applications (hot showers and baths, hot packs or compresses, moist heating pads)
  5. Weight control or weight loss can lessen stress on weight-bearing joints.
  6. Complementary and alternative therapies (topical capsaicin products, acupuncture, acupressure, tai chi, music therapy) and reduce pain can pain perception
  7. Cognitive-behavioral therapies (imagery, prayer, meditation)

Surgical Management

- Surgery may be indicated to manage the pain of OA and to improve mobility.
  1. *Total joint arthroplasty* (TJA) (surgical creation of a joint), also known as *total joint replacement* (TJR), is the most common type of surgery for OA. Almost any synovial joint of the body can be replaced with a prosthetic system that consists of at least two parts, one for each joint surface.
  2. An *osteotomy (bone resection)* may be performed to correct joint deformity, but this procedure is less common because of the success rate of TJR.

- *Total hip arthroplasty* (THA) with a replacement prosthesis can be done by a variety of procedures, including open hip incision or minimally invasive surgery (MIS). The replacement joint consists of four parts, the acetabular component (this has two parts) and the femoral component (this has two parts).
  1. Provide preoperative care.
     a. Assess the patient's level of understanding about the surgery.
     b. Reinforce the surgeon's explanations about the procedure and postoperative expectations.
     c. Ensure that the surgical site is correct.

d. Explain about transfers, positioning, ambulation, and post-operative exercises.

e. Demonstrate assistive-adaptive devices for ADLs.

f. Teach patients how to perform muscle-strengthening exercises before the procedure.

g. Explain the importance of having any necessary dental procedures done before the surgery to decrease the risk for oral bacterial infection resulting in prosthetic site infection.

h. Assess the patient's risk factors for clotting problems and administering any prescribed anticoagulants.

i. Determine whether the patient needs preoperative supplementation to treat anemia or has made an autologous blood donation or is a candidate for autotransfusion.

j. Administer any prescribed antibiotic therapy before the initial surgical incision is made.

2. Provide postoperative care.

a. Prevent operative joint dislocation by:

(1) Maintaining correct positioning (supine position with the head slightly elevated)

(2) Placing and supporting the affected leg in neutral rotation

(3) For the patient who had a *posterior surgical approach*, place a regular or abduction pillow between the legs to prevent adduction beyond the midline of the body according to agency policy or surgeon preference.

(4) Following agency policy or surgeon preference for postoperative turning

(5) Observing for signs of possible hip dislocation (increased hip pain, shortening of the affected leg, and leg rotation)

❗ NURSING SAFETY PRIORITY: Critical Rescue

If manifestations of hip dislocation occur, keep the patient in bed and notify the surgeon immediately.

b. Prevent thromboembolic complications by:

(1) Administering prescribed anticoagulants, such as subcutaneous heparin or low–molecular-weight heparin

(2) Assessing for manifestations of venous thromboembolism (VTE) (leg swelling, pain)

(3) Teaching leg exercises (plantar flexion and dorsiflexion, circles of the feet, gluteal and quadriceps muscle setting, straight-leg raises)

(4) Applying prescribed antiembolic stockings or devices

(5) Collaborating with the PT to promote early ambulation

   c. Prevent infection and detect infection early by:
     (1) Keeping surgical incision clean and covered until the edges of the incision are sealed
     (2) Observing the incision and patient for signs of infection such as discolored or odorous drainage and signs of poor healing at the incision and the presence of fever or elevated WBCs.

! NURSING SAFETY PRIORITY: Critical Rescue

An older patient may not have a fever with infection but instead may experience an altered mental state. Consider infection in any older patient with new-onset confusion or inability to rouse.

   d. Prevent neurovascular (NV) complications by:
     (1) Checking and documenting color, temperature, distal pulses, capillary refill, movement, and sensation
     (2) Comparing these parameters with those of the nonoperative leg
     (3) Reporting any changes to the surgeon

! NURSING SAFETY PRIORITY: Critical Rescue

Check and document color, temperature, distal pulses, capillary refill, movement, and sensation. Remember to compare the operative leg with the nonoperative leg. These assessments are performed at the same time the vital signs are checked. Report any changes in neurovascular assessment to the surgeon, and carefully monitor for changes. Early detection of changes in neurovascular status can prevent permanent tissue damage.

   e. Manage postoperative acute pain by:
     (1) Assessing the patient's pain level
     (2) Ensuring proper use of pain control devices such as epidural analgesia, intraspinal analgesia, patient-controlled analgesia (PCA), and IV opioid analgesia
     (3) Administering prescribed analgesics as needed
   f. Progress activity by assisting the patient with getting out of bed by:
     (1) Standing on the same side of the bed as the affected leg
     (2) Teaching the patient to stand on the unaffected leg and pivot to the chair
     (3) Assisting the patient to a sitting position

(4) Ensuring that the patient does not flex the hips beyond 90 degrees

(5) Preventing hyperflexion of the replaced joint with the use of raised toilet seats, straight-back chairs, and reclining wheelchairs

3. Weight bearing on the affected leg depends on the surgeon, type of prosthesis, and surgical procedure.

4. Work with the PT to teach the patient how to follow weight-bearing restrictions and progress to full weight-bearing (FWB) status.

5. The OT may recommend assistive-adaptive devices to help with ADLs, especially for patients having traditional surgery.

6. For patients who have traditional surgery, the length of stay in the acute care hospital is typically 3 days; those who have MIS procedures may be discharged on the second postoperative day or, in a few cases, on the day of surgery.

7. The interdisciplinary team provides written instructions for posthospital care and reviews them with patients and their family members.

8. Complete recovery may take 6 weeks or more.

- *Total knee arthroplasty* (TKA) can be performed by traditional open surgery or by MIS procedures for some patients.

1. Provide preoperative care.
   a. Care as described for THA
   b. Explanation and demonstration of a continuous passive motion (CPM) machine (if prescribed)

2. Provide postoperative care.
   a. Care to prevent complications as described for THA
   b. Implement the CPM machine as prescribed for ROM and cycles per minute.
   c. Apply ice packs or a Hot/Ice device to decrease surgical site swelling.
   d. Ensure safe use of peripheral nerve blockade (PNB) for pain control.
      (1) If the nerve block is continuous, perform NV assessments every 2 to 4 hours or according to hospital protocol.
      (2) Assess that the patient can plantar flex and dorsiflex the affected foot but does not feel pain in the extremity.
      (3) Check for movement, sensation, warmth, color, pulses, and capillary refill.
      (4) Monitor for symptoms of systemic infusion of the nerve-blocking drug (a metallic taste, tinnitus, restlessness, nervousness, slurred speech, bradycardia, hypotension, or decreased respirations).
   e. Maintain the knee in a neutral position, not rotated internally or externally.

    f. Ensure that the surgical knee is not hyperextended.

    g. Monitor NV status frequently to check for compromise to the distal operative leg every time vital signs are taken.

- *Total shoulder arthroplasty* (TSA) can be performed either as a TJR or as a hemiarthroplasty (replacement of part of the joint, typically the humeral component). These surgeries are most commonly performed using traditional open incisions, but minimally invasive shoulder arthroplasty can be used instead for some patients.

    1. Preoperative care and postoperative care are similar to those for other joint replacement surgeries.

    2. A sling is applied to immobilize the joint and prevent dislocation until therapy begins.

    3. The hospital stay for TSA is usually 1 to 2 days, until pain is controlled.

    4. Rehabilitation with an OT usually takes 2 to 3 months.

- Other joints that can be replaced include:

    1. Elbow (total elbow arthroplasty [TEA])

    2. Hand or foot joints (phalangeal joint, metacarpal, or metatarsal arthroplasty)

    3. Any bone of the wrist

    4. Ankle (total ankle arthroplasty [TAA]), which has more postoperative complications than other arthroplasties

IMPROVING MOBILITY

- Reinforce the techniques and principles of exercise, ambulation, and promotion of ADLs.
- Collaborate with the physical therapist to implement regular exercise.
- Assist the patient in considering recreational activities such as swimming to maintain muscle strength and joint mobility.
- Collaborate with occupational therapist (OT) to provide suggestions and devices for assistance for ADLs.
- Use active rather than active-assist or passive exercise independent activity.

Care Coordination and Transition Management

- Teach patients with arthritis what exercises to do, joint protection techniques, and energy conservation guidelines to avoid impaired mobility.
- Teach patients who have OA or are prone to the disease to lose weight (if obese), avoid trauma, and limit strenuous weight-bearing activities.
- Collaborate with the discharge planner and the primary health care provider to determine the best placement for the patient with OA at discharge, particularly after joint replacement surgery.

- Implement interventions for patients having total TJA to prevent venous thromboembolic complications (e.g., anticoagulants, exercises, sequential compression devices); observe the patient for bleeding when he or she is taking anticoagulants.
- Provide health teaching.

O

   1. Explain the general principles of joint protection.
      a. Use large joints instead of small ones; for example, place a purse strap over the shoulder instead of grasping the purse with a hand.
      b. Turn doorknobs toward the thumb (rather than toward the little finger) to avoid twisting the arm and promoting ulnar deviation.
      c. Use two hands instead of one to hold objects.
      d. Sit in a chair that has a high, straight back.
      e. When getting out of bed, do not push off with the fingers; use the entire palm of both hands.
      f. Do not bend at the waist; instead, bend the knees while keeping the back straight.
      g. Use long-handled devices, such as a hairbrush with an extended handle.
      h. Use assistive-adaptive devices, such as Velcro closures and built-up utensil handles, to protect joints.
      i. Do not use pillows in bed, except a small one under the head.
      j. Avoid twisting or wringing the hands.
   2. Explain the drug protocol, desired and potential side effects, and adverse or toxic effects.
   3. Emphasize the importance of reducing weight and eating a well-balanced diet to promote tissue healing.
   4. Refer the patient to the Arthritis Foundation for up-to-date information about new treatments and helpful complementary and alternative practices.
   5. Provide written instructions about the required care, regardless of whether the patient goes home or to another inpatient facility.
   6. Refer the patient to the nutritionist, counselor, home health nurse, rehabilitation therapist, financial counselor, and local and state support groups as needed.

OSTEOMALACIA

OVERVIEW

- Osteomalacia is a softening of the bone tissue related to vitamin D deficiency, causing inadequate deposits of calcium and phosphorus in the bone matrix.
- Vitamin D deficiency can occur as a result of inadequate exposure to sunlight, poor dietary intake, abnormal metabolism, chronic use of many drugs, or the presence of chronic disease.
- Older adults are most at risk for osteomalacia.

INTERPROFESSIONAL COLLABORATIVE CARE

- Obtain patient information about:
  1. Age
  2. Exposure to sunlight and skin pigmentation (darker skin reduces vitamin D activation)
  3. Dietary habits
  4. Current prescribed and OTC drug use
     a. Chronic GI inflammatory disease or gastric or intestinal bypass surgery
  5. Renal or liver dysfunction
  6. History of bone fracture
- Assess for and document:
  1. Muscle weakness (causing a waddling and unsteady gait) and cramping
  2. Bone pain (aggravated by activity and worse at night)
  3. Bone tenderness to palpation (especially tibia or rib cage)
  4. Skeletal misalignment (long-bone bowing or spinal deformity)
  5. Hypocalcemia or hyperphosphatemia
  6. Presence of radiolucent bands (Looser's lines or zones) on x-ray
- The major intervention for osteomalacia is vitamin D.
  1. Teach patients to take the amount of vitamin D supplementation prescribed by their primary health care provider.
  2. Teach patients to choose foods that are fortified with vitamin D (milk and dairy products) or are rich in vitamin D (eggs, swordfish, chicken, and liver), in addition to enriched cereals and bread products.

OSTEOMYELITIS

OVERVIEW

- Osteomyelitis is an infection in bone caused by bacteria, viruses, or fungi.
- Osteomyelitis is difficult to treat and can result in chronic recurrence of infection, loss of function and mobility, amputation, and even death.
- The pathologic processes that occur in infected bone tissue include inflammation, blood vessel thromboses, and necrosis.
- Categories of osteomyelitis include:
  1. *Exogenous osteomyelitis,* in which infectious organisms enter from outside the body, as in an open fracture
  2. *Endogenous osteomyelitis,* also called *hematogenous osteomyelitis,* in which organisms are carried by the bloodstream from other areas of infection in the body
  3. *Contiguous osteomyelitis,* in which bone infection results from skin infection of adjacent tissues as with surgical site infection or soft tissue infections from penetrating trauma

- Common causes include bacteremia, pre-existing conditions that interfere with immune health or wound healing such as diabetes, trauma, long-term IV therapy, hemodialysis, *Salmonella* infection of the GI tract, sickle cell disease, poor dental hygiene, periodontal infection, and infections with multi-drug resistant organisms (MDROs) like MRSA.

Considerations for Older Adults

The most common cause of contiguous spread in older adults is slow healing foot ulcers in patients with diabetes or peripheral vascular disease.

INTERPROFESSIONAL COLLABORATIVE CARE
Assessment: Noticing
- Assess for and document:
  1. Bone pain described as a constant, localized, pulsating sensation that worsens with movement
  2. Fever, usually greater than 101°F (38°C) during acute presentation
  3. Swelling, tenderness, erythema, and heat around the site of infection
  4. Ulcerations on the feet or hands
  5. Sinus tract formation and drainage with chronic infection
  6. Elevated WBC, neutrophils, and erythrocyte sedimentation rate (ESR)
  7. Positive blood or wound cultures

Interventions: Responding
NONSURGICAL MANAGEMENT
- Nonsurgical interventions include:
  1. Early, acute diagnosis and appropriate management to avoid the conversion of acute osteomyelitis to chronic status
  2. Administering IV antibiotic therapy for several weeks, followed by oral antibiotic therapy for weeks or months

❗ NURSING SAFETY PRIORITY: Drug Alert

Even when symptoms of osteomyelitis appear to be improved, teach the patient and family that the full course of IV and/or oral antimicrobials must be completed to ensure that the infection is resolved.

  3. Irrigating the wound either continuously or intermittently, with one or more antibiotic solutions
  4. Packing the wound with beads made of bone cement that have been impregnated with an antibiotic

5. Administering drugs for pain control
6. Covering the wound to prevent infection spread
7. Administering hyperbaric oxygen (HBO) therapy for patients with chronic, unremitting osteomyelitis to improve oxygenation via perfusion and promote healing

SURGICAL MANAGEMENT

- Surgery is reserved for patients with chronic osteomyelitis and may include revascularization and:
    1. Sequestrectomy with excision of dead and infected bone to allow revascularization of tissue
    2. Application of bone grafts to repair bone defects
    3. Reconstruction with microvascular bone transfers if excision is extensive
    4. Closure of the defect with muscle flaps and skin grafts
    5. Amputation of the affected limb if the infection cannot be controlled or revascularization is not successful
- Provide postoperative care and:
    1. Perform frequent NV assessments of:
        a. Pain
        b. Movement
        c. Sensation
        d. Warmth
        e. Temperature
        f. Distal pulses
            Capillary refill

 NURSING SAFETY PRIORITY: Critical Rescue

Immediately report to the surgeon any of these signs of neurovascular compromise: pain that cannot be controlled, paresis or paralysis (weakness or inability to move), paresthesias (abnormal tingling sensation), pallor, and pulselessness.

2. Elevate the affected extremity to increase venous return and control swelling.

OSTEOPOROSIS: CELLULAR REGULATION EXEMPLAR

OVERVIEW

- Osteoporosis is a chronic disease of CELLULAR REGULATION that results in loss of trabecular (spongy) and cortical (compact) bone.
- Osteoporosis occurs when the bone remodeling process (a type of cellular regulation) changes such that osteoclastic (bone resorption) activity is greater than osteoblastic (bone building) activity.

- Altered bone remodeling results in decreased bone mineral density and a thin fragile bone tissue that is at risk for fracture, most often at the spine, hip and wrist.
- Osteoporosis can be classified as generalized or regional.
  1. Generalized osteoporosis involves many structures in the skeleton and is further divided into two categories.
     a. *Primary osteoporosis,* which is more common and occurs in postmenopausal women and in men in their sixth or seventh decade of life
     b. *Secondary osteoporosis,* which results from other medical conditions, such as hyperparathyroidism, long-term drug therapy (such as with corticosteroids), or prolonged immobility
  2. Regional osteoporosis occurs when a limb is immobilized related to a fracture, injury, or paralysis for longer than 8 to 12 weeks.
- Risk factors for primary osteoporosis are caused by a combination of genetic, lifestyle, and environmental factors.
  1. Nonmodifiable factors include older age, parental history of osteoporosis, history of fracture after age 50, and genetics that determine bone turnover or remodeling.
  2. Modifiable factors include sedentary lifestyle; chronic low intake of protein, calcium, and vitamin D, or malabsorption syndromes; high phosphorus intake (i.e., 40 ounces of carbonated beverages daily over several years); low body weight or thin build; alcohol and tobacco use; and long-term use of certain drugs, especially corticosteroids.

Genetic/Genomic Considerations Patient-Centered Care

The genetic and immune factors that cause osteoporosis are very complex. Strong evidence demonstrates that genetics is a significant factor, with a heritability of 50% to 90% (Chang, et al., 2010). Many genetic changes have been identified as possible causative factors, but there is no agreement about which ones are most important or constant in all patients. For example, changes in the vitamin D_3 receptor *(VDR)* gene and calcitonin receptor *(CTR)* gene have been found in some patients with the disease. Receptors are essential for the uptake and use of these substances by the cells.

Gender Health Considerations

Primary osteoporosis most often occurs in women after menopause as a result of decreased estrogen levels. Women lose about 2% of their bone mass every year in the first 5 years after natural or surgical (ovary removal) menopause.

Men also develop osteoporosis after the age of 50 because their testosterone levels decrease. Testosterone is the major sex hormone that builds bone tissue. Men are often underdiagnosed, even when they become older adults.

INTERPROFESSIONAL COLLABORATIVE CARE
Assessment: Noticing
- Obtain patient information about:
  1. Age, gender, race, body build, weight
  2. Loss of height (indicating loss of vertebrae integrity)
  3. Back pain after bending, lifting, or stooping (worse with activity, relieved with rest)
  4. Mobility or function
  5. Current drugs
- Assess for and document:
  1. Features of the spinal column, particularly presence of classic "dowager's hump," or kyphosis of the dorsal spine
  2. Location of all painful areas and signs of fracture such as swelling and misalignment. Back pain accompanied by tenderness and voluntary restriction of spinal movement suggests one or more compression vertebral fractures—the most common type of osteoporotic or fragility fracture.
  3. Constipation, abdominal distention from immobility related to fracture
  4. Respiratory compromise
  5. Body image disturbance
  6. Changes in quality of life and sexuality
- Diagnostic tests may include:
  1. Levels of serum calcium, vitamin D, phosphorus, and protein
  2. Imaging to determine bone density:
     a. Dual-energy x-ray absorptiometry (DXA or DEXA)
     b. CT-based absorptiometry (qualitative computed tomography [qCT])
     c. MRI or magnetic resonance spectroscopy (MRS)

Analysis: Interpreting
- The priority problem for patients with osteoporosis or osteopenia is the potential for fractures due to weak, porous bone tissue.

Planning and Implementation: Responding
NONSURGICAL MANAGEMENT
Nutrition Therapy
- Coordinate health teaching and nutrition planning with the dietitian.
  1. Teach patients to eat a diet that includes:
     a. Calcium and vitamin D; if lactose intolerant suggest soy and mineral-fortified foods

   b. Low-fat protein sources
   c. Moderation in alcohol intake (fewer than three drinks daily)
   d. Low soda intake; phosphorus in soda reduces calcium absorption

Lifestyle Changes

- Assist with a plan to provide regular, weight-bearing exercise.
   1. Coordinate health teaching with the PT for exercises to improve posture, support, and pulmonary capacity; strengthen core and extremity muscles; and improve ROM.
      a. Strengthen core muscles of abdomen and back to reduce risk for vertebral fractures.
      b. Use resistive and ROM exercise in extremities to reduce fracture risks.
      c. Walk for 30 minutes three to five times a week.
   2. Teach patients to avoid high-impact recreational activities.
- Teach about other lifestyle changes including:
   1. Smoking cessation and avoiding secondhand tobacco smoke
   2. Preventing falls

Drug Therapy

- Administer drug therapy for prevention and management.
   1. Bisphosphonates to slow bone reabsorption
      a. Alendronate (Fosamax) (oral drug)
      b. Ibandronate (Boniva) (oral and IV)
      c. Risedronate (Actonel) (oral drug)
      d. Zoledronic acid (Reclast) (IV; given once annually)
      e. Pamidronate (Aredia) (IV; given once annually)
   2. Estrogen agonist/antagonist: raloxifene (Evista)
   3. Calcium and vitamin D supplementation; these supplements alone are not sufficient to prevent or treat osteoporosis but are important to bone health
   4. Denosumab (Prolia), a monoclonal antibody against a protein (RANKL) that prevents osteoclast activation
   5. *Teriparatide* (Forteo), an anabolic (bone building) drug, is given subcutaneously and can only be used up to 2 years
   6. Salmon *calcitonin* (Miacalcin or Fortical), a hormone used for postmenopausal women when first-line drug therapy is not appropriate

---

❗ NURSING SAFETY PRIORITY: Drug Alert

Osteonecrosis of the jaw is a rare but serious complication of bisphosphonate therapy, especially long-acting preparations. Teach patients to have an oral assessment and preventive dentistry before beginning any bisphosphonate therapy. To promote safety, instruct them to inform any dentist who is planning invasive treatment, such as a tooth extraction or implant, that they are taking a bisphosphonate.

Care Coordination and Transition Management

- Patients with osteoporosis are typically managed in the community and at home.
- Collaborate with members of the interprofessional health team to ensure that the patient's home is safe and hazard-free to help prevent falling.
- Teach patients about diet and lifestyle interventions to slow bone loss.
- Teach patients about drugs used to manage osteoporosis and about the need for ongoing and follow-up with their provider.

OTITIS MEDIA: SENSORY PERCEPTION CONCEPT EXEMPLAR

OVERVIEW

- Otitis media is an inflammation or infection of the middle ear mucosa that can temporarily or permanently impair auditory SENSORY PERCEPTION.
- The inflammation leads to swelling and irritation of the small bones (ossicles) within the middle ear, a purulent exudate, pain, and temporary hearing loss.
- If otitis media progresses or recurs without treatment, permanent conductive hearing loss may occur.
- Otitis media can be acute, chronic, or serous.

INTERPROFESSIONAL COLLABORATIVE CARE

Assessment: Noticing

- Assess for manifestations of acute or chronic otitis media.
  1. Ear pain with or without movement of the external ear (which is relieved when the eardrum ruptures)
  2. Sensation of fullness in the ear
  3. Reduced or distorted hearing
  4. Tinnitus
  5. Headaches
  6. Dizziness or vertigo
  7. Systemic symptoms of fever, malaise, or nausea and vomiting
  8. Otoscopic examination findings
     a. Dilated and red eardrum blood vessels
     b. Red, thickened, or bulging eardrum
     c. Decreased eardrum mobility
     d. Eardrum perforation with pus present in the canal

Analysis: Interpreting

- The priority collaborative problems for patients with otitis media include:
  1. Infection due to otitis media
  2. Pain due to ear infection

Planning and Implementation: Responding
ELIMINATING INFECTION WHILE REDUCING PAIN
Nonsurgical Management
- Evaluate the frequency, duration, and contributing factors of middle ear infection.
  1. Administer oral or topical antibiotics if a bacterial infection is suspected.
  2. Reduce exposure to smoke (cigarettes, environment) and secondhand smoke.
  3. Administer analgesics for mild to moderate pain such as aspirin, ibuprofen (Advil), and acetaminophen (Tylenol, Abenol).
  4. Apply low heat to reduce pain.
  5. Administer antihistamine or decongestant to decrease fluid in middle ear.

Surgical Management
- Surgical management with a myringotomy (surgical opening of the eardrum), often combined with tube insertion (to provide ongoing drainage), may be needed to drain fluid.
  1. Standard preoperative care.
  2. Postoperative care
     a. Teach the patient to keep the external ear and canal free of other substances.
     b. Instruct the patient to avoid washing the hair or showering for 48 hours.

Care Coordination and Transition Management
1. Avoid prolonged immersion in water (swimming, bath tub) if myringotomy is performed.
2. Teach family members to avoid smoking around individuals with recurrent ear infections.
3. Teach ear drop administration.

PAIN: COMFORT CONCEPT EXEMPLAR

OVERVIEW
- Pain is a universal, complex, and personal experience that disrupts comfort.
- Self-report is always the most reliable indication of pain.
  1. *Acute pain* results from trauma, surgery, or tissue injury. It is usually temporary, has a sudden onset, and is localized.

2. *Chronic* or *persistent pain* persists for longer than 3 months, is often poorly localized, and is hard to describe. It is often associated with depression, interference with personal relationships, and inability to maintain activities of daily living (ADLs).
   a. Chronic cancer pain is associated with:
      (1) The cancer itself
      (2) Nerve compression
      (3) Invasion of tissue
      (4) Bone metastasis
      (5) Cancer treatments (e.g., chemotherapy, radiation therapy)
3. Chronic noncancer pain can be associated with nerve damage or chronic conditions such as arthritis or spinal stenosis.

- Pain is also categorized as:
  1. Nociceptive or visceral-somatic, with normal processing of pain signals. This type of pain can be acute or chronic.
  2. Neuropathic, originally the result of nerve injury or the abnormal processing of pain signals. Processing abnormalities may be generated either in the peripheral or central nervous systems. Neuropathic pain is usually chronic.

! NURSING SAFETY PRIORITY: Action Alert

Although many characteristics of chronic pain are similar in different patients, be aware that each situation is unique and requires an individualized plan of care.

- The attitudes of health care professionals toward pain influence the way they perceive and interact with patients in pain.
- Factors such as age, gender, sociocultural background, and genetics influence the patient's ability to process and react to pain.

Considerations for Older Adults

Pain is treated inadequately in almost all health care settings. Populations at the highest risk in medical-surgical nursing are older adults, patients with substance use disorder, and those whose primary language differs from that of the health care professional. Older adults in nursing homes are at especially high risk because many residents are unable to report their pain. In addition, there often is a lack of staff members who have been educated to manage pain in the older-adult population.

Gender Considerations

Certain chronic painful conditions are more common in women; other conditions are more common in men. Women have more migraine headaches, tension headaches, rheumatoid arthritis and osteoarthritis, fibromyalgia, and multiple sclerosis. Men are more likely to experience pain with diagnoses of cluster headaches, back pain, gout, peripheral vascular disease, and postherpetic neuralgia.

INTERPROFESSIONAL COLLABORATIVE CARE

Assessment: Noticing

* Assess and record pain history information:
    1. Pain experience, including precipitating and relieving factors, localization, character and quality of pain, and duration of pain
    2. Beliefs about the cause of the pain and what should be done about it (patient's expectations)
* Assess for signs and symptoms of pain:
    1. Patient's statement or description
        a. All accepted guidelines identify the patient's self-report as the gold standard for assessing the existence and intensity of pain (Pasero & McCaffery, 2011).
    2. Tachycardia and increased or decreased blood pressure (HR and blood pressure less likely to be altered with chronic pain)
    3. Altered movement, such as splinting or listlessness
    4. Functional and cognitive status or situational impairment
    5. Location of pain
        a. Localized (pain is confined to the site of origin)
        b. Projected (pain occurs along a specific nerve or nerves)
        c. Radiating (diffuse pain occurs around the site of origin that is not well localized)
        d. Referred (pain is perceived in an area distant from the site of painful stimuli)
    6. Intensity and quality of pain
        a. Pain intensity (e.g., number rating scale of 0 to 10, with 10 being the worst possible pain) for verbal patients and *Checklist of Nonverbal Pain Indicators* or *Pain Assessment in Advanced Dementia Scale* for nonverbal or cognitively impaired patients
        b. Verbal descriptions to convey the quality of pain such as stabbing, burning, crushing

🌐 Cultural and Spiritual Considerations

Patient-Centered Care

If the chronic pain is associated with a progressive disease such as cancer, rheumatoid arthritis, or peripheral vascular disease, the patient may have worries and concerns about the consequences of the illness. People with cancer-related pain may fear death or body mutilation. Some may think they are being punished for some wrongdoing in life. Others may attach a religious or spiritual significance to lingering pain. Ask open-ended questions (e.g., "Tell me how your pain has affected your job or your role as a mother.") to allow the patient to describe personal attitudes about pain and its influence on life. This opportunity can help someone whose life has been changed by pain. However, some patients choose not to share their private information or fears. As a patient-centered nurse, always respect patients' preferences and values.

Interventions: Responding
NONSURGICAL MANAGEMENT

- Multimodal therapy. Best practices in pain management suggest a combination of interventions including pharmacologic and non-pharmacologic strategies.
  1. Drug therapy
     Selection of drugs is based on level of pain, drug effects and adverse effects, and knowledge of the advantages and disadvantages for each route of administration.
     a. The nonopioid analgesics are the first-line therapy for mild to moderate pain. They are typically available without a prescription and administered orally, rectally, or topically. Examples of nonopioid analgesics:
        (1) Acetaminophen (Tylenol)

❗ NURSING SAFETY PRIORITY: Drug Alert

Teach patients to take no more the 4000 mg daily (2400 mg for older adults) of acetaminophen and for no longer than 4 weeks without informing their primary health care provider about the amount of acetaminophen they take each day. Remind them to have liver and renal function laboratory tests done on a regular basis as prescribed to monitor for early indicators of adverse drug events.

        (2) Nonsteroidal anti-inflammatory drugs (NSAIDs) such as:
            i. Ibuprofen (Motrin, Novo-Profen)
            ii. Naproxen (Naprosyn, Nu-Naprox)
            iii. Celecoxib (Celebrex)

! NURSING SAFETY PRIORITY: Drug Alert

NSAIDs can cause gastrointestinal (GI) disturbances and decrease platelet aggregation (clotting), which can result in bleeding. Therefore observe the patient for gastric discomfort or vomiting and for bleeding or bruising. Tell the patient and family to stop taking these drugs and report these effects to the primary health care provider immediately if any of these problems occur. Celecoxib has no effect on bleeding time and produces less GI toxicity compared with other NSAIDs.

P

   b. Opioid analgesics are used to manage moderate-to-severe pain. They can be administered by any route. Examples include:
      (1) Hydromorphone (Dilaudid)
      (2) Morphine
      (3) Fentanyl (Sublimaze)
      (4) Hydrocodone
      (5) Oxycodone
      (6) Methadone (Dolophine)
      (7) Codeine

! NURSING SAFETY PRIORITY: Critical Rescue

Watch the rise and fall of the patient's chest to determine depth and regularity of respirations in addition to counting the respiratory rate for 60 seconds. For accuracy, respiratory assessment is done before arousing the sleeping patient. *If a patient is difficult to arouse, always stop the opioid, stay with the patient, continue vigorous attempts to arouse, and call for help!* Listening to the sound of the patient's respiration is critical as well—*snoring indicates airway obstruction and must be attended to promptly* with repositioning, including placing the patient in a sitting position. Depending on severity, collaborate with the respiratory therapist for consultation and further evaluation.

- Collaborate with the provider and patient to provide safe, effective care when opioids are used.
   1. Monitor and prevent complications from side effects. Side effects, in order of seriousness, can include respiratory depression, sedation, constipation, nausea and vomiting, urinary retention, and pruritus (itching).
      a. Monitor RR and depth, especially when the patient is sleeping.

❗ NURSING SAFETY PRIORITY: Drug Alert

Respiratory depression is managed with an opioid antagonist, naloxone (Narcan). It is a fast-acting drug given IV to reverse the opioid effect. The respiratory-depressant effect of the opioid is usually longer acting than naloxone. Continue to monitor the patient after giving the drug because respiratory depression can recur, necessitating additional naloxone.

   b. Sedation occurs before opioid-induced respiratory depression, so nurse-monitored sedation levels are recommended by use of a sedation scale for opioid-naive (not currently on an opioid) patients or those receiving opioids intravenously (IV) or epidurally. The key to assessing sedation is determining how easily the patient is aroused.
   c. Prevent constipation with concurrent administration of a stool softener or bowel stimulant.
   d. When opioids are prescribed for longer than 3 to 7 days, consider risk for dependence, tolerance, or addiction.
      (1) *Addiction* is a primary, chronic neurobiologic disease with one or more of the following: impaired control over drug use, compulsive use, continued use despite harm, and craving.
      (2) *Tolerance* is a state of adaptation in which exposure to a drug induces changes that result in a decrease in one or more of the drug's effects over time.
      (3) *Physical dependence* is adaptation manifested by a drug class-specific withdrawal syndrome that can be produced by abrupt cessation, rapid dose reduction, decreasing blood level of the drug, or administration of an antagonist. It occurs in everyone who takes opioids over a period of time.
      (4) *Withdrawal* or *abstinence syndrome* results when a patient who is physically dependent on opioids abruptly ceases using them.
• Collaborate with the provider to deliver safe, effective care when patient-controlled analgesia (PCA) is used to deliver an opioid or xylocaine.
   1. PCA delivers a set amount of drug through IV access, allowing the patient to control the dosage of opioid received, improving pain relief and increasing patient satisfaction.
   2. Morphine, fentanyl, and hydromorphone are the most commonly used drugs for PCA.
   3. Drug security is achieved through a locked syringe pump system or locked drug reservoir system.

4. When the patient presses the button or pendant (on ambulatory pumps), the appropriate bolus or demand dose is delivered. A basal rate may also be continuously administered.

5. Teach patients how to use PCA and to report side effects, such as dizziness, nausea and vomiting, and inability to void.

6. Monitor the patient's vital signs, particularly respirations, and check his or her sedation level at least every 2 hours initially or per agency protocol.

7. Do not allow a proxy or staff to administer a bolus or push the button. If the patient is unable to use the PCA device effectively, discontinue PCA and use another mode of drug delivery.

- Collaborate with the provider to provide safe, effective care when epidural or intraspinal analgesia are used.

1. Epidural analgesia is the instillation of a pain-blocking agent, usually an opioid analgesic alone or in combination with a local anesthetic, such as bupivacaine, into the epidural space.

2. Epidural analgesia is most commonly used for the management of acute pain.

3. Morphine (preservative-free), hydromorphone (Dilaudid), and fentanyl (Sublimaze) are the most commonly used opioids for epidural administration.

4. Pruritus (itching), nausea, and vomiting are common side effects of epidural opioids.

5. A temporary, externalized epidural catheter is used for acute pain control. This device is not sutured to the skin and is easily dislodged. Be sure to tape the catheter in two places to anchor it properly.

6. Complications that occur with epidural analgesia are directly related to catheter placement, catheter maintenance, and the type of analgesic.

7. Infection is rare but can occur as a result of failure to maintain aseptic technique during catheter placement, through direct drug instillation, during infusion of solution and tubing changes, and from a failure to maintain aseptic conditions for indwelling catheters at the site of insertion or at the site of tube junctions.

8. There is a risk for respiratory depression resulting from high plasma or cerebrospinal fluid concentrations of the instilled drug. Monitor the patient's respirations and sedation level at frequent intervals during and after the administration of epidural opioids and immediately report any concerns to the health care provider.

9. Urinary retention is a common problem associated with epidural analgesia and is more likely to occur in men than in women.

P

10. Risk for falls is increased when an epidural local anesthetic is used in combination with an opioid. Assist patients who get out of bed for the first time to determine the degree of leg weakness caused by the epidural analgesic.

- Adjuvant analgesic drugs may be used to relieve pain alone or in combination with other analgesics by potentiating or enhancing the effectiveness of the analgesic.
  1. Antiepileptic drugs (AEDs or anticonvulsants)
     a. Gabapentin (Neurontin)
     b. Pregabalin (Lyrica)
  2. Tricyclic antidepressants
     a. Desipramine (Norpramin)
     b. Nortriptyline (Pamelor)
  3. Other antidepressants
     a. Duloxetine (Cymbalta)
     b. Venlafaxine (Effexor)
  4. Local anesthetics may be given orally (systemic effects), topically, and via epidural routes. Examples include:
     a. Liposomal bupivacaine (Exparel)
     b. Xylocaine
     c. Lidocaine patch (Lidoderm patch)
     d. Lidocaine and prilocaine (EMLA cream)
  5. Local short-acting gels and creams for cryotherapy. Examples include:
     a. Biofreeze
     b. Bengay
- Nonpharmacologic interventions include:
  1. Physical measures
     a. Cutaneous (skin) stimulation strategies
        (1) Application of heat, cold, and pressure
        (2) Therapeutic touch
        (3) Massage
        (4) Vibration
     b. Physical and occupational therapy
        (1) Exercise to strengthen muscles or to provide alternative approaches to avoid painful maneuvers
        (2) Massage or manipulation
        (3) Splinting of joints
     c. Transcutaneous electrical nerve stimulation (TENS)
  2. Cognitive-behavioral strategies
     a. Distraction
     b. Imagery
     c. Relaxation (may be combined with music therapy)
     d. Hypnosis
     e. Mindfulness

3. Complementary and integrative therapies
   a. Music therapy
   b. Acupuncture and acupressure
   c. Prayer and meditation
   d. Massage
   e. Heat or cold applications
4. Invasive techniques for chronic pain
   a. Spinal cord stimulation
5. Referral to a pain clinic or to a palliative care specialist when pain is complex, results in prolonged (more than 3 months) use of opioids, or the patient experience of severe pain is not alleviated with common approaches.

! NURSING SAFETY PRIORITY: Drug Alert

Deceitful administration of a placebo violates informed consent law and jeopardizes the nurse-patient therapeutic relationship. Never administer a placebo to a patient. Promptly contact your nursing supervisor if you are given an order to do so.

Care Coordination and Transition Management

- Pain can be managed in any setting, including the home. Some patients require parenteral pain medications at home, therefore, provide health teaching to ensure continuity of care.
- Refer patients whose pain is difficult to manage to pain specialists and/or pain centers.
- Communicate and coordinate the plan of care for pain management as the patient transfers between health care agencies and home.
- Make appropriate referrals for physical therapy, a clinical nurse specialist in pain management, a social worker, and hospice or palliative care.
- Plan a home care nurse referral for patients who will require assistance or supervision with the patient's pain relief regimen at home.
- Home agency practices and professional support at home are required if patients leave the hospital with infusion therapy for pain management.
- Ensure that the patient, especially one who is on opioids, has enough pain medication to last at least until the first follow-up visit.
- Teach the patient and family about analgesic regimens, including any technical skills needed to administer or deliver the analgesic, the purpose and action of various drugs, their side effects or adverse reactions, and the importance of dosage intervals.
- If the patient is on a flexible analgesic schedule, teach the patient and family how to safely increase and decrease the drug within the prescribed dosing guidelines.

PAIN, BACK

OVERVIEW

- The areas of the back most commonly affected by back pain are the cervical and lumbar vertebrae.
- *Acute low back pain* (LBP) occurs along the lumbosacral area of the vertebral column.
  1. Acute pain is caused by muscle strain or spasm, ligament sprain, disk degeneration, or herniation of the center of the disk (herniated nucleus pulposus).
  2. Acute back pain usually results from injury or trauma such as during a fall, vehicular crash, or lifting a heavy object.
- *Chronic* LBP persists for 3 or more months.
  1. Acute or repeated back injury can contribute to spinal stenosis, a narrowing of the spinal canal, damage to nerve root canals, or intervertebral foramina malformation.
  2. Trauma, arthritis, infection, disk degeneration from aging, and inherited (e.g., ankylosing spondylitis) or congenital conditions like scoliosis can also contribute to chronic LBP.
  3. Back pain may also be caused by *spondylolysis,* a defect in one of the vertebrae, usually in the lumbar spine. Spondylolisthesis occurs when one vertebra slips forward on the one below it, often as a result of vertebral bony defect.

Considerations for Older Adults

Patient-Centered Care

Older adults are at high risk for both acute and chronic LBP. Vertebral fracture from osteoporosis contributes to LBP. Petite, older Euro-American women are at high risk for both bone loss and subsequent vertebral fractures.

- Risk factors for acute and chronic back pain include:
  1. Work environments
  2. Trauma (forceful back movement and lifting)
  3. Obesity
  4. Structural and congenital spinal problems, such as scoliosis or spondylolysis
  5. Smoking (associated with premature disk degeneration)
  6. Poor posture and sedentary lifestyle
     a. Proper posture and exercise can significantly decrease the incidence of low back pain.
     b. The US Occupational Safety and Health Administration (OSHA) mandated that all industries develop and implement a plan to decrease musculoskeletal injuries among their

workers. One way to meet this requirement is to develop an ergonomic plan for the workplace. *Ergonomics* is an applied science in which the workplace is designed to increase worker comfort and reduce injury. An example is a ceiling lift designed to help nurses assist patients to get out of bed.

INTERPROFESSIONAL COLLABORATIVE CARE

Assessment: Noticing

* Assess and document:
  1. Pain location, quality, radiation, severity, and alleviating and aggravating factors
  2. Posture and gait
  3. Vertebral alignment
  4. Muscle tone and strength; limitations or presence of spasm
  5. Tenderness or swelling of the spinal column
  6. Sensory changes: paresthesia, numbness, or tingling
  7. Psychosocial reaction to illness
  8. Vertebral changes seen on an x-ray, computed tomography (CT) scan, or magnetic resonance imaging (MRI) scan
  9. Abnormal electromyography and nerve conduction studies
  10. Medication and other interventions to treat pain, including over-the-counter (OTC) drugs and complementary or alternative care

Interventions: Responding

NONSURGICAL MANAGEMENT

* To treat acute LBP
  1. Use the Williams position when in bed (semi-Fowler's bed position with the knees flexed) if herniated disk is present. In a side-lying position, a pillow between the knees may be helpful.
  2. Collaborate with the physical therapist (PT) to develop an individualized exercise and rehabilitation program to strengthen core and leg muscles after acute pain resolves.
  3. Drug therapy includes NSAIDs (oral and topical) and other drugs to manage acute pain.
  4. Epidural or local corticosteroid injection may be helpful in some cases.
* Approaches for treating chronic back pain
  1. Collaborate with the dietitian to implement a weight loss program if appropriate.
  2. Collaborate with the occupation therapist (OT) for ergonomic and adaptive furniture and aids.
  3. Administer antiepileptic or other drugs to relieve neuropathic pain. Avoid chronic opioid use.
  4. Water therapy combined with exercise is helpful for some patients as is weighted traction.

5. Local electrical stimulation may provide significant pain relief.
6. Adjunctive therapy, such as spinal manipulative therapy, distraction, imagery, and music therapy, can reduce maladaptive responses to chronic pain.

SURGICAL MANAGEMENT
- Conventional open operative procedures include:
  1. *Discectomy,* in which a portion of the disk is removed
  2. *Laminectomy,* which is the removal of one or more vertebral laminae, plus osteophytes, and the herniated nucleus pulposus through a 3 inch (7.5 cm) incision
  3. *Spinal fusion* to stabilize the affected area. Chips of bone are grafted between the vertebrae for support and to strengthen the back. Metal implants (usually titanium pins, screws, plates, or rods) may be required to ensure the fusion of the spine.
  4. Artificial disk replacement may also be part of this type of surgery.
- Minimally invasive operative procedures include *microdiskectomy* or *percutaneous endoscopic discectomy* (PED), a procedure that may be used with *laser thermodiscectomy* to shrink the herniated disk before removal.
- Provide preoperative care as described in Part One and:
  1. Explain to the patient that various sensations may be experienced in the affected leg or both legs (for lumbar surgery) because of manipulation of nerves and muscles during surgery.
  2. Address the need for a postoperative brace and bone grafting if the patient is having a spinal fusion.
- Provide routine postoperative care and:
  1. Perform neurologic assessment with vital signs every 4 hours during the first 24 hours.
  2. Check the patient's ability to void. An inability to void may indicate damage to sacral spinal nerves. Opioid analgesics have been associated with difficulty voiding and constipation.
  3. Maintain vertebral alignment with frequent log roll repositioning and provide venous thromboembolism (VTE) prophylaxis if bed rest is prescribed immediately after surgery

---

! NURSING SAFETY PRIORITY: Action Alert

For the patient after back surgery, inspect the surgical dressing for blood or any other type of drainage. Clear drainage may mean cerebrospinal fluid (CSF) leakage. Blood and CSF may be mixed on the dressing with the CSF being visible as a "halo" around the outer edges of the dressing. The loss of a large amount of CSF may cause the patient to report having a sudden headache. Report signs of any drainage on the dressing to the surgeon immediately. Bulging at the incision site may be due to a CSF leak or a hematoma, both of which should also be reported to the surgeon.

Care Coordination and Transition Management

- After *conventional open back surgery,* the patient may have activity restrictions for the first 4 to 6 weeks, such as:
  1. Limit daily stair climbing.
  2. Restrict or limit driving.
  3. Do not lift objects heavier than 5 pounds.
  4. Restrict pushing and pulling activities (e.g., dog walking).
  5. Take a daily walk.
- Self-management education includes:
  1. Continue with a weight-reduction diet, if needed.
  2. Stop smoking, if applicable.
  3. Perform strengthening exercises as instructed.
- In a few patients, back surgery is not successful. This situation, referred to as failed back surgery syndrome (FBSS), is a complex combination of organic, psychological, and socioeconomic factors.
  1. Nerve blocks, implantable spinal cord stimulators (neuro-stimulators), and other chronic pain management modalities may be needed on a long-term basis to help with comfort.
  2. Ziconotide (Prialt) is a drug that can be given for severe chronic back pain and is given by intrathecal (spinal) infusion with a surgically implanted pump. It is the first available drug in a new class called *N-type calcium channel blockers (NCCBs).*

PAIN, CERVICAL SPINE

OVERVIEW

- Cervical spine or neck pain is often related to herniation of the nucleus pulposus in an intervertebral disk.
- Cervical back pain also may result from muscle strain or ligament sprain, bony spur (from osteoarthritis), arthritis, tumor, infection, poor posture, or history of trauma.

INTERPROFESSIONAL COLLABORATIVE CARE

Assessment: Noticing

- Assess for:
  1. Pain onset, duration, quality, and aggravating and alleviating factors. Classic cervical pain is characterized by numbness and tingling that radiates to the scapula and down the arm.
  2. Vertebral changes seen on CT scan or MRI

3. Electromyography/nerve conduction studies are used to help differentiate cervical radiculopathy, ulnar or radial neuropathy, carpal tunnel syndrome, or other peripheral nerve problems.

Interventions: Responding

NONSURGICAL MANAGEMENT

- Nonsurgical management of cervical spine pain is the same as for back pain, except that the exercises focus on the neck and shoulder.
- A cervical collar may be prescribed for no more than 10 days; prolonged use can lead to increased pain and decreased muscle strength and range of motion (ROM).

SURGICAL MANAGEMENT

- Depending on the causative factors, an anterior or a posterior approach may be used to provide a discectomy and spinal fusion.
- Provide routine preoperative and postoperative care as described in Part One.
  1. Monitor for complications:
     a. CSF leak from the surgical site
     b. Hoarseness or dysphagia resulting from laryngeal injury
     c. Esophageal, tracheal, or vertebral artery injury
     d. Graft extrusion and screw loosening if a fusion was performed

PANCREATITIS, ACUTE: IMMUNITY CONCEPT EXEMPLAR

OVERVIEW

- Acute pancreatitis is a serious and, at times, life-threatening disorder of IMMUNITY caused by premature activation of pancreatic enzymes that destroy ductal tissue and pancreatic cells and results in autodigestion and fibrosis of the pancreas.
- Autodigestion and tissue destruction leads to inflammation and additional tissue destruction ranging from mild involvement, characterized by edema and moderate pain, to severe, necrotizing hemorrhagic damage and diffuse fibrosis and tissue death.
- Many factors can injure the pancreas and contribute to early activation of pancreatic enzymes (lipase, trypsin, elastase), including:
  1. Biliary tract disease and gallstones or pancreatic obstruction
  2. Excessive alcohol ingestion ("binge") or chronic alcoholism
  3. Surgical manipulation after biliary tract, pancreatic, gastric, and duodenal procedures
  4. Blunt or penetrating trauma
  5. Metabolic disturbances: hyperlipidemia, hyperparathyroidism, hypercalcemia
  6. Kidney failure or kidney transplant
  7. Drug toxicities, including opiates, sulfonamides, thiazides, corticosteroids, and oral contraceptives

- Complications include transient hyperglycemia, hypocalcemia, jaundice, pleural effusion, acute respiratory distress syndrome (ARDS), multi-system organ dysfunction, shock, and coagulation defects.

INTERPROFESSIONAL COLLABORATIVE CARE
Assessment: Noticing

- Obtain patient information about:
  1. History of abdominal pain, especially if related to alcohol ingestion or high intake of fat
  2. Individual and family history of alcoholism, pancreatitis, or biliary tract disease
  3. Previous abdominal surgeries or diagnostic procedures
  4. Medical history, including kidney disease, abdominal surgery or procedures, biliary tract diseases, trauma, hyperparathyroidism, and hyperlipidemia
  5. Recent viral infection
  6. Use of prescription and OTC drugs
- Assess for and document:
  1. Abdominal pain (the most frequent symptom), particularly sudden-onset pain in a mid-epigastric or left upper quadrant location with radiation to the back, aggravated by a fatty meal, ingestion of a large amount of alcohol, or lying in the recumbent position
  2. Weight loss, with nausea and vomiting
  3. Jaundice
  4. Gray-blue discoloration of the abdomen and periumbilical area (Cullen's sign)
  5. Gray-blue discoloration of the flanks (Turner's sign)
  6. Absent or decreased bowel sounds
  7. Abdominal tenderness, rigidity, and guarding
  8. Dull sound on abdominal percussion, indicating ascites
  9. Elevated temperature with tachycardia and decreased blood pressure
  10. Adventitious breath sounds, dyspnea, or orthopnea
  11. Elevated serum amylase and lipase levels

❗ NURSING SAFETY PRIORITY: Critical Rescue

For the patient with acute pancreatitis, monitor for significant changes in vital signs that may indicate the life-threatening complication of shock. Hypotension and tachycardia may result from pancreatic hemorrhage, excessive fluid volume shifting, or the toxic effects of abdominal sepsis from enzyme damage. Observe for changes in behavior and level of consciousness (LOC) that may be related to alcohol withdrawal, hypoxia, or impending sepsis with shock.

- Diagnostic studies may include:
  1. Serum lipase, amylase, alkaline phosphatase, alanine amino-transferase (ALT), bilirubin, white blood cell (WBC), hemo-globin, hematocrit, coagulation factors, basic metabolic panel (electrolytes and kidney function), calcium, magnesium, triglycerides, and albumin
  2. Imaging of the pancreas and gallbladder with ultrasound or CT scan

Analysis: Interpreting

- The priority collaborative problems for patients with acute pancreatitis include:
  1. Pain due to pancreatic inflammation and enzyme leakage.
  2. Decreased nutrition due to the inability to ingest food and absorb nutrients.

Planning and Implementation: Responding

MANAGING ACUTE PAIN

- The priority for patient care is supportive care by relieving pain and other symptoms, decreasing inflammation, and an-ticipating or treating complications. As for any patient, con-tinually assess for and support the ABCs (airway, breathing, and circulation).
- Decrease pain with interventions that reduce GI activity (decrease pancreatic synthesis of enzymes).
  1. Initiate NPO status for 24 to 48 hours.
     a. Decrease gastric acid during fasting with administration of a proton pump inhibitor or H_2 (histamine-2) blocker.
  2. Consider nasogastric drainage and suction to manage vomit-ing or biliary obstruction.
- Manage pain with nonopioid and opioid analgesics.
  1. Comfort measures include helping the patient assume a side-lying position to decrease abdominal pain and providing anti-nausea drugs and antiemetics as needed.

! NURSING SAFETY PRIORITY: Action Alert

For the patient with acute pancreatitis, monitor his or her re-spiratory status every 4 to 8 hours or more often as needed, and provide oxygen to promote comfort in breathing. Respira-tory complications such as pleural effusions increase patient discomfort. Fluid overload can be detected by assessing for weight gain, listening for crackles, and observing for dyspnea. Carefully monitor for signs of respiratory failure.

Observe for signs and symptoms of hypocalcemia by as-sessing for Chvostek's and Trousseau's signs. These tests cause muscle spasms after stimulating the associated nerves.

PROMOTING NUTRITION
1. Maintain hydration and electrolyte balance with IV fluids.
2. Provide jejunal enteral or parenteral nutrition early, within 72 hours of admission to the hospital for treatment of pancreatitis.
3. When food is tolerated, provide small-volume, high-carbohydrate, and high-protein feedings with limited fats.

- Administer antibiotics for patients with acute necrotizing pancreatitis.
- Patients with complications such as pancreatic pseudocyst or abscess may require surgical drainage; a procedure to remove gallstones may be needed.

Care Coordination and Transition Management
- Patient and family health teaching is aimed at preventing both future episodes and disease progression to chronic pancreatitis.
  1. Encourage alcohol abstinence to prevent pain and extension of the inflammatory damage.
  2. Teach the patient to notify the physician if he or she is experiencing acute abdominal pain or symptoms of biliary tract disease such as jaundice, clay-colored stools, and dark urine.
  3. Emphasize the importance of follow-up visits with the primary health care provider.
  4. Refer the patient with an alcohol abuse problem to support groups such as Alcoholics Anonymous.
  5. Refer the patient to home health nursing as needed.

PANCREATITIS, CHRONIC

OVERVIEW
- Chronic pancreatitis is a progressive, destructive disease with remissions and exacerbations.
- Inflammation and fibrosis of pancreatic tissue contribute to pancreatic insufficiency and the onset of diabetes.
  1. Pancreatic insufficiency is characterized by the loss of exocrine function resulting in a decreased output of enzymes and bicarbonate and altered digestion.
  2. Diabetes results from loss of endocrine function.

INTERPROFESSIONAL COLLABORATIVE CARE
Assessment: Noticing
- Assess for and document:
  1. Abdominal pain (major clinical manifestation): continuous, burning, or gnawing dullness with intense and relentless exacerbations
  2. Left upper quadrant mass, indicating a pseudocyst or abscess

3. Dullness on abdominal percussion, indicating pancreatic ascites
4. Steatorrhea, foul-smelling stools that may increase in volume as pancreatic insufficiency progresses
5. Family history of pancreatic disorders
6. Weight changes
7. Jaundice and dark urine
8. Signs and symptoms of diabetes mellitus
9. Elevated serum amylase, bilirubin, and alkaline phosphatase levels
10. Identification of calcification of pancreatic tissue in biopsy specimen
11. Fatigue and muscle wasting

Interventions: Responding

NONSURGICAL MANAGEMENT

- Drug therapy includes:
  1. Opioid analgesia (the patient may become dependent on opioids with long-term use)
  2. Nonopioid analgesics
  3. Pancreatic-enzyme replacement therapy (PERT) is the standard of care to prevent malnutrition, malabsorption, and excessive weight loss.

❗ NURSING SAFETY PRIORITY: Drug Alert

Teach the patient to take these drugs with meals and snacks and a glass of water. If needed, open the capsules and spread their contents over applesauce, mashed fruit, or rice cereal. Enzyme preparations should not be mixed with foods containing proteins because the enzymatic action dissolves the food into a watery substance. Be sure that patients drink a full glass of water after taking the drug to ensure that none of the enzymes remain in the mouth. Advise the patient to wipe his or her lips with a wet towel to prevent the skin irritation and breakdown that residual enzymes can cause.

---

  4. Insulin to control diabetes
  5. H_2-blocker or proton pump inhibitor to decrease gastric acid
- Record daily weight and the number and consistency of stools per day to monitor the effectiveness of drug therapy.
- Diet therapy includes:
  1. Fasting to avoid recurrent pain exacerbated by eating
  2. Providing jejunal or total parenteral nutrition (TPN)
  3. Consult with the dietician to provide sufficient calories and protein to maintain health.

- Surgical management of both complications from and precursors to pancreatitis include:
  1. Incision and drainage for abscess or pseudocyst
  2. Laparoscopic cholecystectomy or endoscopic procedures for biliary tract disease
  3. Sphincterotomy (incision of the sphincter) for fibrosis
  4. Pancreatojejunostomy (the pancreatic duct is opened and anastomosed to the jejunum, relieving obstruction) to relieve pain and preserve pancreatic tissue and function
  5. Partial pancreatectomy, which may be performed for advanced pancreatitis or disabling pain
  6. Vagotomy with gastric antrectomy to alter nerve stimulation and decrease pancreatic secretion

Care Coordination and Transition Management
- Health teaching is aimed at preventing further exacerbations.
  1. Avoid known precipitating factors, such as alcohol and foods with a high-fat content.
  2. Comply with diet instructions: high protein, high carbohydrate, and low or no fat.
  3. Follow written instructions and prescriptions for pancreatic enzyme therapy regarding:
     a. How and when to take enzymes
     b. The importance of maintaining therapy
     c. The importance of notifying the physician of increased steatorrhea, abdominal distention, cramping, and skin breakdown
  4. Comply with elevated glucose management, including oral hypoglycemic drugs or insulin injections and monitoring of blood glucose levels.
  5. Keep follow-up visits with the physicians.
- Refer the patient to case management, financial counseling, social services, vocational rehabilitation, home health services, and Alcoholics Anonymous, as needed.

PARALYSIS, FACIAL

OVERVIEW
- Facial paralysis, or Bell's palsy, is an acute paralysis of cranial nerve (CN)VII (7) but may also affect CN V (5) and VIII (8).
- Acute maximum paralysis occurs over 2 to 5 days in almost all patients.

INTERPROFESSIONAL COLLABORATIVE CARE
- Common signs and symptoms are:
  1. Inability to close eyelid, wrinkle the forehead, smile, whistle, or grimace

2. Tearing may stop or become excessive.
3. The face appears mask-like and sags.
4. Taste is usually impaired to some degree, but this symptom seldom persists beyond the second week of paralysis.
5. Tinnitus (ringing in the ears) may also occur.

- Most patients go into remission within 3 months.
- The cause of Bell's palsy is believed to be the result of inflammation triggered by a formerly dormant herpes simplex virus type 1 (HSV-1).
- Treatment includes:
  1. Administering corticosteroid and antiviral agents
  2. Administering mild analgesics for pain
  3. Protecting the eye from corneal abrasion or ulceration by patching and administering artificial tears
  4. Teaching the patient to use warm, moist heat; massage; and facial exercises such as whistling, grimacing, and blowing air out of the cheeks three or four times a day

✴ PARKINSON'S DISEASE: MOBILITY CONCEPT EXEMPLAR

OVERVIEW

- Parkinson's disease (PD) is a progressive neurodegenerative disorder involving the basal ganglia and substantia nigra, leading to a decrease of dopamine in the brain. Loss of dopamine results in difficulty with voluntary movement. Loss of dopamine reduces the sympathetic nervous system influence in the cardiovascular system contributing to autonomic dysfunction and neuropsychiatric symptoms like mood disorders.
- The disease is characterized by tremor, muscle rigidity, bradykinesia or akinesia (slow movements), and postural instability.
- The disease involves five stages.
  1. *Stage 1:* mild disease with unilateral limb involvement
  2. *Stage 2:* bilateral limb involvement
  3. *Stage 3:* significant gait disturbances and moderate generalized disability
  4. *Stage 4:* severe disability, akinesia, and muscle rigidity
  5. *Stage 5:* complete dependency in all aspects of ADLs

INTERPROFESSIONAL COLLABORATIVE CARE

Assessment: Noticing

- Obtain patient information about:
  1. Time and the progression of symptoms such as tremors, and slowed voluntary and automatic movements such as a change in handwriting
  2. Family history related to neurologic disorders

    3. History of head injury that can damage central nervous system (CNS) structures

    4. Use of drugs to treat serious mental illness; some anti-psychotic medications can have Parkinson-like adverse effects

- Assess for and document:
  1. Rigidity, which is present early in the disease process and progresses over time
     a. Cogwheel rigidity manifested by a rhythmic interruption of muscle movement.
     b. Plastic rigidity defined as mildly restrictive movements.
     c. Lead-pipe rigidity defined as total resistance to movement.
  2. Posture and appearance
     a. Stooped posture, flexed trunk
     b. Fingers adducted and flexed at the metacarpophalangeal joint
     c. Wrists slightly dorsiflexed
  3. Gait
     a. Slow and shuffling with short, hesitant steps
     b. Propulsive gait
     c. Difficulty stopping quickly
  4. Speech
     a. Change in voice volume, phonation, or articulation; a soft, low-pitched voice
     b. Echolalia, or automatic repetition of what another person says
     c. Repetition of sentences
     d. Change in voice volume, phonation, or articulation
  5. Motor dysfunction
     a. Bradykinesia or akinesia
     b. Tremors, especially at rest
     c. "Pill-rolling" movement
     d. Mask-like face
     e. Difficulty chewing and swallowing
     f. Difficulty getting into and out of bed
     g. Little arm swinging when walking
  6. Autonomic dysfunction
     a. Orthostatic hypotension
     b. Excessive perspiration and oily skin
     c. Flushing, changes in skin texture
     d. Blepharospasm
     e. Uncontrolled drooling, especially at night
     f. Bowel and bladder dysfunction
  7. Psychosocial effects
     a. Emotional lability, easily upset, rapid mood swings
     b. Depression

P

    c. Paranoia
    d. Cognitive impairments
    e. Delayed reaction time
    f. Sleep disturbances

Analysis: Interpreting

- The priority collaborative problems for patients with PD include:
  1. Decreased mobility due to muscle rigidity, tremors, and postural instability.
  2. Decreased self-esteem due to impaired cognition, tremors, and decrease in self-care ability.

Planning and Implementation: Responding

PROMOTING MOBILITY

   Nonsurgical Interventions

- Provide drug therapy.
  1. Administer drug therapy on time to maintain continuous therapeutic drug levels.
     a. Dopamine agonists like apomorphine (Apokyn), pramipexole (Mirapex), and ripinirole (Requip)

❗ NURSING SAFETY PRIORITY: Drug Alert

Dopamine agonists are associated with adverse effects such as orthostatic (postural) hypotension, hallucinations, sleepiness, and drowsiness. Remind patients to avoid operating heavy machinery or driving if they have any of these symptoms. Teach them to change from a lying or sitting position to standing by moving slowly. The primary health care provider should not prescribe drugs in this class to older adults because of their severe adverse drug effects.

---

    b. Levodopa combinations are less expensive than the dopamine agonists and are better at improving motor function, but long-term use leads to dyskinesia.
    c. Catechol *O*-methyltransferase (COMT) inhibitors to interfere with the breakdown of dopamine in the CNS
    d. Anticholinergic drugs if the patient's primary symptom is tremor
    e. Monoamine oxidase inhibitors
    f. Variety of other drugs and drug combinations

❗ NURSING SAFETY PRIORITY: Drug Alert

Teach patients taking Monamine oxidase inhibitors (MAOIs) about the need to avoid foods, beverages, and drugs that contain tyramine, including cheese and aged, smoked, or cured foods and sausage. Remind them to also avoid red wine and beer to prevent severe headache and life-threatening hypertension (Burchum & Rosenthal, 2016). Patients should continue these restrictions for 14 days after the drug is discontinued.

   2. Monitor the patient for drug toxicity and adverse effects such as delirium, and decreased effectiveness of the drug.
      a. Drug toxicity can be treated with a decrease in drug dose or frequency or a drug holiday of about 10 days.
- Manage mobility impairment with:
   1. Nontraditional exercise such as yoga and tai chi
   2. Collaborate with PT and OT to maintain patient flexibility, prevent falling, and promote out-of-bed activity.
   3. Encourage the patient to participate as much as possible in self-management, including ADLs.
   4. Make the environment conducive to independence, including using adaptive or assistive devices.
   5. Collaborate the dietitian and speech-language pathologist to ensure sufficient oral intake and avoid injury from swallowing difficulties.
   6. Together with the interprofessional team, develop a communication plan if the patient has speech difficulties.

Surgical Interventions

- Care of the patient undergoing surgical interventions for PD is similar to general perioperative care and specifically to care of the patient undergoing a craniotomy. The procedures most commonly used are:
   1. Deep brain stimulation (DBS) is used to manage PD symptoms. Electrodes are implanted into the brain and connected to a small electrical device called a *pulse generator* (placed in the chest similar to a cardiac pacemaker) that delivers electrical current. The generator is externally programmed to deliver an electrical current to decrease involuntary movements.
   2. Fetal tissue transplantation is an experimental and highly controversial ethical and political treatment. Fetal substantia nigra tissue, either human or pig, is transplanted into the caudate nucleus of the brain.
   3. DBS involves placing a thin electrode in the thalamus or subthalamus and connecting it to a "pacemaker" that delivers electrical current to interfere with "tremor cells." The electrodes are connected to an implantable pulse generator that is placed underneath the skin in the patient's chest, something like a cardiac pacemaker.

PROMOTE SELF-ESTEEM
- Teach the family to emphasize the patient's abilities or strengths and provide positive reinforcement when he or she meets expected outcomes.
- The patient, the family or significant other, and the rehabilitation team mutually set realistic expected outcomes that can be achieved.

Care Coordination and Transition Management
- The long-term management of PD presents a special challenge in the home care setting.
- A case manager may be required to coordinate interprofessional care and provide support for the patient and family.
- Teach patients and their families about the need to follow instructions regarding the safe administration of drug therapy.
- Remind them to immediately report adverse effects of medication such as dizziness, falls, acute confusion (delirium), and hallucinations.
- Collaborate with the social worker or case manager to help the family with financial and health insurance issues, as well as respite care or permanent placement if needed.
- Refer the patient and family to social and state agencies, as well as support groups.

 PELVIC INFLAMMATORY DISEASE: SEXUALITY CONCEPT EXEMPLAR

OVERVIEW
- Pelvic inflammatory disease (PID) is a complex infectious process that can alter the structural and functional traits associated with SEXUALITY.
- PID occurs when organisms from the lower genital tract migrate from the endocervix upward through the uterine cavity into the fallopian tubes.
- It is a major cause of infertility and ectopic pregnancies.
- It is most often caused by sexually transmitted organisms, especially *Chlamydia trachomatis* and *Neisseria gonorrhoeae.* Other organisms may include *Gardnerella vaginalis, Haemophilus influenzae, Staphylococcus, Streptococcus,* and *Escherichia coli.*
- The infection may spread to other organs and tissues. Resultant infections include:
  1. Endometritis (infection of the endometrial cavity)
  2. Salpingitis (inflammation of the fallopian tubes)
  3. Oophoritis (ovarian infection)
  4. Parametritis (infection of the parametrium)
  5. Peritonitis (infection of the peritoneal cavity)
  6. Tubal or tubo-ovarian abscess

- Sepsis and death can occur, especially if treatment is delayed or inadequate.
- Although common signs and symptoms include tenderness in the tubes and ovaries (adnexa) and low, dull abdominal pain, some patients have only mild discomfort or menstrual irregularity, and others experience no symptoms at all. These variations can make the diagnosis of PID challenging.

INTERPROFESSIONAL COLLABORATIVE CARE
Assessment: Noticing
- Obtain patient information about:
  1. Menstrual history
  2. Obstetric and sexual history, including whether unprotected sex or sexual abuse occurred
  3. Results of cultures or serum analysis congruent with infection or infecting organism
  4. Results of pelvic examination, particularly the presence of purulent cervical discharge or friable cervical tissue
  5. Previous reproductive surgery
  6. Abnormal vaginal bleeding
  7. Dysuria (painful urination)
  8. Increase or change in vaginal discharge
  9. Dyspareunia (painful sexual intercourse)
  10. Risk factors, including:
     a. Age younger than 26 years
     b. Multiple sexual partners
     c. Intrauterine device (IUD) in place within the previous 3 weeks
     d. Smoking
     e. Previous episodes of sexually transmitted infection or PID
- Assess for and document:
  1. Pain, especially lower abdominal pain
  2. Fever, chills, generalized aches
  3. Hunched-over gait
  4. Abdominal tenderness, rigidity, or rebound tenderness
- Assess for psychosocial issues, such as:
  1. Anxiety and fear
  2. Need for reassurance and support during the physical examination
  3. Embarrassment
  4. Discomfort when discussing symptoms or sexual history
- Diagnosis is made based on history, physical symptoms and signs, cervical or vaginal mucopurulent discharge, presence of WBCs on saline microscopy of vaginal secretions, and positive culture or nucleic acid test (e.g., laboratory identification of *N. gonorrhoeae*

or *Chlamydia* in urine or genital secretions/discharge). Other tests that may be helpful include ultrasonography, MRI, and endometrial biopsy.

Analysis: Interpreting

- The priority collaborative problem for patients with PID is:
    1. Infection due to invasion of pelvic organs by sexually-transmitted pathogens.

Planning and Implementation: Responding

MANAGING INFECTION

- Uncomplicated PID is usually treated with oral antibiotics.
- Hospitalization for PID for treatment with intravenous antibiotics is recommended if the patient has a complicated history or presentation (such as pregnancy or tubo-ovarian abscess), does not respond to oral antibiotic therapy, or has severe illness.
- Drug therapy includes oral and/or parenteral antibiotics for 14 days.
- In a small number of patients, a laparotomy may be needed to remove a pelvic abscess.
- Provide nonjudgmental emotional support, and allow time for her to discuss her feelings.

Care Coordination and Transition Management

- If not hospitalized, be seen by the primary health care provider within 72 hours after starting the antibiotics and then at 1 and 2 weeks from the time of the initial diagnosis.
- Counsel the patient to contact her sexual partner(s) for examination and treatment.
- Teach the patient about the need to:
    1. Abstain from sexual intercourse during treatment
    2. Check her temperature twice a day
- Discuss contraception and the patient's need or desire for it. This discussion includes the use of condoms that can decrease the risk for future episodes of PID.
- Provide referral for follow-up related to serious psychosocial reactions. A patient who has PID may exhibit a variety of feelings (guilt, disgust, anger) about having a condition that may have been transmitted to her sexually. These feelings may affect her relationship with significant others and future sexual partners.

PERICARDITIS

OVERVIEW

- Pericarditis is an inflammation or alteration of the pericardium, the membranous sac enclosing the heart. Alterations include fibrotic, serous, hemorrhagic, purulent, and neoplastic changes to the sac or fluid in the pericardial space.

- There are two types of pericarditis.
  1. *Acute pericarditis* is most commonly associated with infective organisms (bacteria, viruses, fungi), malignant neoplasms, post-myocardial infarction syndrome, postpericardiotomy syndrome, systemic connective tissue diseases, kidney failure, and idiopathic causes.
  2. *Chronic constrictive pericarditis* is caused by tuberculosis, radiation therapy, trauma, kidney failure, connective tissue disorders, and metastatic cancer, with the pericardium becoming rigid, preventing adequate ventricular filling, and resulting in cardiac failure.

INTERPROFESSIONAL COLLABORATIVE CARE

- Obtain patient information about:
  1. History of cardiac disease, cardiac surgery, chest trauma, or recent systemic infections
  2. History of chest radiation, connective tissue diseases, or cancer
- Assess for and document:
  1. The nature of chest discomfort; pericardial pain is typically substernal, worse on inspiration and lessens when the patient leans forward
  2. Pericardial friction rub
  3. Acute pericarditis
     a. Elevated WBC count
     b. Nonspecific ST-T wave elevation on electrocardiogram (ECG)
     c. Fever (infectious cause)
     d. Signs or symptoms of cardiac tamponade, particularly paradoxical pulse (increased SBP by 10 mm Hg or more on inspiration compared with exhalation) and sudden jugular venous distension
  4. Chronic constrictive pericarditis
     a. Right-sided heart failure, including dyspnea, exertional fatigue, and orthopnea
     b. Pericardial thickening on echocardiogram and CT scan
     c. Inverted or flat T waves on ECG
     d. Atrial fibrillation
- Treatment depends on the type of pericarditis.
- Acute pericarditis is treated by:
  1. Administering NSAIDs, corticosteroids, and antibiotics
  2. Encouraging rest
- Chronic pericarditis is treated by:
  1. Radiation or chemotherapy if it is associated with malignant disease
  2. Hemodialysis if it is associated with uremia from kidney disease

3. Surgical excision of the pericardium if the chronic pericarditis is constrictive. (e.g., *pericardial window* or *pericardectomy*)
- Complications of pericarditis include pericardial effusion and cardiac tamponade resulting in decreased cardiac output similar to heart failure.

PERIOPERATIVE CARE: SAFETY CONCEPT EXEMPLAR

- Patient care before (**preoperative**), during (**intraoperative**), and after (**postoperative**) surgery is the **perioperative** experience. Patient SAFETY throughout the perioperative period is the number one priority and requires teamwork and interprofessional collaboration.
- Research identifies communication—the critical component of teamwork and collaboration—as a critical element in maintaining patient safety in the perioperative environment. Lack of communication contributes to adverse events and unexpected negative outcomes.
- Perioperative quality improvement efforts focus on measures that prevent wrong-site surgery, patient falls, hospital-acquired pressure ulcers, infection, serious cardiac events, VTE or deep vein thrombosis (DVT), and maintain normothermia.
- Ensuring patient-centered care includes strategies to avoid surgery-related harm from adverse drug and anesthesia effects or complications from hypoventilation, hemodynamic instability, hypothermia, and infection.

PREOPERATIVE MANAGEMENT

OVERVIEW

- The preoperative period begins when the patient is scheduled for surgery and ends at the time of transfer to the surgical suite.
- The nurse prepares the patient for surgery and ensures patient safety.
- *Inpatient* refers to a patient who is admitted to a hospital the day before or the day of surgery and requires hospitalization after surgery.
- *Outpatient* and *ambulatory* refer to a patient who goes to the surgical area the day of the surgery and returns home on the same day (same-day surgery [SDS]).
- The primary reasons for surgery are:
  1. Diagnostic
  2. Curative
  3. Restorative
  4. Palliative
  5. Cosmetic

- The urgency of surgery may be:
  1. Elective
  2. Urgent
  3. Emergency
- Surgery can be considered minor or major.
  1. Minor surgery can include cautery, curettage, dermal excisions, and other minor incisions. Major body cavities are not opened and vital organs are not stressed. Local, regional, or general anesthesia may be required.
  2. Major surgery involves opening the abdomen, chest, skull, or other body cavity. Major surgery can stress vital organs like brain, lungs, kidney, or heart. Generally major surgery is more complicated and requires general anesthesia.
- The extent of surgery can be:
  1. Simple
  2. Radical
  3. Minimally invasive surgery (MIS)

INTERPROFESSIONAL COLLABORATIVE CARE
Assessment: Noticing
- Obtain a history that includes the following:
  1. Age
  2. Use of tobacco, alcohol, prescribed or over-the-counter drugs, or illicit and alternative substances, including marijuana
  3. Use of complementary or integrative health therapies, such as herbal therapies, folk remedies, or acupuncture
  4. Medical history, including prior surgical procedures and how these were tolerated
  5. Prior experience with anesthesia, pain control, and management of nausea or vomiting
  6. Autologous or directed blood donations
  7. Allergies, including sensitivity to latex products
  8. General health and family history
  9. Type of surgery planned
  10. Knowledge about and understanding of events during the perioperative period
  11. Adequacy of the patient's support system

> **! NURSING SAFETY PRIORITY: Action Alert**
>
> Ask about a history of joint replacement and document the exact location of any prostheses. Communicate this information to operating room personnel to ensure that electrocautery pads, which could cause an electrical burn, are not placed on or near the area of the prosthesis. Other areas to avoid

| Chart 2-16 | Selected Factors that Increase Risk for Surgical Complications |

Age
- Older than 65 years

Medications
- Antihypertensives
- Tricyclic antidepressants
- Anticoagulants
- NSAIDs
- Immunosuppressives

Medical History
- Decreased immunity
- Diabetes
- Pulmonary disease
- Cardiac disease
- Hemodynamic instability
- Multi-system disease
- Coagulation defect or disorder
- Anemia
- Dehydration
- Infection
- Hypertension
- Hypotension
- Any chronic disease

Prior Surgical Experiences
- Less-than-optimal emotional reaction
- Anesthesia reactions or complications
- Postoperative complications

Health History
- Malnutrition or obesity
- Drug, tobacco, alcohol, or illicit substance use or abuse
- Altered coping ability
- Herbal use

Family History
- Malignant hyperthermia
- Cancer
- Bleeding disorder
- Anesthesia reactions or complications

Type of Surgical Procedure Planned
- Neck, oral, or facial procedures (airway complications)
- Chest or high abdominal procedures (pulmonary complications)
- Abdominal surgery (paralytic ileus, venous thromboembolism)

electrocautery pad placement include on or near bony prominences, scar tissue, hair, tattoos, weight-bearing surfaces, pressure points, or metal piercings.

- Take and record VS; report VS that may indicate it is unsafe to perform surgery:
  1. Hypotension or hypertension
  2. Heart rate less than 60 or more than 120 beats/min
  3. Irregular heart rate

    4. Chest pain
    5. Shortness of breath or dyspnea
    6. Tachypnea
    7. Pulse oximetry reading of less than 94%
- Assess for and report any signs or symptoms of infection, including:
    1. Fever
    2. Purulent sputum
    3. Dysuria or cloudy foul-smelling urine
    4. Red, swollen, draining wound or vascular access site
    5. Increased white blood cell count
- Assess for and report factors that may contraindicate surgery, including:
    1. Increased prothrombin time (PT), international normalized ratio (INR), or activated partial thromboplastin time (aPTT)
    2. Abnormal electrolytes, particularly hypokalemia or hyperkalemia
    3. Patient report of possible pregnancy or positive pregnancy test
    4. New or worsening kidney function, including altered urine characteristics, decreased urine output, reduced glomerular filtration rate (GFR), and increased serum creatinine or blood urea nitrogen
- Assess for and report clinical conditions that may need to be evaluated by a provider before proceeding with the surgical plans, including:
    1. Change in mental status
    2. Vomiting
    3. Rash
    4. Recent administration of an anticoagulant drug
    5. Family or personal history of malignant hyperthermia with anesthesia
    6. Risk for falling related to impaired cognition, reduced muscle strength, unsteady gait, or dependence in activities of daily living (ADLs)
    7. Skin conditions or the presence of prosthetics that may require special positioning or surveillance in the perioperative suite
- Use a standardized form to ensure the following items are available before surgery starts:
    1. History and physical
    2. Signed, dated, and witnessed procedure consent form
    3. Nursing assessment
    4. Preanesthesia assessment
    5. Labeled diagnostic and radiology test results. Two common but not required tests are chest x ray and electrocardiogram (ECG). Tests specific to the condition or surgical procedure (e.g., CT scan, magnetic resonance image [MRI] scans, abdominal films, orthopedic films) should also be noted.

6. Banked blood products, implants, devices, and/or special equipment for the procedure and patient preferences about blood product transfusion

Chart 2-17	Specific Considerations When Planning Care for the Older Preoperative Patient

- Greater incidence of chronic illness (hypertension, diabetes, cardiac, etc.)
- Greater incidence of malnutrition and dehydration
- More allergies
- Increased abnormal lab values (anemia, low albumin level)
- Increased incidence of impaired self-care abilities
- Inadequate support systems
- Decreased ability to withstand the stress of surgery and anesthesia
- Increased risk for cardiopulmonary complications after surgery
- Risk for a change in mental status when admitted (e.g., related to unfamiliar surroundings, change in routine, drugs)
- Increased risk for a fall and resultant injury
- Impaired mobility

Analysis: Interpreting
- The priority collaborative problems for preoperative patients are:
  1. Knowledge deficit due to unfamiliarity with surgical procedures and preparation.
  2. Anxiety due to new or unknown experience, possibility of pain, and possible surgical outcomes.

Planning and Implementation: Responding
PROVIDING INFORMATION
- Explore the patient's level of knowledge and understanding of the planned surgery by having the patient explain in his or her own words the purpose and expected results.
- As required by The Joint Commission, ensure the correct site is selected and the wrong site is avoided. A licensed independent practitioner marks the site and, whenever possible, involves the patient.
- Ensure proper patient identification including placement of identification bands. Use at least two appropriate identifiers.
- Ensure informed consent is obtained from the patient (or legal designee) by the surgeon before sedation is given and before surgery is performed. Consent implies that the patient has sufficient information to understand:
  1. The nature of and reason for surgery
  2. Who will perform the surgery and whether others will be present during the procedure

3. All available options and the risks associated with each option
4. The risks associated with the surgical procedure and its potential outcomes
5. The risks associated with the use of anesthesia

! NURSING SAFETY PRIORITY: Action Alert

If you believe that the patient has not been adequately informed, contact the surgeon and request that he or she sees the patient for further clarification. Document this request in the electronic health record.

- Preoperative care includes:
  1. Determining the existence and nature of the patient's advance directives.
  2. Implementing and evaluating adherence to oral or dietary restrictions.
     a. Recommendations include NPO status (no eating or drinking), typically for 6 or more hours for easily digested solid food and 2 hours for clear liquids.
     b. Failure to adhere to NPO status can result in cancellation of surgery or increase the risk for aspiration during or after surgery.
  3. Ensuring intestinal preparation.
     a. Before abdominal, bowel, or intestinal surgery, a simple enema, "enemas until clear," or mild or potent laxatives (polyethylene glycol electrolyte solution [GoLYTELY] is an example of a potent laxative) may be prescribed to empty the large intestine to reduce the potential for contamination of the surgical field.
     b. Antibiotics may be administered immediately before orthopedic and abdominal surgery to reduce bacterial load.
  4. Performing skin preparation.
     a. Confirm or assist the patient in the use of an antiseptic solution while showering and removal of oil and skin debris. This intervention reduces the number of organisms on the skin and the potential for a site infection.
     b. Remove hair at the surgical site with clippers.
  5. Teaching the patient about the potential use of tubes, drains, and vascular access.
     a. Reassure the patient that these are temporary and that efforts will be made to reduce discomfort.
     b. Common devices include:
        (1) Foley catheter
        (2) NGT

       (3) Drains (e.g., Penrose, Jackson-Pratt, Hemovac)

       (4) Vascular access

6. Teaching about postoperative interventions to prevent respiratory complications.
   a. Deep diaphragmatic and expansion breathing, splinting during cough, and position changes
   b. Incentive spirometry
   c. Turning and positioning

7. Teaching about identification and prevention of cardiovascular complications.
   a. Teach that DVT (a type of VTE) is swelling in one leg, the presence of calf pain that worsens with ambulation, or worsening shortness of breath.
   b. Use antiembolic stockings (TEDs or Jobst stockings), elastic (Ace) wraps, or pneumatic compression devices to prevent superficial venous stasis and VTE.
   c. Use leg exercises and early ambulation to prevent VTE and promote venous return.

8. Reviewing the plans for pain management postoperatively.
   a. If the patient is receiving sedation or general anesthesia, stress the importance of having another adult drive the patient home after the procedure.

9. Communicating during handoff to the operating room (OR) personnel all care that has been provided and what care may still be needed.

10. Ensuring appropriate clothing removal and storage of valuables.
    a. Removal and safekeeping of dentures, dental prostheses (e.g., bridges, retainers), jewelry (including body piercing), eyeglasses, contact lenses, hearing aids, wigs, and other prostheses

11. Correctly administer prescribed preoperative drugs, including cardiovascular drugs and antibiotics.
    a. Many oral drugs are held the morning before surgery or given via IV preoperatively.
    b. Others, especially for cardiac disease, respiratory disease, seizures, and hypertension, are usually allowed before surgery with a sip of water.

12. Keeping the side rails up, the bed in the low position, and the call system within easy reach of the patient, especially after administering preoperative sedatives.

MINIMIZING ANXIETY

- Assess the patient's knowledge about the surgical experience.
- Allow ample time for questions.
- Respond to questions accurately or facilitate communication with the knowledgeable care provider.

- Incorporate family or supportive adults in communications.
- Provide prescribed antianxiety drugs.
- Provide opportunity for distraction, rest, or relaxation.
- Communicate to the perioperative team any of the patient's concerns, fears, or preferences.

INTRAOPERATIVE MANAGEMENT

OVERVIEW

- The intraoperative period begins when the patient enters the surgical suite (OR) and ends at the time of transfer to the postanesthesia recovery area, SDS unit, or ICU.
- Perioperative nursing priorities are *safety* and health care organization designed to reduce, control, and manage many hazards.

  1. *Construction and design* of the OR suite centers on preventing infection by reducing contaminants through controlled air exchanges in the room, maintaining recommended temperature and humidity levels, and limiting the traffic and activities in the OR by means of sliding door closures and designated traffic patterns.

  2. *Electrical and fire safety* is an integral part of the design process. The nurse ensures safety through the use of electrical equipment that meets specific standards.

     a. Multiple outlets on separate circuits are required to avoid overloads preventing short circuits and the potential loss of power.

     b. Proper placement of grounding pads, inspection of the electrosurgical devices, and avoiding patient contact with metal components of the OR table, other electrical equipment, or pooling prep solutions helps to prevent surgical burns and injury.

  3. *Patient safety devices* and nursing interventions are used to manage risk during surgical procedures. In the OR, the patient is at risk for infection, impaired TISSUE INTEGRITY, impaired COMFORT from pain or anxiety, inadequate thermoregulation and altered body temperature, and injury related to falls, positioning, and other intraoperative interventions.

     a. Safety straps are required for the patient, and the OR bed is locked in place.

     b. Blankets or warming units are used to prevent hypothermia from inadequate thermoregulation.

     c. Positioning devices, gel pads, and frames are used to prevent skin breakdown and injury during the positioning process.

  4. The OR setting presents multiple occupational hazards that can put the surgical team at risk for injury and disability from lifting and transferring of patients; carrying heavy instrument

sets; moving equipment; and exposure to sharps, bloodborne pathogens, anesthetic gases, radiation, chemicals, and other environmental hazards.

  a. The use of patient transfer equipment, personal protective equipment (gowns, gloves, masks, and eye protection), on-going monitoring of the environment for trace anesthetic gases, and monitoring of radiation badges worn by personnel (for exposure levels to radiation) and lead shielding are basic SAFETY precautions utilized in the OR to manage personnel safety and minimize known risk factors.

  b. Constant awareness of the environment and adherence to practice standards will reduce staff injuries from slips, trips, and falls related to clutter in the room, cords on the floor, or wet surfaces.

- Surgical team members include:

  1. The *surgeon*, a physician who assumes responsibility for the surgical procedure and any surgical judgments about the patient

  2. One or more *surgical assistants* who might be another physician (or resident or intern), an advanced practice nurse, physician assistant, certified registered nurse first assistant (CRNFA), or surgical technologist

  3. The *anesthesia provider*, who gives anesthetic drugs to induce and maintain anesthesia and delivers other drugs as needed to support the patient during surgery

     a. The *anesthesiologist*, a physician who specializes in giving anesthetic agents

     b. The *certified registered nurse anesthetist (CRNA)*, who is a registered nurse with additional education and credentials who delivers anesthetic agents under the supervision of an anesthesiologist, surgeon, dentist, or podiatrist

  4. *Perioperative nursing staff,* who may undergo orientation for 6 to 12 months

     a. The *holding area nurse*, who coordinates and manages the care of the patient in the presurgical holding area next to the main OR. This nurse assesses the patient's physical and emotional status, gives emotional support, answers questions, and provides additional education as needed.

❗ NURSING SAFETY PRIORITY: Action Alert

Once the patient has been moved into the holding area or the OR, do not leave him or her alone.

     b. The *circulating nurse*, who is responsible for coordinating all activities within that particular OR. He or she sets up the OR and ensures that supplies, including blood products and diagnostic support, are available as needed. This nurse positions the patient, assists the anesthesia provider, inserts a Foley catheter if needed, and scrubs the surgical site before the patient is draped with sterile drapes. In the absence of a holding area nurse, the circulating nurse also provides holding area tasks. Other responsibilities include:

(1) Monitoring traffic in the room
(2) Assessing the amount of urine and blood loss
(3) Reporting findings to the surgeon and anesthesia provider
(4) Ensuring that sterile techniques and a sterile field are maintained
(5) Communicating information about the patient's status to family members
(6) Documenting care, events, interventions, and findings
(7) Completing documentation in the OR and nursing records about the presence of drains or catheters, the length of the surgery, and a count of all sponges, "sharps" (needles, blades), and instruments

c. The *scrub nurse* sets up the sterile field, drapes the patient, and hands sterile supplies, sterile equipment, and instruments to the surgeon and the assistant. The scrub nurse also maintains an accurate count of sponges, sharps, instruments, and amounts of irrigation fluid and drugs used. An OR technician may also perform these tasks.

d. The *specialty nurse* may be in charge of a particular type of surgical specialty (e.g., orthopedic, cardiac, ophthalmologic) and is responsible for nursing care specific to patients needing that type of surgery.

- Types of surgery
  1. *Minimally invasive surgery (MIS)* is planned when one or more small incisions are made in the surgical area and an endoscope (a tube that allows viewing and manipulation of internal body areas) is placed through the opening.
     a. MIS may include injecting gas or air into the cavity (insufflation) before the surgery to separate organs and improve visualization; insufflation may contribute to complications and patient discomfort.
     b. *Robotic technology* during MIS consists of the use of a console, surgical arm cart, and video cart to improve control and dexterity.
        (1) This new technology requires additional education for the perioperative nurse.

        (2) Mechanical trauma and thermal injury are two types of injury that a patient can incur during MIS and robotic surgery.

2. Open techniques
   a. Open surgery is a traditional approach where a long incision is made through which instruments can be inserted and the anatomy can be viewed.
   b. Skin and tissue closures include sutures, staples, special tape, and tissue adhesive (surgical "glue") and are used to close the incision. A dressing may then be applied to prevent contamination from the environment while the site heals.
      (1) *Absorbable sutures* dissolve over time via body enzymes.
      (2) *Nonabsorbable sutures* become encapsulated in the tissue during the healing process and remain in the tissue unless they are removed.

- Types of anesthesia and complications
  1. *General anesthesia* is a reversible loss of consciousness induced by inhibiting neuronal impulses in several areas of the central nervous system (CNS). The patient is unconscious and unaware and has loss of muscle tone and reflexes. Agents are administered by inhalation and IV injection. Complications include:
     a. Malignant hyperthermia (MH), an acute life-threatening complication of certain drugs used for general anesthesia.
        (1) The reaction begins in skeletal muscles exposed to the drugs, causing increased calcium levels in muscle cells and increased muscle metabolism. Serum calcium and potassium levels are increased, as is the metabolic rate, leading to acidosis, cardiac dysrhythmias, and a high body temperature.
        (2) MH is a genetic disorder with an autosomal dominant pattern of inheritance and is most common in young, well-muscled men.
        (3) Drugs most associated with MH are halothane, enflurane, isoflurane, desflurane, sevoflurane, and succinylcholine.
        (4) When MH occurs, the treatment is intravenous dantrolene.

! NURSING SAFETY PRIORITY: Critical Rescue

Recognize that you must monitor patients for the cluster of elevated end-tidal carbon dioxide level, decreased oxygen saturation, and tachycardia to identify symptoms of MH. If these changes begin, respond by alerting the surgeon and anesthesia provider immediately.

   b. Adverse effects from anesthesia can occur when the patient's metabolism and elimination are slower than expected, such as an older adult or one with liver or kidney dysfunction.

   c. Unrecognized hypoventilation with failure to exchange gases adequately can lead to cardiac arrest, permanent brain damage, and death.

   d. Intubation complications from improper neck extension or anatomic differences in a patient can lead to broken or injured teeth and caps, swollen lips, or vocal cord trauma.

   e. Hemodynamic instability from medications, fluid loss, or dysrhythmias can contribute to brain or other organ damage.

2. *Local or regional anesthesia* disrupts sensory nerve impulse transmission providing a risible loss of sensation in a predetermined area of the body undergoing surgery. The patient remains conscious and able to follow instructions.

   a. Local anesthesia is delivered topically (applied to the skin or mucous membranes of the area to be anesthetized) and by local infiltration.

   b. Regional anesthesia is a type of local anesthesia that blocks multiple peripheral nerves and reduces sensation. Regional anesthesia includes field block, nerve block, spinal, and epidural.

   c. Complications of local or regional anesthesia are related to patient sensitivity to the anesthetic agent (anaphylaxis), incorrect delivery technique, systemic absorption, and overdose.

3. *Moderate sedation*, also called conscious sedation, is the IV delivery of sedative and opioid drugs to reduce the level of consciousness but allow the patient to maintain a patent airway and to respond to verbal commands.

   a. The nurse monitors the patient during and after the procedure for response to the procedure and the drugs, including airway, level of consciousness, oxygen saturation, capnography (measure of carbon dioxide level), ECG status, and VS every 15 to 30 minutes until the patient is awake, oriented, and VS have returned to baseline levels.

   b. The patient is expected to be sleepy but arousable for several hours after the procedure. Oral intake is not permitted until 30 minutes after the patient received the last dose of sedation or according to the physician's orders.

INTERPROFESSIONAL COLLABORATIVE CARE
Assessment: Noticing

• Correct identification of the patient is the responsibility of every member of the health care team. Verify with closed loop communication

the patient's identity with two types of identifiers (e.g., name, birth date, telephone number, medical record number).
1. Use the patient's identification bracelet.
2. Ask the patient, "What is your name?" and "What is your birth date?"
- Validate that the surgical consent form has been signed and witnessed.
- Ask the patient, "What kind of operation are you having today?"
- Compare patient responses to the information on the operative permit and the operative schedule.
- When the procedure involves a specific site, validate the side on which a procedure is to be performed.

! NURSING SAFETY PRIORITY: Patient-Centered Care

The Joint Commission now recommends that the patient and the licensed independent practitioner who is ultimately accountable for the procedure and will be present during the procedure (usually the surgeon performing the surgery) mark the surgical site with an indelible marker, preferably when the patient is able to confirm accurate marking.

- Investigate any discrepancy and notify the surgeon.
- Validate that all aspects of the checklist are complete.
  1. Ask the patient about any allergies.
  2. Determine whether autologous blood was donated.
  3. Check the patient's attire to ensure adherence with facility policy.
  4. Ensure that all prostheses have been removed, including dentures, dental bridges or retainers, jewelry, contact lenses, and wigs.
- The circulating nurse and anesthesia provider review the patient's electronic health record in the perioperative holding area or the OR. This record provides information to identify patient needs during surgery and allows the nurse to assess and plan specific care during and after surgery, including:
  1. Advance directives (be prepared to implement do-not-resuscitate orders)
  2. Allergies or adverse reactions especially to anesthesia, blood transfusion, iodine, drugs, and latex
  3. Laboratory and diagnostic test results
  4. Medical history and physical examination findings
  5. Anesthesia evaluation
     a. Patient's previous responses and reactions to anesthesia
     b. The physical status of a patient is ranked according to a classification system developed by the American Society of

Anesthesiologists (ASA) assigning the patient to one of six categories based on current health and the presence of diseases and disorders.

(1) A totally healthy patient has an ASA ranking of 1; a patient who is brain dead receives a ranking of ASA 6.

(2) This system is used to estimate potential risks during surgery and patient outcomes.

P

❗ NURSING SAFETY PRIORITY

Correct identification of the patient is the responsibility of every member of the health care team to avoid mistakes in surgery. Make sure that a least two methods are used to identify the patient.

Analysis: Interpreting
- The priority collaborative problems for patients during surgery are:
  1. Potential for injury due to improper perioperative positioning.
  2. Potential for infection due to invasive procedure.
  3. Compromised gas exchange due to anesthesia, pain, and reduced respiratory effort.

Planning and Implementation: Responding
PREVENTING INJURY
- Ensure proper positioning and prevent injury or pressure ulcer formation by:
  1. Padding the operating bed with foam or silicone gel pads, or both
  2. Properly placing the grounding pads
  3. Assisting the patient to a comfortable position
  4. Modifying the patient's position according to the patient's safety and special needs
  5. Avoiding excessive joint abduction
  6. Securing the arms firmly on an armboard, positioned at shoulder level
  7. Supporting the wrist with padding and not overtightening wrist straps
  8. Placing safety straps above or below the nerve locations
  9. Maintaining minimal external rotation of the hips
  10. Not placing equipment on lower extremities
  11. Urging OR personnel to avoid leaning on the patient's lower extremities
  12. Maintaining the patient's extremities in good anatomic alignment by slightly flexing joints and supporting the patient with pillows, trochanter rolls, or pads

- Observe for complications of special positioning, such as wrist-drop or footdrop, loss of sensation, changes in extremity temperature or circulation, and inflammation.

PREVENTING INFECTION
- Identify patients with pre-existing health problems such as diabetes mellitus, immunodeficiency, obesity, and renal failure.
- Perform prescribed skin preparation.
- Protect the patient's exposure to cross-contamination.
- Ensure the use of sterile surgical technique, protective drapes, skin closures, and dressings.
- Administer preoperative antibiotics within 30 to 60 minutes of the first incision.

QSEN EVIDENCE-BASED PRACTICE

Aseptic technique must be strictly practiced by all operating room (OR) personnel.

PREVENTING HYPOVENTILATION
- The purpose of interventions is to prevent respiratory and circulatory complications resulting from the effect of anesthesia on breathing and gas exchange.
  1. Continuously monitor the patient according to established standards, including:
     a. Breathing
     b. Cardiac rhythm
     c. Blood pressure
     d. Heart rate
     e. Oxygen saturation
- Respect the patient's privacy and dignity by minimizing body exposure as a component of ethical care.
- Communicate information about the patient's status to waiting family members.
- Communicate clearly and accurately information about patient's surgical experience when handing off the patient to the postanesthesia care nurse.

POSTOPERATIVE MANAGEMENT

OVERVIEW
- Postoperative care begins at the completion of surgery and transfer of the patient to the postanesthesia care unit (PACU) or other area for specialized monitoring and continues until all activity restrictions have been lifted. The purpose of a PACU (recovery room) is the ongoing direct evaluation and stabilization of patients to anticipate, prevent, and manage complications after surgery.

- Postoperative and postanesthesia care is divided into three phases based on the level of care needed, not the physical setting. Not every patient will need all three phases.
  1. Phase 1 includes close monitoring of airway, VS, and indicators of recovery every 5 to 15 minutes. This phase typically lasts 1 to 2 hours.
  2. Phase 2 focuses on preparing the patient for care in another setting such as an acute care unit, ICU, SNF, or home.
  3. Phase 3 occurs in the extended care environment (e.g., hospital, residence) with assisted and self-management.

P

Chart 2-18 | **Postoperative Hand-Off Report**

Best Practice for Patient Safety and Quality Care

- Type and extent of the surgical procedure
- Type of anesthesia and length of time the patient was under anesthesia
- Allergies (especially to latex or drugs)
- Any health problems or pathophysiologic conditions
- Any relevant events/complications during anesthesia or surgery such as a traumatic intubation
- If intraoperative complications, how were they managed and patient responses (e.g., laboratory values, excessive blood loss, injuries)
- Status of vital signs, including temperature and oxygen saturation
- Intake and output, including current IV fluid administration and estimated blood loss
- Type and amount of IV fluids or blood products
- Medications administered and when last dose of pain med given
- When the next dose of medications are due especially antibiotics, cardiac drugs
- Primary language, any sensory impairments, any communication difficulties
- Special requests that were verbalized by the patient preoperatively including communications with family
- Preoperative and intraoperative respiratory function and dysfunction
- Location and type of incisions, dressings, catheters, tubes, drains, or packing
- Prosthetic devices

- Joint or limb immobility while in the operating room, especially in the older patient
- Other intraoperative positioning that may be relevant in the postoperative phase

INTERPROFESSIONAL COLLABORATIVE CARE
Assessment: Noticing
- The initial assessment of the patient immediately after surgery includes the respiratory status (including peripheral oxygenation [Spo_2]), level of consciousness, temperature, pulse, and blood pressure.

■ NURSING SAFETY PRIORITY: Critical Rescue

During the postoperative period, all patients remain at risk for pneumonia, shock, cardiac arrest, respiratory arrest, clotting and VTE, and gastrointestinal (GI) bleeding. These serious complications can be prevented or the consequences reduced with collaborative care. Nursing observations and interventions are part of critical rescue management for patient safety and quality care.

- Examine the surgical area for bleeding and drainage.
- Assess VS on admission and then follow agency protocol for frequency. Changes in heart rate, blood pressure, respiratory rate, or peripheral oxygenation (oximetry, Spo_2) that are concerning need to be communicated urgently to the provider or rapid response team.
- Increase the frequency of VS assessment whenever VS increase or decrease, particularly when there is clinical concern around maintaining a narrow range of values. High or low values in VS can be early indicators of adverse reaction to operative drugs, blood or volume loss, and postoperative complications including myocardial infarction or stroke.

■ NURSING SAFETY PRIORITY: Action Alert

Respiratory assessment is the most critical assessment to perform after surgery for any patient who has undergone general anesthesia or moderate sedation or has received sedative or opioid drugs.

- Routine postoperative monitoring and assessment include:
  1. Respiratory status
     a. Evaluate airway patency and adequacy of gas exchange by oxygen saturation, end-tidal carbon dioxide levels, respiratory rate, pattern, and effort.
     b. Ensure security and placement (e.g., depth) of an artificial airway (endotracheal tube, nasal trumpet, oral airway).
     c. Maintain type of oxygen delivery device and the concentration of oxygen delivered.
     d. Auscultate lung fields for breath sounds.
     e. Examine the degree of symmetry of breath sounds and chest movement.
     f. Determine the presence of snoring and stridor.

! NURSING SAFETY PRIORITY: Critical Rescue

If you recognize that your patient's oxygen saturation drops below 95% (or below his or her presurgery baseline), immediately respond by notifying the surgeon or anesthesia provider. If the patient's condition continues to deteriorate or he or she becomes symptomatic, an emergency response is imperative.

  2. Cardiovascular status
     a. Evaluate heart rate, quality, and rhythm.
     b. Carefully monitor blood pressure values.
     c. Monitor electrocardiography for dysrhythmias.
     d. Compare distal pulses, color, temperature, and capillary refill on extremities.
     e. Examine feet and legs for manifestations of DVT (e.g., redness, pain, warmth, swelling).
     f. Maintain prescribed compression devices or antiembolic stockings applied in the preoperative or operative suite.
  3. Neurologic status
     a. Trending level of consciousness or awareness:
        (1) Presence of lethargy, restlessness, or irritability
        (2) Patient responses to stimuli (calling the patient's name, touching the patient, and giving simple commands such as "Open your eyes" and "Take a deep breath")
        (3) Degree of orientation to person, place, and time by asking the conscious patient "What is your name?" (person), "Where are you?" (place), and "What day is it?" (time)
     b. Compare the patient's baseline preoperative neurologic status with postoperative findings.

4. Motor and sensory function status
   a. Ask the patient to move each extremity.
   b. Assess the strength of each limb and comparing the results on both sides.
   c. Gradually elevate the patient's head and monitor for hypotension.
5. Fluid, electrolyte, and acid-base balance
   a. Measure intake and output (including IV fluid intake, emesis, urine, wound drainage, NGT drainage).
   b. Check hydration status (e.g., inspecting the color and moisture of mucous membranes; the turgor, texture, and tenting of the skin; the amount of drainage on dressings; and the presence of axillary sweat).
6. Kidney and urinary status
   a. Measure intake and output.
   b. Assess for urine retention by inspection, palpation, percussion of the lower abdomen for bladder distension, or use of a bladder scanner.
   c. Perform prescribed intermittent catheterization.
   d. Assess urine for color, clarity, and amount.
7. GI status
   a. Listen for bowel sounds in all four abdominal quadrants and at the umbilicus.
   b. Assess for nausea and vomiting; postoperative nausea and vomiting are common with general anesthesia.
   c. Administer prescribed antiemetic drugs.
   d. Assess for manifestations of paralytic ileus (few or absent bowel sounds, distended abdomen, abdominal discomfort, vomiting, and no passage of flatus or stool).
   e. Assess and recording the color, consistency, and amount of the NGT drainage.
   f. Check NGT placement.

! NURSING SAFETY PRIORITY: Action Alert

After gastric surgery, do not move or irrigate the tube without an order from the surgeon.

8. Skin status
   a. Assess the incision (if visible) for redness, increased warmth, swelling, tenderness or pain, and the type and amount of drainage; be sure to look under the patient for pooling, collection, or drainage and blood.
   b. Condition of the sutures or staples.
   c. Presence of open areas.

9. Dressings and drains
   a. Document color, amount, consistency, and odor of drainage.
   b. Examine for leakage around or under the patient.
   c. Determine patency of drains.
   d. Perform neurovascular checks to identify restriction of circulation or sensation.
10. Altered comfort: pain
    a. Pain usually reaches its peak on the second day after surgery when the patient is active and the intraoperative anesthetic agents and drugs have been eliminated.
    b. Follow best practices for surgical pain management described in the following text.
11. Anxiety or fear: Age and medical history, the surgical procedure, and the impact of surgery on recovery, body image, roles, and lifestyle can contribute to anxiety following surgery.
12. Fluid and electrolyte balance: NPO status preoperatively and IV fluid administration intraoperatively can affect hydration and electrolyte values, resulting in either deficit or excess.
13. Acid-base balance can be affected by both the respiratory status (hypoventilation leading to hypercarbia and respiratory acidosis) and hydrations status (dehydration leading to metabolic acidosis).

Analysis: Interpreting
- The priority collaborative problems for patients in the immediate postoperative period are:
  1. Potential for compromised gas exchange due to the effects of anesthesia, pain, opioid analgesics, and immobility
  2. Potential for infection and delayed healing due to wound location, decreased mobility, drains and drainage, and tubes
  3. Acute pain due to the surgical incision, positioning during surgery, and endotracheal tube (ET) irritation
  4. Potential for decreased peristalsis due to surgical manipulation, opioid use, and fluid and electrolyte imbalances

Planning and Implementation: Responding
IMPROVING GAS EXCHANGE
1. Support a patient airway
   a. Monitor for snoring or stridor, which indicates obstruction.
   b. Insert an oral airway or a nasal airway (nasal trumpet) to pull the tongue forward and hold it down to prevent obstruction.
   c. Keep the manual resuscitation bag and emergency equipment for intubation or tracheostomy nearby.
   d. Position the patient in a side-lying or elevated back rest position to prevent aspiration.

    e. Suction the mouth, nose, and throat to keep the airway clear of mucus or vomitus as needed.

2. Apply prescribed oxygen by face tent, nasal cannula, or mask.
3. Assist the patient to breathe deeply (with the incision splinted) and use the incentive spirometer.
4. Assist the patient to reposition himself or herself every 2 hours and to ambulate as soon as possible.

PREVENTING WOUND INFECTION AND DELAYED HEALING

- Reinforce the dressing, change the dressing, assess the wound for healing and infection, and care for drains, including emptying drainage containers/reservoirs, measuring drainage, and documenting drainage features.

  1. The surgeon usually performs the first dressing change to assess the wound, remove any packing, and advance (pull partially out) or remove drains. However, the facility or unit may have standards or policies that dictate specific protocols for dressing changes and incision care.
  2. An unchanged wet or damp dressing is a source of infection. Change dressings using aseptic technique until the sutures or staples are removed.
  3. Skin sutures or staples are usually removed 5 to 10 days after surgery, although this varies up to 30 days depending on the type of surgery and the patient's health.
  4. Generally, administer antibiotics for no longer than 24 hours after surgery unless the patient has a documented infection.
  5. *Dehiscence* is a wound opening or rupture along the surgical incision. An *evisceration* is a wound opening with protrusion of internal organs and a surgical emergency.

     a. Dehiscence or evisceration may follow forceful coughing, vomiting, or straining and when not splinting the surgical site during movement. The patient may state, "Something popped" or "I feel as if I just split open."
     b. Have the patient lie flat (supine) with knees bent to reduce intra-abdominal pressure; apply sterile nonadherent dressing materials to the wound and notify the surgeon or rapid response team.

MANAGING PAIN

- Drug therapy is commonly used to manage surgical pain, but drugs may mask or increase the severity of symptoms of anesthesia.

  1. Administer opioids as prescribed and closely monitor patient responses with the first dose.
  2. Assess the type, location, and intensity of the pain before and after giving pain medication. Monitor the patient's VS for hypotension and hypoventilation after giving opioid drugs.

3. Use around-the-clock scheduling or use patient-controlled analgesia (PCA) systems for consistent blood levels and more effective surgical pain management.

4. Monitor epidural analgesia effects when administered intermittently by the anesthesia provider or by continuous infusion through an epidural catheter left in place after surgery. Common drugs given by epidural catheter include the opioids fentanyl (Sublimaze), preservative-free morphine (Duramorph), and bupivacaine (Marcaine).

5. Offer prescribed pain medication 30 to 45 minutes before the patient gets out of bed.

6. Use nonopioid drugs to augment pain management; typically, NSAIDs or acetaminophen are used.

- Use adjuvant therapy like distraction, positioning, and relaxation and anxiety-reducing interventions to manage pain.

PROMOTING PERISTALSIS

- Monitoring bowel sounds, rectal output, and abdominal status (distension) with VS
- Ensuring adequate hydration with intravenous fluids, oral fluids, and evaluation of intake and output to achieve hydration or fluid balance goals
- Promoting early and progressive out-of-bed mobility
- *Gum chewing* in the early postoperative period has been suggested to promote intestinal peristalsis. Chewing gum stimulates digestive secretions, including gastric hormones that trigger increased motility, without adding bulk to the GI system.
- Providing drug therapy to maintain or restore intestinal peristalsis
  1. Alvimopan (Entereg) and methylnaltrexone (Relistor) to counteract opioid-induced slowed peristalsis
  2. Prokinetic drugs like metoclopramide (Reglan; Maxeran) are used once an ileus occurs (this drug does not prevent slowed peristalsis).

! NURSING SAFETY PRIORITY: Action Alert

Always ensure that the patient and family receive oral and written discharge instructions to follow at home. Assess the understanding of the patient and family by having them explain the instructions in their own words.

Care Coordination and Transition Management

- If the patient is discharged directly to home, assess information about the home environment for safety and the availability of caregivers.

- Reinforce to the patient and family after surgery the specific interventions to use to prevent complications (e.g., hand hygiene, incision splinting, deep-breathing exercises, range-of-motion exercises).
- Collaborate with the social worker or discharge planner to identify needs related to care after surgery, including meal preparation, dressing changes, drain management, drug administration, physical therapy, and personal hygiene.
- The patient with visible scars after surgery may need more emotional support from and acceptance by his or her family.
- If dressing changes and drain or catheter care are needed, instruct the patient and family members on the importance of proper hand washing to prevent infection. Explain and demonstrate wound care to the patient and family, who then perform a return demonstration.
- Perform a drug reconciliation with the patient before discharge. Ensure that drugs for other health problems are resumed, as needed.
- A diet high in protein, calories, and vitamin C promotes wound healing; vitamin supplementation may be temporarily added to home drugs.
- Teach the patient to increase activity level slowly, rest often, and avoid straining the wound or the surrounding area; healing requires both time and avoidance of stress.

PERIPHERAL ARTERIAL DISEASE

OVERVIEW

- Peripheral arterial disease (PAD) is a result of atherosclerosis, a chronic condition in which partial or total arterial blockage decreases perfusion to the extremities, most commonly the legs.
  1. Inflow PAD obstructions involve the distal end of the aorta and the common, internal, and external iliac arteries, manifested by discomfort in the lower back, buttocks, or thighs.
  2. Outflow PAD obstructions involve the femoral, popliteal, and tibial arteries and typically cause significant tissue damage.
- *Chronic* PD can be divided into four stages:
  1. Asymptomatic
  2. Presence of *claudication* described as pain, cramping or burning with exercise that is relieved by rest (*intermittent claudication*)
  3. Pain while resting; pain that awakens the patient during sleep; relief of pain when extremity is in a dependent position
  4. Occurrence of ulcers, blackened tissue on toes, forefoot, and heel; gangrene infection of tissues
- *Acute* arterial occlusion occurs when there is an acute obstruction by a thrombus or embolus, causing severe, acute pain below the level of the obstruction.

INTERPROFESSIONAL COLLABORATIVE CARE
Assessment: Noticing
* Assessment findings include:
  1. Abnormal ankle-brachial index (ABI): The value can be derived by dividing the ankle blood pressure by the brachial blood pressure. A value of less than 0.9 indicates outflow disease. With inflow disease, pressures taken at the thigh level indicate the severity of disease. Mild inflow disease may cause a difference of only 10 to 30 mm Hg in pressure on the affected side compared with the brachial pressure.
  2. Leg pain (burning, cramping in calves, ankles, feet, and toes with exercise or rest) or discomfort in the lower back, buttocks, or thighs
  3. Ischemic changes of the extremity
     a. Loss of hair on the lower calf, ankle, and foot
     b. Dry, scaly skin
     c. Thickened toenails
     d. Color changes (elevation pallor or dependent rubor)
     e. Mottled and cool or cold extremity
  4. Decreased or absent leg pulses: The most sensitive and specific indicator of arterial function is the quality of the posterior tibial pulse because the pedal pulse is not palpable in a small percentage of people.
  5. Painful arterial ulcers that develop on the toes, between the toes, or on the upper aspect of the foot; PAD ulcers differ from diabetic and venous ulcers.
     a. Diabetic ulcers develop on the plantar surface of the foot, over metatarsal heads, on the heel, or on pressure areas; they may not be painful.
     b. Venous stasis ulcers occur at the ankles, with discoloration of the lower extremity at the ulcer; they cause minimal pain.
* Diagnostic assessment includes:
  1. Blood pressure and ABI measurement
  2. MRI and Doppler/ultrasound to assess blood flow in peripheral arteries

Interventions: Responding
NONSURGICAL MANAGEMENT
* Teach the following methods of increasing arterial blood flow in chronic arterial disease:
  1. Exercising to promote collateral circulation
  2. Positioning to promote circulation and decrease swelling
     a. Elevate legs at rest but not above the level of the heart.
     b. Avoid crossing legs and wearing restrictive clothing.
  3. Promoting vasodilation
     a. Avoid cold exposure to the affected extremity with warm socks and room temperature modulation.

    b. Avoid nicotine, caffeine, and emotional stress.

    c. Comply with drug therapy, including vasodilator and anti-platelet therapy.

    d. Control blood pressure to avoid hypertension.

- Percutaneous vascular intervention may be used to dilate the occluded artery, provide atherectomy, or place an endovascular stent or graft to restore arterial circulation. After endovascular intervention, care of the patient includes:
  1. Observing the puncture site for bleeding
  2. Closely monitoring vital signs for hypotension and hypertension
  3. Checking the neurovascular status of limbs (color, warmth, pulses, sensation, and voluntary movement)
  4. Encouraging the patient to maintain bed rest for 6 to 8 hours or as ordered, with the limb straight
  5. Administering antiplatelet or anticoagulation therapy, which may continue for 3 to 6 months after the procedure
- An acute occlusion may be managed with systemic or local fibrinolytic therapy, such as intravenous administration of atelplase (Activase). If this is done:
  1. Monitor the patient for bleeding and hemorrhagic stroke.
  2. Maintain IV access and fluid infusion.
  3. Avoid hypo- and hypertension.

> **! NURSING SAFETY PRIORITY: Drug Alert**
>
> When *fibrinolytics* are given, assess for signs of bleeding, bruising, or hematoma. For patients receiving any *platelet inhibitor,* monitor platelet counts for the first 3, 6, and 12 hours after the start of the infusion or per agency protocol. If the platelet count decreases to below $100,000/mm^3$, the infusion needs to be readjusted or discontinued. If any of these complications occur, notify the provider or Rapid Response Team immediately.

SURGICAL MANAGEMENT
- An emergency surgical embolectomy is performed on patients who experience an acute peripheral artery occlusion by a thrombosis or embolus.
- Arterial revascularization surgery is used to increase arterial blood flow in an affected limb and includes inflow procedures such as aortoiliac bypass, aortofemoral bypass, and axillofemoral bypass and outflow procedures, including femoropopliteal bypass and femorotibial bypass.

- Grafting materials for bypass surgeries include the autogenous saphenous vein and synthetic graft material such as polytetrafluoroethylene.
- Provide postoperative care.
  1. Monitor for the patency of the graft by checking for changes in the extremity:
     a. Color
     b. Temperature
     c. Pulse quality; mark the site of pulses for consistent evaluation
     d. Sensation and pain intensity (typical pain is described as throbbing pain, which occurs from increased blood flow to the affected limb)
  2. Monitor the patient's blood pressure, notifying the physician about increases and decreases beyond desired ranges.
  3. Avoid bending the knee and hip of the affected limb for 6 to 8 hours.
  4. Monitor for signs and symptoms of vessel re-occlusion at or around the graft and incision sites, such as hardness, tenderness, redness, or coolness or warmth.
- Thrombectomy (removal of the clot) is the most common treatment for acute graft occlusion; thrombolytic therapy may be used.
- Compartment syndrome occurs when tissue pressure within a confined body space becomes elevated and restricts blood flow.
- Use sterile technique when in contact with the incision and observe for symptoms of infection.

! NURSING SAFETY PRIORITY: Critical Rescue

Graft occlusion (blockage) is a postoperative emergency that can occur within the first 24 hours after arterial revascularization. Monitor the patient for and report severe continuous and aching pain, which may be the first indicator of postoperative graft occlusion and ischemia. Many people experience a throbbing pain caused by the increased blood flow to the extremity. Because this alteration in COMFORT is different from ischemic pain, be sure to assess the type of pain that is experienced. Pain from occlusion may be masked by patient-controlled analgesia (PCA). Some patients have ischemic pain that is not relieved by PCA.

Monitor the patency of the graft by checking the extremity every 15 minutes for the first hour and then hourly for changes in color, temperature, and pulse intensity. Compare the operative leg with the unaffected one. *If the operative leg feels cold; becomes pale, ashen, or cyanotic; or has a decreased or absent pulse, contact the surgeon immediately!*

Care Coordination and Transition Management
- Patient and family education includes:
  1. Teaching the patient to monitor tissue perfusion to the affected extremity
     a. Distal circulation, sensation, and motion
     b. Presence of pain, pallor, paresthesias, pulselessness, paralysis, and coolness
  2. Reinforcing the need for individualized positioning and an exercise plan
  3. Providing written and oral foot care instructions, per agency policy
  4. Providing dressing change and incision care instructions, if necessary
  5. Providing instructions concerning discharge medications, particularly to improve safety when using antiplatelet and anticoagulant drugs
  6. Encouraging healthy diet choices to reduce atherosclerotic plaque formation and growth

PERIPHERAL VENOUS DISEASE

OVERVIEW
- Peripheral venous disease (PVD) is a condition that alters the natural flow of blood through the veins of the peripheral circulation. Three health problems result in PVD:
  1. Thrombus (thrombosis) formation (see *Venous Thromboembolism [VTE]*) and thrombophlebitis or clot with associated inflammation
  2. Defective valves leading to venous insufficiency and varicose veins
  3. Reduced skeletal muscle activity when weight bearing is limited or muscle tone decreases
     a. Skeletal muscles help pump blood in veins.
     b. When weight bearing is limited or muscle tone decreases, PVD can develop.

INTERPROFESSIONAL COLLABORATIVE CARE
- For the patient with PVD, assess for:
  1. Serum markers of inflammation or impaired coagulation
  2. Cellulitis, the presence of open wounds, or venous stasis ulcers
  3. The possibility of deep vein thrombosis (DVT):
     a. Lower extremity pain, sudden unilateral leg swelling, and decreased perfusion
     b. Induration along the occluded vein

    c. Results of ultrasonography or Doppler flow studies identifying the presence or location of thrombosis

    d. Serum markers of inflammation and coagulation

- For recovery from PVD complications of thrombosis, phlebitis syndromes, and venous ulcer formation, interventions include:
    1. Positioning the lower extremities to reduce the risk for injury from venous insufficiency
    2. Informing patients of increased risk for VTE events, to monitor for symptoms, and to follow up with their primary health care provider at regular intervals
    3. Having the patient wear compression stockings during the day and evening
    4. Avoiding bed rest or prolonged periods of inactivity such as standing still or sitting
    5. Treating open venous ulcers with occlusive dressings and topical agents, with or without antibiotics to chemically débride the ulcer, and using a zinc oxide paste in a gauze compression bandage (e.g., Unna boot) to promote venous stasis ulcer healing

PERTUSSIS

OVERVIEW

- Pertussis is also known as whooping cough; it is a highly contagious respiratory infection caused by *Bordello pertussis*.
- Pertussis can be prevented with appropriate vaccination (www.cdc.gov)

INTERPROFESSIONAL COLLABORATIVE CARE

- Culture or polymerase chain reaction (PCR) testing of sputum is recommended for individuals with coughing for greater than 3 weeks.
- The disease has three distinct phases:
    1. Catarrhal phase of 1 to 2 weeks with symptoms of a mild cold
    2. Paroxysmal phase of up to 10 weeks with severe coughing "fits" lasting several minutes and bloody, purulent thick exudate in airways is common; coughing can led to cardiovascular complications (e.g., bradycardia, angina, stroke) in infants and older adults
    3. Convalescent phase of several months
- Treatment is with antibiotic, typically a macrolide like azithromycin or clarithromycin.
- Close contacts within 3 weeks of exposure should also receive antibiotic prophylaxis.

PERITONITIS: IMMUNITY CONCEPT EXEMPLAR

OVERVIEW

- Peritonitis is a life-threatening acute INFLAMMATION and infection of the visceral/parietal peritoneum and endothelial lining of the abdominal cavity.
- *Primary peritonitis* is a rare acute bacterial infection that develops as a result of contamination of the peritoneum through the bloodstream.
- *Secondary peritonitis* is caused by bacterial invasion as a result of perforation or a penetrating wound, such as appendicitis, diverticulitis, peptic ulcer, ascending genital infection, or a gunshot injury to the abdomen. Chemical peritonitis is the result of leakage of bile, pancreatic enzymes, and gastric acid.
- Peritonitis is associated with sepsis, hypovolemic and septic shock, respiratory problems, and paralytic ileus or bowel obstruction.

INTERPROFESSIONAL COLLABORATIVE CARE

Assessment: Noticing

- Obtain patient information about:
  1. History of abdominal trauma or surgery
  2. Character of abdominal pain, onset, duration, location, quality, aggravating and alleviating factors; the cardinal signs of peritonitis are abdominal pain, tenderness, and distension; often, pain is aggravated by coughing or movement and relieved by knee flexion
  3. Abdominal distention and presence/absence of bowel sounds
  4. Tachypnea with low peripheral saturation (decreased Spo_2)
  5. Low-grade fever or recent spikes in temperature

❗ NURSING SAFETY PRIORITY: Action Alert

For patients with peritonitis, assess for abdominal wall rigidity, which is a classic finding that is sometimes referred to as a "board-like" abdomen. Monitor the patient for a high fever because of the infectious process. Assess for tachycardia occurring in response to the fever and decreased circulating blood volume. Observe whether he or she has dry mucous membranes and a low urine output seen with edema or third spacing. Nausea and vomiting may also be present. Hiccups may occur as a result of diaphragmatic irritation. Be sure to document all assessment findings.

- Diagnostic tests may include:
    1. CBC; anticipate an elevated WBC count and neutrophilia
    2. Serum electrolytes, blood urea nitrogen (BUN), and creatinine
    3. Abdominal CT scan, x-ray, or ultrasound to determine the presence of dilation, edema, and inflammation of the intestines

❗ NURSING SAFETY PRIORITY: Critical Rescue

A sudden worsening of abdominal pain or a change from localized to generalized abdominal pain may signal perforation or new-onset peritonitis from an abdominal condition. This symptom is a medical emergency and needs to be communicated, along with vital signs, to the primary health care provider immediately to avoid patient progression to vascular and respiratory compromise.

Analysis: Interpreting

- The priority collaborative problems for patients with peritonitis include:
    1. Potential for infection due to peritonitis
    2. Potential for fluid volume shift due to fluid moving into interstitial or peritoneal space
    3. Acute pain due to peritonitis

Planning and Implementation: Responding

DECREASE POTENTIAL FOR INFECTION

Nonsurgical Management

1. Monitor vital signs and peripheral oxygenation (Spo_2) with level of consciousness and report concerning findings (systolic blood pressure [SBP] less than 90 mm Hg, heart rate [HR] greater than 110, respiratory rate [RR] greater than 20, Spo_2 less than 92% on supplemental oxygen or decreased cognition) to the provider urgently.
2. Provide and evaluate pain management with analgesics.
3. Administer oxygen to maintain Spo_2 greater than 92%.
4. Assess for intra-abdominal compartment syndrome.

Surgical Management

- Surgical management may be necessary to identify and repair the underlying cause of the peritonitis.
- Surgery is focused on controlling the contamination, removing foreign material from the peritoneal cavity, and draining fluid collections.
- During surgery, the peritoneum is irrigated with antibiotic solution, and drainage catheters are inserted.

- Provide routine postoperative care, including:
  1. Close monitoring of the patient's cardiovascular stability for early detection of shock (level of consciousness, HR, SBP, Spo_2, and urine output should remain within normal limits for the patient)
  2. Providing meticulous wound care; irrigating and packing the wound, as prescribed
  3. Assisting the patient in gradually increasing his or her activity level

Considerations for Older Adults

The early signs and symptoms of shock, infection, or dehydration in the older adult may consist of a subtle decrease in mental status, such as confusion or lethargy. Do not delay in communicating subtle changes in consciousness or cognition to the primary health care provider.

RESTORE FLUID VOLUME BALANCE
- Administer IV fluids and antibiotics.
- Record intake, output, and daily weight.
- Monitor and record drainage from the nasogastric tube (NGT) used for gastric and intestinal decompression.

MANAGE ACUTE PAIN
- Peritonitis causes significant pain and interventions to manage pain focus on drug therapy.
  1. Administer analgesics and monitor for pain control.

Care Coordination and Transition Management
- The patient may be discharged home or to a transitional care unit to complete antibiotic therapy and recovery.
- If the patient is discharged home, collaborate with the case manager to determine the need for assistance.
- Provide written and oral postoperative instructions, including:
  1. The necessity to report any redness, swelling, tenderness, or unusual or foul-smelling drainage from the wound
  2. Care of the incision and dressing; ensuring that the patient has the necessary equipment to perform wound care (dressings, solutions, catheter-tipped syringe); and stressing the importance of hand washing
  3. The need to report fever (typically 101°F [38°C]) or abdominal pain to the primary health care provider
  4. Administration and monitoring of drugs for pain

PHEOCHROMOCYTOMA

OVERVIEW

* Pheochromocytoma is a catecholamine-producing tumor of the adrenal medulla.
* These tumors are most often benign, but at least 10% are malignant.
* Pheochromocytomas produce, store, and release epinephrine and norepinephrine; these hormones stimulate adrenergic receptors and can have wide-ranging adverse effects mimicking the action of the sympathetic division of the autonomic nervous system.

INTERPROFESSIONAL COLLABORATIVE CARE

Assessment: Noticing

* Obtain patient information about episodes of norepinephrine and epinephrine excess, including:
  1. Severe headaches
  2. Palpitations
  3. Heat intolerance, flushing, profuse diaphoresis
  4. Apprehension or a sense of impending doom
  5. Pain in the chest or abdomen, with nausea and vomiting
* Assess for and document intermittent or recurrent symptoms of sympathetic nervous system stimulation, including:
  1. Hypertension
  2. Tremors
  3. Profuse diaphoresis, flushing
  4. Apprehension, sense of doom

❗ NURSING SAFETY PRIORITY: Action Alert

Do not palpate the abdomen because this action could cause a sudden release of catecholamines and severe hypertension.

* Diagnosis is made based on high urine levels of metanephrine and catecholamines.
* A clonidine suppression test can be used when catecholamine levels are not diagnostic.
* MRI or CT scans can precisely locate tumors.

Interventions: Responding

* Surgery is performed to remove the tumors and the adrenal gland or glands.
* Provide preoperative care.
  1. Monitor blood pressure regularly; place the cuff consistently on the same arm, with the patient in lying and standing positions.

2. Avoid heat and other stressors that may lead to a hypertensive crisis.
3. Teach the patient not to smoke, drink caffeine-containing beverages, or change position suddenly postoperatively.
4. Ensure adequate hydration.
5. Administer prescribed drug therapy (phenoxybenzamine [Dibenzyline]) to stabilize the patient's blood pressure (usually started days before surgery).

- Provide postoperative care and:
  1. Closely monitor for hypertension, hypotension, and hypovolemia
  2. Monitor for adequate tissue perfusion
     a. Vital signs with level of consciousness
     b. Fluid intake and output
  3. Check opioid effects on blood pressure
- If inoperable, tumors are managed with alpha- and beta-adrenergic blocking agents and self-measurement of blood pressure with home monitoring equipment.

PHLEBITIS

OVERVIEW

- Phlebitis is an inflammation of the superficial veins caused by an irritant, commonly IV therapy.
- Phlebitis is manifested as pain with a reddened, warm, swollen area radiating up an extremity.
- Treatment involves application of warm, moist soaks, which dilate the vein and promote circulation. *Do not massage the area.*

PNEUMONIA: GAS EXCHANGE CONCEPT EXEMPLAR

OVERVIEW

- Pneumonia is an excess of fluid in the lungs from an inflammatory process that can impair GAS EXCHANGE.
- It can be caused by many infectious organisms, by inhalation of irritating agents, or aspiration of stomach contents.
- Infectious pneumonias are categorized as *community-acquired pneumonia* (CAP) or *hospital-acquired pneumonia* (HAP), *health care–acquired pneumonia* (HCAP), and *ventilator-associated pneumonia* (VAP).
- Inflammation and infection in the lungs result in local capillary leak, edema, and exudate that interfere with gas exchange leading to hypoxemia that has the potential to cause death.
- Risk factors for pneumonia include:
  1. Being an older adult
  2. The presence of a chronic health problem, particularly a respiratory problem or condition that is associated with immunosuppression

3. Recent exposure to respiratory viral or influenza infections
4. Poor nutritional status

INTERPROFESSIONAL COLLABORATIVE CARE
Assessment: Noticing
- Obtain patient information about:
    1. Age
    2. Living, work, and school environments, including exposure to droplet-based infection
    3. Diet, exercise, and sleep routines
    4. Swallowing problems or presence of a nasogastric tube
    5. Tobacco and alcohol use
    6. Past and current use of drugs, including drug addiction or injection drug use
    7. Acute or chronic respiratory problems
    8. Recent skin rashes, insect bites, or exposure to animals
    9. Home respiratory equipment use and cleaning
    10. Date of last influenza or pneumococcal vaccine

Considerations for Older Adults

Interprofessional Care
The older adult with pneumonia has weakness, fatigue (which can lead to falls), lethargy, confusion, and poor appetite. Fever and cough may be absent, but hypoxemia is often present. The most common symptom of pneumonia in the older adult patient is acute confusion from hypoxia. The WBC count may not be elevated until the infection is severe. Waiting to treat the disease until more typical symptoms appear greatly increases the risk for sepsis and death.

- Assess for and document:
    1. General appearance for signs of flushing and hypoxia-related anxiety
    2. Oxygen saturation, evaluating for hypoxemia or $Spo_2 < 90\%$ to 92%
    3. Abnormal lung sounds, particularly crackles, rhonchi, and wheezing
    4. Respiratory rate and dyspnea or increased effort of breathing such as use of accessory muscles
    5. Cough
    6. Sputum amount and appearance, especially if purulent, blood-tinged, or rust-colored
    7. Chest or pleuritic pain or discomfort
    8. Fever, diaphoresis, chills, and fatigue or weakness
    9. Tachycardia, hypotension
    10. Mental status changes (especially in an older adult)

> **❗ NURSING SAFETY PRIORITY: Action Alert**
>
> Because pneumonia is a frequent cause of sepsis, use a sepsis screening tool to monitor patients who have pneumonia. For patients with pneumonia, always check oxygen saturation with vital signs.

11. Laboratory and imaging results such as elevated WBC, sputum or blood culture results, or consolidation on chest x-ray (CXR)

Analysis: Interpreting

- The priority interprofessional collaborative problems for patients with pneumonia include:
  1. Decreased gas exchange due to decreased diffusion at the alveolar-capillary membrane
  2. Potential for airway obstruction due to excessive pulmonary secretions, fatigue, and muscle weakness
  3. Potential for sepsis due to the presence of microorganisms in a very vascular area and decreased immunity
  4. Potential for pulmonary empyema due to the spread of infectious organisms from the lung into the pleural space

Planning and Implementation: Responding

IMPROVE GAS EXCHANGE

- Monitor rate, rhythm, depth, and effort of breathing and lung sounds.
- Assess pulse oximetry and administer oxygen by nasal cannula or mask to maintain $Spo_2 > 95\%$ prescribed.
- Instruct the patient on cough and deep-breathing technique or the correct use of incentive spirometry (sustained maximal inspiration) and encourage him or her to perform 5 to 10 breaths per session every hour while awake.
- Assess the patient's ability to use incentive spirometry correctly and cough effectively.
- Monitor fluid intake and encourage the alert patient to maintain sufficient intake to dilute mucus; generally this goal also provides a dilute urine output.
- Administer prescribed inhaled bronchodilators, oral mucolytics, and inhaled or systemic corticosteroids.
- Monitor for complications such as cognitive impairment, hypoxemia, ventilatory failure, atelectasis, pleural effusion, and pleurisy.

PREVENT AIRWAY OBSTRUCTION

- Assist patient to cough and deep breathe at least every 2 hours.
- Encourage the alert patient to use the incentive spirometer.
- Encourage the alert patient to drink at least 2 L of fluid daily.

- Monitor intake and output, oral mucous membranes, and skin turgor for hydration status.
- Bronchodilators may be used when bronchospasm is present.

PREVENT SEPSIS

- Administer prescribed anti-infective therapy based on organism sensitivity.
- For pneumonia resulting from aspiration of food or stomach contents, steroids and NSAIDs are used with antibiotics to reduce the inflammatory response.

MANAGE EMPYEMA

- Pulmonary empyema is a collection of pus in the pleural space and is diagnosed from symptoms of poor gas exchange, abnormal breath sounds, CXR or chest CT, and examination of a sample of pleural fluid obtained via thoracentesis.
- Treatment includes draining the empyema cavity, re-expanding the lung with chest tube/closed chest drainage, and controlling the infection with antibiotics.

Care Coordination and Transition Management

- Teach the patient about:
  1. The importance of completing the full course of antibiotic therapy
  2. Notifying the primary health care provider if chills, fever, persistent cough, dyspnea, wheezing, hemoptysis, increased sputum production, chest discomfort, or increasing fatigue recurs or if symptoms fail to resolve
  3. The importance of getting plenty of rest and gradually increasing exercise
  4. Preventing upper respiratory tract infections and viruses by:
     a. Using hand washing
     b. Avoiding crowds and people who have a cold or flu
     c. Avoiding exposure to irritants such as smoke
     d. Obtaining an annual influenza vaccination
     e. Obtaining pneumococcal vaccinations
- Encourage the patient to quit smoking and provide information on smoking cessation because smoking is a risk factor for both onset and severity of pneumonia.

PNEUMOTHORAX

OVERVIEW

- Pneumothorax, also called a *collapsed lung,* is air in the pleural space and a reduction in vial capacity that can lead to lung collapse.
- A common cause of pneumothorax is blunt trauma to the chest. It can also occur as a complication of medical procedures (e.g., central line placement) or spontaneously.

INTERPROFESSIONAL COLLABORATIVE CARE

- Assess for and document:
  1. Reduced breath sounds on auscultation
  2. Hyperresonance on percussion
  3. Prominence of the involved side of the chest, which moves poorly with respirations
  4. Deviation of the trachea away from (closed) or toward (open) the affected side
  5. Pleuritic chest pain
  6. Tachypnea
  7. Subcutaneous emphysema (air under the skin in the subcutaneous tissues)
- An ultrasound examination or a chest x-ray is used for diagnosis.
- A needle thoracostomy followed by chest tube placement may be needed to allow the air to escape and the lung to reinflate. Chest tube placement and water seal drainage without needle thoracostomy may be done when the patient is stable. When the pneumothorax is small, watchful waiting may be the only treatment.

PNEUMOTHORAX, TENSION

OVERVIEW

- Tension pneumothorax is a rapidly developing and life-threatening complication of large amounts of air entering the pleural space from an air leak in the lung or chest wall.
- Air that enters the pleural space during inspiration does not exit during expiration, allowing air to continue to collect under pressure, collapsing the lung, compressing blood vessels, limiting venous return, and reducing cardiac output.
- Immediate large bore needle thoracostomy by the primary health care provider provides emergent treatment. Generally this procedure is followed by chest tube placement and closed chest drainage.

! **NURSING SAFETY PRIORITY: Critical Rescue**

If not promptly detected and treated, tension pneumothorax is quickly fatal.

- Assess for and document similar to pneumothorax. Symptoms occur with rapid onset and respiratory distress with hemodynamic instability also occur rapidly.

POLYNEUROPATHY

OVERVIEW

- The terms *polyneuritis*, *polyneuropathy*, and *peripheral* neuropathy may be used interchangeably.

- The disorders are characterized by muscle weakness with or without atrophy; pain that is described as stabbing, cutting, or searing; paresthesia or loss of sensation; impaired reflexes; autonomic manifestations; or a combination of these symptoms.
- The most common type is a symmetric polyneuropathy in which the patient experiences decreased sensation along with a feeling that the extremity is asleep. Tingling, burning, tightness, or aching sensations usually start in the feet and progress to the level of the knee before affecting the hands ("glove and stocking" neuropathy).
- The disorders can result from inflammatory or noninflammatory processes; both can damage cranial and peripheral nerves.
- Factors associated with polyneuropathy include diabetes; kidney or hepatic failure; alcoholism; vascular disease; vitamin B_1, B_6, and B_{12} deficiencies; and exposure to heavy metals or industrial solvents.

INTERPROFESSIONAL COLLABORATIVE CARE

- Assess for and document:
  1. Light touch sensation and pain in the distal extremities
  2. Position sense and kinesthetic sensation
  3. Any signs of injury
  4. Indications of autonomic dysfunction, such as orthostatic hypotension, abnormal sweating, and miosis
- Treatment consists of elimination or treatment of the underlying cause and symptomatic therapy.
  1. Treat the underlying cause.
  2. Supplement the patient's diet with vitamins.
  3. Provide pain management as needed.
  4. Provide health teaching, including the importance of foot care and of inspecting the extremities for injuries.
  5. Stress the importance of wearing shoes at all times and of purchasing well-fitting shoes.
  6. Teach the patient how to recognize potential hazards, such as exposure to extremes of environmental temperature.
  7. Discourage smoking.
  8. Promote glycemic control.

POLYPS, GASTROINTESTINAL

OVERVIEW

- Polyps in the intestinal tract are small growths covered with mucosa that are attached to the surface; polyps have the potential to become malignant.
- Two forms of inherited GI polyps are particularly concerning to the primary health care provider: (1) familial adenomatous polyposis (FAP); and (2) hereditary nonpolyposis colorectal cancer (HNPCC). If these conditions are left untreated, colorectal cancer will occur.

- Polyps are usually asymptomatic but can cause rectal bleeding, intestinal obstruction, and intussusception.
- Polyps can usually be removed with a snare or by electrocautery during colonoscopy. After the procedure, monitor for abdominal distention, pain, and bleeding.
- Teach the patient about the need for regular, routine monitoring (colonoscopy) if polyps were found (removed) during colonoscopy because there is a risk for new/recurrent polyp formation, particularly with a positive family history of polyps. The specific follow-up time frame varies but generally occurs within 3 years.

 PRESSURE INJURY: TISSUE INTEGRITY CONCEPT EXEMPLAR

OVERVIEW

- A pressure injury is a loss of TISSUE INTEGRITY caused when the skin and underlying tissue are compressed between a bony prominence and external surface for an extended period.
- They form most commonly over the sacrum, hips, and ankles but can occur on any body surface.
- Tissue compression from pressure restricts blood flow to the skin, resulting in reduced tissue perfusion and gas exchange leading to cell death.
- Once formed, pressure injuries lead to complications, increased cost for care, and greater risk for mortality.
- Complications include infection, osteomyelitis, and pain.
- The forces that lead to pressure injury formation include:
  1. *Pressure:* A mechanical force occurring as a result of gravity, compressing blood vessels at the point of contact and leading to ischemia, inflammation, and tissue necrosis
  2. *Friction:* A mechanical force occurring when surfaces rub the skin and irritate or tear fragile epithelial tissue as when the patient is dragged or pulled across bed linen
  3. *Shear* or *shearing forces:* Mechanical forces occurring when the skin itself is stationary and the tissues below the skin (e.g., fat, muscle) shift or move, reducing the blood supply to the skin such as when the patient is in a semi-sitting position in bed and slides down

Considerations for Older Adults

Older adults are at particular risk for pressure injuries because of the presence of age-related skin changes.
- Flattening of the cells in the dermal-epidermal junction increases risk for injury from mechanical shearing forces, such as removal of tape or friction from restraints.

- As well, cognitive impairment may interfere with self-management for elimination or self-report of discomfort from inadequate pressure relief.
- Assess older adults with cognitive impairments more frequently for pressure injury formation.
- Avoid prolonged exposure to urine or feces; moisture and irritation from incontinence combining with friction can lead to skin destruction.

P

- Pressure injuries are categorized using the following descriptors:
  1. *Suspected deep tissue injury:* The intact skin area appears purple or maroon and blood-filled blisters may be present. Other changes include a sensation of firmness, mushiness, or bogginess at the site, a cooler or warmer temperature compared with surrounding tissue, and a report of pain at the site.
  2. *Stage I:* The intact skin is red (or darker or lighter than surrounding skin) and does not blanch with external pressure. The site might feel firm or boggy, warm or cool, and be painful or itchy.
  3. *Stage 2:* The skin is not intact, and there is a partial-thickness skin loss of the epidermis or dermis. The superficial ulcer may appear as an abrasion, a blister (open or fluid-filled), or a shallow crater, and bruising is not present.
  4. *Stage 3:* Skin loss is full thickness and subcutaneous tissues may be damaged or necrotic. Bone, tendon, and muscle are not exposed, but the fat may show a deep, crater-like appearance. Undermining and tunneling may be present.
  5. *Stage 4:* Skin loss is full thickness with exposed or palpable muscle, tendon, or bone. Undermining, tunneling, and sinus tracts are often present. Slough and eschar are often present on at least part of the wound.
  6. *Unstageable:* Skin loss is full thickness, and the base is completely covered with slough or eschar, obscuring the true depth of the wound.
- Health promotion and maintenance
  1. Identify patients at risk for pressure injury formation, commonly with a valid and reliable tool such as the Braden Scale. Risk factors include:
     a. Mental status changes
     b. Impaired mobility
     c. Poor nutritional status
     d. Incontinence
  2. Implement aggressive intervention for prevention
     a. Use pressure-relieving or pressure reduction techniques and devices to avoid skin and capillary compression.

    b. Techniques include frequent repositioning, adequate fluid and nutrition intake, skin care to avoid moist or dry skin, and effective skin cleaning.

    c. Devices include specialty beds, mattress replacements, overlays, and assistive devices.

3. Use health care team education and communication to reduce risk and identify pressure injuries early before complications occur.

    a. The dietitian and wound consultant/expert are essential consults in the team.

    b. The patient care assistant is also a key team member to help identify risk and early-stage pressure injuries and to implement aggressive interventions to prevent progression or deterioration of skin injury from compression.

    c. Teach all personnel to use Standard Precautions and to properly dispose of soiled dressings and linens.

INTERPROFESSIONAL COLLABORATIVE CARE

Assessment: Noticing

- Obtain patient information about contributing factors and causes of pressure injuries, including:
  1. Prolonged bed rest
  2. Immobility
  3. Incontinence
  4. Diabetes
  5. Inadequate nutrition or hydration
  6. Cognitive problems or decreased sensory perception
  7. Peripheral vascular disease
- Assess for and document:
  1. Inspection of the entire body for areas of skin injury or pressure
  2. General appearance for body weight and the proportion of weight to height (obesity and underweight contribute to skin problems)
  3. Overall cleanliness of the skin, hair, and nails
  4. Any loss of mobility or range of joint motion
- Assess existing wounds on admission, with each dressing change, and in accordance with the facility policy on ongoing assessment.
  1. Location, size (length, width, and depth), color, and extent of tissue involvement and document this information along with:
     a. Presence of blanching if skin is intact
     b. Exudate
     c. Condition of surrounding tissue, including wound margin
     d. Presence of foreign bodies
     e. Presence or absence of necrotic tissue (eschar)
     f. Presence of undermining and tunneling

g. Comparison of existing wound features with those documented previously to determine the current state of healing or deterioration

h. Inflammation or cellulitis (inflammation of skin and surrounding tissue)

i. Fever or mental status changes associated with acute infection

j. Peripheral edema that can interfere with healing

k. Vascular imaging result indicated poor perfusion to pressure injury, such as ultrasound/Doppler or angiography results

- Assess for psychosocial issues, including:
  1. Altered body image
  2. Coping patterns
  3. Changes in lifestyle and ADLs
  4. Financial resources
  5. Patient's and family's willingness and skill in cleaning the wound and applying a dressing
- Assess laboratory data for:
  1. Culture and sensitivity reports indicating wound colonization, which is the presence of organisms without any manifestation of infection, often manifested by some odor and serous (clear) drainage
  2. Culture and sensitivity reports indicating wound infection manifested by greater odor and pus/purulent drainage
  3. Elevated WBC indicating infection
  4. Laboratory reports indicating malnutrition including low prealbumin, albumin, and total protein

Analysis: Interpreting
- The priority collaborative problems for patients with pressure injuries include:
  1. Compromised tissue integrity due to vascular insufficiency and trauma
  2. Potential for wound deterioration due to insufficient wound management

Planning and Implementation: Responding
MANAGING WOUNDS
  Nonsurgical Management
- Dressing and wound care are the basis for pressure injury management. A well-designed dressing removes surface debris, protects exposed healthy tissues, and creates a barrier until the ulcer is closed. The frequency of dressing changes is dependent on the nature of the pressure injury and the facility's policies or procedures. Common dressing techniques for wound débridement are:
  1. Wet-to-damp saline moistened gauze for surface débridement
  2. Continuous wet gauze to dilute viscous exudate and loosen eschar

  3. Topical enzyme preparations to breakdown adherent eschar and proteins
  4. Moisture-retentive dressing to promote autolysis and separation of necrotic tissue
- When drainage is present or the wound is deep, additional materials may be needed to protect surrounding skin or prevent contamination from the environment.
  1. *Hydrophobic* materials are protective when there is little exudate.
  2. *Hydrophilic* materials draw exudate away, protecting skin from maceration.
- Drug therapy with topical or systemic antibacterial agents may be needed to control bacterial growth.
- Nutrition therapy provides adequate nutritional intake of calories, protein, vitamins, minerals, and water.
  1. Perform a nutritional assessment at least weekly.
  2. Coordinate with the dietitian to encourage the patient to eat a well-balanced diet, emphasizing proteins, vegetables, fruits, whole-grain breads and cereals, and vitamins.
- New technologies may be useful for chronic ulcers that remain open for months.
  1. *Electrical stimulation* is the application of a low-voltage current to a wound area to increase blood vessel growth and promote granulation.
  2. *Negative-pressure wound therapy* uses a suction tube covered by a special sponge ("foam"). Closely monitor patients for bleeding for the first 2 hours after placement and stop suction if bleeding occurs. Suction removes exudate and infectious materials. The foam needs to be changed three times weekly.

❗ NURSING SAFETY PRIORITY: Critical Rescue

Recognize that you do not use a continuous negative pressure wound therapy device with any patient who is on anticoagulant therapy; has reduced tissue health near the wound (e.g., with radiation therapy, poor nutrition); or has any exposed blood vessels, nerves, or organs in the wound area. Respond by consulting with members of the interprofessional team, such as the primary health care provider and wound nurse, for appropriate methods of treatment.

  3. *Hyperbaric oxygen* (HBO) therapy is the administration of oxygen under high pressure, which raises the tissue oxygen concentration.
  4. *Topical growth factors* are biologically active substances that stimulate cell movement and growth and are applied to the wound.

5. *Skin substitutes* are engineered products that aid in the temporary or permanent closure of various types of wounds.

   Surgical Management

- Surgical management includes removal of necrotic tissue (surgical débridement) and skin grafting or use of muscle flaps to close wounds that cannot heal by epithelialization and contraction.

PREVENTING INFECTION AND WOUND DETERIORATION

- Priority nursing interventions focus on preventing wound infections and promoting progression to complete wound healing.
   1. Monitor the ulcer's appearance using objective criteria.
   2. Re-evaluate the treatment plan if an ulcer worsens or shows no progress toward healing within 7 to 10 days.
   3. Check for manifestations of wound infection.
      a. Pain, tenderness, and redness at the wound margins
      b. Purulent and malodorous drainage
      c. Increased size or depth of the wound
      d. Changes in the color or texture of the granulation tissue

Care Coordination and Transition Management

- Have the patient or family member demonstrate a dressing change successfully before discharge from acute or home health care.
- Teach the patient and family that most dressing supplies and pressure-relief devices can be obtained at a pharmacy or medical supply store.
- If débridement is needed, a handheld shower or forceful irrigation with a 35-mL syringe can be used.
- Frequent rest periods with leg elevation may be needed to reduce peripheral edema and promote healing.
- Explain the manifestations of wound infection, and remind the patient and family to report these to the primary health care provider or wound care clinic.
- Work with the social worker or case manager to obtain special beds or mattress overlays for the home and assistance for complex care.
- Ensure an accurate hand-off to home care services regarding the wound description and plan for management.
- Encourage the patient to eat a balanced diet with frequent high-protein snacks.
- Monitor patient weight to ensure nutrition and hydration goals are sustained.
- Emphasize the need to keep the skin of an incontinent patient clean and dry; adult absorbent underwear can wick away moisture.

- Make referrals for home care nursing visits, if needed, to monitor wound progress or provide assistance with activity or rehabilitation.

PROLAPSE, PELVIC ORGAN

OVERVIEW

- The pelvic organs are supported by a sling of muscles and tendons, which sometimes become weak and are no longer able to hold an organ in place.
- *Uterine prolapse* is the downward displacement of the uterus. It can be caused by neuromuscular damage of childbirth; increased intra-abdominal pressure related to pregnancy, obesity, or physical exertion; or weakening of pelvic support due to decreased estrogen.
- A *cystocele* is a protrusion of the bladder through the vaginal wall (urinary bladder prolapse), which can lead to stress urinary incontinence (SUI) and urinary tract infections (UTIs).
- A *rectocele* is a protrusion of the rectum through a weakened vaginal wall (rectal prolapse).

INTERPROFESSIONAL COLLABORATIVE CARE

- Assessment findings include:
  1. Patient's report of feeling as if "something is falling out"
  2. Dyspareunia (painful intercourse)
  3. Backache
  4. Feeling of heaviness or pressure in the pelvis
  5. Protrusion of the cervix when the woman is asked to bear down
  6. Bowel or bladder problems, such as urinary incontinence, constipation, hemorrhoids, or fecal impaction
- Interventions are based on the degree of prolapse.
  1. Nonsurgical management may include:
     a. Teaching women to improve pelvic support and tone by pelvic floor muscle exercises (*Kegel exercises*)
     b. Using space-filling devices such as a pessary or sphere worn intravaginally to elevate the uterine prolapse
     c. Administering intravaginal estrogen therapy
     d. Promoting bladder training and attention to complete emptying
     e. Promoting bowel elimination with high-fiber diet and a stool softener or laxative
  2. Surgical management may be recommended for severe symptoms.
     a. Transvaginal repair can be completed using vaginal mesh or tape and is minimally invasive.
     b. Anterior colporrhaphy (anterior repair) tightens the pelvic muscles for better bladder support.

    c. Posterior colporrhaphy (posterior repair) reduces rectal bulging.

    d. A hysterectomy may cure uterine prolapse.

3. Nursing care is similar to that for a woman undergoing a vaginal hysterectomy (see *Surgical Management* under *Leiomyomas [Uterine Fibroids]*):

    a. Warn the patient to avoid lifting anything heavier than 5 pounds, strenuous exercises, and sexual intercourse for 6 weeks.

    b. Instruct her to notify her surgeon if she has signs of infection, such as fever, persistent pain, or purulent, foul-smelling discharge.

✦ PROSTATIC HYPERPLASIA, BENIGN: ELIMINATION CONCEPT EXEMPLAR

OVERVIEW

- When the prostate gland enlarges, it extends upward into the bladder and inward, causing bladder outlet obstruction impairing urinary ELIMINATION.

1. The patient has an increased residual urine (stasis) or acute or chronic urinary retention.

2. Increased residual urine causes overflow urinary incontinence in which the urine "leaks" around the enlarged prostate, causing dribbling.

3. Urinary stasis can result in urinary tract infections, hydroureter, hydronephrosis, bladder calculi (stones), and contribute to chronic kidney disease.

- With aging and increased dihydrotestosterone (DHT) levels, the glandular units in the prostate undergo nodular tissue hyperplasia (an increase in the number of cells).

1. Testosterone and DHT are the major androgens (male hormones) in the adult male.

2. Testosterone is produced by the testis and circulates in the blood. DHT is a testosterone derivative produced in the prostate gland.

INTERPROFESSIONAL COLLABORATIVE CARE

Assessment: Noticing

- Evaluate for presence of risk factors, including:

1. Older age
2. Family history
3. Obesity
4. Diabetes mellitus
5. Testosterone and other androgen supplements
6. Decreased physical activity

- Use a standardized tool such as the International Prostate Symptom Score (I-PSS) to determine the severity of lower urinary tract symptoms.
- Assess for and document:
  1. Current urinary patterns such as frequency, straining to begin urination, number of voids overnight (nocturia), hesitancy, force and size of urinary stream, sensation of bladder fullness after voiding, and post-void dribbling or leaking
  2. Bladder distention (by palpation or bedside ultrasound)
  3. History or finding by the provider of an enlarged prostate
  4. Psychosocial responses to symptoms or diagnosis, including anxiety, depression, or changes in sexual function
  5. Laboratory diagnostics
     a. Urinalysis or urine culture
     b. Serum prostate-specific antigen (PSA) and a serum acid phosphatase level to rule out prostate cancer
     c. Basic metabolic panel to examine kidney function (BUN and creatinine)
  6. Imaging
     a. Transabdominal ultrasound and/or transrectal ultrasound (TRUS)
     b. MRI

Analysis: Interpreting

- The priority collaborative problems for the patient with benign prostatic hypertrophy (BPH) are:
  1. Urinary retention due to bladder outlet obstruction
  2. Decreased self-esteem due to overflow incontinence and possible sexual dysfunction with or without surgery

Planning and Implementation: Responding

IMPROVE URINARY ELIMINATION

Nonsurgical Management

- "Watchful waiting" observation period with yearly examination.
- Drug therapy is usually a combination of agents from two categories:
  1. A drug to lower DHT; *5-alpha reductase inhibitors (5-ARI)*
     a. Finasteride (Proscar)
     b. Dutasteride (Avodart)

❗ NURSING SAFETY PRIORITY: Drug Alert

Remind patients who are being treated with a 5-ARI for BPH that they may need to take it for as long as 6 months before improvement is noticed. Teach them about possible side effects, which include erectile dysfunction (ED), decreased libido, and dizziness due to orthostatic hypotension. *Remind them to change positions carefully and slowly!*

2. A drug to improve urine outflow: *alpha-1 selective blocking agents*
   a. Tamsulosin (Flomax) (OTC)
   b. Alfuzosin (Uroxatral)
   c. Doxazosin (Cardura)
   d. Silodosin (Rapaflo)

! NURSING SAFETY PRIORITY: Drug Alert

If giving alpha blockers in an inpatient setting, assess for orthostatic (postural) hypotension, tachycardia, and syncope ("blackout"), especially after the first dose is given to older men. If the patient is taking the drug at home, teach him to be careful when changing position and to report any weakness, lightheadedness, or dizziness to the primary health care provider immediately. Bedtime dosing may decrease the risk for problems related to hypotension.

- Prostatic fluid can be released and obstructive symptoms reduced with frequent sexual intercourse.
- Teach the patient about ways to prevent bladder distention, such as:
  1. Avoiding drinking large amounts of fluid in a short period
  2. Avoiding alcohol, diuretics, and caffeine
  3. Voiding as soon as the urge is felt
  4. Avoiding drugs that can cause urinary retention, especially anticholinergics, antihistamines, and decongestants
- Minimally invasive techniques to reduce prostate tissue and relieve urinary symptoms include:
  1. *Transurethral needle ablation* (TUNA), in which low radiofrequency energy shrinks the prostate
  2. *Transurethral microwave therapy* (TUMT), in which high temperatures heat and destroy excess tissue
  3. *Interstitial laser coagulation* (ILC), also called *contact laser prostatectomy* (CLP), in which laser energy coagulates excess tissue
  4. *Electrovaporization of the prostate,* in which high-frequency electrical current cuts and vaporizes excess tissue
  5. *Prostatic stents,* which may be placed into the urethra to maintain permanent patency after a procedure for destroying or removing prostatic tissue
  6. *Prostate artery embolization,* when the interventional radiologist threads a small vascular catheter into the prostate's arteries and injects particles blocking some of the blood flow to shrink the prostate gland

Surgical Management
- The most common surgery for BPH is a *transurethral resection of the prostate* (TURP), in which the enlarged portion of the prostate

is cut into pieces and removed through the urethra by an endoscopic instrument. A similar procedure is the *transurethral incision of the prostate* (TIUP), in which small cuts are made into the prostate to relieve pressure on the urethra.

- Minimally invasive surgical techniques include *holmium laser enucleation of the prostate* (HoLEP), laparoscopic prostatic adenomectomy, and robotic-assisted simple prostatectomy (RASP).

- Provide preoperative care and:
  1. Correct any misconceptions about the surgery such as concerns about the automatic loss of sexual functioning or permanent incontinence.
  2. Inform the patient if he will have an indwelling bladder catheter for at least 24 hours and may have traction on the catheter.
  3. Explain that the patient will feel the urge to void while the catheter is in place.
  4. Reassure the patient that it is normal for the urine to be blood-tinged after surgery.

- Provide postoperative care and:
  1. Monitor the patient's urine output every 2 to 4 hours with vital signs.
  2. Provide aseptic continuous or intermittent urinary bladder irrigation to maintain patency as prescribed. This is typically associated with a TURP procedure.

> **! NURSING SAFETY PRIORITY: Critical Rescue**
>
> If arterial bleeding occurs, the urinary drainage is bright red or ketchup-like with numerous clots. Notify the surgeon immediately, and irrigate the catheter with normal saline solution per surgeon or hospital protocol.

  3. Monitor for severe bleeding, including serum hemoglobin and hematocrit levels, presence of hematuria, and signs of hypovolemia from blood loss in the first 24 postoperative hours.
  4. Administer antispasmodic drugs as prescribed.
  5. Keep the catheter free of obstruction and kinks; monitor for clots and sudden cessation of urine output.
  6. Instruct the patient to maintain fluid intake to keep the urine clear.

IMPROVE SELF-ESTEEM

- The patient with BPH typically has frequent urges to void and may have overflow incontinence at times due to urinary retention.
- Teach the patient to keep the surrounding area clean and dry to prevent skin breakdown.
- Remind him to toilet when he feels the urge, and if needed, wear a small absorbent pad to prevent undergarment soiling.

- Involve the patient's sexual partner, if any, in teaching about the cause of the incontinence and any prescribed treatment.

Care Coordination and Transition Management

- Following TURP, patients are typically discharged with a urinary catheter in place for about a week or longer; a catheter at discharge is not common with minimally invasive techniques.
- Teach patients not to take a bath or swim to prevent a urinary tract infection while the catheter is in place.
- When the urinary catheter is removed, the patient may experience burning on urination and some urinary frequency, dribbling, and leakage. Reassure him that these symptoms are normal and will decrease.
- Instruct him to take in fluid at 2000 to 2500 mL daily to decrease dysuria and keep the urine clear unless a comorbid disease requires fluid restriction (e.g., heart failure).
- Assist the patient and his family in finding ways to keep his clothing dry until sphincter control returns.
- Instruct him to contract and relax his sphincter frequently to re-establish urinary elimination control (pelvic floor or *Kegel* exercises).
- Teach the patient that sexual function should not be affected after surgery, but that retrograde ejaculation is possible.

PSEUDOCYST, PANCREATIC

OVERVIEW

- Pancreatic pseudocysts develop as a complication of acute and chronic pancreatitis or abdominal trauma.
- These "false cysts" do not have an epithelial lining and are encapsulated, sac-like structures that form on or surround the pancreas.
- The pancreatic wall is inflamed, vascular, and fibrotic and contains large amounts of straw-colored or dark brown viscous fluid (enzyme exudate from the pancreas).
- The pseudocyst may be palpated as an epigastric mass.
- The primary symptoms are epigastric pain radiating to the back, abdominal fullness, nausea, vomiting, and jaundice. Serum amylase and lipase levels may be elevated.
- Complications include rupture; hemorrhage; infection; obstruction of the bowel, biliary tract, or splenic vein; abscess or fistula formation; and pancreatic ascites.
- A pseudocyst may spontaneously resolve.
- Surgical intervention with internal drainage is accomplished by creating an ostomy between the pseudocyst and the stomach, jejunum, or duodenum; external drainage is provided by the insertion of a sump drainage tube to remove pancreatic exudate and secretions.

PSORIASIS
OVERVIEW
- Psoriasis is a chronic, autoimmune scaling skin disorder that has exacerbations and remissions characterized by inflammation.
- Langerhans (immune) cells in the skin activate T-lymphocytes resulting in increased cell division of keratinocytes. Normally, cells at the basement membrane of the epidermis take about 28 days to reach the outermost layer where they are shed. In a person with psoriasis, the rate of cell division is speeded up so that cells are shed every 4 to 5 days.
- Triggering factors can contribute to the onset and severity of psoriasis. These factors can be local or systemic and include trauma, sunburn, infection, hormonal changes (adolescence, aging), stress, drugs, obesity, and the comorbidity of diabetes.
- Some patients can develop a debilitating arthritis or joint deterioration.

INTERPROFESSIONAL COLLABORATIVE CARE
Assessment: Noticing
- Obtain patient information about:
  1. Any family history of psoriasis
  2. Current status
     a. Age at onset
     b. Description of the disease progression
     c. Pattern of recurrences
     d. Whether fever and itching are present
     e. Exposure to precipitating factors, including skin trauma or surgery
- Assess for and document the appearance of psoriasis and its course.
  1. *Psoriasis vulgaris* is the most common type of psoriasis.
     a. Thick, reddened papules or plaques covered by silvery white scales
     b. Sharply defined borders between the lesions and normal skin
     c. Lesions are usually present in the same areas on both sides of the body
     d. Common lesion sites are the scalp, elbows, trunk, knees, sacrum, and outside surfaces of the limbs
  2. *Exfoliative psoriasis* (erythrodermic psoriasis) has generalized erythema and scaling that do not form obvious lesions.
Interventions: Noticing
- Teach the patient about the disease and its treatment, and provide emotional support for the changes in body image often experienced with psoriasis.

- Three therapeutic approaches are used to manage psoriasis.
  1. Topical therapy includes:
     a. Corticosteroid creams or gels with warm moist dressings or occlusive wraps to enhance absorption
     b. Tar preparations applied to the skin lesions as solutions, ointments, lotions, gels, and shampoos
     c. Anthralin (Anthraforte, Drithocreme, Lasan) application alone or in combination with coal tar baths and ultraviolet (UV) light
     d. Calcipotriene (Dovonex), a synthetic form of vitamin D that regulates skin cell division
     e. Tazarotene (Tazorac), a vitamin A derivative that can cause birth defects
  2. UV radiation therapy decreases dermal growth rates.
     a. Ultraviolet B (UV-B) light therapy
     b. Ultraviolet A (UV-A) light exposure following ingestion of an oral sensitizing agent
     c. Psoralen and UV-A (PUVA) treatments involve the ingestion of a photosensitizing agent (psoralen) 2 hours before exposure to UV-A light
  3. Systemic therapy
     a. Oral vitamin A derivatives
     b. Biologic or immunologic modulating agents that contribute to immune suppression and are administered parenterally (IV, IM, or subcutaneously).
- Provide emotional support when the patient suffers because of the presence of skin lesions and the unpleasantness of some of the treatments.
  1. Encourage the patient and family members to express their feelings about having an incurable skin problem that can alter appearance and seek additional support through community-based groups.
  2. Use touch to communicate acceptance; avoid the use of gloves during an introductory handshake or other social interaction.
- Teach women of childbearing age who are taking vitamin A derivatives and immunosuppressive or immunomodulating drugs to use a reliable method of contraception because these agents can cause birth defects when taken during pregnancy.

PULMONARY ARTERIAL HYPERTENSION

OVERVIEW

- Primary pulmonary arterial hypertension (PAH) is a problem of the pulmonary blood vessel constriction in the absence of lung disease.
- Primary PAH is considered idiopathic because the causes of this life-threatening disorder are unclear, although exposure to some drugs increases the risk.

- Primary PAH is rare and occurs mostly in women between the ages of 20 and 40 years.
- Secondary PAH can occur as a complication of other lung disorders.
- As PAH increases, blood flow decreases, leading to poor lung perfusion and gas exchange. Eventually, the right side of the heart fails *(cor pulmonale)* because of the continuous workload of pumping against the high pulmonary pressures.

INTERPROFESSIONAL COLLABORATIVE CARE
Assessment: Noticing
- Assess for and document:
  1. Dyspnea and fatigue in an otherwise healthy adult
  2. Angina-like chest pain
- Diagnosis is made from the results of right-sided heart catheterization showing elevated pulmonary pressures.

Interventions: Responding
- Drug therapy can reduce pulmonary pressures and slow the development of *cor pulmonale* by dilating pulmonary vessels and preventing clot formation.
  1. Endothelin-receptor antagonists (e.g., bosentan [Traceleer]) induce blood vessel relaxation.
  2. Natural and synthetic prostacyclin agents dilate pulmonary blood vessels (e.g., epoprostenol [Flolan], treprostinil [Remodulin]).
  3. Antiplatelet agents and warfarin (anti-clotting) can decrease clot formation that occurs with vessel constriction.

❗ NURSING SAFETY PRIORITY: Critical Rescue

Although IV prostacyclin therapy is very effective, deaths have been reported if intravenous drug delivery is interrupted for even a few minutes. Teach the patient to always have backup drug cassettes and battery packs. If these are not available or the line is disrupted the patient should go to the emergency department immediately.

- Secondary pulmonary hypertension is usually managed by treating the underlying lung pathology. When lung pathology is terminal or untreatable, then management of symptoms or palliative care becomes the focus of care.
- Teach patients about the need to:
  1. Use strict aseptic technique in all aspects of manipulating the drug delivery system.
  2. Notify the pulmonologist at the first sign of any respiratory or systemic infection.

- Surgical management of PAH involves single-lung or whole-lung transplantation.
- If *cor pulmonale* also is present, the patient may need combined heart-lung transplantation.

PULMONARY CONTUSION

OVERVIEW

- Pulmonary contusion most often follows injuries caused by rapid deceleration during vehicular accidents. Hemorrhage and edema occur in and between the alveoli, decreasing lung movement and reducing the area for gas exchange.
- Respiratory failure often develops over time rather than immediately after the trauma.

INTERPROFESSIONAL COLLABORATIVE CARE

- Signs and symptoms include:
  1. Dyspnea
  2. Hypoxemia
  3. Bloody sputum
  4. Decreased breath sounds
  5. Crackles and wheezes
  6. Hazy opacity on chest x-ray in the lobes or parenchyma
- Management is aimed at maintenance of ventilation and oxygenation.
  1. Use central venous pressure (CVP) to monitor response to fluid therapy and limit overhydration.
  2. Provide oxygen therapy and mechanical ventilation with positive end-expiratory pressure (PEEP) to maintain open alveoli.
  3. Monitor the work of breathing and maintain vigilance for early detection of the onset of ARDS, a relatively common complication of extensive lung contusion.

PULMONARY EMBOLISM: GAS EXCHANGE CONCEPT EXEMPLAR

OVERVIEW

- Pulmonary embolism (PE) is a collection of particulate matter (solids, liquids, or air) that enters venous circulation and lodges in pulmonary vessels leading to reduced GAS EXCHANGE.
- Large emboli obstruct pulmonary blood flow, leading to reduced oxygenation, pulmonary tissue hypoxia, decreased perfusion, and potential death.
- Most often a PE occurs when inappropriate blood clotting forms a venous thromboembolism (VTE; deep vein thrombosis) in a leg or pelvic vein and a clot breaks off, traveling through the vena cava to the right side of the heart lodging in the pulmonary artery or one of its branches.

- The local response includes blood vessel constriction and pulmonary hypertension that impair GAS EXCHANGE and tissue perfusion.
- Major risk factors for VTE, leading to PE are:
  1. Prolonged immobility
  2. Central venous catheters
  3. Surgery (especially pelvic or leg surgery)
  4. Obesity
  5. Older age
  6. Conditions that increase blood clotting
  7. History of thromboembolism
  8. Smoking
  9. Pregnancy, estrogen therapy, amniotic fluid, and fetal debris
  10. Heart failure
  11. Cancer and circulating tumor cells
  12. Trauma/traumatic injury
  13. Fat, oil, foreign objects (broken catheters), injected particles, and septic clots that enter the vein

INTERPROFESSIONAL COLLABORATIVE CARE
Assessment: Noticing
- Obtain patient information about risk factors for VTE and PE.
- Assess for manifestations, knowing that signs and symptoms can be vague and nonspecific.
  1. Respiratory symptoms can include:
     a. Dyspnea
     b. Pleuritic chest pain (sharp, stabbing pain on inspiration)
     c. Crackles, wheezes, pleuritic rub
     d. Dry or productive cough
     e. Hemoptysis (bloody sputum)
     f. Anxiety related to hypoxia
  2. Cardiac signs and symptoms
     a. Rapid HR
     b. Distended neck veins
     c. Syncope (fainting or loss of consciousness)
     d. Cyanosis
     e. Hypotension
     f. Abnormal heart sounds, such as an S_3 or S_4
     g. ECG abnormalities (nonspecific and transient T-wave and ST-segment)

! NURSING SAFETY PRIORITY: Critical Rescue

Monitor patients at risk to recognize signs and symptoms of PE (e.g., shortness of breath, chest pain, hypotension without an obvious cause). If such symptoms are present, respond by notifying the Rapid Response Team. If PE is strongly suspected, prompt categorization and management are started before diagnostic studies have been completed.

- Diagnosis is most commonly made with chest CT scan using a PE protocol or CT angiography.
- Laboratory studies can include a metabolic panel, troponin, b-natriuretic peptide (BNP), and d-dimer (fibrin split product).

Analysis: Interpreting
- The priority collaborative problems for patients with PE include:
  1. Hypoxemia due to mismatch of lung perfusion and alveolar gas exchange with oxygenation
  2. Hypotension due to inadequate circulation to the left ventricle
  3. Potential for excessive bleeding due to anticoagulation or fibrinolytic therapy causing inadequate clotting
  4. Anxiety due to hypoxemia and life-threatening illness

Planning and Implementation: Responding
MANAGING HYPOXEMIA
- Increase gas exchange, improve lung perfusion, reduce the risk for further clot formation, and prevent complications.
  - ***Nonsurgical Management***
- Oxygen therapy
  1. Apply oxygen by nasal cannula or by mask in less severe cases.
  2. Institute intubation and mechanical ventilation for the severely hypoxemic patient.
  3. Monitor:
     a. Oxygen saturation continually
     b. Vital signs, lung sounds, and cardiac status hourly
  4. Assess for and document increasing or decreasing:
     a. Dyspnea
     b. Dysrhythmias
     c. Distended neck veins
     d. Abnormal lung sounds
     e. Peripheral perfusion
- Drug therapy
  1. Anticoagulants keep the embolus from enlarging and prevent the formation of new clots.
     a. Heparin initially for 5 to 10 days, with oral anticoagulants started and overlapping with heparin around day 2 of heparin therapy.
     b. Fibrinolytic drugs

2. Review the patient's coagulation profile before therapy is started and thereafter according to facility policy.

Surgical Management

- *Embolectomy* is the surgical removal of the embolus from pulmonary blood vessels using special thrombectomy catheters that can mechanically break up clots (e.g., AngioJet).
- *Inferior vena cava filtration* with placement of a retrievable vena cava device prevents further emboli from reaching the lungs in some patients with ongoing risk for PE.

MANAGING HYPOTENSION

- Hypotension is related to inadequate circulation to the left ventricle and/or reduced circulation from bleeding due to anticoagulant or antifibrinolytic therapy.
- IV fluid therapy involves giving crystalloid solutions to restore plasma volume and prevent shock.
- Drug therapy with vasopressors is used when hypotension persists despite fluid resuscitation. Common IV agents are norepinephrine, epinephrine, and dopamine.
  1. Continuously monitor:
     a. Pulse rate and blood pressure to achieve normal values
     b. Urine output to at least 0.5 to 1.0 mL/kg/hour

MINIMIZING BLEEDING

- Monitor the patient's response to anticoagulant and antifibrinolytic therapy to reduce the risk for unintended hemorrhage from excess anticoagulation or recurrent clot formation from inadequate anticoagulation therapy.
  1. Inspect skin and mucous membranes for bleeding and petechiae.
  2. Assess hemoglobin, hematocrit, platelets, and coagulation test results; maintain values in safe range.
  3. Examine stools, urine, drainage, and vomit for gross blood and test for occult blood in hemoglobin drops.

MINIMIZING ANXIETY

- Provide oxygen therapy and monitor patient response.
- Communicate to allay fears; speak calmly while sharing the plan or rationale for interventions.
- Acknowledge the patient's perception of a life-threatening situation.
- Identify and use supportive coping strategies.
- Drug therapy with an antianxiety drug may be prescribed if the patient's anxiety prevents adequate oxygenation and rest.

Care Coordination and Transition Management

- The patient with PE is discharged after hypoxemia and hemodynamic instability have been resolved and adequate anticoagulation has been achieved.

- Anticoagulation therapy usually continues after discharge.
- Patients with extensive lung damage may have reduced activity tolerance.
- Teach the patient and family about:
  1. Bleeding precautions
  2. Activities to reduce the risk for VTE
  3. Need for follow-up care

PULMONARY EMPYEMA

P

OVERVIEW

- Pulmonary empyema is a collection of pus in the pleural space; the fluid is thick, opaque, exudative, and foul smelling.
- The most common cause is pulmonary infection (pneumonia), lung abscess, or infected pleural effusion that can spread across the pleura, obstructing lymph nodes and leading to a retrograde (backward) flood of infected lymph into the pleural space.
- Other causes include liver or abdominal abscesses that spread infection through the lymphatic system into the lung area, thoracic surgery, and chest trauma.

INTERPROFESSIONAL COLLABORATIVE CARE

Assessment: Noticing

- Obtain patient information about:
  1. Recent febrile illness (including pneumonia)
  2. Chest pain
  3. Dyspnea
  4. Cough and sputum
  5. Chest trauma
  6. Fever, chills, night sweats
- Assess for and document:
  1. Reduced chest wall motion
  2. Decreased or abnormal breath sounds
  3. Dyspnea, labored breathing, or tachypnea
  4. Weight loss
  5. Hypotension
  6. Hypoxia, decreased SpO_2
- Diagnosis is made by chest x-ray and analysis of pleural fluid is obtained by thoracentesis.

Interventions: Responding

- Therapy for empyema is focused on emptying the empyema cavity, re-expanding the lung, and controlling the infection.
- Antibiotics that are appropriate for the identified organism are prescribed.
- Closed–chest drainage is used to promote lung expansion.

- Open thoracotomy and removal of a portion of the pleura may be needed for thick pus or marked pleural thickening.
- Nursing care is the same as for patients with a pleural effusion, pneumothorax, or infection.

PYELONEPHRITIS: ELIMINATION CONCEPT EXEMPLAR

OVERVIEW
- Pyelonephritis is a bacterial infection of the kidney and renal pelvis and interferes with urinary ELIMINATION.
- Pyelonephritis can be acute or chronic.
  1. Acute pyelonephritis is an active bacterial infection.
  2. Chronic pyelonephritis results from repeated or continued upper UTIs, usually in patients with anatomic abnormalities of the urinary tract, urinary stasis, or obstruction with reflux.

INTERPROFESSIONAL COLLABORATIVE CARE
Assessment: Noticing
- Obtain patient information about:
  1. History of urinary tract and kidney infections
  2. History of diabetes mellitus or other conditions associated with immunocompromise
  3. History of stone disease or other structural or functional abnormalities of the genitourinary tract
- Assess for:
  1. Pregnancy because pyelonephritis is associated with early onset of labor, compromising fetal health
  2. Flank or abdominal discomfort
  3. Hematuria, cloudy urine
  4. Systemic signs of infection: general malaise, fever, chills
  5. Asymmetry, edema, or erythema at the costovertebral angle
  6. Presence of leukoesterase, nitrogen, WBCs, or bacteria in the urine
- Diagnostic testing may include:
  1. Urinalysis and urine for culture and sensitivity
  2. WBC count with differential, basic metabolic panel for kidney function
  3. X-ray, CT, or cystourethrogram to diagnose stones or obstruction. *Ensure that the patient is not pregnant before any imaging study is performed.*

Analysis: Interpreting
- The priority collaborative problems for the patient with pyelonephritis are:
  1. Pain (flank and abdominal) due to inflammation and infection
  2. Potential for chronic kidney disease (CKD) due to kidney tissue destruction

Planning and Implementation: Responding

MANAGING PAIN

Nonsurgical Interventions

- Acetaminophen is preferred over NSAIDs because it does not interfere with kidney autoregulation of blood flow.
- Prevent CKD and progression of acute kidney injury.
  1. Administer antibiotics. Drug therapy begins with broad-spectrum antibiotics. With urine and blood culture sensitivity results, a narrow-spectrum antibiotic may be ordered.
  2. Maintain sufficient perfusion to the kidneys (a typical goal is mean arterial pressure > 65 mm Hg) to prevent hypotensive or hypertensive kidney injury.
  3. Maintain sufficient fluid intake to promote urine output greater than 1 mL/kg/hr.
  4. Assess for signs of acute kidney injury, such as increasing BUN or creatinine level or decreased urinary output.
  5. For the patient with a chronic need for indwelling urinary catheter, replace the catheter and closed drainage system to reduce bioburden.

Surgical Procedures

1. Pyelolithotomy (removal of a stone from the renal pelvis)
2. Nephrectomy (removal of a kidney)
3. Ureteral diversion or reimplantation of the ureter to restore the bladder drainage mechanism

PREVENTING CHRONIC KIDNEY DISEASE

- Specific antibiotics are prescribed to treat the infection.
  1. Stress the importance of completing drug therapy as directed.
- Stress regular follow-up examinations.
- Monitor BP carefully because blood pressure control slows the progression of kidney dysfunction.
- Encourage the patient to drink sufficient fluid to prevent dehydration, which can reduce kidney function.

Care Coordination and Transition Management

- Health teaching includes:
  1. Information about pyelonephritis, its causes, and therapy
  2. Antibiotic self-administration including effects, side effects, and importance of following the prescribed duration of therapy
  3. Planning and implementing healthy choices for fluid intake
  4. Describing the plan for post-treatment follow-up, including knowledge of recurrent symptoms
  5. Management of an indwelling urinary catheter if needed for a chronic condition or following a surgical intervention

R

RAYNAUD'S PHENOMENON AND RAYNAUD'S DISEASE

OVERVIEW

- *Raynaud's phenomenon* is caused by vasospasm of the arterioles and arteries of the upper and lower extremities, usually unilaterally.
- *Raynaud's disease* occurs bilaterally. It is more common in women and occurs between the ages of 17 and 50 years.
- The pathophysiology is the same for both entities: vasospasm of the arterioles and arteries of the upper and lower extremities.
- Cutaneous vessels are constricted, causing blanching of the extremities followed by cyanosis.
- When the vasospasm is relieved, the tissue becomes reddened or hyperemic.
- Patients often have an associated systemic connective tissue disease (CTD) such as systemic lupus erythematosus (SLE) or progressive systemic sclerosis.

INTERPROFESSIONAL COLLABORATIVE CARE

- Assess for:
  1. Color changes in the extremity or digits, ranging from blanched to reddened to cyanotic
  2. Numbness of the extremity or digits
  3. Coldness of the extremity or digits
  4. Pain
  5. Swelling
  6. Ulcerations
  7. Aggravation of symptoms by cold or stress
  8. Gangrene of digits in severe cases
- Interventions include:
  1. Drug therapy to prevent vasoconstriction, including calcium channel blockers
  2. Lumbar sympathectomy to relieve severe symptoms in the feet
  3. Sympathetic ganglionectomy to relieve severe symptoms in the upper extremities
- Health teaching emphasizes methods to minimize vasoconstriction.
  1. Smoking cessation and caffeine reduction
  2. Minimizing exposure to cold by wearing warm clothes, socks, and gloves and maintaining a warm indoor ambient temperature
  3. Stress management

RESPIRATORY FAILURE, ACUTE

OVERVIEW

* Acute respiratory failure can be defined in three ways, based on the underlying problem.
  1. *Ventilatory failure* occurs when air movement into/out of the lungs is inadequate. As a result, too little oxygen reaches the alveoli and carbon dioxide is retained. Problems include respiratory center depression (e.g., sedation, anesthesia, opioid overdose, brain damage), a lung problem (e.g., adult respiratory distress syndrome, severe pneumonia), or poor function of respiratory muscles (e.g., chronic degenerative neurologic disorders like amyotrophic lateral syndrome [ALS] or diaphragmatic injury). In addition to reduced arterial oxygen, this type of acute respiratory failure is characterized by significant hypercarbia ($Paco_2$ greater than 50 mm Hg) and acidemia (pH less than 7.35).
  2. *Oxygenation failure* is a problem in which air moves in and out of lungs without difficulty but does not oxygenate the pulmonary blood sufficiently. Generally, lung blood flow (PERFUSION) is decreased. Problems leading to this type of failure include impaired diffusion of oxygen at the alveolar level (e.g., lung fibrosis), right-to-left shunting of blood in the pulmonary vessels (e.g., atelectasis), and failure of hemoglobin to bind oxygen (e.g., inherited hemoglobin disorders, carbon monoxide poisoning).
  3. *Combined ventilatory and oxygenation failure* involves hypoventilation and impairment of oxygenation at the alveolar-capillary membrane. This type of respiratory failure leads to a more profound hypoxemia than either ventilatory failure or oxygenation failure alone. It is seen in patients who have abnormal lungs (chronic bronchitis, emphysema, or during asthma attacks) and in patients who have both cardiac failure and respiratory disease.
* Regardless of the underlying cause, the patient in acute respiratory failure is always hypoxemic.

INTERPROFESSIONAL COLLABORATIVE CARE

Assessment: Noticing

* Assess for and document:
  1. Dyspnea (the hallmark of respiratory failure)
  2. Changes in the respiratory rate or pattern
  3. Abnormal lung sounds
  4. Manifestations of hypoxemia
     a. Pallor or cyanosis
     b. Tachypnea
     c. Restlessness, anxiety, or confusion

R

5. Hypoxia (arterial oxygen levels [Pao_2], 60 mm Hg or peripheral oxygenation [Spo_2]) less than 90%
6. Hypercarbia (arterial carbon dioxide levels [$Paco_2$] or end-tidal CO_2 [$EtCO2$]) levels greater than 45 mm Hg) with acidemia (pH less than 7.35)

Interventions: Responding

- Management of acute respiratory failure of any origin includes:
  1. Applying oxygen therapy to keep the Spo_2 92% or greater and Pao_2 greater than 60 mm Hg. These values may be modified if the patient has a lung condition like chronic obstructive pulmonary disease (COPD).
  2. Implementing invasive or noninvasive mechanical ventilation if other measures do not increase oxygenation
  3. Reducing hypercarbia to patient baseline. Patients with chronic respiratory conditions that include carbon dioxide retention may have a baseline $Paco_2$ greater than 45 mm Hg.
  4. Assisting the patient to find a position of comfort that allows easier breathing, usually a more upright position
  5. Assisting the patient to use relaxation, diversion, and guided imagery to reduce anxiety
  6. Instituting energy-conserving measures of minimal self-care and no unnecessary procedures
  7. Administering drug therapy given systemically or by metered dose inhaler (MDI) to resolve bronchoconstriction contributing to poor air exchange
  8. Encouraging deep-breathing techniques or incentive spirometer use to increase oxygen intake or reduce carbon dioxide retention

REHABILITATION NURSING CARE

OVERVIEW

- Rehabilitation is a philosophy of practice and an attitude toward caring for people with disabilities and chronic health problems.
  1. A *disabling health condition* is any physical or mental health/behavioral health problem that can cause disability.
  2. A *chronic health condition* is one that has existed for at least 3 months.
- Patients with chronic and disabling health conditions need the integration of rehabilitation nursing concepts into their care, regardless of setting, to prevent further disability, maintain function, and restore individuals to optimal functioning in their community. This desired outcome requires care coordination and collaboration with the interprofessional health care team.
- Rehabilitation care occurs on a continuum.
- Services decrease across the continuum from the inpatient rehabilitation facility (IRF) or skilled nursing facility (SNF) to home health to outpatient ambulatory programs,

Veterans' Health Considerations

Patient-Centered Care and Health Care Disparities

Combat in war is another major source of major disability. Many military men and women who served in recent wars such as those in Iraq and Afghanistan have one or more physical or mental health disabilities, most commonly traumatic brain injury (TBI), single or multiple limb amputations, and post-traumatic stress disorder (PTSD). There is also a large population of veterans living with disabilities from wars of the past. These disabilities require months to years of follow-up rehabilitation after returning to the community.

Rehabilitation nurses in the inpatient setting coordinate the collaborative plan of care and function as the patient's case manager. Nurses also create a rehabilitation milieu, which includes:

* Allowing time for patients to practice self-management skills
* Encouraging patients and providing emotional support
* Protecting patients from embarrassment (e.g., bowel training)
* Making the inpatient unit a more homelike environment

In addition to the patient, family, and/or significant others, members of the interprofessional health care team in the rehabilitation setting include:

* Nurses and nursing assistants
* Rehabilitation nurse case managers
* Physicians and physicians' assistants
* Advanced practice nurses (APNs), such as nurse practitioners and clinical nurse specialists
* Physical therapists and assistants
* Occupational therapists and assistants
* Speech-language pathologists and assistants
* Rehabilitation assistants/restorative aides
* Recreational or activity therapists
* Cognitive therapists or neuropsychologists
* Social workers
* Clinical psychologists
* Vocational counselors
* Spiritual care counselors
* Registered dietitians (RDs)
* Pharmacists

INTERPROFESSIONAL COLLABORATIVE CARE

Assessment: Noticing

* An essential component of rehabilitation assessment and evaluation is the assessment of functional ability.
    1. *Functional ability* refers to the ability to perform **activities of daily living (ADLs),** such as bathing, dressing, eating, using the toilet, and ambulating.

2. **Instrumental activities of daily living (IADLs)** refer to activities necessary for living in the community, such as using the telephone, shopping, preparing food, and housekeeping. Functional assessment tools are used to assess a patient's abilities.

Chart 2-19 Assessment of Patients in Rehabilitation Settings	
Body System	**Relevant Data**
Cardiovascular system	Chest pain
	Fatigue
	Fear of heart failure
Respiratory system	Shortness of breath or dyspnea
	Activity tolerance
	Fear of inability to breathe
Gastrointestinal system and nutrition	Oral intake, eating pattern
	Anorexia, nausea, and vomiting
	Dysphagia
	Laboratory data (e.g., serum prealbumin level)
	Weight loss or gain
	Bowel elimination pattern or habits
	Change in stool (constipation or diarrhea)
	Ability to get to toilet
Renal-urinary system	Urinary pattern
	Fluid intake
	Urinary incontinence or retention
	Urine culture and urinalysis
Neurologic system	Motor function
	Sensation
	Perceptual ability
	Cognitive abilities
Musculoskeletal system	Functional ability
	Range of motion
	Endurance
	Muscle strength
Integumentary system	Risk for skin breakdown
	Presence of skin lesions

Considerations for Older Adults

Patient-Centered Care

Older adults who need rehabilitation often have other chronic diseases that need to be managed, including diabetes mellitus, coronary artery disease, osteoporosis, and arthritis. These health problems, added to the normal physiologic changes associated with aging, predispose older adults to secondary complications such as falls, pressure injuries, and pneumonia. When discharged from the acute care setting, some older patients are undernourished, which causes weakness and fatigue. The longer the hospital stay, the more debilitated the older adult can become. For some patients severe undernutrition results in decreased serum albumin and prealbumin, causing third spacing. Assess the older adult for generalized edema, especially in the lower extremities. Be sure to collaborate with the RD to improve the patient's nutritional status, with a focus on increasing protein intake that is needed for healing and decreasing edema.

Health teaching may be challenging because some older patients may have beginning changes in COGNITION, including short-term memory loss. Sensory loss, like vision and hearing, may also affect their ability to give an accurate history or grasp new information.

R

Analysis: Interpreting
- Regardless of age or specific disability, these priority patient problems are common. Additional problems depend on the patient's specific chronic condition or disability. The priority collaborative problems for patients with chronic and disabling health conditions typically include:
  1. Decreased mobility related to neuromuscular impairment, sensory-perceptual impairment, and/or chronic pain
  2. Decreased functional ability related to neuromuscular impairment and/or impairment in perception or cognition
  3. Risk for pressure injury related to altered sensation and/or altered nutritional state
  4. Urinary incontinence or urinary retention related to neurologic dysfunction and/or trauma or disease
  5. Constipation related to neurologic impairment, inadequate nutrition, or decreased mobility

Planning and Implementation: Responding
INCREASING MOBILITY
- Most problems requiring rehabilitation relate to decreased or impaired mobility.
- Before assisting patients with mobility nurses must understand the importance of safe patient handling and mobility practices (SPHM).
  1. Maintain a wide, stable base with your feet.
  2. Put the bed at the correct height—waist level while providing direct care, and hip level when moving patients.
  3. Keep the patient or work directly in front of you to prevent your spine from rotating.
  4. Keep the patient as close to your body as possible to prevent reaching.

- Encourage the patient to be as independent as possible when performing ADLs and safe mobility skills.
- Collaborate with rehabilitation therapists to teach patients how to transfer, increase bed mobility, and gait training techniques.
- In collaboration with the rehabilitation therapists, evaluate the ability of patients to use assistive/adaptive devices to promote independence.
- Prevent complications of immobility for patients and teach them how to avoid complications (e.g., pressure ulcers, urinary calculi, venous thromboembolism [VTE]).
- Use SPHM practices, as well as using mechanical lifts and working with other team members, when assessing and moving patients to prevent injury and improve mobility.

INCREASING FUNCTIONAL ABILITY
- ADLs, or self-care activities, include eating, bathing, dressing, grooming, and toileting.
  1. Encourage the patient to perform as much self-care as possible.
  2. Collaborate with the occupational therapist (OT) to identify ways in which self-care activities can be modified so the patient can perform them as independently as possible and with minimal frustration.
  3. Most facilities have developed restorative nursing programs and have coordinated these programs with rehabilitation therapy and activities therapy.
  4. A variety of devices are available for patients with chronic conditions and disabilities for assisting with self-care (Chart 2-20).

PREVENTING PRESSURE INJURY
- The best intervention to prevent pressure injury and maintain tissue integrity is frequent position changes in combination with adequate skin care and sufficient nutritional intake.
  1. Teach staff to assist with turning and repositioning at least every 2 hours if the patient is unable to reposition independently.
  2. Patients who sit for prolonged periods in a wheelchair need to be repositioned at least every 1 to 2 hours.
  3. Adequate skin care is an essential component of prevention.
     a. If a patient is incontinent, use topical barrier creams or ointments to help protect the skin from moisture.
  4. Use pressure-relieving devices and adequate nutrition to prevent new skin breakdown.

ESTABLISHING URINARY CONTINENCE
- Neurologic disabilities often interfere with successful bladder control. These disabilities result in two basic functional types of neurogenic bladder: overactive (e.g., reflex or spastic bladder) and underactive (e.g., hypotonic or flaccid bladder).
  1. *Overactive bladder* causes incontinence with sudden voiding.

| Chart 2-20 | Examples and Uses of Common Assistive/Adaptive Devices |

Device	Use
Buttonhook	Threaded through the buttonhole to enable patients with weak finger mobility to button shirts
	Alternative uses include serving as pencil holder or cigarette holder
Extended shoehorn	Assists in the application of shoes for patients with decreased mobility
	Alternative uses include turning light switches off or on while patient is in a wheelchair
Plate guard and spork (spoon and fork in one utensil)	Applied to a plate to assist patients with weak hand and arm mobility to feed themselves; spork allows one utensil to serve two purposes
Gel pad	Placed under a plate or a glass to prevent dishes from slipping and moving
	Alternative uses include placement under bathing and grooming items to prevent them from moving
Foam buildups	Applied to eating utensils to assist patients with weak hand grasps to feed themselves
	Alternative uses include application to pens and pencils to assist with writing or over a buttonhook to assist with grasping the device
Hook and loop fastener (Velcro) straps	Applied to utensils, a buttonhook, or a pencil to slip over the hand and provide a method of stabilizing the device when the patient's hand grasp is weak
Long-handled reacher	Assists in obtaining items located on high shelves or at ground level for patients who are unable to change positions easily
Elastic shoelaces or Velcro shoe closure	Eliminates the need for tying shoes

2. *Underactive bladder* causes urinary retention and overflow (dribbling).
- Teach bladder management techniques, including triggering techniques, intermittent catheterization, and consistent toileting (timed voiding).
- Mild overactive bladder may be treated with antispasmodics such as oxybutynin (Ditropan XL, Apo-Oxybutynin), solifenacin (VESIcare), or tolterodine (Detrol LA).

Considerations for Older Adults

Patient-Centered Care

When urinary antispasmodic drugs are used in older adults, observe for, document, and report hallucinations, delirium, or other acute cognitive changes caused by the anticholinergic effects of the drugs.

ESTABLISHING BOWEL CONTINENCE
- Neurologic problems often affect the patient's bowel pattern by causing a reflex (spastic) bowel, a flaccid bowel, or an uninhibited bowel.
  1. Establish a bowel retraining program with adequate fluid intake, a consistent toileting schedule, dietary modification, time for bowel evacuation, and, if needed, drug therapy such as a laxative (bisacodyl [Dulcolax]) or stool softener.
  2. Collaborate with patients with a chronic condition to schedule bowel elimination as close as possible to their previous routine.

Considerations for Older Adults

Many rehabilitation patients are at high risk for constipation, especially older adults. Encourage fluids (at least 8 glasses a day) and 20 to 35 g of fiber in the diet. Teach patients to eat two to three daily servings of whole grains, legumes, and bran cereals, and five daily servings of fruits and vegetables. Do not offer a bedpan when toileting. Instead, be sure that the patient sits upright on a bedside commode or bathroom toilet to facilitate defecation.

Care Coordination and Transition Management
- Care coordination and transition management begin at the time of the patient's admission. If the patient is transferred from a hospital to an IRF or SNF, orient him or her to the change in routine and emphasize the importance of self-care. When the patient is admitted, a case manager and/or OT/PT should assess his or her current living situation at home.
  1. Before discharge, the home must be assessed to ensure accessibility for the patient, given a new mobility impairment. If a patient will use a wheelchair after discharge, the patient may need home modifications.
  2. The OT and PT should teach the patient to perform ADLs independently.

3. After discharge to the home, various health care resources (e.g., physical therapy, home care nursing, vocational counseling) are available to the patient with chronic conditions and disabilities.
4. Assess the need for additional care and support throughout the hospitalization and coordinate with the case manager and health care provider in arranging for home services.

RETINAL HOLES, TEARS, AND DETACHMENTS
OVERVIEW
* A *retinal hole* is a break in the retina, usually caused by trauma or aging.
* A *retinal tear* is a jagged and irregularly shaped break, often caused by traction on the retina.
* A *retinal detachment* is the separation of the retina from the epithelium. Detachments are classified by the nature of their development.

INTERPROFESSIONAL COLLABORATIVE CARE
Assessment: Noticing
* Subjective manifestations are sudden:
  1. Bright flashes of light *(photopsia)* or floating dark spots in the affected eye
  2. The sensation of a curtain being pulled over part of the visual field
  3. No pain
* Ophthalmoscopic manifestations
  1. Gray bulges or folds in the retina that quiver
  2. Possibly a hole or tear at the edge of the detachment
Interventions: Noticing
* For detachment, surgical repair is needed to place the retina in contact with the underlying structures. A common repair procedure is scleral buckling.
  1. Preoperative care includes applying prescribed topical drugs to inhibit pupil constriction and accommodation and allaying fears about visual loss.
  2. Standard postoperative care and:
     a. Monitor the patient's vital signs and check the eye patch and shield for any drainage.
     b. If gas or oil has been placed in the eye, teach the patient to keep his or her head in the position prescribed by the surgeon to promote reattachment.
     c. Remind the patient to avoid activities that increase intraocular pressure (IOP).
     d. Teach the patient to avoid reading, writing, and close work such as sewing during the first week after surgery because these activities cause rapid eye movements and promote detachment.

R

    e. Teach the patient the manifestations of infection and detachment (sudden reduced visual acuity, eye pain, pupil that does not respond to light by constricting) and the need to notify the provider immediately if symptoms occur.

ROTATOR CUFF INJURIES

OVERVIEW

- The function of the rotator cuff is to stabilize the head of the humerus during shoulder abduction.
- It may be injured by substantial trauma or the accumulation of many small tears related to aging, repetitive motions, or falls.

INTERPROFESSIONAL COLLABORATIVE CARE

- Symptoms include shoulder pain and the inability to achieve or maintain abduction of the arm at the shoulder.
- Conservative management involves the use of nonsteroidal anti-inflammatory drugs (NSAIDs), physical therapy, sling or immobilizer support, and ice or heat applications while the injury heals.
- Surgical cuff repair may be needed for patients who do not respond to conservative treatment over a 3- to 6-month period and for those who have a complete tear.

S

SARCOIDOSIS

OVERVIEW

- Sarcoidosis is a granulomatous disorder of unknown cause that can affect any organ, especially the lung.
- It develops over time as an autoimmune disorder in which the normally protective T-lymphocytes increase and cause damaging actions in lung tissue.
- Alveolar inflammation (alveolitis) results from the presence of immune cells in the alveoli and the chronic inflammation causes fibrosis that reduces lung compliance (elasticity) and the ability to exchange gases.
- *Cor pulmonale* (right-sided cardiac failure) is often present because the heart can no longer pump effectively against the stiff, fibrotic lung.
- The disease usually affects young adults.
- Manifestations include enlarged lymph nodes in the hilar area of the lungs, lung infiltrate on chest x-ray, skin lesions, eye lesions, cough, dyspnea, hemoptysis, and chest discomfort.

- The disease may resolve permanently or may lead to progressive pulmonary fibrosis and severe systemic disease.
- The goal of therapy is to lessen symptoms and prevent fibrosis and includes immunomodulation drugs such as corticosteroids and cytokine mediators.

SEIZURE DISORDERS
OVERVIEW
- A seizure is an abnormal, sudden, excessive, uncontrolled electrical discharge of neurons within the brain that may result in alterations in consciousness, motor or sensory ability, or behavior.
- Epilepsy is defined as two or more seizures experienced by a person.
- Three major categories and associated subclasses of seizures are:
  1. *Generalized seizures* that involve both cerebral hemispheres
     a. *Tonic-clonic seizure* (formerly called a *grand mal seizure*) is characterized by stiffening or rigidity of the muscles (tonic phase), followed by rhythmic jerking of the extremities (clonic phase). Immediate unconsciousness occurs, and the patient may be incontinent of urine or feces and may bite his or her tongue.
     b. *Clonic* seizures last several minutes and cause muscle contraction and relaxation.
     c. *Tonic* seizures are characterized by stiffening of the muscles, loss of consciousness, and autonomic changes lasting 30 seconds to several minutes.
     d. The *myoclonic seizure* causes a brief jerking or stiffening of the extremities that may occur singly or in groups. Lasting for just a few seconds, the contractions may be symmetric (both sides) or asymmetric (one side).
     e. In an *atonic (akinetic) seizure,* the patient has a sudden loss of muscle tone, lasting for seconds, followed by **postictal** (after the seizure) confusion. In most cases, these seizures cause the patient to fall, which may result in injury. This type of seizure tends to be most resistant to drug therapy.
  2. Partial (also called *focal* or *local*) seizures that begin in one cerebral hemisphere
     a. The patient with a *simple partial seizure* remains conscious throughout the episode.
        (1) An **aura** (unusual sensation) may occur before the seizure takes place. Such as a "déjà vu" (already seen) phenomenon, perception of an offensive smell, or sudden onset of pain.
        (2) During the seizure, the patient may have one-sided movement of an extremity, experience unusual sensations, or have autonomic symptoms. Autonomic

S

changes include a change in heart rate, skin flushing, and epigastric discomfort.

b. *Complex partial seizures* may cause loss of consciousness (**syncope**), or "black out," for 1 to 3 minutes.

(1) Characteristic automatisms (e.g., lip smacking, patting) may occur as in absence seizures. The patient is unaware of the environment and may wander at the start of the seizure. In the period after the seizure, he or she may have **amnesia** (loss of memory).

(2) Because the area of the brain most often involved in this type of epilepsy is the temporal lobe, complex partial seizures are often called *psychomotor* seizures or *temporal lobe* seizures.

3. **Unclassified,** or **idiopathic, seizures** account for about half of all seizure activity. They occur for no known reason and do not fit into the generalized or partial classifications.

- *Status epilepticus* is a seizure that lasts longer than 10 minutes or repeated seizures over the course of 30 minutes. It is a neurologic emergency and must be treated promptly, or brain damage and possibly death from anoxia, cardiac dysrhythmias, or lactic acidosis may occur. The most common cause is abrupt or sustained cessation of antiepileptic drugs in a person with a diagnosed seizure disorder.

- Seizures caused by head injury, substance abuse, high fever, metabolic disorders, or electrolyte derangements are not considered epilepsy.

- Genetic, structural, and metabolic abnormalities contribute to seizure occurrence.

Considerations for Older Adults

Complex partial seizures are most common among older adults. These seizures are difficult to diagnose because symptoms appear similar to dementia, psychosis, or other neurobehavioral disorders, especially in the postictal stage (after the seizure). New-onset seizures in older adults are typically associated with conditions such as hypertension, cardiac disease, diabetes mellitus, stroke, dementia, and recent brain injury.

INTERPROFESSIONAL COLLABORATIVE CARE
Assessment: Noticing

- Obtain patient information about:
  1. Frequency, duration, and pattern of occurrence for seizure activity

2. Description of preictal symptoms and postictal activity (aura, motor activity, sequence of progression, eye signs, consciousness, respiratory patterns) and events surrounding the seizure
3. Current drugs, including dosage, frequency of administration, and the time at which the drug was last taken
4. Compliance with the antiepileptic drug schedule and reasons for noncompliance, if a diagnosis of epilepsy has been made

• Note whether an observed seizure is new (first occurrence) or recurrent. Seizures occurring in greater intensity, number, or length than the patient's usual seizures are considered *acute*. New or acute seizures may also appear in clusters that are different from the patient's typical seizure pattern.

Interventions: Responding

NONSURGICAL MANAGEMENT

• Administer antiepileptic drugs and monitor the patient's response with serum levels for effectiveness. Anticipate multiple drug-drug interactions with antiepileptic drugs and other medications.
• When providing care for the patient during a seizure:
  1. Protect the patient from injury by removing environmental hazards.
  2. Do not force anything into the patient's mouth.
  3. Turn the patient to the side.
  4. Loosen any restrictive clothing.
  5. Maintain the airway, and suction as needed.
  6. Do not restrain the patient; rather, guide the patient's movements.
  7. Document onset and cessation of seizure activity: date, time, and duration.
  8. Report sequence and type of movement and whether more than one activity occurs to the neurologist.
  9. At the completion of the seizure:
     a. Take vital signs.
     b. Perform neurologic assessment.
     c. Allow the patient to rest.
• Drug therapy is the major component of management; the health care provider introduces one anticonvulsant at a time to achieve seizure control.
  1. Serum drug levels are monitored for the first 3 days after the start of anticonvulsants and thereafter as needed.
  2. An initial or sustained seizure may be managed with intravenous (IV) lorazepam (Ativan, Apo-Lorazepam) or possibly diazepam (Valium) to stop motor movement, followed by phenytoin (Dilantin) or fosphenytoin (Cerebyx) to prevent recurrence. General anesthesia may be used as a last resort to stop the seizure activity.

> **! NURSING SAFETY PRIORITY: Critical Rescue**
>
> Convulsive status epilepticus must be treated promptly and aggressively! Establish an airway and notify the health care provider or Rapid Response Team immediately if this problem occurs! Establishing an airway is the priority for this patient's care. Intubation by an anesthesia provider or respiratory therapist may be necessary. Administer oxygen as indicated by the patient's condition. If not already in place, establish IV access with a large-bore catheter, and start 0.9% sodium chloride. The patient is usually placed in the intensive care unit for continuous monitoring and management.

- Follow agency policy for the implementation of seizure precautions.
  1. Keep oxygen, suctioning equipment, and an airway available at the bedside.
  2. Maintain IV access (a saline lock) for patients at risk for tonic-clonic seizures.
  3. Padded tongue blades do not belong at the bedside; nothing should be inserted into the patient's mouth after a seizure begins.
  4. Keep the bed in the low position. Use of padded side rails is controversial; side rails are rarely the source of significant injury and the use of padded side rails may embarrass the patient and family.
  5. Notify the health care provider immediately.

> **! NURSING SAFETY PRIORITY: Critical Rescue**
>
> Ensure that oxygen and suction are available at the bedside of any patient who is at risk for seizure activity. Maintaining oxygen/gas exchange can prevent brain injury during a seizure.

SURGICAL MANAGEMENT
- Several procedures may be performed when traditional methods fail to maintain seizure control.
  1. Vagal nerve stimulation involves surgically implanting a vagal nerve–stimulating device below the left clavicle to control partial seizures.
  2. Conventional surgical procedures include a craniectomy and removal of the area of the brain if vital areas of the brain will not be affected.

3. A partial corpus callosotomy involves severing the corpus callosum to prevent neuronal discharges from passing through the two hemispheres of the brain. It is used to treat tonic-clonic or atonic seizures.

- Routine perioperative care, with the addition of assessing neurologic status with vital signs postoperatively

Care Coordination and Transition Management

- Promote self-management with education for patient and family.
    1. Emphasize the importance of taking all drugs consistently as prescribed (even if seizures have stopped) and monitoring for effects and side effects; dosage or effectiveness may change over time or with the occurrence of comorbid conditions.
    2. Explain the great risk of drug-drug and drug-herb interactions with most anticonvulsant drugs; advise not to add drugs to health care without notifying the health care provider.
    3. Review components of a balanced diet and that alcohol should be avoided.
    4. Discuss the role of rest, time management, and stress management in health promotion.
    5. Explore the utility of keeping a seizure diary to determine whether there are factors that tend to be associated with seizure activity.
    6. Review restrictions (if any), such as driving or operating dangerous equipment and participating in certain physical activities or sports.
    7. Teach the value of follow-up visits with the health care provider.
    8. Offer information about a medical alert bracelet or necklace.
- Inform the patient that state laws prohibit discrimination against people who have epilepsy.
- Refer the patient to the state Vocational Rehabilitative Services, Epilepsy Foundation of America, National Epilepsy League, National Association to Control Epilepsy, and local support groups.

 ## SHOCK, HYPOVOLEMIC: PERFUSION CONCEPT EXEMPLAR

OVERVIEW

- Shock is a widespread abnormal cellular metabolism that occurs when gas exchange with oxygenation and tissue PERFUSION are not sufficient to maintain cell function. All body organs are affected by shock.
- Any problem that impairs oxygen delivery to tissues and organs can start the condition of shock and lead to a life-threatening emergency.

- The basic problem of hypovolemic shock is a loss of vascular volume, resulting in a decreased mean arterial pressure (MAP) and, in some cases, a loss of circulating red blood cells (RBCs). The reduced MAP slows blood flow, decreasing tissue perfusion.
- Decreased tissue perfusion and oxygenation lead to anaerobic cellular metabolism, with subsequent increases in serum lactate.
- Uncorrected hypovolemic shock progresses in four stages as poor cellular oxygenation continues.
  1. *Initial stage of shock (early shock)* occurs when the patient's baseline MAP is decreased by less than 10 mm Hg. Adaptive (compensatory) mechanisms are effective at returning MAP to normal levels, and oxygenated blood flow to all vital organs is maintained. Heart and respiratory rates are increased from the patient's baseline level; peripheral vasoconstriction (slowed capillary refill, decreased pulses) are present.
  2. *Nonprogressive stage (compensatory stage)* occurs when MAP decreases by 10 to 15 mm Hg from baseline. Kidney and hormonal compensatory mechanisms are activated, triggering release of norepinephrine, epinephrine, renin, vasopressin (antidiuretic hormone [ADH]), and aldosterone. Urine output decreases and widespread vasoconstriction is present. Targeted interventions at this stage can reduce the cellular effects of hypoxic tissue damage and stop the progression of shock when the signs and symptoms (described previously) are recognized early.
  3. *Progressive stage of shock (intermediate stage)* occurs when there is a sustained decrease in MAP of more than 20 mm Hg from baseline. Compensatory mechanisms are functioning but can no longer provide adequate perfusion. There is a worsening of signs and symptoms, including a rising plasma lactate.

! NURSING SAFETY PRIORITY: Action Alert

The progressive stage of shock is a life-threatening emergency. Vital organs tolerate this situation for only a short time before developing multiple organ dysfunction syndrome (MODS) with permanent damage. Immediate interventions are needed to reverse the effects of this stage of shock. The patient's life usually can be saved if the conditions causing shock are corrected within 1 hour or less of the onset of the progressive stage. Continuously monitor vital signs, physical signs, urine output, and laboratory results and compare with earlier findings to assess therapy effectiveness and determine when therapy changes are needed.

4. *Refractory stage of shock (irreversible stage)* occurs when cell death and tissue damage results from too little oxygen reaching the tissues combined with the build-up of toxic metabolites and destructive enzymes that are not removed due to poor perfusion. The body can no longer respond effectively to interventions, and shock continues. Despite aggressive interventions, MODS occurs and death is an expected outcome.

INTERPROFESSIONAL COLLABORATIVE CARE
Assessment: Noticing

* Assess patient history for risk factors associated with hypovolemic shock (fluid intake, urine output, recent illness or trauma)
* Assess for:
  1. Cardiovascular changes
     a. Decreased cardiac output
     b. Decreased systolic blood pressure (SBP) and MAP
     c. Narrowed pulse pressure
     d. Postural hypotension (positive orthostatic blood pressure)
     e. Slow capillary refill in nail beds and reduced peripheral pulses
  2. Respiratory changes
     a. Increased respiratory rate
     b. Shallow depth of respirations
     c. Decreased Pao_2 or peripheral oxygenation (Spo_2)
  3. Neuromuscular changes
     a. Early
        (1) Anxiety and restlessness
        (2) Increased thirst
     b. Late
        (1) Lethargy to coma
        (2) Generalized muscle weakness
        (3) Sluggish pupillary response to light
     c. Kidney changes
        (1) Decreased and concentrated urine output
  4. Skin and mucous membrane changes
     a. Cool, pale, mottled, or cyanotic changes

! NURSING SAFETY PRIORITY: Action Alert

Assign a registered nurse rather than a licensed practical nurse/licensed vocational nurse (LPN/LVN) or unlicensed assistive personnel (UAP) to assess the vital signs of a patient who is at risk for or suspected of having hypovolemic shock.

Analysis: Interpreting
- The priority collaborative problems for patients with hypovolemic shock are:
  1. Hypoxia due to hypovolemia
  2. Inadequate perfusion due to active fluid volume loss and hypotension
  3. Anxiety due to potential for death and decreased cerebral perfusion
  4. Decreased cognition due to decreased cerebral perfusion

Planning and Implementation: Responding
NONSURGICAL MANAGEMENT
- The purposes of shock management are to maintain tissue gas exchange, increase vascular volume, and support compensatory mechanisms. Oxygen therapy, fluid replacement therapy, and drug therapy are useful. See Chart 2-21 for care of the patient in hypovolemic shock.
- Oxygen therapy is useful whenever shock is present. It can be delivered by mask, hood, nasal cannula, nasopharyngeal tube, endotracheal tube, or tracheostomy tube.
- IV fluid resuscitation is initiated as prescribed.
  1. Crystalloid solutions are first-line treatment and include normal saline or lactated Ringer's.
  2. If the patient is bleeding, anticipate infusing packed RBCs, plasma, plasma fractions, and clotting factors.
  3. Drug therapy is used when the patient does not respond to the replacement of fluid volume and blood products and can include intravenous vasoconstricting agents like norepinephrine (Levophed).

Chart 2-21	Best Practice for Patient Safety & Quality Care: The Patient in Hypovolemic Shock

- Ensure a patent airway.
- Insert an IV catheter or maintain an established catheter.
- Administer oxygen.
- Elevate the patient's feet, keeping his or her head flat or elevated to no more than a 30-degree angle.
- Examine the patient for overt bleeding.
- If overt bleeding is present, apply direct pressure to the site.
- Administer drugs as prescribed.
- Increase the rate of IV fluid delivery.
- Do not leave the patient.

- Additional nursing interventions include assessing the patient's response to therapy.
  1. Until shock is controlled, monitor the following every 15 to 60 minutes:
     a. Blood pressure, pulse pressure, and MAP
     b. Heart rate and pulse quality
     c. Skin and mucosal color
     d. Urine output
     e. LOC
     f. Respiratory rate and Spo_2

SURGICAL MANAGEMENT

- Surgical intervention in addition to nonsurgical management may be needed to correct the cause of shock.
  1. Such procedures include vascular repair, surgical hemostasis of major wounds, closure of bleeding ulcers, and chemical scarring (chemosclerosis) of varicosities.

Care Coordination and Transition Management

- Hypovolemic shock is a complication of another condition and is resolved before patients are discharged from the acute care setting.
- Because surgery and many other invasive procedures now occur on an ambulatory care basis, more patients at home are at increased risk for hypovolemic shock.
- Teach patients and family members the early indicators of shock (increased thirst, decreased urine output, light-headedness, sense of apprehension) and to seek immediate medical attention if they appear.

SHOCK, SEPTIC: IMMUNITY CONCEPT EXEMPLAR

OVERVIEW

- Sepsis leading to septic shock is a complex type of distributive shock that usually begins as a bacterial or fungal infection and progresses to a critical emergency over a period of days.
- As progression occurs, the pathologic problems occur faster and to a greater degree.
- Control of sepsis and prevention of severe sepsis and septic shock are easier to achieve early in the process.
- Failure to recognize and intervene in early sepsis is a major factor for progression to septic shock and death.
- Sepsis resulting from widespread infection, triggers an inflammatory response when infectious microorganisms are present in the blood.
- As infectious organisms increase, widespread inflammation, known as *systemic inflammatory response syndrome (SIRS)*, is triggered as a

Chart 2-22	Sepsis with Systemic Inflammatory Response Syndrome (SIRS) Criteria

Suspected or identified infection with some of the following:
- Temperature of more than 101°F (38.3°C) or less than 96.8°F (36°C)
- Heart rate of more than 90 beats per minute
- Respiratory rate of more than 20 breaths per minute
- Abnormal WBC count ($>$12,000/mm^3 or $<$4000/mm^3)
- Normal WBC count with $>$10% bands
- Plasma C-reactive protein $>$2 standard deviations above normal
- Plasma prolactin $>$2 standard deviations above normal
- Arterial hypotension (SBP $<$90 mm Hg; MAP $<$70 mm Hg)
- Arterial hypoxemia (Pao$_2$/Fio$_2$ $<$300)
- Urine output $<$0.5 mL/kg/hr for 2 hours despite adequate fluid resuscitation
- Creatinine increase $>$0.5 mg/dL
- INR $>$1.5 or aPTT $>$60
- Absent bowel sounds
- Platelet count $<$100,000/mm^3
- Total bilirubin $>$4 mg/dL
- Elevated lactic acid (lactate) levels
- Decreased capillary refill or presence of mottling
- Hyperglycemia (plasma glucose $>$140 mg/dL or 7.7 mmol/L) in absence of diabetes
- Unexplained change in mental status
- Significant edema or positive fluid balance

aPTT, Activated partial thromboplastin time; *Fio$_2$,* fraction of inspired oxygen; *INR,* international normalized ratio; *MAP,* mean arterial pressure; *Pao$_2$,* partial pressure of arterial oxygen; SBP, systolic blood pressure; *WBC,* white blood cell.
Adapted from Dellinger, R.P., Levy, M., Rhodes, A., et al. (2013). Surviving Sepsis Campaign. (2015). Updated bundles in response to new evidence. Retrieved December 2015 from: http://www.survivingsepsis.org/SiteCollectionDocuments/SSC_Bundle.pdf

result of infection escaping local control (see chart 2-22). With the organisms and their toxins in the bloodstream and entering other body areas, inflammation becomes an enemy, leading to extensive hormonal, tissue, and vascular changes and oxidative stress that further impair gas exchange and tissue perfusion.
- When SIRS becomes amplified, all tissues are involved and are hypoxic to some degree. Some organs are experiencing cell death and dysfunction at this time. Microthrombi formation is widespread, with clots forming where they are not needed. This process uses up (consumes) many of the available platelets and clotting factors, a condition known as *disseminated intravascular coagulation (DIC)*.

- Septic shock is sepsis-induced hypotension persisting despite adequate fluid resuscitation. It is the stage of sepsis and SIRS when MODS with organ failure is evident and poor clotting with uncontrolled bleeding occurs.

INTERPROFESSIONAL COLLABORATIVE CARE
Assessment: Noticing

- Signs and symptoms of sepsis and septic shock occur over many hours, and some change during the progression.
- Obtain patient information about:
  1. Recent illness, trauma, procedures, allergies, infections, or chronic health problems that may contribute to decreased perfusion
  2. Document:
     a. Swelling, skin discoloration, or severe localized pain that may indicate an internal hemorrhage or infection
     b. Appearance of any wounds, particularly wounds with surrounding inflammation, pus, or odor
     c. Communicate trend information regularly to the provider about cardiovascular changes, particularly blood pressure (SBP, MAP, and pulse pressure), heart rate, peripheral pulse quality, and presence of coolness in extremities
  3. Record respiratory changes
     a. Increased rate
     b. Decreased depth
     c. Spo$_2$
     d. Acute respiratory distress syndrome (ARDS) can occur in septic shock.
  4. Record and communicate urine changes
     a. Decreased urine output
     b. Increased urine concentration
     c. Serum creatinine rises
  5. Document skin perfusion changes
     a. Cool or clammy sensation
     b. Pallor or cyanosis, especially oral mucous membranes
     c. Slow or sluggish capillary refill
     d. Blood may ooze from the gums or other mucous membranes
  6. Recognize and communicate central nervous system (CNS) changes
     a. Decreasing alertness, orientation, or cognition and increasing confusion (level of consciousness [LOC])
     b. Restlessness or apprehension
  7. Identify and communicate significant laboratory changes
     a. Hallmarks of sepsis are a rising serum procalcitonin level, an increasing serum lactate level, a normal or low total

S

white blood cell (WBC) count, and a decreasing segmented neutrophil level with a rising band neutrophil level

Analysis: Interpreting

- The priority interprofessional collaborative problems for patients with sepsis and septic shock are:
  1. Widespread infection due to inadequate immunity
  2. Potential for myocardial dysfunction due to inappropriate clotting, poor perfusion, and poor gas exchange from widespread infection and inflammation

Planning and Implementation: Responding

- Interventions for sepsis and septic shock focus on identifying the problem as early as possible, correcting the conditions causing it, and preventing complications.

DRUG THERAPY

- The use of a sepsis resuscitation bundle for treatment of sepsis within 6 hours is the standard of practice.
- *Oxygen therapy* is useful whenever poor tissue perfusion and poor gas exchange are present.
  1. The patient with septic shock is more likely to be mechanically ventilated.
- Antibiotic therapy within 1 to 2 hours of suspected septic shock; antibiotics are administered intravenously and are broad spectrum.
- The stress of severe sepsis can cause adrenal insufficiency. Adrenal support may involve providing the patient with low- dose corticosteroids during the treatment period.
- *Blood replacement therapy* is used when poor clotting with hemorrhage occurs and may include clotting factors, platelets, fresh frozen plasma (FFP), or packed red blood cells.
- During severe sepsis, patients have microvascular abnormalities and form many small clots. Heparin therapy with fractionated heparin is used to limit inappropriate clotting and prevent the excessive consumption of clotting factors.

Care Coordination and Transition Management

- Identified sepsis should be resolved before patients are discharged from the acute care setting.
- Because more patients are receiving treatment on an ambulatory care basis and are being discharged earlier from acute care settings, more patients at home are at increased risk for sepsis.
- Protecting frail patients from infection and sepsis at home is an important nursing function.
- Teach about the importance of self-care strategies, such as good hygiene, hand washing, balanced diet, rest and exercise, skin care, and mouth care.

✳ SICKLE CELL DISEASE AND TRAIT: PERFUSION CONCEPT EXEMPLAR

OVERVIEW

- *Sickle cell disease* (SCD) is a genetic disorder that results in chronic anemia, pain, disability, organ damage, increased risk for infection, and early death as a result of poor PERFUSION.
- The disorder is the result of formation of abnormal hemoglobin chains (HbS) that distort the cell into an abnormal (sickle-shape) form during low oxygen stated. RBCs affected by abnormal hemoglobin chairs are also fragile and sticky, leading to a reduced circulating time and clumping in small vessels.
  1. SCD is an autosomal recessive genetic disorder. Inheritance of two sickle-type alleles results in more than 80% to 100% of hemoglobin chain formed abnormally.
  2. *Sickle cell trait* (AS) is the inheritance of one normal and one abnormal gene for hemoglobin formation. The symptoms of AS are milder when precipitating conditions (hypoxemia-causing situations) are present because less hemoglobin is abnormal.
- Episodes of vascular occlusion from sickled, clumped RBCs cause poor perfusion, leading to potential organ damage from ischemia and infarction.
- Conditions that cause sickling include hypoxia, dehydration, infections, venous stasis, pregnancy, alcohol consumption, high altitudes, low environmental or body temperatures, acidosis, strenuous exercise, and anesthesia.
- Episodes of severe sickling are called *crisis*.
- SCD is a painful, life-threatening disorder that can be passed to one's children.

INTERPROFESSIONAL COLLABORATIVE CARE

Assessment: Noticing

Obtain patient information about:

- Family history
- Previous sickling occurrences and crises with precipitating events, and treatments
- Onset of pain and events leading to current symptoms
- Signs and symptoms from RBC destruction or anemia
  1. Skin changes (jaundice, pallor, or cyanosis)
  2. Priapism, a prolonged penile erection, can occur in men with SCD.
  3. Organ damage or systemic dysfunction from poor perfusion such as acute or chronic kidney disease, heart failure, lung damage, cirrhosis/liver damage, jaundice from RBC destruction (elevated serum bilirubin), joint swelling, bone necrosis,

muscle damage, disability (dependent activities of daily living [ADLs]), open wounds, stroke, or seizure
- Symptoms related to acute chest syndrome, a life-threatening condition associated with respiratory infection, fat embolism, and pulmonary debris from sickled cells. Symptoms are cough, dyspnea, abnormal lung sounds, and CXR infiltrate similar to pneumonia.
- The diagnosis of SCD is based on the percentage of hemoglobin S (HbS) on electrophoresis.

Analysis: Interpreting
- The priority collaborative problems for the patient with sickle cell disease include:
  1. Pain due to poor tissue oxygenation and joint destruction
  2. Potential for infection, sepsis, multiple organ dysfunction, and death

Planning and Implementation: Responding
MANAGING PAIN
- Severe pain can cause/prolong crisis.
  1. Morphine and hydromorphone (Dilaudid) are common agents used to manage pain with sickle cell crisis for the first 48 hours.
  2. Patients are often managed with daily opioids in the community; pain management can be complicated by issues of tolerance or addiction.
     a. Seek expert pain management consultation for the patient who regularly takes opioids.
     b. Complementary and integrative therapies to manage pain can be used.
  3. Administer hydroxyurea (Droxia) to reduce sickling episodes and pain.
  4. Provide hydration by the oral or IV route to reduce the duration of pain episodes.

PREVENTING SEPSIS, MULTIPLE ORGAN DYSFUNCTION, AND DEATH
- Monitor vital signs, temperature, and other indicators of perfusion impairment regularly to detect early signs of organ damage.
  1. Monitor temperature, complete blood count (CBC) with differential, along with lung sounds and urine output characteristics for early indicators of infection.
  2. Anoxic damage to the spleen can contribute to immunosuppression and risk for infections.
  3. Use oxygen therapy and optimize perfusion to prevent or minimize multiorgan dysfunction because of occlusion and ischemia during sickling episodes.
  4. Administer therapeutic or prophylactic antibiotics and evaluate patient response to drugs.

Chart 2-23	Patient and Family Education: Preparing for Self-Management Prevention of Sickle Cell Crisis

- Drink at least 3 to 4 liters of liquids every day.
- Avoid alcoholic beverages.
- Avoid smoking cigarettes or using tobacco in any form.
- Contact your health care provider at the first sign of illness or infection.
- Be sure to get a "flu shot" every year.
- Ask your primary health care provider about taking the pneumonia vaccine.
- Avoid temperature extremes of hot or cold.
- Be sure to wear socks and gloves when going outside on cold days.
- Avoid planes with unpressurized passenger cabins.
- Avoid travel to high altitudes (e.g., cities like Denver and Santa Fe).
- Ensure that any health care professional who takes care of you knows you have sickle cell disease, especially the anesthesia provider and radiologist.
- Consider genetic counseling.
- Avoid strenuous physical activities.
- Engage in mild, low-impact exercise at least 3 times a week when you are not in crisis.

S

Care Coordination and Transition Management

- Provide and reinforce self-management education, including:
  1. Avoiding activities that lead to hypoxia and hypoxemia (Chart 2-23)
  2. Recognition of early symptoms of crisis and steps to seek help or intervene
  3. Implications of an inheritable condition
  4. Opportunities for social and other support and community resource

SJÖGREN'S SYNDROME

OVERVIEW

- Sjögren's syndrome (SS) is a group of problems that often appear with other autoimmune disorders, typically rheumatoid arthritis or fibromyalgia. Inflammation and autoimmune responses obstruct certain secretory ducts and glands.
- Problems include dry eyes (sicca syndrome), dry mucous membranes of the nose and mouth (xerostomia), and vaginal dryness.
  1. Insufficient tears cause ulceration of the cornea. Other manifestations include blurred vision, burning and itching of the eyes, and thick mattering in the conjunctiva.

2. Insufficient saliva decreases digestion of carbohydrates, promotes tooth decay, and increases the incidence of oral and nasal infections. Difficulty swallowing food, changes in taste sensation, nosebleeds, and upper respiratory infections may also occur.

3. Vaginal dryness may cause pain during sexual intercourse and increase risk for infection.

- There is no cure, and management focuses on slowing the intensity and the progression of the disorder by suppressing immune and inflammatory responses.
- Dry eye and mouth symptoms may be managed with artificial tears and saliva.
- Use of water-soluble vaginal lubricants or moisturizers can increase patient comfort.

SKIN INFECTIONS

OVERVIEW

- Skin infections can be bacterial, viral, fungal, or parasitic. Most are bacterial, caused by *Staphylococcus* or *Streptococcus* microorganisms.
- *Folliculitis* is a superficial infection involving only the upper portion of the follicle. It usually manifests as a raised, red rash with small pustules.
- *Furuncles* (boils) are deeper follicle infections with a large, sore-looking, raised bump that may or may not have a pustular "head" at its point.
- *Cellulitis* is a generalized infection and involves the deeper connective tissue.
- The major cause of bacterial skin infection is minor skin trauma.
- Viral skin infections are commonly caused by the herpes simplex virus (HSV) and include type I infections (common cold sore) and type II infections (genital herpes). A second viral infection manifested in skin but that is actually an infection of the nerve is herpes zoster (shingles). Viral infections differ from bacterial infections in two ways.
  1. After the first infection, the virus remains in the body in a dormant state in the nerve ganglia and the patient has no symptoms.
  2. Re-activation stimulates the virus to travel the pathways of sensory nerves to the skin, where lesions reappear.
- Many fungal infections also affect the skin.
  1. Superficial dermatophyte infections include:
     a. Tinea pedis ("athlete's foot")
     b. Tinea manus (hands)
     c. Tinea cruris (groin, "jock itch")
     d. Tinea capitis (head)
     e. Tinea corporis (ringworm)

2. *Candida albicans,* also known as *yeast infection,* is another common superficial fungal infection of skin and mucous membranes.
   a. Risk factors include immunosuppression, long-term antibiotic therapy, diabetes mellitus, and obesity.
   b. The incidence is higher in hot, humid climates.
   c. Infected skin (most often in skin folds such as under the breasts) has a moist, red, irritated appearance, usually with itching and burning.
- Parasitic skin infections include lice, scabies, and bedbugs.
   1. Lice infestation or pediculosis can occur in the scalp or pubic area as well as be generalized on the body. Both the parasite and eggs must be destroyed.
      a. The most common manifestation is itching.
      b. Treatment is chemical killing of lice with topical sprays, creams, and shampoos with an active ingredient of permethrin or malathion.
      c. Oral agents such as ivermectin can be used.
      d. Clothing and bed linens that have touched the infected body part should be washed in hot water and detergent.
      e. Social contacts may also need treatment.
   2. Scabies is a mite infestation passed on by close personal contact or contact with infested bedding. Intense itching and curved or linear ridges on the skin are the common manifestations. Egg and mites can be seen under a microscope from skin scrapings.
      a. Treatment involves the use of a topical scabicide with permethrin, malathion, or benzyl benzoate as an active ingredient.
      b. Laundry of clothes, personal items, and linen with hot water and detergent is also necessary to eliminate mites.
   3. Bedbugs are a parasite that lives on human blood but do not cause infection. The bite can itch but it is NOT an infection. Humans do not harbor or carry the mite.
      a. Management can include a topical antihistamine for itch relief. Topical insecticides are not used.
      b. The environment in which the bites occurred (home, hotel, transport) will need extensive pest control by experts to eradicate this parasite.
- Prevention of skin infections, especially bacterial and fungal infections, involves avoiding the offending organism and good personal hygiene to remove the organism before infection can occur.

S

! NURSING SAFETY PRIORITY: Action Alert

Hand washing and not sharing personal items with others are the best ways to avoid contact with some of the most easily transmitted organisms.

INTERPROFESSIONAL COLLABORATIVE CARE
Assessment: Noticing
- Obtain patient information about:
  1. Recent history of skin trauma
  2. Living conditions, home sanitation, personal hygiene habits, and leisure or sport activities
  3. Whether fever and malaise are also present
  4. Lesion locations, especially skin folds, lips, mouth, or genital region
  5. History of similar lesions in the same location
  6. Presence of burning, tingling, or pain
  7. Recent contact with an infected person
  8. Whether the patient has ever had chickenpox or shingles
  9. Whether the patient has received Zostavax, the shingles prevention vaccine
  10. Social and environmental factors
      a. Direct contact with an infected person
      b. Personal hygiene practices
      c. Frequent contact with animals
      d. Type and frequency of athletic activities
- Assess for and document the condition of the skin, including local or general:
  1. Redness
  2. Warmth
  3. Edema
  4. Tenderness
  5. Pain
  6. Itching
  7. Stinging
  8. Location of areas of inflammation, rash, or infection
  9. Presence of:
      a. Blisters or vesicles
      b. Pustules
      c. Papules
      d. Scaling
      e. Single or multiple lesions

Interventions: Noticing
- Most skin infections heal well with nonsurgical management, but surgery may be required if an infectious agent is present in deep tissue layers.
- Nursing interventions include:
  1. Skin care instructions
     a. Showering daily with soap; chlorhexidine gluconate showers or dilute bleach baths can reduce bacterial load
     b. Not squeezing any pustules or crusts but removing them gently

    c. Applying warm compresses twice a day to furuncles or areas of cellulitis

    d. Avoiding constricting garments that might rub the lesions

    e. Keeping the skin dry between treatments

    f. Positioning for optimal air circulation to the area

  2. Prevention of transmission

    a. Using hand washing and antimicrobial hand solutions to prevent cross-contamination

    b. Isolating the patient if infections are colonized with bacteria resistant to antibiotic therapy (e.g., *methicillin-resistant staphylococcus*)

    c. Teaching patients to avoid sharing personal items such as hairbrushes, articles of clothing, or footwear

    d. Teaching patients to avoid skin-to-skin and sexual contact when infectious skin lesions are present

- Drug therapy includes:
  1. Topical agents for superficial infections and mild bacterial infections
  2. Systemic antibiotic therapy for extensive infections, especially if fever or lymphadenopathy is present
  3. Antiviral agents such as acyclovir (Zovirax), valacyclovir (Valtrex), or famciclovir (Famvir)
  4. Antifungal agents such as ketoconazole (Nizoral) or fluconazole

SPINAL CORD INJURY: MOBILITY CONCEPT EXEMPLAR

OVERVIEW

- Spinal cord injury (SCI), often results in loss of or impaired MOBILITY, sensory perception, and bowel and bladder control.
- SCI is classified as:
  1. *Complete* if the spinal cord is damaged in a way that eliminates all innervation below the level of injury, and total motor and sensory loss occurs
  2. *Incomplete* (more common), allowing some function or movement below the level of injury
- Trauma is the leading cause of SCI.
- The causes of SCI can be divided into primary and secondary mechanisms of injury. Five primary mechanisms may result in an SCI:
  1. Hyperflexion: a sudden and forceful acceleration (movement) of the head forward causing extreme flexion of the neck. Examples: Motor vehicle or diving accident
  2. Hyperextension: the head is suddenly accelerated and then decelerated. Examples: Motor vehicle collisions where the

vehicle is struck from behind of during falls when the patient's chin is struck.

3. Axial loading or vertical compression: injuries resulting from diving accidents, falls onto the buttocks, or a jump in which a person lands on the feet.

4. Excessive rotation: results from injuries that are caused by turning the head beyond the normal range.

5. Penetrating trauma: classified by the speed of the penetrating object. Low speed injuries cause damage directly at the site or local damage to the spinal cord. In contrast, high-speed injuries, such as a gunshot wound, cause both direct and indirect damage.

- Secondary injury worsens the primary injury. Secondary injuries include:
  1. Hemorrhage
  2. Ischemia
  3. Hypovolemia
  4. Local edema
- Complications of SCI include pressure ulcers, contractures, and deep vein thrombosis (DVT) or pulmonary emboli. Muscle spasticity and bone loss can occur over time.

INTERPROFESSIONAL COLLABORATIVE CARE
Assessment: Noticing
- Obtain information about:
  1. How the injury occurred and the probable mechanism of injury
  2. The patient's position and location immediately after the injury
  3. Symptoms that occurred after the injury and what changes have occurred since
  4. Prehospital rescue personnel should be questioned about:
     a. Problems encountered during the extrication and transport
     b. Type of immobilization devices used
     c. Medical treatment given at the scene
  5. Medical history, with particular attention to a history of arthritis of the spine, congenital deformities, osteoarthritis or osteomyelitis, cancer, previous back or SCI, and respiratory problems
- Assess for and document:
  1. Adequacy of airway, breathing, and circulation
     a. The patient with a cervical SCI is at high risk for respiratory compromise because the cervical spinal nerves (C3 to C5) innervate the phrenic nerve controlling the diaphragm.
  2. Vital signs and indication of hemorrhage or other non-CNS injury
  3. Indications of a head injury, such as a change in LOC, abnormal pupil size and reaction to light, and change in behavior or ability to respond to directions

4. For spinal shock recognizing that neurogenic shock and spinal shock are NOT interchangeable terms. Spinal shock is characterized by complete but temporary loss of motor, sensory, reflex, and autonomic function that often lasts less than 48 hours but may continue for several weeks.

5. Sensory perception and mobility, to determine the level of injury and establish baseline data for future assessment.

   a. The level of injury is the lowest neurologic segment with intact or normal motor and sensory function. **Tetraplegia** (also called *quadriplegia*) (paralysis) and **quadriparesis** (weakness) involve all four extremities, as seen with cervical cord and upper thoracic injury. **Paraplegia** (paralysis) and **paraparesis** (weakness) involve only the lower extremities, as seen in lower thoracic and lumbosacral injuries or lesions.

❗ NURSING SAFETY PRIORITY: Critical Rescue

In *acute* SCI, monitor for a decrease in SENSORY PERCEPTION from baseline, especially in a proximal (upward) dermatome and/or new loss of motor function and MOBILITY. The presence of these changes is considered an emergency and requires immediate communication with the health care provider using SBAR or other agency-approved protocol for notification. Document these assessment findings in the electronic health record.

6. Change in thermoregulatory capacity, with the patient's body tending to assume the temperature of the environment (hypothermia)

7. Breathing problems resulting from an interruption of spinal innervation to the respiratory muscles, assessing for atelectasis and/or pneumonia symptoms; *patients with injuries at or above thoracic vertebra #6 (T6) are especially at risk for respiratory complications and pulmonary embolus during the first 5 days after injury*

8. Evaluation of the patient's abdomen for manifestations of internal bleeding, distention, or paralytic ileus; paralytic ileus is manifested by decreased or absent bowel sounds and distended abdomen, usually 72 hours or longer after injury

9. Bladder fullness and/or urinary tract infection. Autonomic dysfunction initially causes an areflexic (neurogenic) bladder (no reflex ability for bladder contraction), which later

leads to urinary retention. The patient is at risk for urinary tract infection (UTI) from an indwelling urinary catheter, intermittent catheterizations, or bladder distention, stasis, and/or overflow.

   a. **Autonomic dysreflexia (AD)**, sometimes referred to as *autonomic hyperreflexia,* is a potentially life-threatening condition in which noxious visceral or cutaneous stimuli (such as from a full bladder or bowel) cause a sudden, massive, uninhibited reflex sympathetic discharge in people with high-level SCI.

10. Coping strategies used to deal with illness, difficult situations, or disappointments; initial hospitalization after SCI lasts for 3 or more months to include rehabilitation

Analysis: Interpreting

- The priority collaborative problems for patients with an acute SCI include:

   1. Potential for respiratory distress/failure related to aspiration or decreased diaphragmatic innervation
   2. Potential for cardiovascular instability (e.g., shock, autonomic dysreflexia) related to loss or interruption of sympathetic innervation or hemorrhage
   3. Potential for secondary SCI related to hypoperfusion, edema, or delayed spinal column stabilization
   4. Decreased mobility and sensation related to spinal cord damage and edema

Planning and Implementation: Responding

MANAGING THE AIRWAY AND IMPROVING BREATHING

- Manage the airway and improve breathing related to risk for aspiration or lack of diaphragmatic innervation.

   1. Manage respiratory secretions with assisted coughing, positioning, and suctioning.
   2. Implement strategies to prevent ventilator-associated injury.
   3. Coordinate the cough effort of the tetraplegic patient with an assistant who uses an upward thrust to the diaphragm during forceful exhalation ("quad cough" or "assist cough").

❗ NURSING SAFETY PRIORITY: Action Alert

Assess breath sounds every 2 to 4 hours during the first few days after SCI, and document and report any adventitious or diminished sounds. Monitor vital signs with pulse oximetry. Watch for changes in respiratory pattern or airway obstruction. Intervene per agency or primary health care provider (PHCP) protocol when there is a decrease in oxygen saturation (Spo_2) to below 95%.

MONITORING FOR CARDIOVASCULAR INSTABILITY
- Monitor for cardiovascular instability (e.g., shock, AD) related to loss or interruption of sympathetic innervation or hemorrhage.
  1. Maintain adequate hydration via IV and oral intake to sustain urine output of more than 30 mL/kg/hour and avoid serum lactate levels less than 2 mg/dL.
  2. Reduce risk for AD by preventing bladder and bowel distention, managing pain and room temperature, and monitoring for early signs of sympathetic stimulation including hypertension.

! NURSING SAFETY PRIORITY: Critical Rescue

Monitor the patient with acute SCI at least hourly for:
- Pulse oximetry (Spo$_2$) <90% or symptoms of aspiration (e.g., stridor, garbled speech, inability to clear airway)
- Symptomatic bradycardia, including reduced level of consciousness and deceased urine output
- Hypotension with systolic blood pressure (SBP) <90 mm Hg or mean arterial pressure (MAP) <65 mm Hg

Notify the physician immediately if these symptoms occur because this problem is an emergency!

! NURSING SAFETY PRIORITY: Critical Rescue

If the patient experiences AD, raise the head of the bed *immediately* to help reduce the blood pressure. Notify the PHCP immediately for drug therapy to quickly reduce blood pressure as indicated. Determine the cause of AD and treat it promptly. For example, if the bladder is distended, catheterize the patient to relieve the urinary retention. Check the room temperature and bed coverings, and adjust as needed for patient comfort. Lack of sensory perception may prevent the patient from noticing temperature variations.

PREVENTING SECONDARY SPINAL CORD INJURY
  1. Prevent secondary SCI associated with hypoperfusion, edema, or delayed spinal column stabilization.
     a. Assess the patient's mobility (motor) and sensory perception function, vital signs, pulse oximetry, and altered comfort every 1 to 4 hours.
     b. Keep the patient in proper body alignment to prevent further cord injury or irritability.
     c. Support immobilizing supports like traction, halo device, or early surgical vertebral fusion to prevent further spinal cord damage.

2. For the patient with a chronic disability related to an established (non-acute) SCI, implement measures related to decreasing risk for or treating pressure ulcers, contractures, venous thromboembolism (VTE, DVT, and/or pulmonary embolus), and fractures related to osteoporosis. Patients with high SCIs are also at risk for orthostatic hypotension.

   a. Provide safe, effective positioning and re-positioning.

   b. Use pressure-relieving devices early and at all times (e.g., chair-sitting).

   c. Assist with slow transitions to upright posture, especially after a period of supine positioning because patients with high SCIs are also at risk for orthostatic hypotension.

   d. The patient may have spastic or flaccid bladder and bowel related to direct neurologic damage or disruption in nerve impulses.

      (1) The type of bladder emptying program depends on the usual elimination pattern and whether the injury involved upper motor neurons (UMNs) or lower motor neurons (LMNs).

      (2) Use a bedside bladder residual volume and determine effectiveness of bladder emptying strategies.

      (3) Teach the patient that the essential elements of a bowel program include stool softeners, increased fluid intake (unless medically contraindicated), high-fiber diet, and a consistent time for elimination.

      (4) Evaluate for UTI, particularly foul-smelling urine; the SCI patient may not develop flank pain, urgency, frequency, or other signs of UTI.

Drug Therapy for SCI

a. Centrally-acting skeletal muscular relaxants, such as *tizanidine* (Zanaflex, Sirdalud), may help control severe muscle spasticity.

b. These drugs cause severe drowsiness and sedation in most patients and may not be effective in reducing spasticity.

c. As an alternative to these drugs, *intrathecal baclofen (ITB) (Lioresal)* therapy may be prescribed.

   (1) This drug is administered through a programmable, implantable infusion pump and intrathecal catheter directly into the cerebrospinal fluid. The pump is surgically placed in a subcutaneous pouch in the lower abdomen. Monitor for common adverse effects, which include sedation, fatigue, dizziness, and changes in mental status. *Seizures and hallucinations may occur if ITB is suddenly withdrawn.*

Surgical Management for SCI

a. Surgery within 24 hours of injury to stabilize the vertebral spinal column, particularly if there is evidence of spinal cord compression, results in decreased secondary complications.

b. Emergent surgery also removes bone fragments, hematomas, or penetrating objects such as a bullet. Typical procedures include wiring and spinal fusion for cervical injuries and the insertion of steel or metal rods (e.g., Harrington rods) to stabilize thoracic and lumbar spinal injuries.

!   **NURSING SAFETY PRIORITY: Action Alert**

After surgical spinal fusion, assess the patient's neurologic status and vital signs at least every hour for the first 4 to 6 hours and then, if the patient is stable, every 4 hours. Assess for complications of surgery, including worsening of motor or sensory function at or above the site of surgery.

MANAGING DECREASED MOBILITY

- Patients with SCI are especially at risk for pressure ulcers, thromboembolism, contractures, orthostatic hypotension, and fractures related to osteoporosis. The following interventions may be used to decrease risks:

  1. Frequent and therapeutic positioning not only helps prevent complications but also provides alignment to prevent further SCI or irritability.

  2. Assess the condition of the patient's skin, especially over pressure points, with each turn or repositioning.

  3. Turning may be performed manually or the patient may be placed on an automatic rotating bed.

  4. Reduce pressure on any reddened area, and monitor it with the next turn.

  5. Reposition patients frequently (every 1 or 2 hours). When sitting in a chair, the patient is repositioned or taught to reposition himself or herself more often than every hour.

  6. Paraplegic patients usually perform frequent "wheelchair push-ups" to relieve skin pressure.

  7. Use a pressure-reducing mattress and wheel chair or chair pad to help prevent skin breakdown.

  8. Prevent VTE, including using interventions of intermittent pneumatic compression stockings and low–molecular-weight heparin (LMWH).

  9. Collaborate with the rehabilitation team to teach or reinforce mobility skills.

Care Coordination and Transition Management
- Most patients are discharged to a rehabilitation setting where they learn processes to enable self-care, mobility, and bladder and bowel management.
  1. Psychosocial adaptation is a crucial factor in determining the success of rehabilitation.
     a. Assist the patient to verbalize feelings and fears about body image, self-concept, role performance, and self-esteem.
     b. Talk to the patient about the expected reactions of those outside the hospital environment.
     c. Help to set and reinforce realistic goals for managing self-care while promoting independence and decision making daily.
     d. Provide opportunities for emotional and spiritual support.
     e. Sexuality can be a major concern; work closely with the rehabilitation interprofessional team to address concerns about intercourse and reproduction.
  2. Collaborate with the case manager or discharge planner for a review of the patient's insurance and financial status to plan for rehabilitation because this phase of care can last 3 or more months.
  3. Collaborate with the patient, family, case manager, and rehabilitation professionals to assess the home environment to ensure accessibility access and plan for vocational adaptation or education.
  4. Ensure that the patient can correctly use all adaptive devices ordered for home use.
  5. Ensure that adaptive equipment is installed in the home before discharge.
  6. Teach the patient and family, in collaboration with health care team members:
     a. Mobility skills
     b. Pressure ulcer prevention
     c. ADL skills
     d. Bowel and bladder program
     e. Education about sexuality and referral for counseling to promote sexual health
     f. Prevention of AD with appropriate bladder, bowel, and skin care practices and recognition of early signs or symptoms of autonomic dysreflexia

STENOSIS, RENAL ARTERY
OVERVIEW
- Renal artery stenosis involves narrowing of the lumen and reduced blood flow to the kidney tissues. Uncorrected stenosis leads to ischemia and atrophy of kidneys.

- Renal artery stenosis is suspected when a sudden onset of hypertension occurs. Low renal blood flow from stenosis results in neurohormonal changes (such as activation of the renin-angiotensin-aldosterone system) that elevate blood pressure in a compensatory response to improve renal blood flow.
- Pathology may be fibrotic, atherosclerotic, or both.
- Treatment includes:
  1. Antihypertensive drugs
  2. Percutaneous transluminal balloon angioplasty or stent placement in the renal artery
  3. Renal artery bypass surgery

STOMATITIS: TISSUE INTEGRITY CONCEPT EXEMPLAR

- Stomatitis is a broad term that refers to inflammation within the oral cavity that impairs TISSUE INTEGRITY of the protective lining of the mouth.
- It can result from infection, allergy, vitamin deficiency, systemic disease, and irritants like tobacco and alcohol.
- Primary stomatitis includes noninfectious aphthous ("canker sores"), herpes simplex lesions, and traumatic ulcers.
- Secondary stomatitis results from infection by opportunistic viruses, fungi, or bacteria in patients who are immunocompromised.
  1. A common type of secondary stomatitis is caused by *Candida albicans.*
  2. Long-term antibiotic therapy destroys other normal flora and allows the *Candida* to overgrow. The result can be **candidiasis,** also called *moniliasis,* a fungal infection that is very painful. Candidiasis is also common in those undergoing immunosuppressive therapy, such as chemotherapy, radiation, and corticosteroids.
  3. Oral hygiene can discourage the frequency and severity of stomatitis, although it may not completely prevent all occurrences.

! NURSING SAFETY PRIORITY: Action Alert

When assessing the patient with stomatitis, be alert for signs and symptoms of dysphagia, such as coughing or choking when swallowing, a sensation of food "sticking" in the pharynx, or difficulty initiating the swallowing process. If dysphagia is suspected, document all findings and report these to the health care provider because dysphagia can cause numerous problems, including airway obstruction, aspiration pneumonia, and malnutrition.

INTERPROFESSIONAL COLLABORATIVE CARE
Assessment: Noticing
- Assess for:
  1. History of recent infection
  2. Nutritional changes
  3. Oral trauma
  4. Hygiene habits
  5. Stress
- Document the course of the current outbreak, and determine if stomatitis has occurred frequently.
- Ask the patient if the lesions interfere with swallowing, eating, or communicating.
- While examining the mouth, wear gloves, use a penlight to ensure adequate lighting, and use a tongue blade to aid examining the oral cavity.
- Assess the mouth for lesions, coating, and cracking.
- Document characteristics of the lesions, including their location, size, shape, odor, color, and drainage.
- For definitive diagnosis, the provider may order swallowing studies.

Analysis: Interpreting
- The priority collaborative problems for the patient with stomatitis include:
  1. Compromised tissue integrity due to oral and/or esophageal lesions
  2. Alteration in COMFORT related to oral and/or esophageal lesions

Planning and Implementation: Responding
PRESERVING TISSUE INTEGRITY
- Instruct the patient to:
  1. Use a soft-bristled brush to gently clean teeth, gums, and the oral cavity.
  2. Rinse the mouth often with sodium bicarbonate solution, warm saline, or hydrogen peroxide solution. Avoid alcohol-based commercial mouthwashes.
  3. Take antimicrobials (antivirals, antifungals, and antibacterials) or immune modulators as prescribed.

MINIMIZING ALTERATIONS IN COMFORT
- Manage oral pain by teaching the patient to:
  1. Use topical agents (with benzocaine or lidocaine).
  2. Modify diet to avoid salty, spicy, acidic, and other irritating foods.

! NURSING SAFETY PRIORITY: Drug Alert

Teach patients to use viscous lidocaine with extreme caution because its anesthetizing effect may cause burns from hot liquids in the mouth and/or increase the risk for choking.

Care Coordination and Transition Management

- Teach appropriate administration of home medications such as swish and swallow versus swish and spit (rinse only).
- Teach the patient about dietary choices that will not irritate the oral cavity.

✳️ STROKE (BRAIN ATTACK): PERFUSION CONCEPT EXEMPLAR

OVERVIEW

- Stroke is caused by an interruption of PERFUSION to any part of the brain. The National Stroke Association uses the term *brain attack* to describe a stroke to convey the urgency for activation of the emergency medical system for care.
- Strokes may be classified as:
  1. *Acute ischemic stroke,* which is caused by the occlusion of a cerebral artery; types of ischemic strokes include:
     a. A *thrombotic stroke* is commonly associated with the development of atherosclerosis of the blood vessel wall. Rupture of one or more atherosclerotic plaque exposes foam cells to clot-promoting elements in the blood. The result is clot formation. The artery becomes occluded, and blood flow to the area is markedly diminished, causing transient ischemia and then complete ischemia and infarction of brain tissue. Signs and symptoms occur over minutes to hours.
     b. An *embolic stroke* is caused by a thrombus or group of thrombi that travel to the cerebral arteries through the carotid artery and block the artery, resulting in ischemia. Sudden and rapid development of focal neurologic deficits occurs. Cerebral hemorrhage may result if the vessel wall is damaged. Embolic strokes are associated with atrial fibrillation, coronary disease, and heart valve disease or repair.
     c. Ischemic stroke may be preceded by warning signs of brief neurologic impairment, including *transient ischemic attack* (TIA).
        (1) A TIA is a temporary neurologic dysfunction resulting from a *brief* interruption in cerebral blood flow is easy to ignore or miss, particularly if symptoms resolve by the time the patient reaches the emergency department (ED).
        (2) Typically, symptoms of a TIA resolve within 30 to 60 minutes and symptoms may be ignored or missed.
  2. *Hemorrhagic stroke,* in which the integrity of the vessel wall is interrupted and bleeding occurs into the brain tissue (intracerebral) or spaces surrounding the brain (ventricular, subdural,

S

subarachnoid); causes include hypertension, ruptured aneurysm, and arteriovenous malformation (AVM).

a. An *aneurysm* is the abnormal ballooning of an artery that may become stretched or thinned and rupture.

b. *AVM* is a thin-walled, dilated vessel which results in an abnormal communication between the arterial and venous vessels without a capillary network.

c. *Vasospasm,* a sudden and periodic constriction of a cerebral artery, often follows a cerebral hemorrhage caused by aneurysm or AVM rupture. Blood flow to distal areas of the brain supplied by the affected artery is markedly diminished, leading to cerebral ischemia and infarction and further neurologic dysfunction.

INTERPROFESSIONAL COLLABORATIVE CARE

- Although an accurate history is important in the diagnosis of a stroke, *the first priority is to ensure the patient is transported to a stroke center.* A stroke center is designated by The Joint Commission (TJC) for its ability to rapidly recognize and effectively treat strokes. TJC designates two distinct levels of stroke center certification: The *primary* stroke center is *not* required to provide advanced diagnostic testing or stroke therapy; the *advanced* stroke center provides timely and life-saving interventions such as fibrinolytic therapy that can prevent long-term disability.

Assessment: Noticing
- Obtain patient information about:
  1. Time of symptom onset
  2. Progression and severity of symptoms, including the presence of TIA previously
  3. LOC, orientation, and other measures of cognitive function
  4. Motor status: gait, balance, reading and writing abilities
  5. Sensory status: speech, hearing, vision
  6. Medical history with attention to identifying risk factors such as hypertension, hyperlipidemia, cardiovascular disease, diabetes, smoking, sedentary lifestyle, alcohol use, obesity, high fat diet, conditions that alter coagulation, and the presence of atrial fibrillation (dysrhythmia)
  7. Social history, with attention to identifying sources of support
  8. Current drugs and non-prescribed drugs, especially anticoagulants, aspirin, vasodilators, and illegal drugs
- For the patient in the ED, assess symptoms within 10 minutes of arrival and determine disposition (e.g., transport to a Stroke Center or to diagnostic computerized tomography [CT] scan).

- Assess for and document:
  1. Neurologic function using a standard stroke screening tool such as the National Institutes of Health Stroke Scale (NIHSS), including:
     a. LOC
     b. Orientation
     c. Motor ability
     d. Pupil size and reaction to light, extraocular movement, visual field deficits, ptosis (drooping eyelid)
     e. Speech and language
  2. Vital signs
  3. Blood glucose
  4. Additional assessment for ongoing care includes:
     a. Cognition, memory, judgment, and problem-solving and decision-making abilities
     b. Ability to concentrate and attend to tasks
     c. Range of motion (ROM), proprioception, head and trunk control, balance, gait, coordination, bowel and bladder control
     d. Sensory status (response to touch and painful stimuli; ability to distinguish between two tactile stimuli presented simultaneously; ability to read, write, and follow verbal directions; and ability to name objects and use them correctly)
     e. Speech pattern (rhythm, clarity, aphasia)
     f. Visual system (homonymous hemianopsia, bitemporal hemianopsia, amaurosis fugax)
     g. Cranial nerve function
     h. Cardiac system (dysrhythmias and murmurs)
     i. Coping mechanisms or personality changes
  5. Emotional lability and screen for depression
  6. Nutritional status
  7. Social support, financial status, and occupation
- Diagnostic tests
  1. CT scan of the head without contrast is performed within 30 minutes after arrival at the emergency department. This study is essential to determine patient eligibility for fibrinolytic therapy.
  2. Magnetic resonance imaging (MRI) and related multimodal imaging demonstrate ischemia earlier than CT scan and are used to identify the presence of hemorrhage or a cerebral aneurysm. Results also help differentiate stroke from other pathologic changes that mimic a stroke.
  3. CBC, serum electrolytes, and coagulation factors
  4. Carotid ultrasound
  5. ECG and echocardiography to determine whether cardiac disease or dysrhythmia is a contributing factor to stroke

Analysis: Interpreting
- Depending on stroke severity and/or response to immediate management, the priority collaborative problems for patients with stroke may include:
  1. Inadequate perfusion to the brain due to interruption of arterial blood flow and a possible increase in intracranial pressure (ICP)
  2. Decreased mobility and ability to perform ADLs due to neuromuscular or cognitive impairment
  3. Aphasia or dysarthria due to decreased circulation in the brain or facila muscle weakness
  4. Sensory perception deficits due to altered neurologic reception and transmission

Planning and Implementation: Responding
IMPROVING CEREBRAL PERFUSION
   Nonsurgical Management
- Management includes either fibrinolytic therapy or endovascular procedures.

> **❗ NURSING SAFETY PRIORITY: Drug Alert**
>
> In addition to frequent monitoring of vital signs, carefully observe for signs of intracerebral hemorrhage and other signs of bleeding during administration of fibrinolytic drug therapy.

- Monitor for neurologic changes or complications before, during, and after medical interventions.
  1. Perform a neurologic assessment at least every 2 to 4 hours, checking:
     a. Verbal ability, orientation
     b. Eye opening, pupil size, and reaction to light
     c. Motor response
  2. Monitor vital signs with neurologic checks.
     a. Ask the physician for acceptable limits for blood pressure.
     b. A typical goal is to sustain a SBP at 140 to 150 mm Hg and avoid pressures above 180 mm Hg or below 120 mm Hg.

> **❗ NURSING SAFETY PRIORITY: Critical Rescue**
>
> Be alert for symptoms of increased ICP and report any deterioration in the patient's neurologic status to the health care provider immediately. The first sign of increased ICP is a declining LOC.

3. Perform a cardiac assessment.
   a. Monitor the patient for dysrhythmias; auscultate the heart and palpate peripheral pulses to identify new irregular heart rhythms in the absence of a cardiac monitor.
4. Position the backrest to promote cerebral perfusion. In the presence of ischemic stroke, a flat backrest may be preferred initially.
5. Avoid activities that may increase ICP.
   a. Maintain the patient's head in a midline neutral position.
   b. Position the patient to avoid extreme hip or neck flexion.
   c. Avoid clustering of nursing procedures.
   d. Provide a quiet environment; room lights should be low.
   e. Assess the need for suctioning; hyperoxygenate the patient before suctioning.
- Drug therapy
1. Fibrinolytic therapy may be used for an acute ischemic stroke.
   a. Alteplase (tPA [tissue plasminogen activator], Activase) is approved for administration within 3 to 4.5 hours of stroke onset.
      (1) Patients who have had a stroke or serious head trauma in the past 3 months, a hemorrhagic stroke, recent MI, increased partial thromboplastin time (PTT), anticoagulant therapy, or who are pregnant are not candidates for this therapy.
   b. Catheter-directed fibrinolytic therapy may be performed as an alternative treatment for up to 6 hours after initial symptoms.
2. Anticoagulant therapy and antiplatelet therapy may be prescribed depending on the health care provider's preference following ischemic stroke or TIA.
   a. Oral drugs to manage ischemic stroke include aspirin and other antiplatelet drugs like clopidogrel and dabigatran or warfarin to prevent progression or future thrombotic and embolic strokes.
3. Other drugs used to treat symptoms associated with stroke include:
   a. Calcium channel blockers (nimodipine [Nimotop]), which may be administered to treat vasospasm or chronic spasm of the vessel that inhibits blood flow to the area
   b. Stool softeners, analgesics for pain, and antianxiety drugs
   c. Antihypertensives to maintain blood perfusion within prescribed limits
- Monitor the patient for complications such as:
1. Vasospasm, or narrowing of the cerebral arteries, which leads to cerebral ischemia and infarction and is manifested by a

decreased LOC, motor and reflex changes, and increased neurologic deficits (cranial nerve deficits, aphasia)
2. Bleeding following fibrinolytic therapy or rebleeding with hemorrhagic stroke
3. Bleeding caused by thrombolytic, anticoagulant, or antiplatelet therapy; observe for blood in the urine and stool, epistaxis (nosebleed), bleeding gums, and easy bruising
4. Hydrocephalus-enlarged ventricles manifested by a change in the LOC, gait disturbances, and behavior changes
- Carotid artery angioplasty is a nonsurgical intervention used to treat certain types of ischemic stroke. A distal protection device may be placed beyond the stenosis to catch any debris that breaks off during the angioplasty or stenting procedure.

Surgical Management
- Two surgical procedures that may be used for ischemic stroke are:
  1. Carotid endarterectomy to remove atherosclerotic plaque from the inner lining of the carotid artery
  2. Extracranial-intracranial bypass to bypass the occluded area and re-establish blood flow to the affected area
- Surgical and interventional radiologic procedures to treat intracranial aneurysm or AVM are:
  1. Surgical ligation or resection, removing involved vessels through stereotactic, gamma knife, or conventional approaches
  2. Placing a coil or clip to clamp the base or neck of an aneurysm
  3. Creating flow diversion with stent-like devices delivered under fluoroscopy
  4. Using liquid polymer embolization, generally before surgical ligation

PROMOTING MOBILITY AND ADL ABILITY
1. In collaboration with the rehabilitation therapists, assess the patient's functional ability for bed MOBILITY skills and ADL ability and implement early progressive rehabilitation.
2. Follow agency guidelines for screening for swallowing difficulties; this may be a component of the stroke care protocol.
3. Provide nutrition and avoid aspiration when dysphagia occurs in collaboration with the speech-language pathologist and interprofessional team members.
4. Implement VTE prophylaxis.
5. Collaborate with physical therapist (PT) and occupational therapist (OT) to manage flaccid or spastic limbs.

PROMOTING EFFECTIVE COMMUNICATION
1. Present one idea or thought in a sentence (e.g., "I am going to help you get into the chair.").

2. Use simple one-step commands rather than ask patients to do multiple tasks.
3. Speak slowly but not loudly; use cues or gestures as needed.
4. Avoid "yes" and "no" questions for patients with expressive aphasia.
5. Use alternative forms of communication if needed, such as a computer, handheld mobile device, communication board, or flash cards (often with pictures).

MANAGING CHANGES IN SENSORY PERCEPTION
1. Unilateral neglect, or neglect syndrome, occurs most commonly in patients who have had a right cerebral stroke.
   a. Help the patient adapt to these disabilities by using frequent verbal and tactile cues and by breaking down tasks into discrete steps.
   b. *Always approach the patient from the unaffected side, which should face the door of the room!*
2. Hemianopsia, in which the vision of one or both eyes is affected, places the patient at additional risk for injury, especially falls.
   a. Teach the patient to turn his or her head from side to side to expand the visual field.
   b. The scanning technique is also useful when the patient is eating or ambulating.
3. With a right sided stroke, there may be an inability to recognize his or her physical impairment or a lack of proprioception (position sense).
   a. Teach the patient to touch and use both sides of the body.
   b. When dressing, remind the patient to dress the affected side first.
4. The patient with a left hemisphere lesion generally has memory deficits and may show significant changes in the ability to carry out simple tasks.
   a. Assist with memory problems, re-orient the patient to the month, year, day of the week, and circumstances surrounding hospital admission.
   b. Establish a routine or schedule that is as structured, repetitious, and consistent as possible.
   c. Provide information in a simple, concise manner.

Care Coordination and Transition Management
- Provide a detailed plan of care at the time of discharge for patients to be transferred to a rehabilitation center or long-term care facility.
- If possible, a case manager should be assigned to help coordinate plans for the patient discharged to the home setting. The case

manager should collaborate with the home health agency and with physical and occupational therapists to:

1. Identify and suggest corrections of hazards in the home before discharge.
2. Ensure that the patient and family can correctly use all adaptive devices ordered for home use.
3. Arrange follow-up appointments as needed.

- Teaching for self-management includes:
  1. Providing drug information as needed
     a. Discharge with antithrombotic therapy is a core measure of the Joint Commission for patients with ischemic stroke.
     b. Provide both written and verbal instruction at discharge.
  2. Reinforcing mobility skills (in collaboration with other therapists) such as:
     a. How to safely climb stairs, transfer from bed to chair, and get into and out of a car
     b. How to use adaptive equipment
  3. Teaching the family that depression and emotional or mood changes may occur
     a. Depression is usually self-limited but counseling or antidepressants may be needed.
     b. Advise the family to avoid being overprotective.
     c. Assist the family and patient to develop realistic and achievable goals.
  4. Patients who have had a TIA or stroke are at risk for another stroke. Teach family members to observe for and act on signs of a new stroke using the **F.A.S.T.** pneumonic:
     Face drooping
     Arm weakness
     Speech or language difficulty
     Time to call 9-1-1
     a. Refer the family to a social worker and community resources for further support and counseling. Family members may need a referral for respite care.
     b. Provide the patient and family with information (including written materials) about ongoing therapy that alters coagulation.

Teamwork and Collaboration

Hand-off errors lead to patient harm. Be sure that clear, consistent communication and complete documentation are available when the patient transfers between in-hospital care units or procedural suites or to rehabilitative or home care.

SUBCLAVIAN STEAL

OVERVIEW

* Subclavian steal occurs in the upper extremities from a subclavian artery occlusion or stenosis and results in altered blood flow and ischemia in the arm.
* The disorder can occur at any age but is more common when the patient also has risk factors for atherosclerosis.

INTERPROFESSIONAL COLLABORATIVE CARE

* Assess for:
  1. Paresthesias
  2. Light-headedness
  3. Dizziness
  4. Pain and discomfort when the arms are elevated
  5. Difference in blood pressure between arms
  6. Subclavian bruit or decreased pulse on the occluded side
  7. Edema, redness or cyanosis, and delayed capillary refill of the affected arm
* Surgical intervention involves one of three procedures.
  1. Endarterectomy of the subclavian artery
  2. Carotid-subclavian bypass
  3. Dilation of the subclavian artery

SYNDROME OF INAPPROPRIATE ANTIDIURETIC HORMONE

OVERVIEW

* Syndrome of inappropriate antidiuretic hormone (SIADH) occurs when ADH (also known as vasopressin) is secreted even when plasma osmolality is low or normal.
* Water is retained, which results in dilutional hyponatremia (a decreased serum sodium level) and expansion of the extracellular fluid volume.
* SIADH occurs with many pathologic conditions and some drugs, including:
  1. Malignancies and cancer treatment, including small cell lung cancer; pancreatic, duodenal, and genitourinary carcinomas; thymoma; and Hodgkin's lymphoma and non-Hodgkin's lymphoma
  2. Pulmonary disorders, including pneumonia, lung abscesses, active tuberculosis, pneumothorax, and chronic lung diseases
  3. CNS disorders including brain trauma, infection, tumors, and strokes
  4. Drugs including selective serotonin reuptake inhibitors, quinolone antibiotics, some antiepileptics, and opioids

INTERPROFESSIONAL COLLABORATIVE CARE

Assessment: Noticing

- Obtain patient information about:
  1. Recent head or brain trauma
  2. Cerebrovascular disease or stroke
  3. Tuberculosis, pneumonia, or other pulmonary disease
  4. Cancer
  5. All past and current drug use
  6. Loss of appetite, nausea, and vomiting
  7. Recent weight gain
- Assess for fluid overload, electrolyte derangements, pulmonary edema, and heart failure.
  1. Increased pulse quality (bounding central and peripheral pulses)
  2. Increased neck vein distention
  3. Presence of crackles in lungs
  4. Increasing peripheral edema
  5. Altered serum sodium, potassium, calcium, phosphate, and magnesium levels
  6. Reduced and concentrated urine output
  7. Lethargy or decreased mental status
  8. Neuromuscular changes related to electrolyte imbalance, especially hyponatremia

---

! **NURSING SAFETY PRIORITY: Critical Rescue**

Pulmonary edema can occur very quickly and can lead to death. Notify the health care provider about any change that indicates the fluid overload from SIADH is not responding to therapy or is becoming worse.

Interventions: Responding

- Fluid restriction; intake may be restricted to 500 to 1000 mL/24 hr.
- Assess therapy for fluid excretion and sodium replacement.
  1. Measure intake and output; anticipate a goal that output is greater than intake.
  2. Weigh the patient daily.
  3. Monitor serum electrolytes and osmolality.
- Drug therapy may include:
  1. Administering ADH antagonists to promote water loss without urinary sodium excretion: tolvaptan (oral) (Samsca) or conivaptan (IV) (Vaprisol)

! NURSING SAFETY PRIORITY: Drug Alert

Administer tolvaptan or conivaptan only in the hospital setting, so serum sodium levels can be monitored closely for the development of hypernatremia.

2. Using loop diuretics if heart failure results from fluid overload
3. Hypertonic saline (i.e., 3% sodium chloride [3% NaCl]) infusions
4. Demeclocycline (Declomycin), an antibiotic with ADH antagonist properties
- Provide a safe environment when serum sodium is below 120 mEq/L.
  1. Initiate seizure precautions.
  2. Increase patient surveillance to prevent falls or harm during a period of disorientation.
- Include comfort measures during oral fluid restriction, including saliva substitute or stimulant.

SYPHILIS

OVERVIEW

- Syphilis is a complex sexually transmitted disease (STD) that can become systemic and can cause serious complications, including death.
- The causative organism is a spirochete called *Treponema pallidum.*
- Syphilis progresses through four stages: primary, secondary, latent, and tertiary.
  1. In *primary syphilis* a chancre develops within 10 to 90 days after exposure at the site of entry (inoculation) of the organism. Without treatment, the chancre disappears within 6 weeks; however, the organism spreads throughout the body, and the patient is highly infectious.
  2. *Secondary syphilis* develops 6 weeks to 6 months after the onset of primary syphilis. Manifestations are typical of systemic infections: fever, malaise, and generalized aches; and a rash, often manifested on palms and soles, that progresses to contagious pustules.
  3. *Latent syphilis* is a later stage of the disease and has two phases.
     a. *Early latent syphilis* occurs during the first year after infection, and infectious lesions can recur.
     b. *Late latent syphilis* is a disease occurring more than 1 year after infection. It is not infectious except to the fetus of a pregnant woman.

4. *Tertiary syphilis* or *late syphilis* occurs after 4 to 20 years in untreated cases. Any organ system can be affected, and manifestations vary widely. Manifestations include benign lesions (gummas) of the skin, mucous membranes, and bones; aortic valvular disease and aortic aneurysms; and neurosyphilis with CNS problems (e.g., meningitis, hearing loss, generalized paresis).

- Men who have sex with men (MSM) are at greatest risk for contracting primary and secondary syphilis and made up 75% of cases of these diseases in 2012.

Gender Health Considerations

Patient-Centered Care

Unique needs regarding sexual health and prevention and treatment of sexually transmitted infections for lesbian, gay, bisexual, transgender, and questioning (LGBTQ) patients should be identified and addressed by the nurse. Because of discrimination, health care disparities, and health care provider lack of understanding, the overall health status of people in these populations may be poor. LGBTQ people may have difficulty finding health care that identifies and addresses their particular risks and concerns. Taking a health history that provides opportunity for the patient to identify his or her sexual orientation, gender identity, and sexual activity is crucial. Especially among transgender people, opportunities for physical examination are avoided or missed by both the patient and care provider because of fears of being misunderstood or inadequately prepared to give or receive appropriate care.

INTERPROFESSIONAL COLLABORATIVE CARE

- Diagnosis of primary or secondary syphilis is confirmed by a finding of *T. pallidum* on microscopic examination, by a positive Venereal Disease Research Laboratory (VDRL) serum test, or by a positive rapid plasma reagin (RPR) test result.
- Latent and tertiary syphilis may be confirmed by the fluorescent treponemal antibody absorption (FTA-ABS) test or the microhemagglutination assay for *T. pallidum* (MHA-TP).
- Antibiotic therapy with penicillin G given intramuscular (IM) is the treatment for all stages of syphilis. A prolonged course of intravenous antibiotics for the late latent stage may be required.

! NURSING SAFETY PRIORITY: Drug Alert

Discuss with the patient the importance of partner notification and treatment, including the risk for re-infection if the partner goes untreated. All sexual partners must be prophylactically treated as soon as possible, preferably within 90 days of the syphilis diagnosis.

* Provide education about safe sex practices.
* It is essential to teach patient to follow up at 6, 12, and 24 months after initial treatment.
* Inform the patient that the disease will be reported to the local health authority and that all information will be held in strict confidence.
* Encourage the patient to provide accurate information for this follow-up to ensure that all at-risk partners are treated appropriately.
* Provide a setting that offers privacy and encourages open discussion.

SYSTEMIC LUPUS ERYTHEMATOSUS

OVERVIEW

* There are two main classifications of lupus:
  1. *Systemic lupus erythematosus* (SLE) is a chronic, progressive, inflammatory connective tissue disease that can cause major body organs and systems to fail.
     a. The main mechanism of organ damage is the formation of immune complexes in organ tissues and in blood vessels, which deprive the organ of essential oxygen.
     b. It is classified as an autoimmune disease and has periods of spontaneous remissions and exacerbations (flares) with a wide variation in symptoms. However, most patients with SLE have kidney involvement because the immune complexes tend to aggregate in that system.
  2. *Discoid lupus erythematous* (DLE) affects only the skin.
     a. The cause is unknown, although like many autoimmune disorders, a genetic predisposition with environmental interactions is likely.
     b. Only a small percentage of patients with lupus have the DLE type.

Gender and Cultural Considerations

Lupus affects women 10 times more often than men; women of color are affected far more often than Euro-Americans. The reason for this difference is unknown.

INTERPROFESSIONAL COLLABORATIVE CARE
Assessment: Noticing
- Assess for and document:
  1. Dry, scaly, raised nonscarring rash on the face (butterfly rash) or upper body for SLE or round (discoid, coin-like) scarring skin lesions of DLE
  2. Joint involvement
     a. Initial changes are similar to rheumatoid arthritis.
     b. Later changes may include joint deformity.
  3. Muscle aches and atrophy
  4. Fever
  5. Various degrees of weakness, fatigue, anorexia, and weight loss
  6. Kidney disease characterized by reduced urine output, proteinuria, hematuria, and fluid retention
  7. Pulmonary effusions or pneumonia
  8. Pericarditis (the most common cardiovascular change)
     a. Tachycardia
     b. Chest pain
     c. Myocardial ischemia
  9. Neurologic changes
     a. Psychoses
     b. Seizures
     c. Paresis
     d. Migraine headaches
     e. Cranial nerve palsies
  10. Raynaud's phenomenon or other manifestations of vasculitis
  11. Abdominal pain from peritoneal and blood vessel inflammation
  12. Body image changes
  13. Social isolation
  14. Fear, anxiety
- Diagnostic tests include:
  1. Skin biopsy for DLE
  2. Positive blood tests for immune dysregulation or dysfunction
     a. Rheumatoid factor
     b. Antinuclear antibodies
     c. Erythrocyte sedimentation rate or C-reactive protein
     d. Serum complement (especially C3 and C4 and immunoglobulins)
     e. Anti-SS-A (Ro), anti-SS-B (La), anti-Smith (anti-SM), anti-DNA, extractable nuclear antigens (ENA)
     f. Serum protein electrophoresis
  3. CBC to evaluate pancytopenia

4. Complete metabolic panel to evaluate kidney function
5. Cardiac and liver enzymes to asses organ function or damage

Interventions: Responding

- Drug therapy may include:
  1. For DLE
     a. Topical or oral corticosteroid therapy for skin rash
     b. Hydroxychloroquine (Plaquenil) to reduce inflammatory skin responses
  2. For SLE
     a. Immunosuppressive agents, such as methotrexate (Rheumatrex) or azathioprine (Imuran)
     b. Anti-inflammatory corticosteroid (also called glucocorticoid) especially during disease flare or exacerbation
     c. Antineoplastic drugs, such as cyclophosphamide (Cytoxan, Procytox)
     d. Belimumab (Benlysta), an intravenous agent to reduce B-lymphocyte activity and the production of autoantibodies

S

> ### ❗ NURSING SAFETY PRIORITY: Action Alert
>
> When patients are taking immunosuppressant or corticosteroid agents, stress the importance of avoiding large crowds and people who are ill. Teach patients to report any early sign of infection to their health care provider. Observe for side effects and toxic effects of these drugs and report their occurrence immediately. Remind patients to take their medication early in the morning before breakfast because that is the time when the body's natural corticosteroid level is the lowest.

- Teach the patient how to protect the skin by:
  1. Minimizing exposure to sunlight and other forms of ultraviolet light by:
     a. Wearing long sleeves and wide-brimmed hats
     b. Using sun-blocking agents with a sun protective factor of at least 30
  2. Cleaning the skin with a mild soap and avoiding harsh, perfumed products
  3. Using moisturizers and sun protectants
  4. Using mild protein shampoo and avoiding hair bleaching agents, permanents, and dyes

- Reinforce measures for joint protection and energy conservation (see *Arthritis, Rheumatoid*).
- Help the patient identify coping strategies and support systems that can help him or her deal with the unpredictable nature of the exacerbations.
- Teach the patient about:
  1. Informing his or her provider at the onset of symptoms signaling exacerbation
  2. Monitoring for infection, particularly the onset of fever
  3. Protecting joints and conserving energy
  4. Risks related to pregnancy and for contraception options
  5. Resources such as the Lupus Foundation and the Arthritis Foundation
  6. Drug therapy information for scheduling, side effects, and any precautions

SYSTEMIC SCLEROSIS

OVERVIEW

- Systemic sclerosis (SSc), also called *scleroderma,* is a chronic, inflammatory, autoimmune connective tissue disease that usually first manifests with hardening of the skin.
- The disease is often confused with SLE but is less common, and not always progressive.
- The manifestations vary widely from person to person.
- It is classified as:
  1. *Diffuse cutaneous SSc,* with skin thickening on the trunk, face, and proximal and distal extremities (over most of the body); the first symptom is hand and forearm edema, which may exist with bilateral carpal tunnel syndrome
     a. When scleroderma progresses, swelling is replaced by tightening, hardening, and thickening of skin tissue with loss of elasticity and greatly decreased ROM.
     b. Ulcerations and joint contractures may develop, and the patient may be unable to perform ADLs.
  2. *Limited cutaneous SSc,* with thick skin limited to sites distal to the elbow and knee but also involving the face and neck; patients have the *CREST syndrome.*
     a. *C*alcinosis (calcium deposits)
     b. *R*aynaud's phenomenon
     c. *E*sophageal dysmotility
     d. *S*clerodactyly (scleroderma of the digits)
     e. *T*elangiectasia (spider-like hemangiomas)
- Women are affected more often than men and usually are between 25 and 65 years old.

INTERPROFESSIONAL COLLABORATIVE CARE

Assessment: Noticing

- Asses skin and joints.
- Assess for major organ involvement:
  1. GI tract changes with dysphagia, gastroesophageal reflux disease (GERD) and diminished peristalsis leading to constipation or obstruction; a small, sliding hiatal hernia may be present
  2. Cardiovascular system changes
     a. Raynaud's phenomenon with potential for digit perfusion abnormalities leading to pain, necrosis, and amputation
     b. Myocardial fibrosis may be present with cardiac dysrhythmias and chest pain.
     c. Vascular involvement may lead to hypertension and stenotic renal artery–induced malignant hypertension.
  3. Lung changes resulting in restrictive airway disease (fibrosis of the alveoli and interstitial tissues); pulmonary hypertension may develop

Interventions: Responding

- Administer drug therapy
  1. Systemic corticosteroids and immunosuppressants are used, often in combination.
  2. Teach about scheduling, dosing, and adverse reactions.
- Protect skin by:
  1. Teaching the patient to use mild soap and lotions and gentle cleaning techniques
  2. Inspecting the skin for further changes or open lesions
  3. Caring for skin ulcers according to their type and location
  4. Adjusting room temperature to prevent vasoconstriction (Raynaud's phenomenon)
  5. Teaching patients to avoid or minimize cigarette smoking with associated vasoconstriction
- Promote gas exchange in fibrotic lungs by:
  1. Providing positioning to expand lungs
  2. Administering oxygen therapy if prescribed
- Promote nutrition by:
  1. Providing small, frequent meals
  2. Instructing the patient to avoid foods that may exacerbate GERD (caffeine, alcohol)
  3. Teaching the patient to keep the head elevated for 1 to 2 hours after a meal
- Reduce pain and maintain joint mobility using interventions similar to those for rheumatoid arthritis.
- Referr patients and families to community resources.

S

T

THROMBOCYTOPENIA

OVERVIEW

- Thrombocytopenia is a reduction in platelets; platelets are essential in clotting.
- Some conditions associated with low platelets include hematopoietic disease (anemia, leukemia, and myelodysplastic syndromes), thrombotic thrombocytopenic purpura (an abnormality of platelet clumping associated with inadequate clumping during trauma or surgery), heparin-induced thrombocytopenia (an immune-mediated response that targets platelets after heparin exposure), and autoimmune thrombocytopenia purpura.
- Treatment is generally focused on preventing bleeding, reducing modifiable factors (such as drug toxidromes), and close monitoring and replacement of platelets or blood products during bleeding.

THROMBOCYTOPENIA PURPURA, AUTOIMMUNE

OVERVIEW

- Autoimmune thrombocytopenic purpura, also called *idiopathic thrombocytopenic purpura* (ITP), is characterized by reduced circulating platelets even though platelet production is normal.
- Antibodies (auto-antibodies) are produced that target the surface of platelets, leading to platelet destruction by macrophages in the spleen.
- The problem is most common among women who are 20 to 50 years old and among people who have other autoimmune disorders.

INTERPROFESSIONAL COLLABORATIVE CARE

- Assess for and document:
  1. Large bruises or petechial rash on the arms, legs, upper chest, and neck
  2. Mucosal bleeding
  3. Anemia
  4. Neurologic impairment as a result of an intracranial bleeding-induced stroke
  5. Laboratory findings: decreased platelet count, large numbers of megakaryocytes in the bone marrow, presence of antiplatelet antibodies in the blood, low hematocrit and low hemoglobin levels, and abnormalities in the structure of the spleen
- Interventions include:
  1. Drug therapy to suppress immune function
     a. Corticosteroids
     b. Immunomodulators like azathioprine (Imuran), eltrombopag, rituximab (Rituxan), and romiplostim

2. Platelet transfusions when platelet counts are less than $10,000/mm^3$ or patient is actively bleeding
3. Preventing or minimizing injury to avoid bleeding
4. A splenectomy (the site of platelet destruction) if there is no response to drug therapy

TOXIC SHOCK SYNDROME

OVERVIEW

- Toxic shock syndrome (TSS) is a form of septic shock caused by *Staphylococcus aureus* or *Streptococcus* infection and is related to menstruation and tampon use.
- Other conditions associated with TSS include internal contraceptive devices, surgical wound infection, nonsurgical infections, and gynecologic surgeries.
- In menstrual-related infection, menstrual blood provides a growth medium for the bacteria, which produces endotoxins that cross the vaginal mucosa to the bloodstream. Tampon insertion or prolonged use can cause vaginal dryness and microabrasions that provide an entry for the microorganisms.

INTERPROFESSIONAL COLLABORATIVE CARE

- Assess for:
  1. Abrupt onset of a high fever
  2. Headache, myalgia, and flu-like symptoms
  3. Severe hypotension
  4. Sunburn-like rash with broken capillaries in the eyes and on the skin
- Management includes:
  1. Removal of the infection source
  2. Management of fluids and electrolyte imbalances, avoiding hypotension
  3. Intravenous (IV) antibiotics and other measures included in the management of sepsis and septic shock
- Patient education focuses on prevention by teaching all women about the proper use of tampons, internal contraceptive devices such as vaginal sponges and diaphragms, and prompt treatment of gynecologic infections.

TRACHEOSTOMY: GAS EXCHANGE CONCEPT EXEMPLAR

OVERVIEW

- A tracheostomy is a stoma (opening) that results from a surgical incision into the trachea to create an airway to maintain gas exchange.
- Tracheostomies can be emergent or planned and temporary or permanent.

- Indications for tracheostomy include acute airway obstruction, the need for airway protection, laryngeal or facial trauma or burns, and airway involvement during head or neck surgery.
- They also are used for prolonged unconsciousness, paralysis, or the inability to be weaned from mechanical ventilation.

INTERPROFESSIONAL COLLABORATIVE CARE
Assessment: Noticing
See details in chart 2-24 below for assessing the patient with a Tracheostomy.

Chart 2-24	Focused Assessment: The Patient with a Tracheostomy

- Note the quality, pattern, and rate of breathing:
  - Within patient's baseline?
- Tachypnea can indicate hypoxia.
- Dyspnea can indicate secretions in the airway.
- Assess for any cyanosis, especially around the lips, which could indicate hypoxia.
- Check the patient's pulse oximetry reading.
- If oxygen is prescribed, is the patient receiving the correct amount, with the correct equipment and humidification?
- Assess the tracheostomy site:
  - Note the color, consistency, and amount of secretions in the tube or externally.
- If the tracheostomy is sutured in place, is there any redness, swelling, or drainage from suture sites?
- If the tracheostomy is secured with ties, what is the condition of the ties? Are they moist with secretions or perspiration? Are the secretions dried on the ties? Is the tie secure?
- Assess the condition of the skin around the tracheostomy and neck for tissue integrity. Be sure to check underneath the neck for secretions that may have drained to the back. Check for any skin breakdown related to pressure from the ties or related to excess secretions.
- Assess behind the faceplate for the size of the space between the outer cannula and the patient's tissue. Are any secretions collected in this area?
- If the tube is cuffed, check cuff pressure.

* Auscultate the lungs.
* Are a second (emergency) tracheostomy tube and obturator available?

Analysis: Interpreting
* The priority interprofessional problems for patients requiring tracheostomy include:
  1. Decreased gas exchange due to weak chest muscles, obstruction, or other physical problems that interfere with ventilation and diffusion of gases
  2. Inadequate communication due to tracheostomy or intubation
  3. Potential for weight loss due to inadequate nutrition from presence of endotracheal tube
  4. Potential for infection related to invasive procedures or problems with the normal protective mechanisms of the respiratory tract
  5. Potential for loss of tracheal tissue integrity due to pressure and trauma from tracheostomy tubes

Interventions: Responding
PROVIDING TRACHEOSTOMY CARE
* Monitor breath sounds hourly in the immediate postoperative phase.
* Prevent complications of tube obstruction with vigilant assessment for difficulty breathing or noisy respirations and provision of inner cannula care, suctioning, and humidifying oxygen. See Chart 2-25 for best practice in tracheostomy care.
* Avoid tube dislodgement by securing the tube to reduce movement and traction.
* Ensure that a replacement tracheostomy tube is at the bedside in acute care settings.
* Use sterile technique for tracheal suctioning to prevent respiratory infection.

! NURSING SAFETY PRIORITY: Critical Rescue

Monitor the patient for tube placement. When you recognize that the tube is dislodged on an immature tracheostomy, respond by ventilating the patient using a manual resuscitation bag and facemask while another nurse calls the Rapid Response Team.

MAINTAINING COMMUNICATION
* A tracheostomy always disrupts verbal communication; plan perioperative information about and strategies for pictorial or written communication.

Chart 2-25	**Best Practice for Patient Safety & Quality Care: Tracheostomy Care**

1. Assemble the necessary equipment.
2. Wash hands. Maintain Standard Precautions.
3. Suction the tracheostomy tube if necessary.
4. Remove old dressings and excess secretions.
5. Set up a sterile field.
6. Remove and clean the inner cannula. Use half-strength hydrogen peroxide (if prescribed) to clean the cannula and sterile saline to rinse it. If the inner cannula is disposable, remove the cannula and replace it with a new one.
7. Clean the stoma site and then the tracheostomy plate with half-strength hydrogen peroxide followed by sterile saline. Ensure that none of the solutions enters the tracheostomy.
8. Change tracheostomy ties if they are soiled. Secure new ties in place before removing soiled ones to prevent accidental decannulation. If a knot is needed, tie a square knot that is visible on the side of the neck. Only one finger should be able to be placed between the tie tape and the neck.
9. Remove gloves and wash hands.
10. Document the type and amount of secretions and the general condition of the stoma and surrounding skin tissue integrity. Document the patient's response to the procedure and any teaching or learning that occurred.

ENSURING NUTRITION
- Swallowing can be a major problem for the patient with a tracheostomy tube in place.
- In a normal swallow, the larynx lifts and moves forward to prevent food and saliva from entering. The tracheostomy tube sometimes tethers the larynx in place, making it unable to move effectively. The result is difficulty in swallowing.
- Refer to Chart 2-26 for best practice to prevent aspiration during swallowing.

PREVENTING TISSUE DAMAGE
- Loss of tissue integrity can occur at the point where the inflated cuff presses against the tracheal mucosa.
- Mucosal ischemia occurs when the pressure exerted by the cuff on the mucosa exceeds the capillary perfusion pressure.
- To reduce the risk for tracheal damage, keep the cuff pressure between 14 and 20 mm Hg or 20 and 30 cm H_2O (ideally, 25 cm H_2O or less).

Chart 2-26	Preventing Aspiration During Swallowing

- Avoid serving meals when the patient is fatigued.
- Provide smaller and more frequent meals.
- Provide adequate time; do not "hurry" the patient.
- Provide close supervision if the patient is self-feeding.
- Keep emergency suctioning equipment close at hand and turned on.
- Avoid water and other "thin" liquids, as well as the use of straws.
- Thicken all liquids, including water.
- Avoid foods that generate thin liquids during the chewing process, such as fruit.
- Position the patient in the most upright position possible.
- When possible, completely (or at least partially) deflate the tube cuff during meals.
- Suction after initial cuff deflation to clear the airway and allow maximum comfort during the meal.
- Feed each bite or encourage the patient to take each bite slowly.
- Encourage the patient to "dry swallow" after each bite (known as "double swallowing") to clear residue from the throat.
- Avoid consecutive swallows of liquids.
- Provide controlled small volumes of liquids, using a spoon.
- Encourage the patient to "tuck" his or her chin down and move the forehead forward while swallowing.
- Allow the patient to indicate when he or she is ready for the next bite.
- If the patient coughs, stop the feeding until he or she indicates that the airway has been cleared.
- Continuously monitor tolerance to oral food intake by assessing respiratory rate, ease, pulse oximetry, and heart rate (HR).

- Check cuff pressure at least once during each shift.
- Inadequate humidity can cause tracheal damage. Humidify the air as prescribed.

Care Coordination and Transition Management

- By the time of discharge, the patient should be able to provide self-care, including tracheostomy care, nutrition care, suctioning, and communication.
- Instruct the patient to use a shower shield over the tracheostomy tube when bathing to prevent water from entering the airway.

- Teach the patient to cover the opening loosely during the day with a small cotton cloth to protect the opening and filter the air entering the stoma.

Considerations for Older Adults

Patient-Centered Care

Self-managing tracheostomy care and oxygen therapy can be difficult for the older patient who has vision problems or difficulty with upper arm movement. Teach him or her to use magnifying lenses or glasses to ensure the proper setting on the oxygen gauge. Assess his or her ability to reach and manipulate the tracheostomy. If possible, work with a family member who can provide assistance during tracheostomy care.

TRANSPLANT REJECTION

OVERVIEW

- Rejection is a complex series of responses that change over time and involve different components of immunity.
- Transplant rejection is caused by general and specific immunity functions of a host directed against tissues and organs transplanted from other people.
- Host natural killer (NK) cells and cytotoxic/cytolytic T cells are the major cells responsible for the destructive attacks on transplanted organs (*grafts*) leading to host rejection of these helpful tissues. Because the solid organ transplanted into the recipient (host) is seldom a perfectly identical match of human leukocyte antigens (HLAs) (unless the organ is obtained from an identical sibling) between the donated organ and the recipient host, the patient's immune system cells recognize a newly transplanted organ as non-self.
- Transplant rejection can be:
  1. Hyperacute, occurring as antigen-antibody complexes form immediately in blood vessels of the transplanted organ
  2. Acute, occurring 1 week to 3 months after transplant as a result of antibody-mediated vasculitis and recipient NK and cytotoxic T cells entering and killing the transplanted organ
  3. Chronic, occurring over more than 4 months' time as a result of chronic inflammation and scarring of blood vessels and transplanted organ tissues

INTERPROFESSIONAL COLLABORATIVE CARE

- *Maintenance therapy* is the continuous immunosuppression used after a solid organ transplant. The drugs used for routine therapy after solid organ transplantation are combinations of a calcineurin inhibitor, a corticosteroid, and an antiproliferative agent.

- *Rescue therapy* is used to treat acute rejection episodes. The drug categories for this purpose are the monoclonal and polyclonal antibodies.
- Corticosteroids are also used to manage acute and recurrent episodes of rejection and can be used for maintenance therapy.

TRAUMA, ABDOMINAL
OVERVIEW
- Abdominal trauma is an injury to the structures located between the diaphragm and the pelvis that occurs when the abdomen is subjected to blunt or penetrating force.
  1. Blunt trauma is also caused by motor vehicle crashes, falls, assaults, and contact sports.
  2. Penetrating trauma is most often caused by bullets, knives, or other objects that open the abdomen.
- Organs that may be injured include the large and small bowel, liver, spleen, duodenum, pancreas, kidneys, and urinary bladder.

INTERPROFESSIONAL COLLABORATIVE CARE
Assessment: Noticing
- Assess for airway, breathing, and circulation (ABCs).
- Identify the mechanism (force and type) of injury.
  1. The spleen is vulnerable to blunt trauma and contributes to significant blood loss.
  2. The liver is the most commonly injured organ with penetrating trauma.
- Evaluate for symptoms of hypovolemia and shock. The key assessment factors related to early shock detection are decreased mental status, hypotension, tachycardia, tachypnea, decreased peripheral oxygenation (Spo_2), and decreased skin perfusion (see *Shock* for discussions of hemorrhagic and hypovolemic forms of shock).
- Assess for and document:
  1. Mental status, vital signs (HR, blood pressure [BP], respiratory rate [RR], and Spo_2), bowel sounds, urinary output, and changes in clinical findings every 15 to 30 minutes until stable, then hourly; report any deterioration immediately to the physician
  2. The patient's report about the presence, location, and quality of pain, including referred pain (e.g., right shoulder) and nausea
  3. Inspection of the abdomen, back, flanks, genitalia, and rectum for contusions, abrasions, lacerations, ecchymosis, penetrating injuries, and symmetry. Ecchymosis around the umbilicus (Cullen's sign) and ecchymosis in either flank (Turner's sign) may indicate retroperitoneal bleeding into the abdominal wall. Be aware that a large volume of blood can accumulate in the

abdominal cavity before there is a change in the size or color during inspection.

4. Auscultation of the abdomen for absent or diminished bowel sounds and bruits

5. Percussion for abnormal sounds such as resonance over the liver or dullness over the stomach or intestines (Ballance's sign)

6. Results from light palpation of the abdomen to identify areas of tenderness, guarding, rigidity, and spasm

7. Kehr's sign, indicating splenic injury, which is left shoulder pain resulting from diaphragmatic irritation

8. Blood in peritoneal lavage, NG tube output, or emesis

Interventions: Responding

NONSURGICAL MANAGEMENT

- Interventions include:
  1. Placing two peripheral IV catheters to provide rapid fluid resuscitation
  2. Infusing IV fluids at a rapid rate, as ordered, and monitoring patient response
  3. Inserting an indwelling Foley catheter and monitoring urine output hourly for at least 24 hours
  4. Inserting an NG tube to prevent vomiting and reduce intra-abdominal pressure
  5. Monitoring intra-abdominal pressure (in some facilities) to detect compartment syndrome, which is compression of structures in the abdominal cavity (see *Compartment Syndrome*)

- Diagnostic studies may include:
  1. Abdominal ultrasound in the presence of blunt trauma
  2. Peritoneal lavage
  3. Abdominal computerized tomography (CT) scan
  4. Chest x-ray
  5. ECG and ongoing ECG monitoring
  6. Serum analyses: CBC, basic metabolic panel, coagulation factors, tests for liver function and blood typing with antibody screening for possible transfusion
  7. Continuous intra-abdominal pressure monitoring

- Analgesics are used for pain, with careful attention to maintaining airway and breathing.

SURGICAL MANAGEMENT

- For patients with severe abdominal trauma, an exploratory laparotomy with rcpair of abdominal injuries is performed.

- Most patients with gunshot or stab wounds require an exploratory laparotomy to assess for internal damage.

- Standard perioperative care is performed (Refer to Perioperative Care).

- A colostomy, either temporary or permanent, may be required.

TRAUMA, BLADDER
OVERVIEW
- Bladder trauma occurs as a result of blunt or penetrating injury to the lower abdomen. And can include sexual assault.
- The most common cause is a fractured pelvis (bone fragments puncture the bladder).

INTERPROFESSIONAL COLLABORATIVE CARE
- Assess:
  1. Urinary output, particularly the presence of hematuria and anuria
  2. Bloody urinary meatus
  3. Results of cystogram and voiding cystourethrogram
- Patients with bladder trauma other than a simple contusion require surgical intervention, including closure repair of the bladder wall and peritoneal membrane.
- Recovery may include prolonged use of a urinary ureteral or suprapubic catheter while the repaired bladder heals.

TRAUMATIC BRAIN INJURY: COGNITION CONCEPT EXEMPLAR
OVERVIEW
- A traumatic brain injury (TBI) is damage to the brain from an external mechanical force that leads to impaired COGNITION, mobility, sensory perception, or psychosocial function.
  1. Examples of mechanical force include a blow to the head or penetration of the brain by a bullet; injury is not caused by neurodegenerative or congenital conditions.
  2. Impairment can be temporary or permanent.
- In a *closed* brain injury, the integrity of the skull remains intact.
- In an *open* brain injury, the skull is fractured or penetrated by an object (e.g., bullet, projectile, knife), exposing meninges or brain tissue to extracranial contaminants.
- Primary injury occurs at the time force occurs with potential for additional primary injury from countercoup forces when the intracranial tissue "bounces" against the skull opposite the site of direct injury. Primary TBI involves the frontal or temporal lobes.
- Secondary brain injury can occur from physiologic, vascular, and biochemical events that extend the area of the primary injury and involve cellular changes that contribute to tissue injury. The most common causes of secondary injury are hypotension, hypoxia, hemorrhage, cerebral edema, and elevated intracranial pressure. Prevention of secondary injury is a major focus of acute care.

- Damage to brain tissue depends on the location, degree, and mechanism of injury.
  1. Brain injury can be classified as mild, moderate, or severe, depending on the initial Glasgow Coma Scale (GCS) score, which has implications for both treatment and prognosis.
  2. It may be also described by the degree of apparent damage to the brain.
     a. A *concussion* is a brain injury that temporarily changes how the brain functions as a result of mechanical force or trauma. It may or may not be associated with a brief loss of consciousness. Typically, no brain tissue damage is visible by CT.
     b. A *contusion* causes bruising of the brain tissue.
     c. A *laceration* causes tearing of the cortical surface vessels and may lead to secondary hemorrhage.
     d. A *diffuse axonal injury* occurs when axons of the central nervous system (CNS) neurons are stretched and damaged, resulting in widespread inflammation and neuron damage or death.
- Types of skull fractures associated with open brain injuries include:
  1. *Linear,* a simple, clean break
  2. *Depressed,* in which bone is pressed inward into brain tissue
  3. *Open,* in which the scalp is lacerated along with the skull fracture
  4. *Comminuted,* in which the skull is fragmented and bone is depressed into the brain tissue
  5. *Basilar,* which occurs at the base of the skull, usually along the paranasal sinus, and which may result in a cerebrospinal fluid (CSF) leak from the nose or ear and potential damage to cranial nerves I, II, VII, and VIII
- The types of hemorrhage that occur after a TBI are epidural, subdural, intracerebral, and subarachnoid.

! NURSING SAFETY PRIORITY: Critical Rescue

After the initial interval, symptoms of neurologic impairment from hemorrhage can progress very quickly with potentially life-threatening ICP elevation and irreversible structural damage to brain tissue. Monitor the patient suspected of epidural bleeding frequently (every 5 to 10 minutes) for changes in neurologic status. The patient can become quickly and increasingly symptomatic. *A loss of consciousness from an epidural or subdural hematoma is a neurosurgical emergency!*

- In the presence of increased intracranial pressure (ICP), the brain tissue may shift (herniate), creating additional neuron damage.
    1. Intracranial hypertension is manifested by decreased consciousness.
    2. Notify the provider immediately with a decrease in a GCS of 2 or more points; all herniation syndromes are potentially life-threatening.

INTERPROFESSIONAL COLLABORATIVE CARE
Assessment: Noticing

- Obtain patient information about:
    1. When, where, and how the injury occurred
    2. The patient's level of consciousness (LOC) immediately after the injury and on admission to the hospital or unit and whether there have been any changes or fluctuations
    3. Presence of seizure activity at the scene of injury
    4. Medical and social history, especially presence of alcohol or drug use
    5. Hand dominance

! NURSING SAFETY PRIORITY: Critical Rescue

The upper cervical spinal nerves innervate the diaphragm to control breathing. Monitor all TBI patients for respiratory problems and diaphragmatic breathing, as well as diminished or absent reflexes in the airway (cough and gag). Hypoxia and hypercapnia are best detected through arterial oxygen levels (partial pressure of arterial oxygen [Pao_2]), oxygen saturation (Spo_2), and end-tidal volume carbon dioxide measurement ($EtCO_2$). Observe chest wall movement and listen to breath sounds. Report any sign of respiratory problems immediately to the physician!

- Assess for:
    1. Airway patency and breathing pattern: RR, depth, and quality with Spo_2
    2. Signs and symptoms of hypovolemic shock or hemorrhage, which may indicate additional traumatic injuries such as abdominal bleeding or bleeding into soft tissue around major fractures
    3. HR and rhythm, BP, peripheral pulses, and core temperature
    4. Baseline and ongoing neurologic status with a standard assessment tool such as the GCS
        a. Decreased or garbled verbal response to auditory or tactile stimulus; new aphasia
        b. Inability to follow commands; confusion

    c. Pupils that are large, pinpoint, or ovoid, and nonreactive to light (indicates cranial nerve dysfunction, especially III, IV, and VII; may indicate brain stem dysfunction)

    d. Decreased or absent motor strength in the extremities; hemiparesis or hemiplegia

    e. Complaints of severe headache, nausea, or vomiting

    f. Seizure activity

    g. Drainage of CSF from the ear or nose ("halo sign")

5. Indications of post-traumatic sequelae in the patient who experienced a brain injury (symptoms may persist for weeks or months)

    a. Persistent headache

    b. Weakness

    c. Dizziness

    d. Loss of memory

    e. Personality and behavioral changes

    f. Problems with perception, reasoning abilities, and concept formation

6. Changes in personality, behavior, and abilities, such as:

    a. Increased incidence of temper outbursts, risk-taking behavior, depression, and denial of disability

    b. Becoming more talkative and developing a very outgoing personality

    c. Decreased ability to learn new information, to concentrate, and to plan

    d. Impaired memory, especially recent or short-term memory; this should not be confused with problems of aphasia

- Assess family dynamics. Family members may be angry with the patient for being injured, especially if the patient's behavior resulted in an injury that could have been prevented, or they may feel guilty that they could not prevent the injury.

- Diagnostic studies may include:

    1. CBC, basic metabolic panel, coagulation studies, arterial blood gases (ABGs), and toxicology screen

    2. CT scan

    3. Chest x-ray and abdominal x-ray to evaluate for the presence of additional injuries

> ## ❗ NURSING SAFETY PRIORITY: Critical Rescue
>
> LOC is the most sensitive and specific indicator of neurologic deterioration. Immediately inform the physician about changes in mentation, orientation, or behavior. A decrease in the GCS score of 2 points or more should be reported to the provider immediately.

Analysis: Interpreting

- The priority collaborative problems for patients with TBI vary greatly depending on the severity of the event. The most common problems include:
  1. Potential for decreased cerebral tissue PERFUSION due to primary event and/or secondary brain injury
  2. Potential for decreased memory, sensation, and/or mobility due to primary or secondary brain injury

Planning and Implementation: Responding

MAINTAINING CEREBRAL TISSUE PERFUSION

1. Assess vital signs with a standard neurologic assessment every 1 to 2 hours to detect early signs of decreased levels of consciousness, poor perfusion, hypovolemia, and dangerous elevations of BP that may cause further brain damage. Cardiac monitoring to detect cardiac dysrhythmias may be implemented. Report derangements immediately.

2. Therapeutic hypothermia may be started regardless of the presence of fever; fever may extend the area of brain damage during the acute phase. The purpose of therapeutic hypothermia is to rapidly cool the patient to a core temperature of 89.6°F and 93.2°F (32°C to 34°C).

3. The patient may be placed in systemic or local (cranial) hypothermia devices (blanket, helmet) to slow brain metabolism during the acute phase.

4. Position the patient to avoid extreme flexion or extension of the neck, which interferes with CSF outflow. Maintain the head in a midline, central position; log roll the patient and elevate the back rest 30 degrees unless contraindicated; use reverse Trendelenburg position if spinal cord injury is still being evaluated.

5. Maintain the Pao_2 at 80 to 100 mm Hg and Spo_2 at greater than 92% to maintain sufficient oxygen to brain cells, preventing secondary brain injury.

6. The patient receiving mechanical ventilation may have settings to maintain the $Paco_2$ at 35 to 38 mm Hg after the 24 hours to promote cerebral vasoconstriction and reduce intracranial hypertension.

7. Monitor ICP with a specialized device in the intensive care unit (ICU) if the patient presents with coma; manage ICP and cerebral perfusion pressure to maintain adequate blood flow to brain tissue. Maintain infection control/prevention processes specific to the use of ICP monitoring devices to prevent secondary brain injury from infection.

8. Monitor brain tissue oxygenation with jugular venous oxygen apparatus (Sjo_2).

9. Administer drug therapy.
   a. Administer hypertonic saline or osmotic diuretics (manni-tol) to reduce cerebral edema.
      (1) Use a filter to eliminate microscopic crystals when removing mannitol from its vial.
      (2) Osmotic diuretics are most effective when given as a bolus rather than a continuous infusion.
   b. Use opioids or sedatives if the patient is mechanically ventilated to control restlessness and agitation that causes increased ICP.

MAINTAINING COGNITION, SENSORY PERCEPTION, AND MOBILITY

- **Cognitive rehabilitation** is a way of helping brain-injured pa-tients regain function in areas that are essential for a return to independence and a reasonable quality of life, but these services are not widely available.
- Always introduce yourself before any interaction.
- Keep explanations of procedures and activities short and simple, and give them immediately before and throughout patient care.
- To the extent possible, maintain a sleep-wake cycle with scheduled rest periods.
- Orient the patient to time (day, month, and year) and place, and explain the reason for the hospitalization.
- Sensory stimulation is done to facilitate a meaningful response to the environment. Present visual, auditory, or tactile stimuli one at a time, and explain the purpose and the type of stimulus presented.

SURGICAL MANAGEMENT

- A craniotomy may be indicated to:
  1. Evacuate a subdural or epidural hematoma
  2. Treat uncontrolled increased ICP by removing a portion of the skull (craniectomy) or removing ischemic brain tissue
     a. After a craniectomy, position the patient so that no pressure is placed on the head where the missing skull section exists, until swelling resolves.
     b. Generally the patient wears a helmet to protect the brain that is not covered by skull once out of bed mobility begins.
     c. It is possible to restore the preserved skull piece at a future date.
  3. Treat hydrocephalus with an external or internal shunt
- An alternative to a craniotomy is surgical burr holes in which a hole is drilled into the skull to expose the dura mater, usually to relieve intracranial hypertension.
- Bedside surgical insertion of an ICP-monitoring device is often performed and some devices allow external drainage of CSF.

Care Coordination and Transition Management

* Most patients with *moderate-to-severe* TBI are discharged with varied long-term physical and cognitive disabilities. Changes in personality and behavior are very common. The family must learn to cope with the patient's increased fatigue, irritability, temper outbursts, depression, loneliness, and memory problems. Patients often require constant supervision at home, and families may feel socially isolated.
   1. Respite care may be needed to help the family cope with feelings of isolation, increased responsibility, financial or emotional stress, or role reversal; refer them to support groups.
   2. The patient may experience a sense of isolation and loneliness because personality and behavior changes make it difficult to resume or maintain pre-injury social contacts; provide referral to counseling and community resources such as the local chapter of the Brain Injury Association of American or the National Brain Injury Foundation.
* Provide a detailed plan of care at the time of transfer to a rehabilitation or long-term care facility:
   1. Drugs, including dosage and possible side effects
   2. Current patient activity
   3. Techniques used to motivate or calm the patient
   4. Successful coping strategies identified by the patient or family
   5. Whether a helmet needs to be used following a craniectomy to prevent injury from a fall
* For patients returning home, consider home care referral and follow-up appointments to promote recovery and adjustment
* Inform the patient and family about resources such as the National Head Injury Foundation or a local brain injury support group.
* Provide the patient and family with information about:
   1. Strategies to adapt to sensory dysfunction and to cope with the personality or behavior problems that may arise
   2. The purpose, dosage, schedule, and route of administration of drugs
   3. Participation in activities as tolerated
* For patients with minor TBI, discuss symptoms of post-traumatic stress disorder and mild cognitive deficit disorder. Inform the patient that these symptoms are common and refer the patient and family to a specialist in brain injury or cognitive therapy and a support group if symptoms persist. Symptoms are similar to *post-traumatic stress disorder* and include:
   1. Personality changes
   2. Irritability

3. Headaches
4. Dizziness
5. Restlessness
6. Nervousness
7. Insomnia
8. Memory loss
9. Depression

TRAUMA, ESOPHAGEAL

OVERVIEW

- Trauma to the esophagus can result from blunt injuries, chemical burns, surgery or endoscopy, or the stress of protracted severe vomiting.
- Trauma may affect the esophagus directly, impairing swallowing and nutrition, or create problems and complications in the lungs or mediastinum.

INTERPROFESSIONAL COLLABORATIVE CARE

- Assess for and document:
  1. Airway patency, breathing
  2. Chest pain
  3. Dysphagia
  4. Vomiting, hematemesis
  5. Results of x-ray examination, CT, and endoscopy
- Treatment includes:
  1. Maintaining NPO status to prevent further leakage of esophageal secretions
  2. Maintaining NG or gastrostomy tube drainage to heal ("rest") the esophagus
  3. Administering total parenteral nutrition (TPN) during esophageal rest (usually for at least 10 days)
  4. Administering broad-spectrum antibiotics, corticosteroids, and analgesics
- Surgery may be needed to remove the damaged tissue. A resection or replacement of the damaged esophageal segment with small bowel tissue may be required.

TRAUMA, FACIAL

OVERVIEW

- Facial trauma is described by the specific bones (e.g., mandibular, maxillary, orbital, or nasal fractures) and the side of the face involved.
- Mandibular (lower jaw) fractures can occur at any point on the mandible and are the most common facial fractures.
- The rich blood supply of the face leads to extensive bleeding and bruising with facial trauma.

INTERPROFESSIONAL COLLABORATIVE CARE

Assessment: Noticing

- The first action to take for a patient with facial trauma is airway assessment.
- Assess for:
  1. Manifestations of airway obstruction
     a. Stridor
     b. Shortness of breath
     c. Anxiety and restlessness or decreased consciousness
     d. Hypoxia and decreased oxygen saturation
     e. Hypercarbia
  2. Soft tissue edema
  3. Facial asymmetry
  4. Pain
  5. Leakage of spinal fluid through the ears or nose
  6. Vision and eye movement
  7. Bruising behind the ears in the mastoid area ("battle sign")

Interventions: Responding

- The priority action is to establish and maintain a patent airway.
  1. Provide suction at the bedside.
  2. Anticipate the need for emergency intubation, tracheotomy, or cricothyroidotomy.
- Other interventions include:
  1. Controlling hemorrhage
  2. Assessing for the extent of injury
  3. Establishing IV access and initiating fluid resuscitation
  4. Assisting in the stabilization of fractures
  5. Administering prescribed antibiotics
  6. For mandibular fixation with plates, teaching the patient about:
     a. Oral care with an irrigating device
     b. Soft diet or dental liquid diet restrictions
     c. How to cut the wires if emesis occurs

> ### ! NURSING SAFETY PRIORITY: Critical Rescue
>
> Instruct the patient with mandibular fixation to keep wire cutters with him or her at all times in case emergent aspiration occurs.

TRAUMA, KIDNEY

OVERVIEW

- Trauma to one or both kidneys may occur with penetrating wounds or blunt injuries to the back, flank, or abdomen or with urologic procedures.

- Traumatic kidney injury is classified into five grades based on the severity of the injury. Grade one consists of low grade injury in the form of kidney bruising, and grade five represents the most severe variety associated with shattering of the kidney and tearing of its blood supply.

INTERPROFESSIONAL COLLABORATIVE CARE
- Obtain patient information about:
  1. The mechanism of injury, including the events surrounding the trauma
  2. History of kidney or urologic disease, including previous surgical intervention
  3. History of diabetes, hypertension, or atherosclerosis
- Assess for and document:
  1. Vital signs, particularly derangements in HR, BP, RR, and Spo_2 indicating poor perfusion or reduced gas exchange that contribute to hypovolemic or hypoxic kidney damage
  2. Abdominal or flank pain, distension, bruising, or asymmetry
  3. Penetrating injuries of the lower thorax, back, or abdomen
  4. Urine output hourly and abnormal urine, especially blood in the urine
  5. Decreased serum hemoglobin and hematocrit values
- Treatment may include fluids and drugs to support perfusion:
  1. Administer fluids, such as crystalloids or packed red blood cells (RBCs), to restore circulatory blood volume.
  2. Assess the need for clotting factors such as vitamin K and platelets.
- Interventional radiology techniques may be used to drain fluid around the urinary tract or to stent or embolize a renal artery.
- Surgical interventions such as nephrectomy or vascular repair may be required.

TRAUMA, LARYNGEAL

OVERVIEW
- Laryngeal trauma occurs with a crushing or direct blow, fracture, or by prolonged endotracheal intubation.
- Manifestations include dyspnea, aphonia, hoarseness, subcutaneous emphysema, and hemoptysis.
- Management consists of assessing the effectiveness of gas exchange.
  1. Monitor vital signs and pulse oximetry every 15 to 30 minutes.
  2. Communicate increased respiratory difficulty immediately to the provider.
     a. Tachypnea, especially rates greater than 28 breaths/minute
     b. Nasal flaring or use of accessory respiratory muscles
     c. Anxiety, restlessness, or a decreased LOC

    d. Dyspnea or new-onset voice weakness or hoarseness
    e. Decreased Spo_2
    f. Stridor

> **!** **NURSING SAFETY PRIORITY: Critical Rescue**
>
> If the patient has respiratory difficulty, stay with him or her and instruct trauma team members or the Rapid Response Team to prepare for an emergency intubation or tracheostomy.

- Surgical intervention is necessary for lacerations of the mucous membranes, cartilage exposure, or paralysis of the cords.
- An artificial airway may be needed.

TRAUMA, LIVER
OVERVIEW
- Common injuries to the liver include simple lacerations, multiple lacerations, avulsions (tears), and crush injuries.
- Because the liver is a vascular organ, blood loss is massive when trauma occurs (see *Shock*, especially the discussion of hemorrhagic and hypovolemic shock). Damage or injury should be suspected whenever any upper abdominal or lower chest trauma is sustained.
- Clinical manifestations of liver trauma include right upper quadrant pain with abdominal tenderness, distention, guarding, rigidity, and abdominal pain aggravated by deep breathing and referred to the right shoulder.
- Ultrasonography or CT determines injury; falling hemoglobin can indicate hemorrhage.
- Anticipate bleeding and prolonged coagulopathy with severe liver injury. The patient with liver trauma may require infusion of multiple blood products, packed RBCs, fresh-frozen plasma, and massive volume replacement to maintain hydration.

TRAUMA, PERIPHERAL NERVE
OVERVIEW
- The peripheral nerves are subject to injuries associated with mechanical or vehicular accidents, sports, the injection of particular drugs, military conflicts, and acts of violence (e.g., knife or gunshot wounds).
- Specific mechanisms of injury include:
    1. Partial or complete severance of a nerve or nerves
    2. Contusion, stretching, constriction, or compression of a nerve or nerves

T

3. Ischemia

4. Electrical, thermal, or radiation injury

- Most commonly affected are the median, ulnar, and radial nerves of the arms and the peroneal, femoral, and sciatic nerves of the legs.
- Nerve damage is characterized by pain, burning, or other abnormal sensations distal to the trauma; weakness or flaccid paralysis; and change in skin color and temperature (a warm phase and a cold phase).
- Nonsurgical treatment consists of immobilization of the area with a splint, cast, or traction followed by physical and occupational therapy.
- Surgery may include resection and suturing to reapproximate the severed nerve ends, nerve grafting, and nerve and tendon transplantation.
- Regeneration of the damaged nerve and return of sensation may occur several years after the injury; motor movement is less likely to recover long after the event.
- Postoperative nursing care is directed toward frequent skin care and assessment, management of pain, and instructing the patient to protect the involved area from new trauma.

TUBERCULOSIS, PULMONARY: IMMUNITY CONCEPT EXEMPLAR

OVERVIEW

- Pulmonary tuberculosis (TB) is a highly communicable disease caused by *Mycobacterium tuberculosis* infection when IMMUNITY fails to prevent infection.
- The organism is transmitted by aerosolization (airborne route) from an infected person during coughing, laughing, sneezing, whistling, or singing.
- When the bacillus is inhaled into a susceptible site in the bronchi or alveoli, it multiplies freely, causing an exudative pneumonitis.
- Initial infection is seen more often in the middle or lower lobes of the lung, and reactivation occurs more in the upper lobes.
- Progression of infection leads to an inflammatory lump that surrounds the bacilli and is filled with collagen, fibroblasts, and lymphocytes. The lump necroses, causing calcification or liquefaction and leading to destruction of lung tissue with cavity formation.
- Cell-mediated immunity develops 2 to 10 weeks after infection and is manifested by a positive reaction to a tuberculin skin test.
- *Miliary,* or *hematogenous,* TB is the spread of TB throughout the body when a large number of organisms enter the blood and can then infect the brain, liver, kidney, or bone marrow.

- Secondary TB is a reactivation of the disease in a previously infected person; this can happen when immunity is reduced (e.g., drug-induced immunosuppression, older age, the presence of multiple chronic diseases).
- An infected individual is not infectious to others until manifestations of disease occur.
- People at greatest risk for developing TB are:
  1. Those in close contact with an individual with active (often undiagnosed) TB
  2. Those who have reduced immunity
  3. Those who live in crowded areas such as long-term care facilities, prisons, and mental health facilities
  4. Older homeless people
  5. Abusers of injection drugs or alcohol, especially if malnutrition is present
  6. Lower socioeconomic groups
  7. Foreign immigrants

INTERPROFESSIONAL COLLABORATIVE CARE
Assessment: Noticing
- Obtain patient information about:
  1. Persistent cough
  2. Unintended weight loss
  3. Anorexia
  4. Night sweats
  5. Fever or chills
  6. Dyspnea or hemoptysis
  7. Past exposure to TB
  8. Country of origin and travel to foreign countries
  9. History of bacillus Calmette-Guérin (BCG) vaccination
- Assess for and document:
  1. Lung sounds: dullness with percussion over involved lung fields, bronchial breath sounds, crackles, wheezes
  2. Fatigue, lethargy, anorexia, weight loss
  3. Fever, night sweats
  4. Cough, with or without purulent sputum that may be streaked with blood
- TB is diagnosed on the basis of manifestations and/or a positive sputum culture using nucleic acid amplification test (NAAT).
- A point of care test, GeneXpert Omni, can be used on a blood sample obtained by pinprick.
- Blood analysis with the QuantiFERON-TB Gold (QFT-G) or T-SPOT TB test show how the patient's immune system responds to the TB bacterium.

- A purified protein derivative (PPD; Mantoux) two-step test is a common, reliable screening test.

❗ NURSING SAFETY PRIORITY: Action Alert

- Do not assume that a positive PPD reaction of 10 mm induration 48 to 72 hours after injection means that active disease is present. It may indicate TB vaccination or the presence of inactive (dormant) disease.
- A PPD skin reaction of < 10 mm at 48 to 72 hours or a negative PPD skin test result does not rule out TB disease or infection in the very old or in anyone who is severely immunocompromised.

Analysis: Interpreting
- The priority collaborative problems for patients with tuberculosis include:
  1. Potential for airway obstructions due to thick secretions and weak cough effort
  2. Potential for development of drug-resistant disease and spread of infection due to inadequate adherence to therapy regimen
  3. Anxiety due to diagnosis
  4. Weight loss due to inadequate intake and nausea from therapy regimen
  5. Fatigue due to lengthy illness, poor gas exchange, and increased energy demands

Planning and Implementation: Responding
PROMOTING AIRWAY CLEARANCE
- Drink plenty of fluids to thin mucus.
- Teach deep breathing to precede cough effort and the use of incentive spirometer.

DECREASING DRUG RESISTANCE AND INFECTION SPREAD
- Administer combination antimicrobial therapy that occurs in an initial phase (8 weeks) and in a continuation phase (18 weeks); drug therapy can last as long as 2 years when a multidrug resistant infecting TB organism is present.
- Teach that strict adherence to the prescribed antimicrobial regimen is crucial for suppressing TB and develop adherence strategies with the patient.
- First line therapy for initiation uses isoniazid (INH, Nidrazid), rifampin (Rifadin), pyrazinamide, and ethambutol (Myambutol).
- Patients with multidrug resistant TB infection or those who are not able to adhere to the therapy independently can be prescribed directly-observed therapy.

> **! NURSING SAFETY PRIORITY: Drug Alert**
>
> The first-line drugs used as therapy for tuberculosis all can damage the liver. Warn the patient to not drink any alcoholic beverages for the entire duration of TB therapy. Bedaquiline fumarate can prolong the QT interval, cause ventricular dysrhythmias, and can lead to sudden death. Patients on this drug need to have regular ECGs and serum electrolyte evaluations.

- Place the hospitalized patient with active TB in airborne (infection control) precautions.
- The community dwelling person will need to stay home, avoid crowds, and ensure others are not exposed to droplets of sputum (e.g., cover mouth, dispose of tissues in dedicated container).
- Encourage household members or other close contacts to undergo TB testing.
- When three consecutive sputum cultures are negative for TB, the individual is no longer consider infectious and can return to former activities.

MANAGING ANXIETY
- Provide information about the disease, prognosis, and treatment to reduce anxiety.
- Refer the patient to social services if he or she does not have sick leave and will lose pay or their position during the time they are homebound for treatment.

IMPROVING NUTRITION
- Conduct a nutrition assessment using an evidence-based tool.
- Determine patient likes/dislikes and ability to buy healthy food and make a plan for meals that are appealing and balance food groups.
- Consult the dietitian when inadequate nutrition is a problem.
- Take once-a-day drugs in the evening to avoid poor intake from nausea.

MANAGING FATIGUE
- Encourage the patient to resume activities slowly and get plenty of rest.
- Implement sleep hygiene strategies to promote night time sleeping.
- Teach the patient and family to anticipate a lengthy convalescence.

Care Coordination and Transition Management
- Ensure that active cases are reported to the local public health department or agency.
- Ensure the patient is discharged to the appropriate environment with continued supervision.
- Teach the patient to follow the drug regimen as prescribed.

- Provide the patient with verbal and written information about TB transmission and how to prevent transmission and the need for ongoing surveillance for 6 months or longer.

TUMORS, BRAIN

OVERVIEW

- Brain tumors can arise anywhere within the brain structures and are named according to the cell or tissue where they are located.
- *Primary tumors* originate within the CNS.
- *Secondary tumors (metastatic tumors)* spread to the brain from cancers in other body areas, such as the lungs, breast, kidney, and GI tract.
- Regardless of brain tumor type or location, the tumor expands and invades, infiltrates, compresses, and displaces normal brain tissue, leading to one or more problems, including:
  1. Cerebral edema/brain tissue inflammation
  2. Increased intracranial pressure, intracranial hypertension
  3. Neurologic deficits: sensory, motor, or cranial nerve dysfunction
  4. Hydrocephalus
  5. Pituitary dysfunction
  6. Seizure activity
- *Supratentorial tumors* are located within the cerebral hemispheres, and *infratentorial tumors* are located in the brain stem structures and cerebellum.
- Some brain tumors are benign (noninvasive), and others are cancerous. Regardless of type, most brain tumors must be treated or death will occur.
- Classification by cell type or tissue type includes tumors arising from:
  1. Neurons, which are responsible for nerve impulse conduction
  2. Neuroglia cells (glial cells), which provide support, nourishment, and protection
     a. Astrocytes (astrocytoma)
     b. Oligodendroglia
     c. Ependymal cells
     d. Microglia (glioma, which is malignant)
  3. Meninges, which are the coverings of the brain (meningioma)
  4. Pituitary (pituitary adenomas)
  5. The sheath of Schwann cells in cranial nerve VII (acoustic neuromas)
- Metastatic, or secondary, tumors from other body areas make up about 30% of brain tumors.
- The exact cause of brain tumors is unknown but may be related to genetic changes, heredity, errors in fetal development, ionizing radiation, electromagnetic fields, environmental hazards, diet, viruses, or injury.

INTERPROFESSIONAL COLLABORATIVE CARE

Assessment: Noticing

- Obtain patient information about general symptoms of a brain tumor, including:
  1. Headaches that are usually more severe on awakening in the morning
  2. Nausea and vomiting
  3. Vision changes (blurred or double vision)
  4. Seizures
  5. Changes in mentation or personality
  6. Papilledema (swelling of the optic disc)
  7. Specific neurologic deficits
     a. Supratentorial (cerebral) tumors usually result in paralysis, seizures, memory loss, cognitive impairment, language impairment, or vision problems.
     b. Infratentorial tumors produce ataxia, autonomic nervous system dysfunction, vomiting, drooling, hearing loss, and vision impairment.
- Diagnosis is based on the history, neurologic assessment, clinical examination, results of neurodiagnostic testing, CT, magnetic resonance imaging (MRI), and skull x-rays. Cerebral angiography, electroencephalography (EEG), lumbar puncture (LP), brain scan, and positron emission tomography (PET) may be also be used to further define the tumor.

Interventions: Responding

NONSURGICAL MANAGEMENT

- Management depends on tumor size and location, patient symptoms and general condition, and whether the tumor is primary or has recurred.
- Drug therapy for symptom management may include:
  1. Analgesics for headache
     a. Codeine
     b. Acetaminophen
  2. Agents to control cerebral edema
     a. Dexamethasone (Decadron)
     b. Corticosteroids
  3. Phenytoin (Dilantin) or other antiepileptic drug for seizure activity
  4. Agents to prevent stress ulcers, typically proton pump inhibitors (e.g., pantoprazole [Protonix])
  5. Institution-specific seizure precautions
- Chemotherapy may be given alone, in combination with radiation therapy and surgery, and with tumor progression. More than one agent may be given orally, IV, intra-arterially, or intrathecally

T

through an Ommaya reservoir placed in a cranial ventricle. Both cytotoxic and targeted therapy agents may be used.

1. An emerging practice is direct drug delivery to the tumor using a disk-shaped drug wafer (polifeprosan 20 with carmustine implant [Gliadel]) placed directly into the cavity created during surgical tumor removal (interstitial chemotherapy).
2. General management issues for care of patients undergoing chemotherapy are presented, under *Cancer.*

- Radiation therapy may be used alone, after surgery, or in combination with chemotherapy and surgery.
  1. Traditional external beam radiation may be used.
  2. A radioactive monoclonal antibody may be directly injected into the cavity from which the tumor was removed.
  3. General management issues for care of patients undergoing radiation therapy are presented under *Cancer.*
- Stereotactic radiosurgery (SRS) is an alternative to traditional surgery. Techniques used may include:
  1. Modified linear accelerator using accelerated x-rays (LINAC)
  2. Particle accelerator using beams of protons (cyclotron)
  3. Isotope seeds implanted in the tumor (brachytherapy)
  4. Gamma knife using a single high dose of ionized radiation to focus 201 beams of gamma radiation produced by the radioisotope cobalt 60
  5. CyberKnife

SURGICAL MANAGEMENT

- Brain biopsy is done to determine the specific pathology. Then a craniotomy (incision into the cranium) may be performed to improve symptoms related to the lesion or to decrease pressure effect from the tumor. Complete removal is possible with some tumors, which results in a "surgical cure."
  1. Minimally invasive surgery (MIS) may involve:
     a. The transnasal approach with endoscopy for pituitary tumors
     b. Stereotactic surgery using burr holes and local anesthesia
     c. Laser surgery
  2. In traditional open craniotomy, the patient's head is placed in a skull fixation device, and a piece of bone (bone flap) is removed to expose the tumor area. The tumor is removed, the bone flap is replaced, and a drain or monitoring device may be inserted.
- Provide preoperative care, including:
  1. Allowing the patient to express anxiety and concerns about:
     a. Surgery into the brain
     b. Possibility of neurologic deficits
     c. Changes in appearance and self-image

2. Teaching the patient and family about what to expect immediately after surgery and throughout the recovery period
3. Ensuring that the patient has refrained from alcohol, tobacco, anticoagulants, or nonsteroidal anti-inflammatory drugs (NSAIDs) for at least 5 days before surgery

! NURSING SAFETY PRIORITY: Action Alert

The focus of postoperative care is to monitor the patient to detect changes in status and to prevent or minimize complications, especially increased ICP.

- Provide postoperative care, including:
  1. Implementing routine postoperative care
  2. Assessing neurologic (LOC) and vital signs every 15 to 30 minutes for the first 4 to 6 hours after surgery and then every hour
  3. Assessing for:
     a. Decreased LOC
     b. Motor weakness or paralysis
     c. Aphasia
     d. Visual changes
     e. Personality changes
  4. Ensuring appropriate positioning
     a. After supratentorial surgery:
        (1) Elevate the head of the bed 30 degrees
        (2) Avoid extreme hip or neck flexion
        (3) Maintain the head in a midline, neutral position
        (4) Place the patient on the nonoperative side
     b. After infratentorial (brain stem) craniotomy:
        (1) Keep the patient flat
        (2) Position the patient on either side for 24 to 48 hours
  5. Maintaining NPO status for at least the first 24 hours after surgery
  6. Administering prescribed drug therapy
     a. Antiepileptic drugs
     b. Proton pump inhibitors
     c. Corticosteroids
     d. Analgesics
  7. Monitoring the dressing every 1 to 2 hours for:
     a. Amount, type, and color of drainage
     b. Suction of drains maintained as prescribed

! NURSING SAFETY PRIORITY: Critical Rescue

Immediately report to the surgeon a saturated head dressing or drainage greater than 50 mL in 8 hours.

8. Applying cold compresses for periorbital edema and ecchymosis of one or both eyes
9. Irrigating the affected eye with warm saline solution or artificial tears
10. Assessing the airway and managing mechanical ventilation
    a. Keeping $Paco_2$ at about 35 mm Hg
    b. Keeping the arterial oxygen levels higher than 95 mm Hg
    c. Hyperoxygenating the patient carefully before suctioning
11. Assessing the cardiac monitor for dysrhythmias
12. Precisely measuring intake and output to maintain a balance, avoiding overhydration and underhydration
13. Implementing any prescribed fluid restriction
14. Ensuring that range-of-motion (ROM) exercises are performed with all extremities at least every 2 to 3 hours
15. Ensuring that the patient turns, coughs, and breathes deeply every 2 hours (if permitted)
16. Maintaining venous thromboembolism (VTE) prophylaxis until the patient ambulates
17. Monitoring laboratory values for changes and abnormalities
    a. CBC
    b. Serum electrolyte levels and osmolality
    c. Coagulation studies
    d. ABGs
18. Assessing for fluid volume overload or syndrome of inappropriate antidiuretic hormone (SIADH)
    a. Irritability
    b. Rapid weight gain
    c. Low serum sodium and potassium values
    d. Low urine output in relation to fluid intake
19. Assessing for diabetes insipidus (DI)
    a. High serum sodium and osmolality
    b. Muscle weakness and restlessness
    c. Extreme thirst and dry mouth
    d. High output of dilute urine
20. Assessing for cerebral salt wasting (CSW)
    a. Low serum sodium and decreased osmolality
    b. No dilution of other electrolytes or of hematocrit and hemoglobin
21. Preventing and assessing for other postoperative complications, including:
    a. Increased ICP
       (1) Severe headache
       (2) Deteriorating LOC
       (3) Restlessness and irritability
       (4) Dilated or pinpoint pupils that are slow to react or nonreactive to light

b. Subdural and epidural hematomas and intracranial hemorrhage
   (1) Severe headache
   (2) Rapid change in LOC
   (3) Progressive neurologic deficits
   (4) Sudden cardiovascular and respiratory arrest
c. Hydrocephalus (increased CSF in the brain)
d. Respiratory complications:
   (1) Atelectasis
   (2) Pneumonia
   (3) Neurogenic pulmonary edema
e. Wound infections:
   (1) Reddened and puffy wound appearance
   (2) Area sensitive to touch
   (3) Area warm
f. Meningitis

Care Coordination and Transition Management
- Assist the family to make the environment safe for prevention of falls (e.g., remove scatter rugs, install grab bars in the bathroom).
- When needed, work with the case manager or discharge planner to help the family select a facility with experience in providing care for neurologically impaired patients.
- Teach patients and families about:
  1. Seizure precautions and what to do if a seizure occurs
  2. Drug therapy and person to call if adverse drug events occur
  3. Avoiding any over-the-counter (OTC) drugs unless approved by the health care provider
  4. The importance of recommended follow-up health care appointments
  5. The need for adequate caloric intake during radiation therapy or chemotherapy
- Refer the patient and family to support groups and community resources such as the American Brain Tumor Association, the National Brain Tumor Foundation, the American Cancer Society, home care agencies, and hospice services or palliative care services (for those who are terminally ill).

ULCERS, PEPTIC: IMMUNITY CONCEPT EXEMPLAR

OVERVIEW
- A peptic ulcer is a mucosal lesion of the stomach or duodenum that can result from impaired IMMUNITY.

- Peptic ulcer disease (PUD) results when mucosal defenses become impaired and no longer protect the epithelium from the effects of acid and pepsin. The term is used to describe both gastric and duodenal ulcers.
- Peptic ulcer development is associated with bacterial infection with *Helicobacter pylori* and physiologic stress. Caffeine, nonsteroidal anti-inflammatory drugs (NSAIDs), corticosteroids, smoking, and radiation therapy also contribute to PUD.
- Types of peptic ulcers include:
  1. *Gastric ulcer,* which occurs when there is a break in the mucosal barrier and hydrochloric acid injures the stomach, usually near the antrum; gastric emptying is often delayed with gastric ulceration, worsening the injury
  2. *Duodenal ulcer,* a chronic break in the duodenal mucosa that extends through the muscularis mucosa and most commonly occurs in the upper portion of the duodenum; it is characterized by high gastric acid secretion and is the most common type of peptic ulcer
  3. *Stress ulcer,* which occurs with acute and chronic diseases or major trauma; bleeding resulting from gastric erosion is the principal manifestation, and multiple lesions occur in the proximal portion of the stomach, beginning with the area of ischemia and evolving into erosions
- Complications of PUD include:
  1. Gastrointestinal (GI) bleeding
  2. Perforation, with the gastroduodenal contents emptying through the anterior wall of the stomach or duodenum into the peritoneal cavity
  3. Pyloric obstruction
  4. Intractable disease, which is characterized by a lack of response to conservative management and with symptoms that interfere with activities of daily living (ADLs)

INTERPROFESSIONAL COLLABORATIVE CARE
Assessment: Noticing
- Obtain patient information about:
  1. Symptoms, including epigastric discomfort, abdominal tenderness, cramps, indigestion, nausea, or vomiting and their onset, duration, location, and frequency, as well as aggravating and alleviating factors, including meal and sleep patterns
     a. Gastric ulcer pain may be relieved by food.
     b. Duodenal ulcer pain occurs 1.5 to 3 hours after eating and often awakens the patient at night.
  2. Tobacco, alcohol, caffeine, and intake of foods known to cause gastric irritation

3. Medical history focusing on GI problems, particularly *H. pylori* infection
4. Prescribed and over-the-counter (OTC) drugs, such as corticosteroids and NSAIDs
5. Recent severe, serious, complex, or traumatic illness
6. Presence of chronic disease and recent changes in flares or medications

- Assess for and document:
  1. Epigastric pain and tenderness; rigid, board-like abdomen accompanied by rebound tenderness (if perforation occurred)
  2. Secretions (emesis, sputum, stool, urine, and nasogastric drainage) for frank or occult blood
  3. Color, amount, and character of stools; note the presence of melena or occult blood
  4. Vital signs, including orthostatic blood pressure indicating hypovolemia or bleeding
  5. Impact of chronic disease on the patient

- Diagnostic studies may include:
  1. Hemoglobin and hematocrit levels to determine occult or severity of GI bleeding
  2. Testing for *H. pylori*
  3. Esophagogastroduodenoscopy (EGD), which is the major diagnostic test for PUD; direct visualization of the ulcer crater by EGD allows the health care provider to take specimens for *H. pylori* testing and for biopsy and cytologic studies for ruling out gastric cancer

Analysis: Responding

- The priority collaborative problems for the patient with peptic ulcer disease include:
  1. Acute pain or chronic noncancer pain due to gastric and/or duodenal ulceration.
  2. Potential for upper GI bleeding due to gastric and/or duodenal ulceration.

Planning and Implementation: Responding

MANAGING ACUTE PAIN OR CHRONIC NONCANCER PAIN

- PUD causes significant discomfort that impacts many aspects of daily living. Interventions to manage pain focus on drug therapy and dietary changes.
  1. Administer drugs to eliminate *H. pylori* infection; a common approach is triple therapy for 10 to 14 days:
     a. Proton pump inhibitor (PPI) such as lansoprazole (Prevacid)
     b. Two antibiotics such as metronidazole (Flagyl, Novonidazol) and tetracycline (Ala-Tet, Panmycin, Nu-Tetra) or clarithromycin (Biaxin, Biaxin XL) and amoxicillin (Amoxil, Amoxil)

2. PPIs may be used alone to heal ulcers. Other drugs to promote healing are:
   a. Histamine-2 (H2) blockers that stop histamine-stimulated gastric acid secretion
   b. Sucralfate (Carafate) binds to and protects the mucosa, preventing further digestive damage from acid and pepsin.
   c. Antacids buffer gastric acid and slow formation of pepsin.
   d. Bismuth subsalicylate (Pepto-Bismol) inhibits *H. pylori* from binding to the mucosal lining and stimulates mucosal protection and prostaglandin production.

❗ NURSING SAFETY PRIORITY: Drug Alert

Teach the patient that to achieve a therapeutic effect, sufficient antacid must be ingested to neutralize the hourly production of acid. For optimal effect, take antacids about 2 hours after meals to reduce the hydrogen ion load in the duodenum. Antacids may be effective from 30 minutes to 3 hours after ingestion. If taken on an empty stomach, they are quickly evacuated. Thus the neutralizing effect is reduced (Lilley et al., 2017).

3. Prevent recurrence with complementary and integrative health therapies that reduce stress including hypnosis and imagery.
- The role of diet in the management of ulcer disease is controversial.
   1. There is no evidence that dietary restriction reduces gastric acid secretion or promotes tissue healing, although a bland diet may assist in relieving pain symptoms.
   2. Food itself acts as an antacid by neutralizing gastric acid for 30 to 60 minutes. An increased rate of gastric acid secretion, called *rebound,* may follow.
- Monitor for gastric outflow or pyloric obstruction caused by edema, spasm, or scar tissue. Obstruction may be manifested by abdominal pain, bloating, distention, tenderness, and reduced bowel sounds.
- Surgery, either in a minimally invasive approach or an open approach, may be used to remove a chronic ulcer or provide a subtotal gastrectomy (partial stomach removal) and/or vagotomy (cutting of the vagus nerve) to reduce acid production.

! NURSING SAFETY PRIORITY: Action Alert

Teach the patient who has peptic ulcer disease to seek immediate medical attention if experiencing any of these symptoms:
- Sharp, sudden, persistent, and severe epigastric or abdominal pain
- Bloody or black stools
- Bloody vomit or vomit that looks like coffee grounds

MANAGING UPPER GI BLEEDING
- For patients with persistent upper GI bleeding, embolization during endoscopy is done. An interventional radiologist may complete a catheter-directed embolization for small or persistent bleeding. For patients with a perforation, a surgical intervention may be needed to remove the ulcer site.
- The patient is at risk for fluid volume deficit (hypovolemia), anemia, and hemorrhagic shock.
  1. Management of hypovolemia and hemorrhage includes:
     a. Monitoring vital signs with urine output to detect hypovolemia manifested by tachycardia, hypotension, increased rate and depth of respirations, decreased SpO_2, reduced LOC, and urine output < 30 mL/Kg/hour for 3 or more hours
     b. Recording intake and output, including output from bleeding or vomiting
     c. Monitoring serum electrolytes, coagulation factors, hematocrit, and hemoglobin and reporting abnormal values to the provider in a timely manner
     d. Replacing fluids with intravenous (IV) fluids such as normal saline or lactated Ringer's solution
     e. Transfusing blood products safely in the presence of symptomatic anemia or hypoxemia from low hemoglobin
     f. Inserting an NG tube to ascertain the presence of blood in the stomach, assess the rate of bleeding, prevent gastric dilation, and provide lavage or removal of blood in the stomach
     g. Keeping the patient NPO during periods of active bleeding

! NURSING SAFETY PRIORITY: Critical Rescue

Recognize that your priority for care of the patient with upper GI bleeding is to maintain airway, breathing, and circulation (ABC). Respond to these needs by providing oxygen and other ventilatory support as needed, starting two large-bore IV lines for replacing fluids and blood, and monitoring vital signs, hematocrit, and oxygen saturation.

Care Coordination and Transition Management

- Instruct the patient about symptoms that should be brought to the attention of the health care provider such as persistent abdominal pain, bloody stools, and signs of hypovolemia.
- Instruct the patient to avoid NSAIDs unless under the care of a health care provider who may prescribe concurrent acid-reducing medication.

> **❗ NURSING SAFETY PRIORITY: Action Alert**
>
> Teach the patient with peptic ulcer disease to avoid substances that increase gastric acid secretion. This includes caffeine-containing beverages (coffee, tea, and cola). Both caffeinated and decaffeinated coffees should be avoided because coffee contains peptides that stimulate gastrin release.

- Teach dietary management to the postoperative patient, especially the patient who has had a partial stomach removal/resection. Management should include:
  1. Eating small-volume meals
  2. Avoiding drinking large volumes of liquids with meals
  3. Abstaining from foods that contribute to discomfort
  4. Receiving vitamin B_{12} injections as appropriate

> **❗ NURSING SAFETY PRIORITY: Action Alert**
>
> Teach the patient who has had surgery for PUD to avoid any over-the-counter (OTC) product containing aspirin or other NSAID. Emphasize the importance of following the treatment regimen for *H. pylori* infection and healing the ulcer. Emphasize the importance of keeping all follow-up appointments. Help the patient identify situations that cause stress, describe feelings during stressful situations, and develop a plan for coping with stressors.

URETHRITIS

OVERVIEW

- Urethritis is inflammation or infection of the urethra.
- Signs and symptoms of urethritis are:
  1. Burning, painful urination similar to cystitis/urinary tract infection (UTI) symptoms
  2. Urgency and frequency
  3. Weak urine stream (men)
  4. Incontinence
  5. Discharge from the urethral meatus, especially in men
  6. Pyuria (cloudy) or foul-smelling urine

- The most common cause of urethritis in males is sexually transmitted infection (STI).
- In postmenopausal women, urethritis may be caused by tissue changes related to low estrogen levels and it is treated with estrogen vaginal cream.
- Noninfectious urethritis may be caused by increased serum urea levels.
- STIs and infectious processes are treated with appropriate antibiotic therapy.

URINARY INCONTINENCE: ELIMINATION EXEMPLAR

OVERVIEW

- Urinary incontinence (UI) is a problem in the urinary tract that disrupts ELIMINATION.
- UI is the transient or permanent involuntary loss of urine severe enough to cause social or hygienic problems.
- UI is *not* a normal change associated with aging and can be stigmatizing, resulting in social isolation.
- Common forms of UI are:
  1. *Stress incontinence,* the loss of small amounts of urine during coughing, sneezing, jogging, or lifting. Patients are unable to tighten the urethra sufficiently to overcome the increased detrusor pressure, and leakage of urine results.
  2. *Urge incontinence,* the involuntary loss of urine associated with a sudden, strong desire to urinate. Patients are unable to suppress the signal for bladder contractions. It is also known as *overactive bladder.*
  3. *Overflow incontinence,* when the bladder becomes overdistended, urine leaks once maximum capacity of the bladder is reached. It is also known as *reflex incontinence* or *underactive bladder* and can be caused by obstruction (e.g., kidney stone) or loss of detrusor muscle/reflex activity (e.g., neurologic condition like spinal cord injury).
  4. *Functional incontinence* is leakage of urine caused by factors other than abnormal function of the bladder and urethra, such as cognitive dysfunction, impaired vision, or inability to reach a toilet.
  5. *Total* or *mixed incontinence,* a combination of two or more types of incontinence.

Considerations for Older Adults

Patient-Centered Care

Many factors contribute to urinary incontinence in older adults. An older adult may have decreased mobility from many causes.

U

In inpatient settings, mobility is limited when the older patient is placed on bed rest. Vision and hearing impairments may also prevent the patient from locating a call light to notify the nurse or assistive personnel of the need to void. Assess for these factors, and minimize them to prevent urinary incontinence. Getting out of bed to urinate is a common cause of falls among older adults in the home and other settings.

INTERPROFESSIONAL COLLABORATIVE CARE
Assessment: Noticing

- Obtain patient information
  1. Determine the presence and severity of incontinence with effective screening questions. Ask the patient to respond with *always*, *sometimes*, or *never* to the following questions:
     a. Do you ever leak urine when you do not want to?
     b. Do you ever leak urine or water when you cough, laugh, or exercise?
     c. Do you ever leak urine on the way to the bathroom?
     d. Do you ever use pads, tissue, or cloth in your underwear to catch urine?
  2. Risk factors for UI
     a. Age, menopausal status
     b. Childbirth, particularly if the first child was delivered after age 30
     c. Urologic procedures
     d. Bowel pattern
     e. Stress or anxiety level
     f. Neurologic like dementia, stroke, Parkinson's disease, or multiple sclerosis
     g. Impaired mobility from injury, paresthesia, pain, or paralysis
     h. Urinary obstruction from prostate enlargement in men and pelvic prolapse in women
     i. Chronic conditions or drugs that affect nerve conduction or elimination like diabetes, diuretic use, obesity, spinal cord or nerve damage
     j. Reduced ability to ambulate and to transfer to a chair or toilet
     k. Inability to communicate the need for toileting
     l. Presence of UTI (cystitis)
- Assess for and document the findings of the following:
  1. Palpate the abdominal area for evidence of bladder fullness and to rule out constipation.
  2. Evaluate the force and character of the urine stream during voiding.

3. Ask the patient to cough while wearing a perineal pad; a wet pad may indicate stress incontinence.
4. Determine the amount of residual urine by portable ultrasound or by catheterizing the patient immediately after voiding.
5. Inspect the external genitalia of women to determine if uterine prolapse, cystocele, or rectocele is present.
6. Describe any secretions or discharge from the genitourinary openings.
7. Query the patient regarding the effects of incontinence on socialization, family relationships, and emotional status.
8. Monitor the urine for color, odor, and presence of sediment or cloudiness, and report abnormal results of a urinalysis in a timely manner to the provider.
9. Review the results of the voiding cystourethrogram or urodynamic testing that detect the anatomic structure and function of the bladder.

Analysis: Interpreting

- The priority collaborative problems for patients with urinary incontinence include:
  1. Stress incontinence due to weak pelvic muscles and structural supports
  2. Urge incontinence due to decreased bladder capacity, bladder spasms, diet, and neurologic impairment
  3. Reflex incontinence due to neurologic impairment
  4. Functional incontinence due to impaired cognition or neuromuscular limitations
  5. Total urinary incontinence (mixed) due to many causes

Planning and Implementation: Responding

REDUCING STRESS INCONTINENCE

- Initial interventions for patients with stress incontinence include keeping a diary, and pelvic muscle exercises (Kegel exercises) (Qaseem et al., 2014). Surgery also may be an option if other interventions are not effective (Testa, 2015).

  Nonsurgical Management

- Nonsurgical management of incontinence may include:
  1. Keeping a diary to record urine leakage, activities, and food eaten
  2. Collaboration with the dietitian to identify and avoid foods that cause bladder irritation and, if needed, to reduce obesity
  3. Pelvic muscle exercises (Kegel exercises) to strengthen the muscles of the pelvic floor (circumvaginal muscles)
     a. Use of weighted vaginal cones in conjunction with pelvic exercises can help strengthen the pelvic muscles.
     b. Biofeedback devices, such as electromyography or perineometers, measure the strength of contraction and provide feedback to the patient during these exercises.

4. Drug therapy with topical estrogen to increase blood flow and muscle tone around the urethra and vagina

5. A *pessary* inserted into the vagina may help with a prolapsed uterus or bladder when this condition is contributing to urinary incontinence

6. Other interventions for stress incontinence include behavior modification, psychotherapy, and electrical stimulation devices to strengthen urethral contraction.

7. Urethral occlusion devices use a tiny balloon that can be manually deflated by the patient to void.

8. Treatment with electrical stimulation to activate sensory nerves, decreasing the sense of urgency

9. Magnetic resonance therapy uses a magnetic device to induce nerve depolarization, reducing urgency.

Surgical Management

- Stress incontinence may be treated by a surgical sling, bladder suspension procedure, or injection of bulking agents into the urethral wall.

  1. A sling procedure uses strips of body tissue or synthetic material (mesh) around the urethra and bladder to support the urinary system. Midurethral sling procedures are particularly effective for stress urinary incontinence.

  2. Bladder suspension procedures use multiple slings to support the bladder and urethra, suturing tissue near the bladder neck to a pubic bone ligament.

  3. Bulking agents provide resistance to urine outflow and these agents include collagen, carbon-coated zirconium beads, and silicone implants.

- Provide preoperative and postoperative care and:

  1. Secure the urethral catheter or suprapubic catheter to prevent traction on the bladder neck and monitor urine output as well as the presence of urine leakage or other drainage.

  2. Catheters are usually in place until the patient can urinate easily and has residual urine volume after voiding of less than 50 mL.

REDUCING URGE INCONTINENCE

- Interventions for urge UI include behavioral interventions such as bladder and habit training and drug therapy to support elimination. Surgery is not recommended.

  1. Bladder training, sometimes called *behavioral training*, requires extensive patient participation.

     a. Start with a bladder diary to determine voiding patterns.

     b. Set interval of toileting (this may be every 45 minutes) based on diary results.

     c. Teach the patient to suppress the urge/not to void between intervals.

    d. If the patient remains dry, then increase voiding intervals by 15 minutes; if not consistently dry, decrease intervals by 15 minutes.

    e. Provide privacy for toileting and praise success with a goal of 3 to 4 hour periods of continence.

    f. *Neuromodulation* therapy, which involves stimulation of the nerves to the bladder, can be used with bladder training.

2. For patients unable to participate in bladder training, use habit training during which caregivers assist the patient in voiding at specific times.

    a. Provide toileting before incontinence occurs, generally every 2 to 3 hours.

    b. Increase timed voiding success by running water in the bathroom and providing privacy.

! NURSING SAFETY PRIORITY: Action Alert

Habit training is undermined when absorbent briefs are used in place of timed toileting. Do not tell patients to "just wet the bed." A common cause of falls in health care facilities is related to patient efforts to get out of bed unassisted to use the toilet. Work with all staff members, including unlicensed assistive personnel (UAP), to implement consistently the toileting schedule for habit training.

3. Drug therapy can relax smooth muscle and increase the bladder capacity and can be used with bladder training.

    a. Anticholinergics (also known as antimuscarinics) inhibit the nerve fibers that stimulate bladder contraction and include darifenacin (Enablex), fesoterodine (Toviaz), oxybutynin (Ditropan and Ditropan XL), propiverdine (Detrunorm), sofenacin (VESIcare), tolterodine (Detrol and Detrol LA), and trospium (Sanctura).

        (1) Some of these drugs are available OTC.

        (2) This class of drugs has serious side effects, particularly for older adults, and is used along with behavioral interventions.

    b. Tricyclic antidepressants with anticholinergic and alpha-adrenergic agonist activity, such as imipramine (Tofranil, Novopramine), have been used successfully in younger patients.

    c. A beta-adrenergic agonist, mirabegron (Myrbetriq) has demonstrated effectiveness in reducing urge incontinence.

    d. Onabotulinum toxin A (Botox) is injected during cystoscopy into multiple areas of the detrusor muscle of the bladder and may relieve incontinence for as long as 6 to 9 months after injection. Side effects may include urinary retention, painful urination, and an increased incidence of urinary tract infections.

REDUCING FUNCTIONAL INCONTINENCE

- Causes of functional incontinence vary greatly. Some are reversible, and others are not. The focus of intervention is treatment of reversible causes. When incontinence is not reversible, urinary habit training is used to establish a predictable pattern of bladder emptying to prevent incontinence.
- Promote strategies that eliminate barriers to elimination, including adapting the environment and teaching the patient behaviors to stay dry.
  1. Alter the environment so the patient can reach the toilet easily.
  2. Implement habit training for the cognitively impaired patient.
  3. Use absorbent pads and briefs to collect urine and keep the patient's skin and clothing dry.
  4. Use an external catheter.

MANAGING TOTAL OR MIXED URINARY INCONTINENCE

- Combine assessment and interventions to reduce problems with elimination and complications from incontinence.
- After identifying the specific types of incontinence an individual patient has, apply the appropriate priority patient problems, interventions, and expected outcomes discussed earlier with each incontinence type.

Care Coordination and Transition Management

- Consider personal, physical, emotional, and social resources, including referral to services that educate and support individuals and families with similar concerns about urinary elimination and incontinence.
- Identify if caregivers need to be involved in planning and delivering interventions and include them in teaching and management strategies.
- Assess the home environment for barriers that impede access to the toileting facilities.
- Assist the patient to identify strategies to manage anxiety related to incontinence while in public.
- Teach the patient and family about the causes of incontinence and treatment options available.
- Review prescribed drugs (purpose, dosage, method, route of administration, and expected and potential side effects).
- Reinforce the value of weight reduction and dietary modification to improve continence.
- Discuss options available for urine containment products, considering the patient's lifestyle and resources.

- If self-catheterization is prescribed, ensure that a return demonstration is correct.

UROLITHIASIS

OVERVIEW

- Urolithiasis is the presence of calculi (stones) in the urinary tract. Stones often do not cause symptoms until they pass into the lower urinary tract, where they can cause excruciating pain. *Nephrolithiasis* is the formation of stones in the kidney. *Ureterolithiasis* is the formation of stones in the ureter.
- The most common condition associated with stone formation is dehydration.
- Formation of stones involves two conditions:
  1. Supersaturation of the urine with the particular element (e.g., calcium, uric acid) that first becomes crystallized and later becomes the stone
  2. Formation of a *nidus* (deposit of crystals that can be the point of infection) along the lining of the kidney and urinary tract
- Calculi may be formed from calcium, phosphate, oxalate, uric acid, struvite, and cystine crystals, but most stones contain calcium as one component.

⬢ Genetic/Genomic Considerations

Family history has a strong association with stone formation and recurrence. More than 30 genetic variations are associated with the formation of kidney stones although single gene disorders are rare. Genetic variation in intestinal calcium absorption, kidney calcium transport, or kidney phosphate transport can contribute to nephrolithiasis. Always ask a patient with a renal stone whether other family members have also had this problem.

U

INTERPROFESSIONAL COLLABORATIVE CARE

Assessment: Noticing

- Obtain patient information about:
  1. Personal and family history of kidney stones
  2. Metabolic disorders and diet history, including fluid intake
- Assess for and document:
  1. The location and duration of pain, which is often described as severe, unbearable, spasmodic (colic), and in the region of the trunk, back, and thighs ("flank" pain)
  2. Nausea and vomiting
  3. Hematuria, oliguria, or anuria
  4. Increased turbidity and odor of urine
  5. Bladder distention

Interventions: Responding

MANAGE ACUTE PAIN

Nonsurgical Management

- Administer drugs to manage severe pain and assess patient response, including:
  1. Opioid agents, such as hydromorphone or morphine to manage severe pain, also known as renal colic
  2. NSAIDs, such as ketorolac (Toradol)
  3. Spasmolytic agents, such as oxybutynin chloride (Ditropan) and propantheline bromide (Pro-Banthine, Propanthel)
  4. Drugs to aid in stone expulsion including a thiazide diuretic and allopurinol
- Assist the patient in finding a comfortable position; distraction or relaxation techniques such as hypnosis, imagery, or acupuncture can be used to relieve pain.
- Encourage ambulation and an upright position to drain the renal calyx and pass renal calculi.
- When infection occurs, a stone has not passed in 1 to 2 months, or when kidney function is at risk, antibiotics or lithotripsy may be used.
- Lithotripsy, or extracorporeal *shock wave lithotripsy* (SWL), is the application of ultrasound or dry shock wave energies to break the stone. The patient receives conscious sedation as the lithotripter and fluoroscope locate and break up the calculus. After lithotripsy, implement routine postoperative care with additional monitoring for urine output (quantity, quality, and presence of sediment or stones).

Surgical Management

- Minimally invasive surgical and open surgical procedures are used if urinary obstruction occurs or if the stone is too large to be passed and include stenting, ureteroscopy, percutaneous ureterolithotomy, and percutaneous nephrolithotomy.
- When other stone removal attempts have failed or when risk for a lasting injury to the ureter or kidney is possible, an *open ureterolithotomy* (into the ureter), *pyelolithotomy* (into the kidney pelvis), or *nephrolithotomy* (into the kidney) procedure may be performed. These procedures are used for a large or impacted stone.
- Preoperative care includes routine care and providing individualized instructions, depending on the procedure to be performed.
- Postoperative care includes routine care and:
  1. Monitoring the urine amount and character (color, presence of sediment or clots, volume) every 1 to 2 hours for 24 hours and preventing urinary obstruction from stone fragments or clots
  2. Monitoring intake to provide adequate hydration
  3. Preventing infection or detecting signs of infection early to avoid complications of surgical site or urinary tract infection
  4. Evaluating effects of intervention with a 24-hour urine collection and chemical analysis

Care Coordination and Transition Management

- Inform the patient that:
  1. Extensive bruising may occur after lithotripsy and may take several weeks to resolve
  2. Urine may be bloody for several days after surgical intervention
- Instruct the patient about:
  1. The importance of following the prescribed drug regimen
  2. The rationale for preventing dehydration, stressing the importance of dilute urine from adequate fluid intake and any dietary restrictions to reduce recurrent stone formation
  3. The importance of reporting symptoms of infection or formation of another stone, such as pain, fever, chills, and difficulty with urination

UTERINE BLEEDING (DYSFUNCTIONAL)

OVERVIEW

- Dysfunctional uterine bleeding (DUB) is abnormal bleeding from the vagina. Most women have menstrual cycles every 24 to 34 days and a cycle that lasts 4 to 7 days. When bleeding or spotting between cycles occurs, when bleeding is very heavy or lasts more than 7 days, or when the time between cycles is less than 21 days, DUB may be diagnosed.
- Most cases of DUB are classified into two types: anovulatory DUB (most common) and ovulatory DUB.
- Risk factors for DUB are obesity, extreme weight loss or gain, age older than 40 years, high stress levels, polycystic ovary disease, long-term use of oral contraceptives, excessive exercise, and anatomic abnormalities including leiomyomas (fibroids) or cancer.

INTERPROFESSIONAL COLLABORATIVE CARE

Assessment: Noticing

- Ask about:
  1. Changes in weight, exercise, and health
  2. Abdominal or pelvic pain
  3. History of contraceptive use
- Determine whether there are systemic symptoms from blood loss (anemia).

Interventions: Responding

NONSURGICAL MANAGEMENT

- Treatment is hormone therapy with progestin or combined estrogen-progestin therapy.
- Evaluate the patient's knowledge about the effects, dosage, and administration schedule of her prescribed hormone therapy.
- Teach the patient the information she needs to know about her prescribed hormone therapy.

SURGICAL MANAGEMENT
- Surgical management includes laser endometrial ablation, uterine artery embolization, dilation and curettage, and hysterectomy.
- Nursing care is similar to that for a woman undergoing a vaginal hysterectomy (see *Surgical Management* under *Leiomyomas [Uterine Fibroids]*).

UTERINE FIBROIDS (LEIOMYOMAS)

- See *Leiomyomas (Uterine Fibroids).*

V

VASCULAR DISEASE, PERIPHERAL
OVERVIEW
- Peripheral vascular disease (PVD) includes disorders that alter the natural flow of blood through the arteries and veins of the peripheral circulation.
- It affects the lower extremities much more commonly than the upper extremities.
- A diagnosis of PVD usually implies arterial disease rather than venous involvement. Some patients have both arterial and venous disease (see *Peripheral Arterial Disease* and *Peripheral Venous Disease*).

VEINS, VARICOSE
OVERVIEW
- Varicose veins are distended, protruding veins that appear darkened or tortuous.
- The vein walls weaken and dilate. Venous pressure increases, and the valves become incompetent. Incompetent valves contribute to venous insufficiency. Both superficial and deep veins can become dilated.
- Varicose veins occur primarily in patients subjected to prolonged standing. They also occur in pregnant women and in patients with systemic problems, such as heart disease or obesity, and a family history of varicose veins.

INTERPROFESSIONAL COLLABORATIVE CARE
- Conservative treatment measures include:
  1. Wearing elastic stockings
  2. Elevating the legs as often as possible
- Surgical management includes endovascular ablation to occlude the bulging vein.
  1. This is generally completed as a same-day surgery with routine perioperative care and restrictions to weight bearing for several days.

   2. Other surgical procedures include:
      a. Sclerotherapy, in which the physician injects a chemical to sclerose the vein, performed on small or a limited number of varicosities
      b. Laser treatment, using a laser to heat and close the main vessel that is contributing to the varicosity
      c. Surgical ligation (tying) and stripping (removal) the affected veins with the patient under general anesthesia
- Collateral veins take over supplying blood to tissues after laser, radiofrequency, or surgical interventions.

✳ VENOUS THROMBOEMBOLISM: CLOTTING CONCEPT EXEMPLAR

OVERVIEW
- Venous thromboembolism (VTE) is one of health care's greatest challenges and includes both thrombus and embolus complications.
- A thrombus (also called a thrombosis) is a blood clot believed to result from an endothelial injury, venous stasis, or hypercoagulability.
- When a thrombus develops, immunity is altered, causing inflammation to occur around the clot, thickening of the vein wall, and possible embolization (the formation of an embolus).
- Pulmonary embolus (PE) is the most common type of embolus.
- Phlebothrombosis is a thrombus without inflammation.
- Thrombophlebitis refers to a thrombus that is associated with inflammation.
- Thrombophlebitis can occur in superficial veins. However, it most frequently occurs in the deep veins of the lower extremities.
- Deep vein thrombophlebitis, commonly referred to as deep vein thrombosis (DVT), is the most common type of thrombophlebitis. It is more serious than superficial thrombophlebitis because it presents a greater risk for PE.
- With PE, a dislodged blood clot travels to the pulmonary artery—a medical emergency!

INTERPROFESSIONAL COLLABORATIVE CARE
Assessment: Noticing
- Obtain patient information about:
  1. History of VTE
  2. Risks associated with development of VTE
     a. Prolonged periods of sitting or bedrest
     b. Recent surgery
     c. Factors affecting coagulation
- Assess for signs and symptoms:
  1. Patients may be asymptomatic.

2. The classic signs and symptoms of DVT are calf or groin tenderness and pain and sudden onset of unilateral leg swelling.
3. Gently palpate the site—observe for induration (hardening) along the blood vessel.
4. Redness may be present.

- The preferred diagnostic test for DVT is venous duplex ultrasonography.
- A D-dimer test is the global marker of coagulation activation and measures fibrin degradation products produced from fibrinolysis (clot breakdown). Used as an adjunct to noninvasive testing.

Analysis: Interpreting

- The priority collaborative problem for most patients with VTE is:
   1. Potential for injury due to complications of VTE and anticoagulation therapy.

Planning and Implementation: Responding
PREVENTING INJURY

- The focus of managing thrombophlebitis is to prevent complications such as pulmonary emboli, further thrombus formation, and an increase in size of the thrombus.

   Nonsurgical Management
- Prevention of DVT and other types of VTE is crucial for patients at risk. Initiate the following interventions to prevent VTE:
   1. Patient education
   2. Leg exercises
   3. Adequate hydration
   4. Graduated compression stockings
   5. Intermittent pneumatic compression, such as sequential compression devices (SCDs)
   6. Venous plexus foot pump
   7. Anticoagulant therapy

   Drug Therapy
- Anticoagulants are the drug of choice for actual DVT and for patients at risk for DVT.
   1. The conventional treatment has been IV unfractionated heparin followed by oral anticoagulation with warfarin (Coumadin).
   2. Unfractionated heparin can be problematic because each patient's response to the drug is unpredictable and hospital admission is usually required for laboratory monitoring and dose adjustments.
   3. The use of low–molecular-weight heparin (LMWH) and the development of novel oral anticoagulants (NOACs, also referred to as direct oral anticoagulants [DOACs]) has changed the management of both DVT and PE. See Chart 2-27 for best practice for the patient receiving anticoagulant therapy.

Chart 2-27	Best Practice for Patient Safety & Quality Care: The Patient Receiving Anticoagulant Therapy

- Carefully check the dosage of anticoagulant to be administered, even if the pharmacy prepared the drug.
- Monitor the patient for signs and symptoms of bleeding, including hematuria, frank or occult blood in the stool, ecchymosis, petechiae, altered mental status (indicating possible cranial bleeding), or pain (especially abdominal pain, which could indicate abdominal bleeding).
- Monitor vital signs frequently for decreased blood pressure and increased pulse (indicating possible internal bleeding).
- Have antidotes available as needed (e.g., protamine sulfate for heparin; vitamin K for warfarin [Coumadin, Warfilone]).
- Monitor aPTT for patients receiving unfractionated heparin. Monitor prothrombin time (PT)/ International normalized ratio (INR) for patients receiving warfarin or LMWH.
- Apply prolonged pressure over venipuncture sites and injection sites.
- When administering *subcutaneous* heparin, apply pressure over the site and do not massage.
- Teach the patient going home while taking an anticoagulant to:
  - Use only an electric razor
  - Take precautions to avoid injury; for example, do not use tools such as hammers or saws, where accidents commonly occur
  - Report signs and symptoms of bleeding, such as blood in the urine or stool, nosebleeds, ecchymosis, or altered mental status
  - Take the prescribed dosage of drug at the precise time that it was prescribed to be taken
  - Do not stop taking the drug abruptly; the physician usually tapers the anticoagulant gradually

! NURSING SAFETY PRIORITY: Critical Rescue

Notify the primary health care provider if the activated partial thromboplastin time (aPTT) value is greater than 70 seconds or follow hospital protocol for reporting critical laboratory values. Assess patient for signs and symptoms of bleeding, which include hematuria, frank or occult blood in the stool, ecchymosis (bruising), petechiae, an altered level of consciousness, or pain. If bleeding occurs, stop the anticoagulant immediately and call the primary health care provider or Rapid Response Team!

> ### ❗ NURSING SAFETY PRIORITY: Drug Alert
>
> For patients taking warfarin, assess for any bleeding, such as hematuria or blood in the stool. Ensure that vitamin K, the antidote for warfarin, is available in case of excessive bleeding. Report any bleeding to the primary health care provider and document in the patient's health record. Teach patients to avoid foods with high concentrations of vitamin K, especially dark green leafy vegetables. These foods interfere with the action of warfarin, which is a vitamin K synthesis inhibitor.

Surgical Management

- Surgical removal of a DVT is rare unless there is a massive occlusion that does not respond to medical treatment.
- A thrombectomy is the surgical procedure used for clot removal.
- For patients with recurrent DVT or pulmonary emboli that do not respond to medical treatment or that cannot tolerate anticoagulation, inferior vena cava filtration may be indicated.
  1. The surgeon or interventional radiologist inserts a filter device into the femoral vein or jugular vein. The device is meant to trap emboli in the inferior vena cava before they progress to the lungs. Holes in the device allow blood to pass through, without interfering with the return of blood to the heart.
  2. Provide standard preoperative care and collaborate with the primary health care provider if the patient has been taking anticoagulants to avoid hemorrhage.
  3. After surgery, inspect the groin insertion site for bleeding and signs or symptoms of infection. Provide standard postoperative care.

Care Coordination and Transition Management

- Patients recovering from thrombophlebitis or DVT are ambulatory when they are discharged from the hospital.
- The primary focus of planning for discharge is to educate the patient and family about anticoagulation therapy.
- Teach patients recovering from DVT:
  1. Stop smoking.
  2. Avoid the use of oral contraceptives.
  3. Discuss alternative methods of birth control.
  4. Most patients are discharged on warfarin (Coumadin) or LMWH.
- The VTE Core Measures and the Joint Commission's National Patient Safety Goals require that patients be given written discharge instructions about anticoagulant therapy that address:
  1. Drug compliance issues (need to take drug as prescribed)
  2. Dietary advice (e.g., foods to avoid)

3. Follow-up monitoring (e.g., Coumadin clinic, INR testing)
4. Information about potential for adverse drug reactions/ interactions (e.g., bleeding, bruising). See Chart 2-27 for best practice for the patient receiving anticoagulants.

VISUAL IMPAIRMENT (REDUCED VISION)
OVERVIEW
- Visual impairment can range from total blindness to various degrees and types of partial impairment of SENSORY PERCEPTION.
- Patients are legally blind if their best visual acuity with corrective lenses is 20/200 or less in the better eye or if the widest diameter of the visual field in that eye is 20 degrees or less.
- Blindness can occur in one or both eyes. When one eye is affected, the field of vision is narrowed, and depth perception is impaired.
- Central vision can be impaired by diseases involving the macula, such as macular edema or macular degeneration.
- Peripheral vision loss affects the patient's ability to drive and awareness of hazards in the periphery.

INTERPROFESSIONAL COLLABORATIVE CARE
Assessment: Noticing
- Test the visual acuity of both eyes immediately of any person who experiences an eye injury or any sudden change in vision.
- Ask the patient about vision problems in any other members of the family because some vision problems have a genetic component.
- Urge all patients to wear eye protection when they are performing yard work, working in a woodshop or metal shop, using chemicals, or are in any environment in which drops or particulate matter are airborne.

Interventions: Responding
- Avoid harm from impaired sensory perception.
  1. Communicate and listen to the patient's preferences for safety.
     a. Stress to hospital staff, family, and friends that changes in item location should not be made without input from the person with reduced vision.
     b. Orient the patient to the immediate environment, including the size of the room. Use one object in the room, such as a chair or hospital bed, as the focal point during your description. Guide the person to the focal point and describe all other objects in relation to the focal point.

V

! NURSING SAFETY PRIORITY: Action Alert

Never leave the patient with reduced vision in the center of an unfamiliar room.

    c. Allow the patient to establish the location of important objects, such as the call light, water pitcher, and clock.

    d. Set up food trays using imaginary clock placement to orient the patient to the location of specific items.

2. Teach safe ambulation.

    a. Allow the patient to grasp your arm at the elbow while keeping the arm close to your body so that he or she can detect your direction of movement.

    b. Alert the patient when obstacles are in the path ahead.

    c. Assist with the correct use of a cane to detect obstacles (the cane is held in the dominant hand several inches off the floor and sweeps the ground where the patient's foot will be placed next).

    d. Go with the patient to other important areas, such as the bathroom. Count steps and highlight landmarks such as the location of the toilet, sink, and toilet paper holder.

3. Promote self-management.

    a. To make better use of existing vision, teach the patient:

       (1) To move the head slightly up and down to enhance a three-dimensional effect

       (2) To line up the object and move toward it when shaking hands or pouring water

       (3) To choose a position that favors the good eye; for example, people with vision in the right eye should position people and items on their right

    b. Knock on the door before entering the room and state your name and the reason for visiting when entering the room. Use a normal tone of voice unless there is a hearing problem.

    c. Encourage mastery of one task at a time and provide positive reinforcement for each success when adapting to visual loss or impairment.

    d. Use local resources that provide adaptive items such as large print books for reduced vision or talking clocks for any impaired vision.

Care Coordination and Transition Management

1. Provide opportunities for the patient and family to express their concerns about deteriorating vision status.

2. Allow the newly blind person a period of grieving for loss of vision.

3. Coordinate care with the case manager to identify community resources for retraining, transportation, and assistance in adapting to reduced vision.

Guide to Head-to-Toe Physical Assessment of Adults

Guide to Head-to-Toe Physical Assessment of Adults

Nursing Activity	Typical Finding	Changes Associated with Aging
NEUROLOGIC SYSTEM		
1. Determine level of consciousness.	1. Awake, alert	1. None
2. Test for orientation.	2. States name, place, and time	2. None
SKIN		
1. Inspect skin.	1. Intact, warm, dry, elastic skin without lesions	1a. Excessive dryness; wrinkles; discolorations from ultraviolet exposure ("age spots") and hemangiomas; inelastic, sagging skin 1b. Ecchymotic areas as a result of increased capillary fragility
HEAD AND FACE		
1. Inspect and palpate the scalp, hair, and skull.	1. No lesions, shiny hair	1. Alopecia, thinning and dullness of hair
2. Inspect the face for symmetry of expression.	2. Symmetric expression	2. None

Continued

Guide to Head-to-Toe Physical Assessment of Adults—cont'd

Nursing Activity	Typical Finding	Changes Associated with Aging
EYE		
1. Inspect the external eye structures.	1. No structural abnormalities	1. Entropion (inverted eyelid) or ectropion (everted eyelid)
2. Inspect the conjunctivae, sclerae, corneas, and irides.	2. No abnormalities; round irides	2. None
3. Use a penlight to test pupillary response (direct and consensual).	3. Pupils are equal and round and react to light and accommodation	3. None
4. Test vision by asking the client to read (if able) or interpret an eye chart.	4. No vision impairment	4. Presbyopia (farsightedness)
NOTE: Be sure that glasses or contact lenses are in place, if used.		
EAR		
1. Inspect the external structure.	1. No structural abnormalities	1. No major change
2. Inspect the auditory meatus for drainage.	2. No drainage; small amount of cerumen may be present	2. None
3. Test hearing by whispering to the client while turning head away.	3. No difficulty in hearing	3. Hearing loss, especially high-frequency sounds
NOTE: Be sure that hearing aid, if used, is in place.		

Guide to Head-to-Toe Physical Assessment of Adults—cont'd

Nursing Activity	Typical Finding	Changes Associated with Aging
MOUTH		
1. Use a penlight to inspect mouth, teeth, and gums.	1. No lesions, extensive dental caries, or gum disease	1. None
NECK		
1. Inspect for symmetry, lesions, pulsations, and JVD.	1. Symmetric, without lesions or JVD	1. None
2. Palpate the carotid pulse, one side at a time; check for bruits.	2. No bruits; pulses equal	2. None
3. Palpate the cervical lymph nodes.	3. Unable to palpate	3. None
4. Test ROM.	4. No limitations	4. Possible reduced flexion and extension at joints in neck; possible crepitus
CHEST (POSTERIOR, ANTERIOR, AND LATERAL)		
1. Inspect the chest for deformity, symmetry, expansion, and lesions; note pulsations or heaves (lifts).	1. Symmetric; without lesions; anteroposterior-lateral ratio of 1:2; no heaves	1. Slight change in anteroposterior-lateral ratio (1:1.5)
2. Palpate any chest lesions.	2. No lesions	2. None
3. Locate the PMI.	3. PMI at the left MCL, fifth ICS	3. None
4. Palpate each vertebra of the spine.	4. No tenderness or bony spurs	4. Thoracic kyphosis
5. Auscultate breath sounds throughout all lung fields.	5. Unlabored excursion of air; no adventitious sounds	5. Shallow respirations
6. Auscultate apical rate and rhythm; auscultate heart sounds.	6. S_1 and S_2 heart sounds	6. Possible S_4 heart sound

Continued

Guide to Head-to-Toe Physical Assessment of Adults—cont'd

Nursing Activity	Typical Finding	Changes Associated with Aging
UPPER EXTREMITIES		
1. Inspect and palpate joints for swelling, tenderness, and deformity.	1. No swelling, tenderness, or deformity	1. Tenderness of one or more joints
2. Palpate brachial and radial arteries; assess for pulse deficit.	2. Pulses equal and within normal limits	2. None
3. Test ROM in all joints and sensation.	3. No restriction	3. Slight decrease in ROM; possible crepitus
4. Test muscle strength of arms, hands, and shoulders.	4. Movement against both gravity and resistance (5/5)	4. None or slight decrease (4+/5)
5. Palpate axillary nodes.	5. Nodes not palpable	5. None
ABDOMEN		
1. Inspect for contour, symmetry, lesions, and pulsations.	1. Symmetric; without lesions or pulsations	1. None
2. Auscultate bowel sounds in all four quadrants.	2. 5–15 sounds/min in each quadrant	2. May be slightly decreased (hypoactive)
3. Auscultate over abdominal aorta for bruit.	3. No bruit	3. None
4. Palpate for liver enlargement.	4. Liver not below costal margin	4. None
LOWER EXTREMITIES		
1. Inspect and palpate for swelling, tenderness, and deformity.	1. No swelling, tenderness, or deformity	1. Tenderness of one or more joints
2. Test ROM in all joints and sensation.	2. No limitation	2. Slight decrease in ROM; possible crepitus

Guide to Head-to-Toe Physical Assessment of Adults—cont'd

Nursing Activity	Typical Finding	Changes Associated with Aging
3. Test muscle strength.	3. Movement against gravity and resistance (5/5)	3. None or slight decrease (4+/5)
4. Palpate femoral, popliteal, and pedal pulses.	4. Pulses equal and within normal range	4. Pedal pulses may be weak or not palpable
5. Palpate inguinal nodes.	5. Nodes not palpable	5. None
GENITALIA		
1. Inspect external genitalia for lesions or drainage.	1. No lesions or drainage	1. None

ICS, Intercostal space; *JVD,* jugular venous distension; *MCL,* mid-clavicular line; *PMI,* point of maximal impulse; *ROM,* range of motion.

*Additional assessments may be needed, depending on the patient's concerns and the medical diagnoses.

For more information on physical assessment, see Ignatavicius, D. D. & Workman, M. L. (2017). *Medical-Surgical Nursing: Patient Centered Collaborative Care* (9th ed.). Philadelphia, PA: Saunders.

Electrocardiographic Complexes, Segments, and Intervals

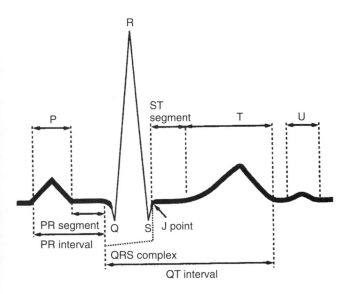

The electrocardiogram (ECG) is the graphic record of electrical activity of the heart. The spread of electrical current in the heart is detected by surface electrodes, and the amplified electrical signals are recorded on calibrated paper.

Cardiac dysrhythmias are abnormal rhythms of the heart's electrical system that can affect its ability to effectively pump oxygenated blood throughout the body. Some dysrhythmias are life threatening, and others are not. They are the result of disturbances of cardiac electrical impulse formation, conduction, or both. When the heart does not work effectively as a pump, perfusion to vital organs and peripheral tissues can be impaired, resulting in organ dysfunction or failure.

Complexes that make up a normal ECG consist of a P wave, a QRS complex, a T wave, and possibly a U wave. Segments include the PR segment, the ST segment, and the TP segment. Intervals include the PR interval, the QRS duration, and the QT interval (see Figure). *Assess the patient to differentiate artifact from actual lethal rhythms! Do not rely only on the ECG monitor!*

P wave represents atrial depolarization.

PR segment represents the time required for the impulse to travel through the atrioventricular (AV) node (where the impulse is delayed).

PR interval represents the time required for atrial depolarization and impulse travel through the AV node, inclusive of the P wave and PR segment. It is measured from the beginning of the P wave to the end of the PR segment, and a normal time in adults is 0.12 to 0.2 second. It is measured from the beginning of the P wave to the beginning of the QRS wave.

QRS complex represents depolarization of both ventricles and is measured from the point at which the complex first leaves the baseline to the end of the last appearing wave (from the end of the PR interval to the J point). This is normally 0.04 to 0.1 second. A wide (i.e., greater than 0.12 second) QRS complex indicates a delay in the conduction time in the ventricles. Delay in ventricular depolarization (i.e., a wide QRS) can be the result of myocardial ischemia, injury, or infarct; it may also result from ventricular hypertrophy or electrolytes imbalances. It is measured from the beginning of the Q or R wave to the end of the R or S wave (not all leads have a Q, R, and S.)

J point represents the junction where the QRS complex ends and the ST segment begins.

ST segment represents early ventricular repolarization. It is measured from the J point to the beginning of the T wave.

T wave represents ventricular repolarization.

U wave represents late ventricular repolarization. It is not normally seen in all leads.

QT interval represents the total time required for ventricular depolarization and repolarization. It is measured from the beginning of the QRS complex to the end of the T wave. It varies with age, gender, and heart rate. It must be corrected to a heart rate of 60 after measurement (QTc). The upper limit of normal QTc is less than 0.43 second in men and less than 0.45 second in women with a normal rate of 60 to 100 beats/min.

Analysis of an ECG rhythm strip requires a systematic approach using an eight-step method:

1. *Determine the heart rate.* The most common method is to count the number of QRS complexes in 6 seconds and multiply that

number by 10 to calculate the rate for a full minute. Normal heart rates fall between 60 and 100 beats/min. A rate less than 60 beats/min is called **bradycardia**. A rate greater than 100 beats/min is called **tachycardia**.

2. *Determine the heart rhythm.* Assess for atrial and/or ventricular regularity. Heart rhythms can be either regular or irregular. Irregular rhythms can be regularly irregular, occasionally irregular, or irregularly irregular. A slight irregularity of no more than three small blocks between intervals is considered essentially regular if the QRS complexes are all of the same shape.

3. *Analyze the P waves.* Ask these questions; a response of yes indicates normality:
   • Are P waves present?
   • Are the P waves occurring regularly?
   • Is there one P wave for each QRS complex?
   • Are the P waves smooth, rounded, and upright in appearance?
   • Do all P waves look similar?

4. *Measure the PR interval.* The normal PR interval is between 0.12 and 0.20 second and should be a constant value in the strip. The PR interval cannot be determined if there are no P waves or if P waves occur after the QRS complex.

5. *Measure the QRS duration.* The QRS duration normally measures between 0.04 and 0.10 second and should be a constant value and consistently shaped throughout the strip. When the QRS is narrow (0.10 second or less), this indicates that the impulse was not formed in the ventricles and is referred to as *supraventricular* or *above the ventricles*. When the QRS complex is wide (greater than 0.10 second), this indicates that the impulse is either of ventricular origin or of supraventricular origin with aberrant conduction. More than one QRS complex pattern or occasionally missing QRS complexes indicates a dysrhythmia.

6. *Examine the ST segment.* The normal ST segment begins at the isoelectric line. ST elevation or depression is significant if displacement is 1 mm (one small box) or more above or below the line and is seen in two or more leads. ST *elevation* may indicate problems such as myocardial infarction, pericarditis, and hyperkalemia. ST *depression* is associated with hypokalemia, myocardial infarction, or ventricular hypertrophy.

7. *Assess the T wave.* Note the shape and height of the T wave for peaking or inversion. Abnormal T waves may indicate problems such as myocardial infarction and ventricular hypertrophy.

8. *Measure the QT interval.* A normal QT interval should be equal to or less than one-half the distance of the R-to-R interval.

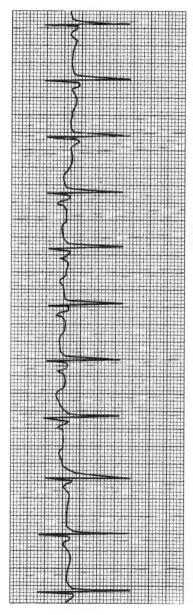

Normal Sinus Rhythm The rate for normal sinus rhythm is 60 to 100 beats/min (bpm) for both atria (i.e., P waves) and ventricles (i.e., QRS waveforms); in this illustration, the rate is 92 bpm. Notice that the atrial and ventricular rhythms are essentially regular (a slight variation in rhythm is normal). One P wave occurs before each QRS complex, and all P waves are of a consistent morphology (shape). The PR interval measures 0.14 second and is constant; the QRS complex measures 0.08 second and is constant. The T waves vary in amplitude because of respirations; they are flat with inspiration and positive with expiration.

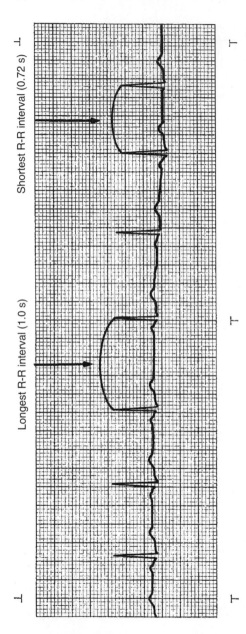

Longest R-R interval (1.0 s)

Shortest R-R interval (0.72 s)

Sinus Arrhythmia or Sinus Dysrhythmia Caused by Respiratory Variation All P waves have the same shape and PR interval, indicating that they are from the sinus node. The rhythm is slightly irregular with the shortest RR interval at 0.74 second and the longest at 1 second. Sinus dysrhythmia most commonly originates from respiratory causes (inhalation/exhalation) and is considered normal. Abnormal causes of RR variation include drugs and acid-base imbalances.

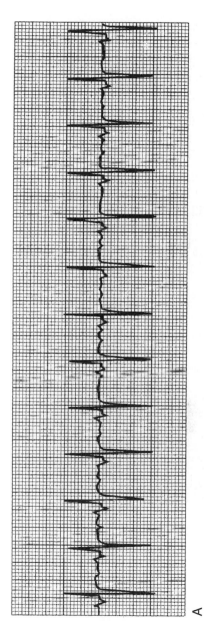

Sinus Rhythm A, Sinus tachycardia is defined as a heart rate (HR) faster than 100 beats/min with normal waves and intervals (HR = 100 beats/min, PR = 0.12 second, QRS = 0.08 second).

A

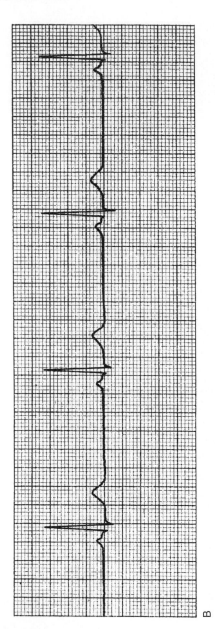

B

Sinus Rhythm—cont'd B, Sinus bradycardia is defined as a heart rate less than 60 beats/min with all other waves and segments within normal values (HR = 35 beats/min, PR = 0.16 second, QRS = 0.10 second).

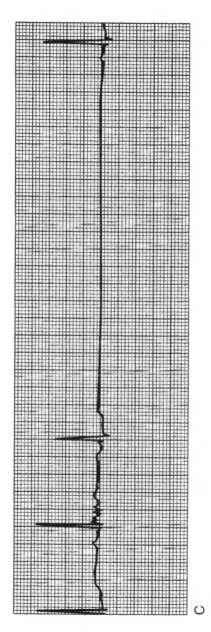

Sinus Rhythm—cont'd C, Sinus pause (underlying HR = 60 beats/min, PR = 0.20 second, QRS = 0.08 second, with just under a 5-second pause.)

C

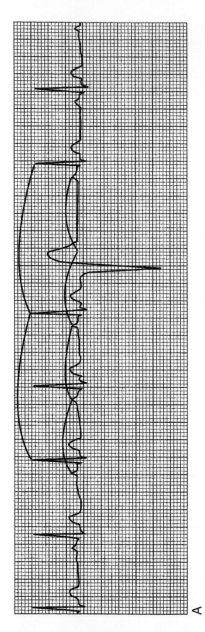

Normal Sinus Rhythm with a Premature Contraction A, Normal sinus rhythm with a premature ventricular contraction (PVC). A complete compensatory pause follows the PVC, indicated by the fact that the sinus P wave after the pause comes exactly when it was due to occur.

A

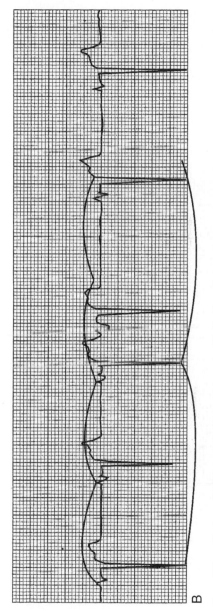

Normal Sinus Rhythm with a Premature Contraction —cont'd B, Normal sinus rhythm with a premature atrial contraction (PAC). An incomplete or noncompensatory pause follows the PAC, indicated by the sinus P wave after the pause coming before it was originally due to occur. The QRS complex also comes before it was due.

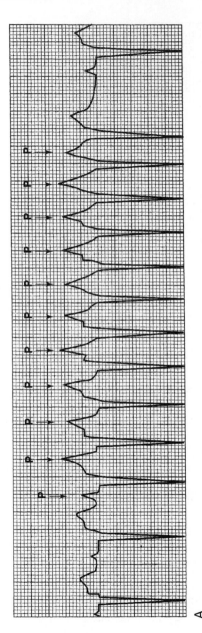

Atrial Dysrhythmias An atrial dysrhythmia implies that the source of the irregular rate or rhythm originates in the atria. **A,** Normal sinus rhythm with an 11-beat run of paroxysmal atrial tachycardia (PAT) with 1:1 conduction.

A

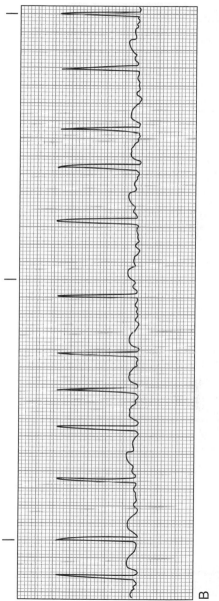

Atrial Dysrhythmias—cont'd B, Atrial fibrillation (AF). Multiple pacemaker sites in the atria cause atrial depolarization at 350 to 600 times per minute. The result is an irregular, wavy baseline between each QRS rather than organized P waves. Atrial fibrillation is often but not universally characterized by an irregular ventricular response, seen in this figure.

B

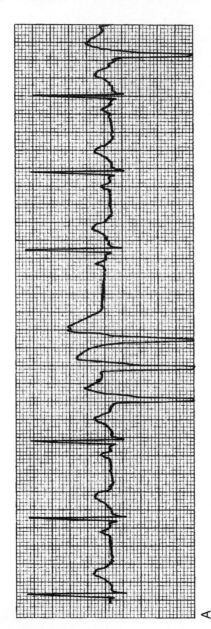

Ventricular Dysrhythmias A, Normal sinus rhythm with a three-beat run of ventricular tachycardia and one unifocal premature ventricular complex.

A

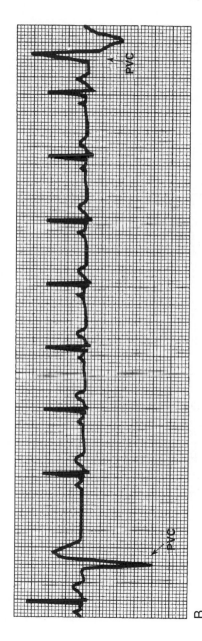

Ventricular Dysrhythmias—cont'd B, Normal sinus rhythm with multifocal PVCs (one negative and the other positive).

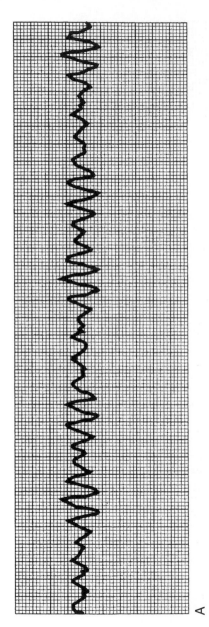

Ventricular Dysrhythmias The dysrhythmia originates in the ventricle. Sustained ventricular tachycardia, ventricular fibrillation, and a systole are all associated with sudden cardiac death they do not support a blood pressure or perfusion. **A,** Coarse ventricular fibrillation.

A

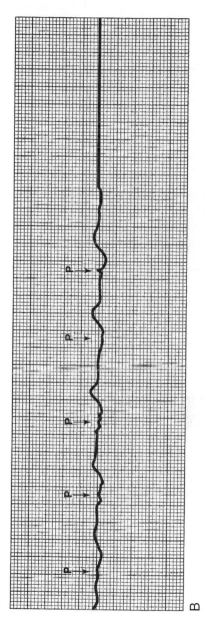

Ventricular Dysrhythmias—cont'd B, Ventricular asystole, initially with five P waves and then with no P waves (arterial and ventricular standstill).

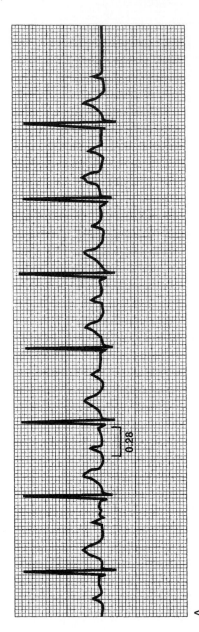

A

Atrioventricular Block A heart block implies a disruption in the normal conduction of a pacemaker signal that originates in the sinoatrial (SA) node. **A,** Normal sinus rhythm with a first-degree AV block (PR interval = 0.28 second). First- and second-degree heart block imply a delay at the AV node.

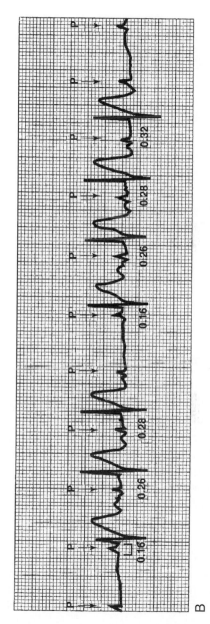

Atrioventricular Block—cont'd B, Second-degree AV block type 1 (Wenckebach) with an irregular rhythm, grouped beating, and progressive prolongation of the PR interval until a P wave is completely blocked and not followed by a QRS complex.

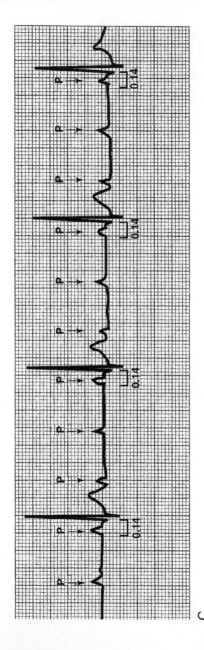

Atrioventricular Block—cont'd C, Second-degree AV block type 2 (Mobitz III) with 3:1 conduction and a constant PR interval. A type 2 second-degree block is more serious and indicates the need for more urgent intervention, such as placing a transcutaneous pacemaker and anticipating the placement of a permanent pacemaker.

C

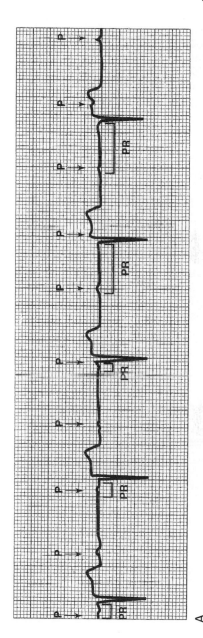

Atrioventricular Block A, Third-degree AV block (complete heart block) with regular atrial and ventricular rhythms. This dysrhythmia indicates no communication between the atria and ventricles at the AV node and is typically treated with a pacemaker. Note the inconsistent PR intervals (AV dissociation) and a junctional escape focus (normal QRS complexes) pacing the ventricles at a rate of 38 beats/min.

A

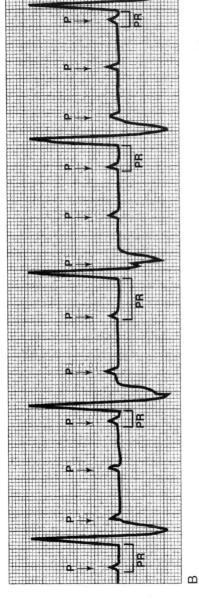

Atrioventricular Block—cont'd B, Third-degree AV block with regular atrial and ventricular rhythms, inconsistent PR intervals (AV dissociation), and ventricular escape focus pacing the ventricles at a rate of 35 beats/min, with wide QRS complexes. Third-degree heart block implies a more serious condition and a delay low in the AV node or along the bundle of His. New onset of this rhythm should be communicated to the physician immediately, and a transcutaneous pacemaker should be placed until the patient can be fully evaluated for possible permanent pacemaker placement.

Communicating Quick Reference for Spanish-Speaking Patients

THE BODY · EL CUERPO (EHL KOO-EHR-POH)

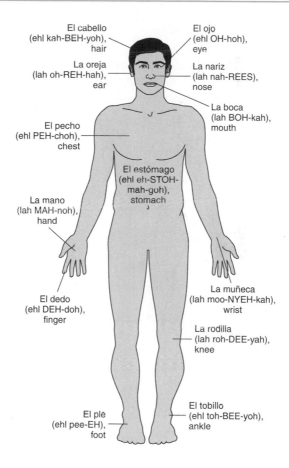

El cabello
(ehl kah-BEH-yoh),
hair

El ojo
(ehl OH-hoh),
eye

La oreja
(lah oh-REH-hah),
ear

La nariz
(lah nah-REES),
nose

La boca
(lah BOH-kah),
mouth

El pecho
(ehl PEH-choh),
chest

El estómago
(ehl eh-STOH-mah-goh),
stomach

La mano
(lah MAH-noh),
hand

La muñeca
(lah moo-NYEH-kah),
wrist

El dedo
(ehl DEH-doh),
finger

La rodilla
(lah roh-DEE-yah),
knee

El pie
(ehl pee-EH),
foot

El tobillo
(ehl toh-BEE-yoh),
ankle

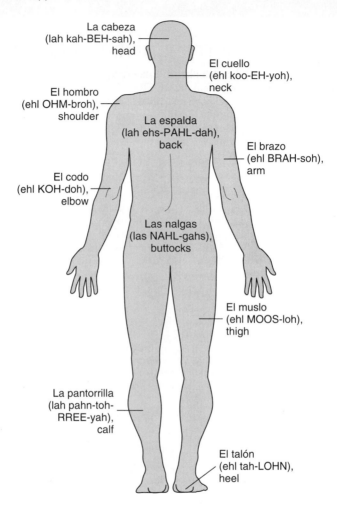

La cabeza
(lah kah-BEH-sah),
head

El cuello
(ehl koo-EH-yoh),
neck

El hombro
(ehl OHM-broh),
shoulder

La espalda
(lah ehs-PAHL-dah),
back

El brazo
(ehl BRAH-soh),
arm

El codo
(ehl KOH-doh),
elbow

Las nalgas
(las NAHL-gahs),
buttocks

El muslo
(ehl MOOS-loh),
thigh

La pantorrilla
(lah pahn-toh-
RREE-yah),
calf

El talón
(ehl tah-LOHN),
heel

COMMON TERMS

Move, mueva (mooh-EH-bah)
Touch, toque (TOH-keh)
Point to, señale (seh-NYAH-leh)

MORE PARTS OF THE BODY

Armpit, la axila (lah ahk-SEE-lah)
Breasts, los senos (lohs SEH-nohs)
Collarbone, la clavícula (lah klah-BEE-koo-lah)
Diaphragm, el diafragma (ehl dee-ah-FRAHG-mah)
Forearm, el antebrazo (ehl ahn-teh-BRAH-soh)
Groin, la ingle (lah EEN-gleh)
Hip, la cadera (lah kah-DEH-rah)
Kneecap, la rótula (lah ROH-too-lah)
Nail, la uña (lah OO-nyah)
Pelvis, la pelvis (lah PEHL-bees)
Rectum, el recto (ehl REHK-toh)
Rib, la costilla (lah kohs-TEE-yah)
Spine, la espina dorsal (lah ehs-PEE-nah dor-SAHL)
Throat, la garganta (lah gahr-GAHN-tah)
Tongue, la lengua (lah LEHN-goo-ah)

ORGANS

Appendix, el apèndice (ehl ah-PEHN-dee-seh)
Bladder, la vejiga (lah beh-HEE-gah)
Brain, el cerebro (ehl seh-REH-broh)
Colon, el colon (ehl KOH-lohn)
Esophagus, el esófago (ehl eh-SOH-fah-goh)
Gallbladder, la vesícula biliar (lah beh-SEE-koo-lah bee-lee-AHR)
Genitals, los genitales (lohs heh-nee-TAH-lehs)
Heart, el corazón (ehl koh-rah-SOHN)
Kidney, el riñón (ehl ree-NYOHN)
Large intestine, el intestino grueso (ehl een-tehs-TEE-noh groo-EH-soh)
Liver, el hígado (ehl EE-gah-doh)
Lungs, los pulmones (lohs pool-MOH-nehs)
Pancreas, el páncreas (ehl PAHN-kreh-ahs)
Small intestine, el intestino delgado (ehl een-tehs-TEE-noh dehl-GAH-doh)
Spleen, el bazo (ehl BAH-soh)
Thyroid gland, la tiroides (lah tee-ROH-ee-dehs)
Tonsils, las amígdalas (lahs ah-MEEG-dah-lahs)
Uterus, el útero (ehl OO-teh-roh)

ESSENTIAL PHRASES

Good morning.	*Buenos días.*	Boo-EH-nohs DEE-ahs.
Good afternoon.	*Buenas tardes.*	Boo-EH-nahs TAHR-dehs.
Good night.	*Buenas noches.*	Boo-EH-nahs NOH-chehs.
Hello.	*Hola.*	OH-lah.
How are you?	*¿Cómo está?*	¿Koh-moh ehs-TAH?
Good (fine)	*Bien.*	Bee-EHN.
Bad, Better, Worse	*Mal, Mejor, Peor*	Mahl, Meh-OHR, peh-OHR
The same	*Igual*	Ee-GOO-ahl
Do you speak English?	*¿Habla inglés?*	¿Ah-blah een-GLEHS?
I don't understand.	*No comprendo.*	Noh kom-PREHN-doh.
Excuse me.	*Discúlpeme.*	Dees-KOOL-peh-meh.
Please speak slowly.	*Por favor, hable más lento.*	Pohr fah-VOHR, AH-bleh mahs LEHN-toh.
Are you in pain?	*¿Está adolorido(a)?*	¿Ehs-TAH ah-doh-loh-REE-doh(dah)?
Yes, No	*Sí, No*	SEE, Noh
Tell me where it hurts.	*Dígame donde le duele.*	DEE-gah-meh DOHN-deh leh doo-EH-leh.
Here, there	*Aquí, ahí*	Ah-KEE, ah-EE

DESCRIPTION OF PAIN

Is your pain ... burning?	*Tiene un dolor ... ¿que arde?*	Tee-EH-neh oon doh-LOHR ... ¿keh AHR-deh?
constant?	*¿constante?*	¿kohns-TAHN-teh?
dull?	*¿amortiguado?*	¿ah-MOHR-tee-goo-AH-doh?
intermittent?	*¿intermitente?*	¿een-tehr-mee-TEHN-teh?
mild?	*¿moderado?*	¿moh-deh-RAH-doh?
severe?	*¿muy fuerte?*	¿MOO-ee foo-EHR-teh?
sharp?	*¿agudo?*	¿ah-GOO-doh?
throbbing?	*¿pulsante?*	¿pool-SAHN-teh?
worse?	*¿peor?*	¿peh-OHR?

Are you allergic to any medication?	*¿Es usted alérgico(a) a algún medicamento?*	¿Ehs oos-TEHD ah-LEHR-hee-koh(kah) ah ahl-GOON meh-dee-kah-MEHN-toh?
I'm here to help you.	*Estoy aquípara ayudarle.*	Ehs-TOH-ee ah-KEE pah-rah ah-yoo-DAHR-leh.
Calm down.	*Cálmese.*	KAHL-meh-seh.
Please.	*Por favor.*	Pohr fah-VOHR.
Thank you.	*Gracias.*	GRAH-see-ahs.
You're welcome.	*De nada.*	Deh NAH-dah.
May I?	*¿Puedo?*	¿Poo-EH-doh?
Who, What, When, Where?	*¿Quién, Qué, Cuándo, Dónde?*	¿Kee-ehn, Keh, Koo-AHN-doh, DOHN-doh?
Zero, one, two, three, four	*Cero, uno, dos, tres, cuatro*	SEH-roh, OO-noh, dohs, trehs, koo-AH-troh
Five, six, seven, eight, nine, ten	*Cinco, seis, siete, ocho, nueve, diez*	SEEN-koh, SEH-ees, see-EH-teh, OH-choh, noo-EH-beh, dee-EHS

PRELIMINARY EXAMINATION

My name is _____, and I am your nurse.	*Me llamo __ , y soy su enfermera(o).*	Meh YAH-moh ___, ee SOH-ee soo ehn-fehr-MEH-rah(roh).
I'm going to ... take your vital signs.	*Le voy a ... tomar los signos vitales.*	Leh VOH-ee ah ... toh-MAHR lohs SEEG-nohs vee-TAH-lehs.
weigh you.	*pesar.*	peh-SAHR.
take your blood pressure.	*tomar la presión.*	toh-MAHR lah preh-see-OHN.
Extend your arm and relax.	*Extienda su brazo y descánselo.*	Ehks-tee-EHN-dah soo BRAH-soh ee dehs-KAHN-seh-loh.
I'm going to take your ... pulse.	*Le voy a tomar ... el pulso.*	Leh voy ah toh-MAHR ... ehl POOL-soh.
temperature.	*su temperatura.*	soo tehm-peh-rah-TOO-rah.
I'm going to count your respirations.	*Voy a contar sus respiraciones.*	VOH-ee ah kohn-TAHR soos rehs-pee-rah-see-OH-nehs.

OBTAINING A BLOOD SAMPLE

I need to draw a blood sample.	*Necesito tomar una muestra de la sangre.*	Neh-seh-SEE-toh toh-MAHR OO-nah MOO-ehs-trah deh lah SAHN-greh.
Please give me your arm.	*Por favor, déme el brazo.*	Pohr fah-VOHR, DEH-meh ehl BRAH-soh.
It may cause a little discomfort.	*Le puede causar alguna molestia.*	Leh poo-EH-deh kah-OO-sahr ahl-GOO-nah moh-LEHS-tee-ah.
I am going to put a tourniquet around your arm.	*Le voy a poner una liga alrededor del brazo.*	Leh VOH-ee ah poh-NEHR OO-nah LEE-gah ahl-reh-deh-DOHR dehl BRAH-soh.
I am going to draw blood from this vein.	*Voy a sacar la sangre de esta vena.*	Voy ah sah-KAHR lah SAHN-greh deh EHS-tah VEH-nah.

OBTAINING BLOOD FROM A FINGER STICK

I need to take a few drops of blood from your finger.	*Necesito sacar unas gotas de sangre de uno de sus dedos.*	Neh-seh-SEE-toh sah-KAHR OO-nahs GOH-tahs deh SAHN-greh deh OO-noh deh soos DEH-dohs.

OBTAINING A URINE SAMPLE

We also need a urine sample.	*También necesitamos una muestra de la orina.*	Tahm-bee-EHN neh-seh-see-TAH-mohs OO-nah moo-EHS-trah deh lah oh-REE-nah.
It has to be from the middle of the stream.	*Tiene que ser de la mitad del chorro.*	Tee-EH-neh keh sehr deh lah mee-TAHD dehl CHOH-rroh.
Put the urine in this cup.	*Ponga la orina en esta tasa.*	POHN-gah lah oh-REE-nah ehn EHS-tah TAH-sah.

OBTAINING A STOOL SPECIMEN

I need a sample of your stool.	*Necesito una muestra de su excremento.*	Neh-seh-SEE-toh OO-nah moo-EHS-trah deh soo ehks-kreh-MEN-toh.
Please put a small amount in this cup.	*Por favor ponga un poco en esta tasa.*	Pohr fah-VOHR POHN-gah oon POH-koh ehn EHS-tah TAH-sah.

OBTAINING A SPUTUM SPECIMEN

I need a sample of your sputum.	*Necesito una muestra de su esputo.*	Neh-seh-SEE-toh OO-nah MOO-ehs-trah deh soo ehs-POO-toh.
Please spit in this cup.	*Por favor, escupa en este vaso.*	Pohr fah-VOHR, ehs-KOO-pah ehn EHS-tah VAH-soh.

ORDERS

You need ... a bandage.	*Necesita ... un vendaje.*	Neh-seh-SEE-tah ... oon behn-DAH-heh.
a blood transfusion.	*una transfusión de sangre.*	OO-nah trahns-foo-see-OHN deh SAHN-greh.
a cast.	*un molde de yeso.*	oon MOHL-deh deh YEH-soh.
gauze.	*la gasa.*	lah GAH-sah.
intensive care.	*cuidado intensivo.*	koo-ee-DAH-doh een-tehn-SEE-boh.
intravenous fluids.	*líquidos intravenosos.*	LEE-kee-dohs een-trah-beh-NOH-sohs.
an operation.	*una operación.*	OO-nah oh-peh-rah-see-OHN.
physical therapy.	*terapia física.*	teh-RAH-pee-ah FEE-see-kah.
a shot.	*una inyección.*	OO-nah een-yehk-see-OHN.
x-rays.	*rayos equis.*	RAH-yohs EH-kees.

Continued

We're going to ... change the bandage.	*Vamos a ... cambiarle el vendaje.*	VAH-mohs ah ... kahm-bee-AHR-leh ehl behn-DAH-heh.
give you a bath.	*darle un baño.*	DAHR-leh oon BAH-nyoh.
take out the IV.	*sacarle el tubo intravenoso.*	sah-KAHR-leh ehl TOO-boh een-trah-beh-NOH-soh.

DESCRIPTION OF TUBES

The tube in your ... arm is for IV fluids.	*El tubo en su ... brazo es para líquidos intravenosos.*	Ehl TOO-boh ehn soo ... BRAH-soh ehs PAH-rah LEE-kee-dohs een-trah-beh-NOH-sohs.
bladder is for urinating.	*vejiga es para orinar.*	beh-HEE-gah ehs PAH-rah oh-ree-NAHR.
stomach is for food.	*estómago es para los alimentos.*	ehs-TOH-mah-goh ehs PAH-rah lohs ah-lee-MEN-tohs.
throat is for breathing.	*garganta es para respirar.*	gahr-GAHN-tah ehs PAH-rah rehs-pee-RAHR.

American Cancer Society. (2017). *Cancer facts and figures—2017. Report No. 00-300M–No. 500817.* Atlanta: Author.

American Heart Association (AHA). (2015). *2015 guidelines highlights.* From https://eccguidelines.heart.org/index.php/guidelines-highlights.

Budd, G., & Peterson, J. (2015). The obesity epidemic, part 2: Nursing assessment and intervention. *American Journal of Nursing, 115*(1), 38–46.

Burchum, J.L.R. & Rosenthal, L.D. (2016). *Lehne's pharmacology for nursing care. (9th Ed.)* St. Louis: Elsevier.

Centers for Disease Control and Prevention (CDC). (2015b). *HIV surveillance report, 2014* (Vol. 26). From http://www.cdc.gov/hiv/pdf/library/reports/surveillance/cdc-hiv-surveillance-report-us.pdf.

Chang, S. F., Yang, R. S., Chung, U. L., Chen, C. M., & Cheng, M. H. (2010). Perception of risk factors and DXA T-score among at-risk females of osteoporosis. *Journal of Clinical Nursing, 19*(13-14), 1795-1802.

Davis, L. (2015). Hypertension: Evidence-based treatments for maintaining blood pressure control. *The Nurse Practitioner, 40*(6), 32–37.

Kidney Disease Improving Global Outcomes (KDIGO). (2013). *KDIGO 2012 clinical practice guideline for the evaluation and management of chronic kidney disease.* Retrieved September 2016 from http://www.kdigo.org/clinical_practice_guidelines/pdf/CKD/KDIGO_2012_CKD_GL.pdf.

Kim, S., Brooks, J., Sheikh, J., Kaplan, M., & Goldberg, B. (2014). Angioedema deaths in the United States: 1979-2010. *Annals of Allergy, Asthma, & Immunology, 113*(6), 630–634.

Lilley, L., Rainforth Collins, S., & Snyder, J. (2017). *Pharmacology and the nursing process* (8th ed.). St. Louis: Elsevier.

McCance, K., Huether, S., Brashers, V., & Rote, N. (2017). *Pathophysiology: The biologic basis for disease in adults and children* (8th ed.). St. Louis: Mosby.

Meziah, O., Kirby, K. A., Williams, B., Yalle, K., Byers, A. L., & Barnes, D. E. (2014). Prisoner of war status, posttraumatic stress disorder, and dementia in older veterans. *Alzheimer's Dementia, 10*(Suppl 3), S236–S241.

Mozaffarian, D., Benjamin, E., Go, A., Arnett, D., Blaha, M., Cushman, M., et al. (2016). Heart disease and stroke statistics—2016 update. *Circulation.* doi:10.1161/CIR0000000000000350.

National Multiple Sclerosis Society. (2016). *Who gets MS.* Retrieved March 2016, from www.nationalmssociety.org/about-multiple-sclerosis/what-we-know-about-ms/index.aspx.

Pasero, C., & McCaffery, M. (2011). *Pain assessment and pharmacologic management.* St. Louis: Mosby.

Qaseem, A., Dallas, P., Forciea, M., Starkey, M., Denberg, T., Shekelle, P., & Clinical Guidelines Committee of the American College of Physicians. (2014). Nonsurgical management of urinary incontinence in women: A clinical practice guideline from the American College of Physicians. *Annals of Internal Medicine, 161*(6), 429–440.

Taal, M. (2016). Risk factors and chronic kidney disease. In K. Skorecki, G. Chertow, P. Marsden, M. Taal, & A. Yu (Eds). *Brenner and Rector's the kidney* (10th ed., pp. 669–692). Philadelphia: Elsevier.

Testa, A. (2015). Understanding adult urinary incontinence. *Urologic Nursing, 35*(2), 82–86.

Vacca, V., & McMahon-Bowen, E. (2013). Anaphylaxis. *Nursing, 43*(11), 16–17.

Wang, L., Jian, Y., Yang, G., Gao, W., Wu, Y., & Zuo, L. (2015). Management of tumor lysis syndrome in patients with multiple myeloma during bortezomib treatment. *Clinical Journal of Oncology Nursing, 19*(1), E4–E7.

World Health Organization (WHO). (2015). *HIV/AIDS Fact Sheet.* From http://www.who.int/mediacentre/factsheets/fs360/en/#.